ANALYTICAL CHEMISTRY

Theory and Practice

Third Edition

R.M. VERMA
Professor
Department of Post-Graduate
Studies and Research in Chemistry
Rani Durgavati University
Jabalpur-482001

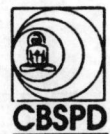

CBSPD

CBS Publishers & Distributors Pvt Ltd

New Delhi • Bengaluru • Chennai • Kochi • Kolkata • Mumbai
Hyderabad • Jharkhand • Nagpur • Patna • Pune • Uttarakhand

Analytical Chemistry
Theory and Practice
(Third Edition)

ISBN: 978-81-239-0266-1

First Edition: 1987
Second Edition: 1991
Third Edition: 1994
    Reprint: 1997, 1998, 1999, 2000, 2001, 2003, 2004, 2005, 2006, 2007, 2008,
        2010, 2012, 2014, 2016, 2018, 2019, 2020, **2025**

Copyright © Author and Publisher

Published by **Satish Kumar Jain** and produced by **Varun Jain** for

CBS Publishers & Distributors Pvt Ltd

4819/XI Prahlad Street, 24 Ansari Road, Daryaganj, New Delhi 110 002, India.
Ph: 011-23266838, 23289259   Website: www.cbspd.com
                                 e-mail: delhi@cbspd.com

Corporate Office: 204 FIE, Industrial Area, Patparganj, Delhi 110 092
Ph: 011-4934 4934   Fax: 011-4934 4935
                         e-mail: publishing@cbspd.com; publicity@cbspd.com

Branches

- **Bengaluru:** Seema House 2975, 17th Cross, KR Road, Banasankari 2nd Stage, Bengaluru 560 070, Karnataka, India
  Ph: +91-80-26771678/79   Fax: +91-80-26771680   e-mail: bangalore@cbspd.com
- **Chennai:** 18/8B, Subbarayan Street, Shenoy Nagar, Chennai 600 030, Tamil Nadu, India
  Ph: +91-44-42032115, 26681266   e-mail: chennai@cbspd.com
- **Kochi:** 42/1325, 1326, Power House Road, Opp KSEB, Power House, Ernakulum Kochi 682 018, Kerala, India
  Ph: +91-484-4059061-65,67   Fax: +91-484-4059065   e-mail: kochi@cbspd.com
- **Kolkata:** 147, Hind Ceramics Compound, 1st Floor, Nilgunj Road, Belghoria, Kolkata-700056, West Bengal, India
  Ph: +033-25633055, 033-25633056   e-mail: kolkata@cbspd.com
- **Lucknow:** Basement, Khushnuma Complex, 7 Meerabai Marg (Behind Jawahar Bhawan), Lucknow-226001, UP India
  Ph: +0522-4000032   e-mail: tiwari.lucknow@cbspd.com
- **Mumbai:** PWD Shed, Gala no 25/26, Ramchandra Bhatt Marg, Next to JJ Hospital Gate no. 2, Opp. Union Bank of India, Noorbaug,
  Mumbai-400009, Maharashtra, India
  Ph: 022-66661880/89
                                 e-mail: mumbai@cbspd.com

Representatives

- Hyderabad   0-9885175004   • Jharkhand   0-9811541605   • Nagpur   0-8692091830
- Patna   0-9334159340   • Pune   0-9664372571   • Uttarakhand   0-9716462459

Printed at   Chaman Enterprises, Daryaganj, Delhi, India

Preface to the Third Edition

The warm reception accorded to the author's *Analytical Chemistry*; *Theory and Practice* by students and teachers all over the country as well as in some other Asian countries is a matter of great satisfaction. A number of suggestions were received for incorporating certain topics. In the light of these the following matter has been included in the third edition of the book.

Chpater 18 has been enlarged to cover the determination of some more functional groups and certain important organic compounds. In order to incorporate the analysis of water, soil, coal oils and fats. urine and blood, a new chapter number 19 has been added. Similary another chapter 20 has been introduced which is devoted to gas analsis and gasometric methods. It is hoped that these additions will help students to learn something about testing of a few commercial and biological samples. The study of analysis of water will be useful to those interested in water-pollution studies.

Comments from teachers and students will be received with thanks and taken care of in later editions.

R.M. VERMA

Preface to the First Edition

Although analytical chemistry has played a decisive role in establishing chemistry as a quantitative experimental science it was rather late that it was recognised as an independent discipline. Perhaps this is the reason that students regard analytical chemistry merely as a collection of empirical instructions for performing qualitative and quantitative analysis. The aim of the present work is to impress upon the fact that analytical chemistry is a distinct subject having its own objectives, methodology and scope.

It has been noticed that while carrying out chemical analysis, a majority of students follow instructions mechanically without understanding the theoretical considerations that underlie various analytical procedures. Attempts have, therefore, been made, as far as possible, to explain the theory behind different steps involved in various analytical schemes. In preparing this book the major emphasis has been on clear and simple presentation in a language that is readily understandable by an average student. This can obviously result in some repetition and at places the langu age may not be refined. But these points have been overlooked in favour of easy and intelligible presentation. It is a well accepted view that in scientific descriptions the clarity and simplicity should overweigh the beauty of the language. Most of the biology group students find the mathematical treatment rather difficult. For the benefit of such students attempt has been made to provide simplified treatment by splitting up a derivation into several simple steps to make it intelligible to students who have had no formal training in mathematics.

The material of the book is mainly concerned with the topics mentioned in the undergraduate syllabi of various Universities. However, at appropriate places some information has been provided which may be useful to post-graduate students as well. Apart from discussing the theoretical aspects of various analytical procedures, a number of experiments have been described in detail which will be helpful to students in carrying out various determinations. The purpose of giving experimental details of some typical determinations is to acquaint the student with various analytical techniques. Once these are properly understood he can successfully perform many more determinations. Keeping in view the recent upsurge in instrumental methods of analysis, basic principles of quantitative analytical procedures based on matter-energy interaction have been discussed along with the classical methods of analysis.

I gratefully acknowledge the suggestions of my colleagues Prof. S.C. Datt, Head Department of Physics and Dean Faculty of Science, R.D. University, Jabalpur, Prof. K.K. Tiwari, Head Department, of Chemistry Institute of Science Education, Jabalpur, and Dr. K.K. Verma, Reader, Department of Chemistry, R.D. University, Jabalpur. Appreciation is expressed to my students Dr. (Miss) Rashmi Saxena, Lecturer, Govt. College of Home Science, Jabalpur and Dr. (Miss) A. Wadhwa for their valuable assistance in the preparation of the manuscript. I am thankful to Mr. Jagdish Ram of UBS Jabalpur and Mr. Satish Kumar Jain of CBS Publishers Delhi for rapid Publication of the book. Help received from Mr. G.P. Chouhan in typing the manuscript and Mr. Rajiv Shrivastava in making the drawings is ' acknowledged. Finally I must recognise the cooperation and patience of my wife and children.

Any suggestions for improving the book will be gratefully received by the author.

R.M. Verma
May 1987

Department of Chemistry
Rani Durgavati Vishwavidyalaya
Jabalpur-482001.

CONTENTS

Preface

PART-I

Fundamental Theoretical Principles

PART-III

Classical Methods of Quantitative Analysis

Experiment 6˙5.

Gravimetric determination of calcium as calcium oxalate.

Experiment 6˙6.

Gravimetric determination of iron as iron (III) oxide.

Experiment 8·1.

Preparation of a 0·1000 M (=0·1000 N) solution of sodium hydroxide.

Experiment 8·2.

Preparation of a 0·1000 M (=0·1000 N) solution of hydrochloric acid.

Experiment 8·3.

Determination of the normality of the given acid solution by alkalimetry.

Experiment 8·4.

Titration of 0·005 M acetic acid iodometrically with a standard thiosulphate solution.

Experiment 8·5.

Quantitative analysis of a mixture of sodium hydroxide and sodium carbonate by titration with hydrochloric acid.

PART-V

Physicochemical or Instrumental Methods of Quantitative Analysis

PART-VI

Elementary Organic Analysis

List of Experiments on Physical Chemistry

Experiment 13.1.
Determination of partition coefficient of iodine between water and carbon tetrachloride.

Experiment 13.2.
Verification of Freundlich adsorption isotherm.

Experiment 14.1.
Potentiometric titration of a given hydrochloric acid solution with an alkali solution.

Experiment 14.2.
Potentiometric titration of a given ferrous sulphate solution with potassium dichromate

Experiment 14.3.
Conductometric titration of hydrochloric acid with sodium hydroxide.

Experiment 14.4.
Conductometric titration of hydrochloric acid with ammonium hydroxide.

Experiment 14.5.
Conductometric titration of acetic acid with ammonium hydroxide

Experiment 14.6.
Amperometric titration of lead nitrate with potassium dichromate.

Experiment 15.1.
Determination of specific rotation of cane sugar.

Experiment 15.2.
Polarimetric determination of cane sugar.

Experiment 17. A 3.
Determination of coefficient of viscosity of a liquid, and finding out percentage composition of a mixture by means of viscosity measurement.

Experiment 17. B. 3.
Determination of surface tension of a liquid and finding out percentage composition of a mixture of liquids by means of surface tension measurements.

Experiment 17.1.
Determination of the heat of neutralisation of a strong acid with a strong base.

Experiment 17 2.
Determination of the heat of dissociation of acetic acid.

PART I
FUNDAMENTAL THEORETICAL PRINCIPLES

1

Importance, Applications, Nature, Growth & Scope of Analytical Chemistry

1.1. THE IMPORTANCE OF ANALYTICAL CHEMISTRY

Analytical chemistry is as old as chemistry itself. In many respects analytical chemistry acts as a foundation for other branches of chemistry. In fact the science of chemistry came into being as a result of human inquisitiveness to understand the nature of an extraordinary variety of matter that surrounded him. And this knowledge was obtained by analysing different types of material. A complex material on analysis can give rise to a number of new and simpler constituents. Each of the constituents can be further analysed and if this process is continued, a stage will come when a constituent will not give any thing new ; such a constituent is called an *element*. Thus the concept of an element, as a substance which cannot be broken down into something simpler by ordinary chemical methods, arose from analytical data on different substances.

The construction of chemical balance provided a quantitative aspect to chemical analysis. With this development the study of analytical chemistry stimulated quantitative approach to various problems of chemistry. Chemical reactions were studied on the basis of qualitative and also quantitative changes that occurred ; this resulted in the discovery of several new compounds and the five laws of chemical combination. In an attempt to theoretically explain these laws, Dalton developed the atomic theory which played a tremendous role in developing chemistry into a quantitative experimental science. Prior to these developments the so called chemical science was mainly preparative in nature centred around empirical synthetic methods. The induction of analytical approach brought about a revolutionary transformation from magic and alchemy to quantitative scientific chemistry.

1`2. APPLICATION OF ANALYTICAL CHEMISTRY TO VARIOUS BRANCHES OF SCIENCE

Analytical chemistry plays a very significant role in chemical research as every chemist uses directly or indirectly data obtained by applying techniques of analytical chemistry. For example, a worker in the field of chemical kinetics has to make use of a suitable analytical procedure for following the course of the reaction under consideration. If one is studying the distribution of solute between two immiscible solvents, say- of iodine between water and chloroform, it is necessary to find out a suitable procedure for determining iodine in the two solvents. Apart from applications to chemical research, analytical techniques are frequently employed in industry in connection with problems such as, quality control and in ascertaining most appropriate experimental conditions for obtaining maximum yield of a particular product. It should be noted that techniques of analytical chemistry find wide applications not only in different branches of chemistry but also in other physical and biological sciences and in many fields of engineering.

Geologists use analytical procedures for analysing ground water, minerals, rocks, ores etc. In agriculture, chemical analysis is used to determine the composition of soils, in the production of fertilizers, insecticides and weed killers. Medical and biological research programmes depend on chemical analysis which provide useful information that enhances our understanding of vital processes and helps in developing medicines to cure various diseases.

In order to safeguard public health there is constant checking of foods, drugs, cosmetics, water supplies etc., and this is done in analytical laboratories. Waste disposals and the composition of air in industrial areas are analysed to know the extent of harm they would cause to public health so that necessary preventive steps can be taken.

There is hardly a branch of national economy which does not make use of analytical techniques. Chemical analysis is important in controlling the quality of raw materials, intermediate and finished products. Hence, to produce high quality products it is essential to have analytical control at all the stages of technological processes. The sale of raw materials by suppliers and their purchase by users is based on the content of the desired constituent which is determined by analysis. Metallurgical products are most essential materials of modern economy. The properties of alloys depend on its composition which is established by analytical methods.

A very large number of examples can be cited where analytical chemistry finds application. It would be no exaggeration if it is said that there is hardly a material related to modern living in which analytical chemistry did not play some part. With the development of sophisticated instruments, analytical techniques can now be used to determine traces of impurities at the part per billion level.

1.3. THE NATURE OF ANALYTICAL CHEMISTRY

Structural information about a complex compound can be obtained either by preparing it from some simple constituents or by breaking it chemically into smaller and simper units and then identifying them. The former approach involves *synthesis* of the compound while the latter is termed *chemical analysis*.

1.3.1. Qualitative and Quantitative Analysis

Chemical analysis can have two aspects ; *qualitative* and *quantitative* Qualitative analysis aims at identifying constituents of a given system such as presence of different compounds in a mixture or of different elements in a compound. Quantitative analysis is concerned with the determination of amounts of different constituents present in a system. Usually the given material is first analysed qualitatively and this is followed by quantitative analysis.

1.3.2. Inorganic and Organic Analysis

Chemical analysis is broadly classified as *inorganic* or *organic* depending upon the nature of the material under examination. *Elemental analysis* deals with the detection and determination of various elements present in a compound. *Functional group* analysis involves the determination of certain groupings of atoms such as carboxyl group ($-COOH$) or hydroxyl group ($-OH$) in an organic material.

1.3.3. Analysis, Determination and Estimation

Some authors make a distinction between *determination* and *analysis*. Determination usually refers to the measurement of a single constituent in a relatively simple specimen ; such as, determination of barium in a given solution of barium chloride. Analysis is referred to a more detailed and complete process which may involve collection of material, preparation of sample solution, identification of its various constituents, planning to determine these constituents keeping in view the composition of the material, separation of the interfering substances and selection of suitable methods for determining different constituents. For example, the analysis of a specimen of a rock or an ore. According to some authors, the term *estimation* implies a rough measurement and they prefer to use the term *determination*. However, in a text book it is not very convenient to adhere rigidly to these restrictions while discussing the theory and methods of analytical chemistry.

1·3·4. Major, Minor and Trace Constituents

A *major constituent* is one whose amount is 1 per cent or more of the sample material. A *minor constituent* is 0·01 to 1 per cent of the sample and a constituent present in quantities smaller than 0·01 per cent is called a *trace constituent*.

1·3·5. Complete and Partial Analysis

Chemical analysis is said to be *complete* when it involves the determination of all the components detected qualitatively in the sample. The analysis is *partial* when it aims at determining only one or a few of the components of the sample such as, determination of copper in a copper ore.

1·3·6. Major Steps of Quantitative Analysis

Quantitative chemical analysis consists of the following four main steps :

(*a*) Sampling, that is, selecting a representative sample of the material to be analysed ;

(*b*) Conversion of the desired constituent into a form suitable for measurement ;

(*c*) Measurement of some property on which the determination is based, such as measurement of weight as in gravimetric analysis or measurement of volume as in volumetric analysis, or measurement of potential as in potentiometric titrations ; and

(*d*) Calculation and interpretation of the result.

Analytical methods are sometimes classified on the basis of the property whose measurement underlie the method of determination.

1·3·7. Classical Chemical Analysis

Quantitative chemical analysis started with the application of techniques of *gravimetric procedures*. In a gravimetric determination, a known volume of sample solution is treated with an excess of a suitable reagent which quantitatively precipitates the desired constituent present in the sample solution. The precipitate which is of known composition is filtered, washed, dried and weighed. Knowing the weight of the precipitate, the amount of the desired constituent in the test solution is calculated. For example, an excess of dilute sulphuric acid is added to a given solution containing barium ions. The precipitate of barium sulphate formed is filtered, washed, dried and weighed. From the weight of barium sulphate, the quantity of barium in the given solution is calculated. Because such determinations are based on the measurement of weight, these are referred to as gravimetric determinations.

In *electrogravimetric analysis*, the constituent to be determined is deposited on an electrode by passing electric current through a suitable electrolytic cell. For example, the amount of copper in given copper sulphate solution can be determined by passing current through the solution and weighing the copper deposited at the negative electrode. Here electric current acts as a precipitating agent.

Gravimetric determination of a volatile constituent can be done by heating the sample and recording the loss of weight. Gravimetric procedures are quite accurate but are lengthy and tedious.

Another group of techniques was soon developed in which quantitative analysis was achieved by measuring volume of solutions, hence it was called *volumetric analysis* (now known as titrimetric analysis). In this type of analysis, to the sample solution of unknown concentration, a reagent solution of known concentration is gradually added till the reaction between them is just complete as shown by some indicator. The volume of the sample and reagent solutions are known, the concentration of the reagent solution is also known so the concentration of the given sample solution can be calculated. For example, a known volume of hydrochloric acid solution whose concentration is to be determined is taken in a conical flask and a few drops of phenolphthalein solution are added as indicator. A solution of sodium hydroxide of known concentration is gradually added through a burette until the solution in the flask becomes just pink. The volume of sodium hydroxide solution added is recorded and from this, the concentration of given hydrochloric acid is calculated. This process is called *titration* and the determination is termed *titrimetric determination*. Earlier such a procedure was called a volumetric procedure but this can mean measurement of volume of a gas also hence the term titrimetric procedure is preferred.

Certain substances, under suitable experimental conditions, quantitatively liberate a gas. The measurement of the volume of the liberated gas can be used as a basis for determining the substance producing the gas. Such analytical procedures are called *"gasometric methods"*. For example, semicarbazide can be decomposed with lead peroxide and the liberated nitrogen can be measured. Knowing the volume of nitrogen, the amount of semicarbazide present in the sample solution can be calculated.

A particular component of a gaseous mixture can be absorbed in a suitable absorbent. The decrease in the volume of the gaseous mixture gives the volume of the constituent absorbed. This method of analysis is called *"gas analysis"*. For example, a mixture of oxygen and carbon dioxide gases can be passed through a solution of potassium hydroxide when carbon dioxide alone is absorbed. Thus the decrease in the volume of the gaseous mixture will be equal to the volume of carbon dioxide present in the mixture.

Gravimetric methods along with titrimetric procedures belong to the *classical methods of chemical analysis*. The titrimetric procedures are much simpler and convenient and hence a large number of titration methods have been worked out for determining a wide variety of inorganic and organic substances. In *direct* titrimetric methods, sample solution is directly titrated with reagent solution. The *indirect* procedure consists of adding a known excess of reagent and titrating back the unused reagent.

1·3·8. Classification of Methods of Quantitative Analysis

The methods of quantitative analysis can be classified from different points of view based on the nature of material under examination, the type of method employed, the amount of desired constituent in sample material and so on.

The analysis can be termed *organic, inorganic, biochemical* etc., depending on the nature of the material analysed.

A much used classification of quantitative analysis is *non-instrumental* and *instrumental*. The former includes gravimetric and titrimetric procedures whereas the latter involves use of instruments such as a colorimeter, a conductivitimeter or a potentiometer and so on. Such a classification is not very much justified because even the so called non-instrumental techniques, such as titrimetry, make use of balances, pipettes, burettes, graduated flasks etc., which though simple but are certainly instruments.

Another classification into *chemical* and *physico-chemical* methods of analysis is also not very sound theoretically although it is quite useful for the sake of convenience. According to this classification, gravimetric and titrimetric methods are termed chemical methods though they are based on the measurement of physical properties, *viz.* weight and volume. The methods of analysis based on such physical properties as potential, conductance, current strength, optical rotation, etc., are generally referred to as physico-chemical methods. But it should be remembered that these so called physical methods involve many chemical operations and that the measurement of a physical property is merely one of the several steps of the analytical procedure. For example, the only difference between a potentiometric titration and an ordinary titration is that the former uses potential measurement rather than a visual indicator for the detection of end-point.

The classical chemical analysis which consists of gravimetric and titrimetric methods is also known as *wet analysis*, sometimes this is referred to as an analysis based on *matter-matter interaction* as it involves a reaction between a substance to be determined and another substance, that is, reagent. There are certain other procedures which are based on *matter-energy interaction* such as, a colorimetric determination which involves passage of light, a form of energy, through solution of the substance, to be determined, which is matter.

The methods of quantitative analysis can also be classified on the basis of the size of the sample for a determination. The term *macroanalysis* is used when the determination involves 0·1 g or more of the sample. If the amount of the sample is approximately 0·01 to 0·1 g, the method is called *semimicro* and for samples weighing 0·001—0·01 g, the term *micromethod* is used. *Ultramicro* analysis involves samples containing less than 0·001 g of material ; some authors have used the term *submicro* analysis also. Certain procedures have been described for analysing quantities smaller than those handled in ultramicro analysis ; these constitute what is known as *supermicro analysis*. The limits mentioned above are not to be considered rigid but only approximate.

Some authors classify quantitative methods of analysis into *centigram, milligram* and *microgam* (or gamma) procedures ; these are applicable to methods in which the weight of the substance to be determined is of the order of a centigram, a milligram or a microgram respectively (See Table 1·1).

According to another classification, macromethods are those in which sample contains more than 2 milliequivalents (meq) of the material and 0·1 N solutions are employed in the determination. In semimicro methods, the sample contains about 1 meq of substance and 0·05 to 0·1 N solutions are used in its titrimetric determination. When the amount of the substance is around 0·1 meq, the method used is called a micromethod ; this generally involves the use of 0·01 N reagent solutions.

1·4. THE GROWTH OF ANALYTICAL CHEMISTRY

Although from earlier times analytical chemistry played an important role in various fields of chemistry, it was only after 1850 that it was regarded as an independent discipline. In India, however, it is only in last few decades that analytical chemistry has acquired the status of a distinct subject.

A remarkable fact about the development of analytical chemistry is that workers in other branches such as inorganic, organic, biochemistry etc., have also contributed significantly to its growth. The difference in approach is that whereas an analytical chemist has his main interest in the methods and techniques themselves, other workers develop analytical procedures for their own specific problems. For example, a worker in the field of chemical kinetics is not primarily interested in various analytical methods and techniques but may develop a method for quantitatively analysing a substance whose concentration is to be determined in order to obtain

Table 1·1. Microchemical Units of Mass and Volume

Name	Definition	Symbol
Gram	10^{-3} kg	g
Centigram	10^{-4} kg	cg
Milligram	10^{-3} g	mg
Microgram	10^{-6} g	μg or γ
Nanogram	10^{-3} μg or 10^{-9} g	ng
Picogram	10^{-6} μg or 10^{-12} g	pg
Millilitre	10^{-3} l	ml
Microlitre	10^{-3} ml or 10^{-6} l	μl
Nanolitre	10^{-3} μl or 10^{-9} l	nl
Picolitre	10^{-6} μl or 10^{-12} l	pl

the necessary kinetic data. On the other hand, the main interest of an analytical chemist is in the development and improvement of an analytical procedure itself and in testing its reliability. He also studies the interference caused by the presence of other substances and attempts to modify the procedure so that such an interference can be eliminated. He also tries to work out conditions when the procedure can be applied to the microdetermination of the substance under consideration. It is necessary to distinguish between an *analytical chemist* and an *analyst*. An analytical chemist carefully chooses a chemical reaction and uses it for developing an analytical procedure taking into account various theoretical considerations. He also studies the effect of different factors that can influence the result of the determination. The job of an analyst is simply to follow the given instructions to perform a determination.

As has already been mentioned, the earlier methods of quantitative analysis were those involving gravimetric procedures. Soon thereafter the technique of volumetric analysis emerged which due to its inherent simplicity and rapidity received preference over gravimetric methods which were lengthy and tedious. One of the earliest volumetric determinations was developed by Margueritte who titrated ferrous iron with potassium permanganate. Such a procedure is now more appropriately called a titrimetric procedure rather than a volumetric method because the latter is a more general term including gasometric methods and gas analysis which are also based on the measurement of volume. Due to their inherent simplicity titrimetric analyses have found and continue to find extensive applications. Both direct and indirect titrimetric procedures have been worked out for the quantitative analysis of wide variety of organic as well as inorganic compounds with the modern accent on micro and submicro analysis.

Over the last 50 years or so there has been a growing tendency to make use of certain instruments to achieve quantitative analysis. For example, instrumental techniques such as potentiometric, conductometric, photometric, amperometric etc., have been applied to locate the end point in a titration or to follow the course of a chemical reaction. It should be noted that in such cases the titrimetric methods are not basically altered from their standard procedures, the instrument simply acts as a substitute for an indicator. Recently such methods commonly known as the instrumental methods of analysis have been increasingly used especially in the field of industrial and commercial quantitative analysis due to their rapidity and sensitivity. But it would be a mistake to conclude that the so called chemical methods of analysis, *i.e.*, gravimetric and titrimetric methods would be totally eliminated from considerations. There are several reasons in favour of this as discussed below :

1. Most instrumental methods depend on calibration curve or calibration data. Solutions needed for this purpose are standardized by chemical methods.

2. Many instrumental methods cannot give precision and accuracy that is readily obtained in most chemical methods.

3. The cost of equipment for chemical analysis is within the reach of every chemical laboratory because such simple equipments as balances, pipettes, burettes, measuring flasks etc., are required. The physico-chemical methods invariably involve costly equipment.

The classical and physico-chemical methods of quantitative analysis should be regarded as complementary. Because once an instrument to be used in quantitative analysis has been properly calibrated, it can be used with great advantage to achieve rapid analysis and due to high sensitivity of physico-chemical procedures, samples at microgram level can be handled.

The advantages of microchemical methods are saving of time, labour and material. Much of the work on vitamines, harmones and other natural products could be done due to the development of microanalytical methods because many of the compounds were present in microquantities.

In about last 50 years there has been increasing sophistication in all areas of chemistry, physics and biological sciences. This created analytical problems which required use of sophisticated instrumentation for their solution. For example, in determining traces of impurities at part per billion level or determining traces of pollutants in the atmosphere of industrial area.

The solution of many such problems have been provided by research workers who are not essentially analytical chemists but are devoted to various other branches of science. A very large proportion of research work in the field of analytical chemistry has been performed in laboratories associated with hospitals, oceanographic institutes, physics departments, agricultural experiment centres and so on. As a result analytical chemistry cannot be bound with sharp lines.

2

Statistical Treatment of
Analytical Data

In any experimental science, experiments are done to measure a quantity. The results so obtained are termed data. The main object of quantitative analytical chemistry is to collect data on the amount of a particular constituent in a given sample. When such a determination is done it is important to know that to what extent it is reliable. This is achieved by measuring the same quantity several times and then making a statistical study of the observed data.

2.1. TRUE, STANDARD AND OBSERVED VALUE

In quantitative analytical work the quantity of a constituent present in a sample is measured or determined.

Example 2(i)

An analyst is interested in finding out the percentage of silver in a given coin and obtains the value to be 99·75% ; this is called the *observed value*. To know how correct his result is, the analyst must know *true* or *correct* or *actual value* for the percentage of silver. Now, true values are known only when we count objects or when a quantity is assigned a particular value, such as, atomic weight of certain isotope of carbon has been given a value of 12·0000. In other cases the true value of a quantity is never known. In the present example, the actual or true value for the percentage of silver can never be known because whosoever attempts to determine it, may make a mistake. However, if an expert using a suitable method and a good quality apparatus carefully determines the percentage of silver in the coin, his value can be regarded as the true value but it is then called *standard value*. Suppose the standard value for the percentage of silver is 100·00%. The difference between the true or standard value and the observed value is called *error*. In our example, the standard value is 100 00% and the observed value is 99·75% hence, the error in the determination is (100·00—99·75) =0·25%.

2·2. ACCURACY AND PRECISION

The term *accuracy* refers to how near the observed value is to true or standard value. In the above determination the error observed is 0·25% hence it can be said that the result is accurate to 0·25%.

In example 2(*i*), the analyst determined the percentage of silver to be 99·75%. He has made only one determination, therefore, he is not sure that his value cannot be challanged. Even if he himself makes a second determination for the percentage of silver in the same coin, he may not get the same value, *i.e.*, 99·75 which he got in the first determination. Thus, if one determines the same quantity a number of times, each value obtained will differ from another by slight or greater amount. The term *precision* refers to nearness between several measurements of the same quantity. The difference between accuracy and precision can be understood by considering the following example.

Example 2(*ii*)

There are two analysts I and II who determine the percentage of silver in the same coin. The standard value for silver in that coin is 100·00%, whereas the two analysts obtained the following results :

Analyst I : 100·00 ; 99·60 ; 99·70 ; 99·10

$$\text{Average value} = \frac{100 \cdot 00 + 99 \cdot 60 + 99 \cdot 70 + 99 \cdot 10}{4} = 99 \cdot 60\%$$

$$\text{Error} = (100 \cdot 00 - 99 \cdot 60) = 0 \cdot 4\%$$

Analyst II : 98·80 ; 98·82 ; 98·84 ; 98·82

$$\text{Average value} = \frac{98 \cdot 80 + 98 \cdot 82 + 98 \cdot 84 + 98 \cdot 82}{4} = 98 \cdot 82\%$$

$$\text{Error} = (100 \cdot 00 - 98 \cdot 82) = 1 \cdot 18\%.$$

The different observed values of analyst I differ quite much among themselves hence the precision is poor but accuracy is fairly good (error=0·4%). On the other hand, the accuracy of the result of analyst II is comparatively poor (error=1·18%) but his observed values do not differ much from each other hence the precision is better as compared to that in the measurements of analyst I.

2·3. SIGNIFICANT FIGURES

The meaning of this term can be understood by considering the following example.

Example 2(*iii*)

Suppose a crucible is weighed on a rough balance which can measure weight up to one tenth of a gram (g) and the result of weighing is 21·3 g. This means that the weight of the crucible is nearer to 21·3 rather than to 21·2 or 21·4 g. Here, three digits have been used to express the result, *i.e.*, three significant figures have been used. The balance is not sensitive enough to record weight up to the second place of decimal hence, only one figure would appear after the demical point. If the same crucible is weighed on an analytical balance which can measure weight up to one tenth of a milligram (mg), the result can now be expressed up to the fourth place after the decimal such as, 21·3182 g. This would mean that the weight of the crucible is closer to 21·3182 as compared to 21·3181 or 21·3183 g. Here six significant figures have been used. Now, it would be wrong to report the weight as 21 3 g because with the analytical balance, one is sure about the figures in the second and third places after the decimal point, which were not known when the rough balance was used for weighing. It is now clear that one has to be careful in expressing the value of the quantity measured.

Significant figures are digits necessary to express the result of a measurement to the precision with which the measurement is made. In example 2(*iii*), the rough balance can read only up to one tenth of a g, hence the weight of an object weighed on it should be expressed in g using only one figure after the decimal point. In the case of an analytical balance the markings are up to one tenth of a mg, hence the weight in g can be reported up to the fourth place of decimal, such as 21·3182 g, using six significant figures. Here the figures 21·318 are known with certainty, the sixth digit has some uncertainty (less than ± 1). That is why we say that the weight of the crucible is closer to 21·3182 than to either 21 3181 or 21·3183 g. Thus all digits which are certain plus one which has some uncertainty are said to be significant figures.

The digit zero may or may not be a significant figure depending upon the meaning it carries, *i.e*, its position.

Example 2(*iv*)

Suppose volume recorded by a burette is 10·04 ml, because here both zeros are measured they are significant. Thus, in all four significant figures have been used. The same volume in litres can be expressed as 0·01004 *l*. The purpose of the zero before the digit 1 is simply to indicate the position of the decimal point hence, it will not be significant. The zero before the decimal point is also not regarded as a significant figure. Thus, although six digits have been used to write the result in litres, only four of them are significant. Terminal zeros, *i.e.*, zeros at the end are significant as in 7·5960.

2·3·1.   Expressing Results in Exponential Form

If the magnitude of a quantity measured is very small or very large it is advisable to express the result in exponential form to avoid any confusion.

Example 2(v)

Suppose the value of a quantity is measured to be 0·000005. It appears that seven significant figures have been used to express the result. But the purpose of zeros before the figure 5 is to locate the position of the decimal point. The zero before the decimal point is also not significant figure. Hence, there is only one significant figure. The same result can be expressed in exponential form (using powers of ten) as 5×10^{-6}. Here it is easily seen that only one significant figure has been used.

Example 2(vi)

The number of molecules in a g mole of any substance is $6·023 \times 10^{23}$. This quantity has only four significant figures, the exponential factor 10^{23} simply indicates the position of the decimal point.

Example 2(vii)

Suppose the volume of a given liquid is reported as 5000 ml. If the digit 5 is considered as the only significant number, it would mean that the volume is closer to 5000 than to 4000 or 6000 ml. But if all the four digits are taken to be significant the meaning would be that the volume is nearer to 5000 rather than to 4999 or 5001 ml. To avoid this confusion, the following method using exponential factors can be used to express the results. Here, the significant numbers can be easily recognized.

	Significant figures used	Means that volume is nearer to
(a) 5×10^3	1	5000 than to 4000 or 6000 ml,
(b) $5·0 \times 10^3$	2	5000 than to 4900 or 5100 ml,
(c) $5·00 \times 10^3$	3	5000 than to 4990 or 5010 ml,
(d) $5·000 \times 10^3$	4	5000 than to 4999 or 5001 ml,

2·3·2.   Absolute and Relative Uncertainty

Absolute uncertainty is expressed directly in units of the measurement.

Example 2(viii)

The volume of a given solution is expressed as 10·1 ml, *i.e.*, the volume is reported to tenths of a ml. It means that the volume is closer to 10·1 rather than to 10·0 or 10·2 ml. Thus the absolute uncertainty is one tenth of a ml. A volume reported as 10·15 ml means that the absolute uncertainty is 0˙01 ml or one hundredth of a ml. (Remember that the last digit has some uncertainity).

Relative uncertainty is expressed in terms of magnitude of the quantity being measured. In example 2(*viii*), the uncertainty is 0˙1 ml in about 10 ml hence, it will be 1 ml if 100 ml volume is considered, *i.e.*, relative uncertainty is 1 part per hundred or 1 per cent. In the second case the uncertainty is 0˙01 ml in 10 ml hence, it will be 0˙1 in 100 ml or 1 in 1000 ml, *i.e.*, the relative uncertainty will be 0˙1 per cent or 1 part per thousand.

Example 2(ix)

The weight of a crucible is reported as 5˙05 g. The last digit is uncertain therefore, the absolute uncertainty is 0˙01 g. Now, in 5˙05 g, uncertainty is 0˙01 g therefore, in 100 g the uncertainty would be 20 times, *i.e.*, 0˙2 g ; the relative uncertainty would be 0˙2 per cent or 2 parts per thousand.

Relative uncertainty (in percentage)

$$= \frac{\text{absolute uncertainty}}{\text{amount of sample}} \times 100 \; ; \; \frac{0˙01}{5˙05} \times 100 = 0˙2\%$$

Relative uncertainty [in part per thousand (ppt)]

$$= \frac{\text{absolute uncertainty}}{\text{amount of sample}} \times 1000 \; ; \; \frac{0˙01}{5˙05} \times 1000 = 2 \text{ ppt.}$$

2˙3˙3.   Significant Figures in Mathematical Operations

In analytical calculations, it is often required to add two or more results or subtract one from another and so on.

(A) Addition or Subtraction. Let us consider the following two results :

Example 2(x)

Weight of bottle+substance=21˙2169 g

Weight of bottle   =20˙8114 g

Weight of substance   = 0˙4055 g

This is quite simple because both the quantities are measured to the same degree of accuracy, *i.e.*, up to one tenth of a mg. Now consider that the weight of the bottle and substance is determined up to the fourth place of decimal but that of the bottle only up to the second place as given below :

Weight of bottle+substance=21˙2169 g

Weight of bottle   =20˙81   g

Weight of substance   =0˙4069 g (improper result)

The weight of the substance should not be written as 0˙4069 g because if one of the quantities is known only up to the second place of decimal, it cannot give result which will be accurate up to the fourth place. The rule, in such operations, is that only as many figures after the decimal point should be considered as appear in the least accurately known quantity and the values should be suitably rounded off. In this example, the least accurately measured quantity is the weight of bottle which is 20˙81 g, using only two digits after the decimal. The first weight which is 21˙2169 g should, therefore, be rounded off to 21˙22 g so that it also contains only two digits after the decimal point. Now, the subtraction can be carried out as follows :

Weight of bottle+substance=21˙22 g

Weight of bottle　　　　=20˙81 g

Weight of substance　　　= 0˙41 g (proper result)

The quantities should be rounded off in a manner shown below :

Observed value	Rounded off value (upto the third place)
0˙2638	0˙264
0˙2632	0˙263
0˙2634	0˙263
0˙2636	0˙264
0˙2635	0˙264

Thus, in addition or subtraction of different observed values one should consider only as many figures after the decimal as contained by the least accurately known quantity.

Example 2(xi)

139˙21+3˙427+0˙6512 should be written as

139˙21+3˙43+0˙65=143˙29.

The first quantity contains only two digits after the decimal point (this is the smallest number of digits after the decimal) hence, all the other quantities should be rounded off in such a manner that they also have only two digits after the decimal point. Note that 3˙427 has been rounded off to 3˙43 and 0˙6512 to 0˙65.

If in a calculation many quantities are involved, it is advised to measure them with the same degree of accuracy. There is no point in doing lot of labour to measure some quantities very accurately when others are not known to the same degree of accuracy.

(B) Multiplication or division. In these operations one must take into consideration the relative uncertainties of different

·quantities involved. The general practice is that the product or ·quotient should be expressed with sufficient significant figures so that its relative uncertainty is comparable to that of the quantity with the greatest relative uncertainty.

Example 2(xii)

Suppose we have to calculate the product $9˙678234 \times 0˙12$. Here, out of the two quantities, $0˙12$ is least accurately known (it is measured only up to second place after the decimal). Hence, it will have greater relative uncertainty. In $0˙12$, the absolute uncertainty is $0˙01$ or relative uncertainty is 1 part in 12. The result of multiplication should, therefore, contain only as many significant figures which will show a similar relative uncertainty. Hence, the result would be written as $1˙2$ and not as $1˙16138808$. Note that in $1˙2$, the relative uncertainty is 1 part in 12.

2˙4. ERRORS

The object of an analyst is to obtain a result as near to the true value as possible. If the analyst has no idea about the accuracy and precision of the method used by him and the possible sources of error, he will not know how correct his results can be or he will have a poor level of confidence regarding the results that he has obtained. A quantitative analytical procedure is not only a collection of operations such as filtration, weighing, titration etc. The person carrying out the determination must know the theoretical principles on which the method is based, the possibility of interference due to presence of other substances and the possible sources of error.

The term *error* is used to show the difference between measured and true value. When a measurement is made, it is not possible to completely eliminate the error, even when the person making the measurement is an expert working with apparatus of best quality. However, attempts are made to minimise the error. To do so one first must know the magnitude of error in his measurement, which is the difference between the observed value and the true value. Since true values are never known one has to make use of the most probable or standard value. The standard value can be obtained by following methods.

(*i*) *Absolute method*. In this method, the sample in question is synthesized using known quantities of the constituents and thus a primary standard is obtained. Hence, the true values for the amount of **different** constituents are known. Now, the sample is analysed by some method, the observed values for the quantities of the constituents are recorded. Knowing the true and the observed· values, the error of the method can be calculated.

(*ii*) *Comparative method*. In some cases, as in the case of a mineral or an ore, it is not possible to prepare the synthetic sample. In such a case, the analytical data provided by some standard agency is obtained. The values provided in that data are the standard values for the quantities of the different constituents present in the sample. The difference in the observed and the standard value gives the error of the method used for analysis.

With the help of the two methods described above one can find out how much error is involved in his procedure of determination. In order to keep the value of error as small as possible it is necessary to know the types of error and their possible causes.

2˙4˙1. Types of Errors

Errors are broadly classified as : (a) determinate or systematic and (b) inderminate or random errors.

(A) **DETERMINATE ERROR.** There are certain errors whose causes, atleast in principle, can be known ; these are usually one sided and by proper planning and careful working can be avoided or kept at a minimum. The most important kinds of determinate errors are :

(i) **Personal error.** These are due to improper working of the person carrying out a determination.

Example 2(xiii)

A person is unable to judge the colour change of the indicator at the end point in a titration. He always adds little more titrant than actually needed and hence would always get a positive error, i.e., his measured value will always be more than the standard value.

Similarly, one may not wash the precipitate properly in a gravimetric determination or may not heat the precipitate to a proper temperature. Such defects can be pointed out and by properly following the procedure this type of error can be eliminated or minimised.

(ii) **Instrumental or Reagent error.** These are due to defect in the equipment say faulty construction of a balance, a wrongly calibrated pipette or burette etc.

Example 2(xiv)

Suppose a 25 ml pipette is used to take a sample solution for analysis. If the pipette is not of a good quality it may take out only 24˙5 ml. Thus an error of 0˙5 ml will be introduced and this will always be on the negative side.

Similarly, if reagents used are impure, the result of analysis will be wrong. These errrors can be removed by using good quality apparatus and pure reagents.

(iii) **Errors of method.** These may be due to incomplete reaction, solubility of a precipitate in gravimetric analysis, decomposition of the precipitate during ignition etc.

Example 2(xv)

Calculations are based on the assumption that the chemical reaction used in the analytical method goes to completion. If the reaction is only 95 per cent complete, the results will not be as expected. The error caused will be one sided and can be removed by creating experimental conditions so that the reaction goes to completion.

Example 2(xvi)

In a gravimetric determination, along with the desired precipitate another substance is also precipitated. This would give rise to an error which can be avoided if the precipitation of another substance is controlled by some means.

(iv) **Additive error.** Sometimes the value of error is constant in a series of determination and is independent of the amount of sample taken for analysis ; these are termed additive errors.

Example 2($xvii$)

In a titration, 0·1ml extra titrant has to be added to see the colour change clearly at the end point, *i.e.*, end point error is 0·1 ml. Therefore, if the standard value is 10·0 ml, the observed value will be 10·1 ml, thus an error of 0·1 ml will be noted. If the sample taken for the titration is doubled, the standard value will be 20·0 ml. But in the titration the value will come out to be 20·1 ml due to the end-point error of 0·1 ml. It should be noted that the error remains the same, *i.e.*, 0·1 ml even when the sample size is doubled.

(v) **Proportional error.** In this type of error the magnitude of the error depends upon the sample size.

Example 2($xviii$)

In the titration of 10·0 ml of 0·1 N hydrochloric acid, 10·0 ml (standard value) of 0·1 N sodium hydroxide solution should be required. But the sodium hydroxide used is impure so the observed titre value (volume of the titrant) comes out to be 10·2 ml. The error in the determination is (10·2−10·0)=0·2 ml. Now, if 20·0 ml of 0·1 N hydrochloric acid solution is titrated with the same impure sodium hydroxide solution, the observed titre value will be 20·4 ml, whereas the standard value is 20·0 ml. Thus, this time, the error is 0·4 ml. It means that on doubling the sample the error has also doubled. Hence, the error observed is a proportional error which can be minimized by using pure sodium hydroxide for the titration.

(B) **INDETERMINATE ERRORS.** These are also known as random or accidental errors. The cause of a random error may or may not be known. We have already seen that determinate errors are one sided and they can be more or less eliminated by careful work. On the other hand, the indeterminate errors are not one sided and they cannot be eliminated even when the analysis is done with great care using high quality apparatus and reagents. Hence, indeterminate or random errors are due to causes over which the analyst has no control.

When the same quantity is measured several times, the different observed values will not be exactly similar. These values differ from each other slightly even if these different measurements are made very carefully by the same person under as identical conditions as possible. These values very frequently will differ from the standard value also and this difference is called indeterminate or random error.

Example 2(xix)

A ball of 10 g is weighed on an analytical balance and we want to know its weight to the nearest of a g, i.e., whether it is 8 or 9 or 10 or 11 g. Here, the weight in different weight readings will always be 10 g, i.e., replicate results will be obtained. But if we want to know the weight of the ball up to the fourth place of decimal, the different weight readings will not be identical but will vary slightly from one another and also from the standard value of the weight of the ball. Thus, random errors will be observed which cannot be avoided. Such errors may be due to reasons like variation in temperature, vibrations in the laboratory building due to passing traffic etc. Some personal judgement is always involved in measuring a property, this also gives rise to random errors. There are two important points that can be noted about random errors :

(i) The number of readings with smaller errors is more than the readings with larger errors, i.e., frequency of results with larger errors is small as compared to that with smaller errors.

Example 2(xx)

Suppose the standard value of a property is 0˙3629. If several measurements of this property are made, most of the readings will be nearer to 0˙3629 and only a few readings will differ much from 0˙3629.

(ii) If a very large number of measurements of a particular quantity is made, the number of readings showing positive error is equal to that of readings showing negative error, i.e., the frequency of positive and negative error is equal.

In example 2(xx), if a very large number of measurements are made, say 100,000 readings are taken, then it will be found that 50,000 readings will have value greater than 0˙3629 and 50,000 reading will have value smaller than 0˙3629.

The above two observations about random errors can be graphically represented as shown in Fig. 2˙1 on page 27.

2·4·2.   Minimisation of Errors

Every analytical chemist attempts to know how much error is present in his determination and tries to minimise it. Determinate errors can be minimised by taking the following precautions.

(i) *Proper calibration of apparatus*. Weights, burettes, pipettes, measuring flasks etc., should be properly calibrated. The chemicals used should also be pure.

(ii) *Running a blank determination*. A blank determination means carrying out one more determination identically in which sample is omitted.

Example 2(xxi)

Ten ml of an acid solution is titrated with a known solution of alkali. The observed titre value is 10·2 ml. The titration is repeated taking 10·0 ml of water in place of the acid solution ; the titre value this time is 0·1 ml. The corrected titre reading will, therefore, be (10·2−0·1)=10·1 ml.

By carrying out a blank determination, the errors due to impure reagents can be minimised. The end point error can also be avoided.

(iii) *Carrying out a control determination*. A parallel determination is carried out, by taking nearly same amount of the constituent that is present in the sample, under identical conditions. The weight of the constituent in the sample is calculated using the following relationship :

$$\frac{\text{Result found for known sample}}{\text{Result found for unknown sample}}$$

$$= \frac{\text{Wt. of constituent in known sample}}{\text{Wt. of constituent in unknown sample}}.$$

Example 2(xxii)

With a known sample, the titration reading is 10·0 ml and with the unknown it is 9·0 ml. If the weight of the desired constituent in the known sample is X g, the weight of the same constituent in the unknown sample will be 0·9 X g.

(iv) *Use of independent method*. Here the determination is done by some other method also and the two results are compared. If the other method also gives similar result as obtained by method under consideration, the result can be regarded as reliable.

Example 2(xxiii)

The amount of sulphuric acid present in a given solution can be determined by treating it with an excess of barium chloride and weighing the precipitate of barium sulphate formed after washing and drying. Now, we want to know whether the result obtained is reliable. The amount of sulphuric acid can also be determined by titration with alkali. If the two results are similar, the gravimetric determination will be considered to be reliable.

Indeterminate errors cannot be avoided. They can be kept at a minimum by choosing a reliable method, using good quality equipment and making the measurement carefully.

2·5 ABSOLUTE AND RELATIVE ERROR

The absolute error is the numerical difference between the observed and ture or standard value.

Example 2(*xxiv*)

In 10·0000 g of a coin, the amount of silver is determined to be 5·2000 g (observed value). Suppose the standard value for silver in 10·0000 g of the same coin is 5·0000 g. The absolute error in the determination will be (observed value—standard value)=(5·2000—5·0000) g =0·2000 g. If it is said that the error is 0·2000 g we can not find out whether this error is large or small. (Because if it is the error in 100 g of silver it is small but if it is the error in 1 g of silver then it is quite large). It means that when error is expressed as absolute error it is necessary to mention the amount of the constituent determined.

The errors are generally expressed relative to the size of the sample such as part per hundred or part per thousand. This is then called *relative error*.

In example 2(*xxiv*), there is an absolute error of 0·2000 g in 5·0000 g of silver hence, if 100 g of silver is considered, the error will also increase 20 times, *i.e.*, 0·2000×20=4·0 g. Then we can say that there is an error of 4·0 g in 100 g of silver or error is 4 parts in 100 parts of silver or the error is 4%. Thus,

Relative error in parts per hundred

$$= \frac{\text{Absolute error}}{\text{Amount of constituent}} \times 100$$

$$= \frac{0\cdot2000}{5\cdot0000} \times 100 = 4\cdot0\% \text{ or 4 parts per hundred.}$$

Now, sometimes results are expressed in percentage, *e.g.*, observed percentage of silver in a coin is 22·50%, whereas the standard value for silver in that coin is 22·00%. The absolute error, therefore, will be (22·50—22·00)=0·50%. Because the value of error is in terms of percentage it may raise doubt that it might be relative error. To avoid this confusion, the relative error can be better expressed in terms of parts per thousand or ppt.

In example 2(*xxiv*), the absolute error is 0·2000 g in 5·000 g, hence if 1000 g of silver is considered, the error will be 200 times, *i.e.*, 0·2000 × 200 = 40 g. The relative error will, therefore, be 40 g per 1000 g or 40 parts per thousand. Thus,

Relative error in part per thousand (ppt)

$$= \frac{\text{Absolute error}}{\text{Amount of constituent}} \times 1000$$

$$= \frac{0·2000}{5·0000} \times 1000 = 40 \text{ ppt.}$$

2·6. MEAN DEVIATION AND RELATIVE MEAN DEVIATION

In order to know errors and minimise their effects upon the final result, a determination should not be done only once but it should be repeated a number of times. The different values so obtained are not all alike but differ among themselves to a greater or lesser extent. These different values are then examined statistically to get the final result.

Average is a measure of central tendency, *i.e.*, other values are around the average value. The average is the arithmatic mean of different values obtained by measuring the same quantity several times.

Example 2(*xxv*)

A silver coin was analysed four times and the values for the percentage of silver obtained in these four determinations are :

(*i*)	22·64%	(x_1)
(*ii*)	22·54%	(x_2)
(*iii*)	22·61%	(x_3)
(*iv*)	22·53%	(x_4)

the sum is, 90·32%

The arithmatic mean is given by :

$$\frac{\text{Sum of different values}}{\text{Number of times determination is made}} = \frac{(x_1 + x_2 + x_3 + \cdots)}{n} = \bar{x}.$$

Thus the average value in the above case will be :

$$\frac{90·32}{4} = 22·58\% \text{ of silver } (\bar{x}).$$

Deviation (*d*), in a particular measurement, is the difference between the measured value and the average value, *i.e.*, $x_1 - \bar{x} = d_1$; d_1 is the deviation in the first determination.

The *average* or *mean deviation* $(\bar{d})$, is the arithmatic mean of the different deviations observed in several measurements of the same quantity. Thus,

$$\bar{d} = \frac{d_1 + d_2 + d_3 + d_4 + \cdots}{n}$$

where d_1, d_2, d_3, d_4 etc., are the magnitude of deviations noted in different measurements and 'n' is number of times the measurement is made.

Relative mean deviation is given as :

$$\frac{\text{Mean deviation}}{\text{Amount of constituent}} \times 100$$

In example 2($xxvi$), given below, the relative mean deviation will be :

$$\frac{0\cdot04 \times 100}{22\cdot58} = 0\cdot18\%.$$

In calculating mean deviation, the positive or negative sign of individual deviations is disregarded.

The *standard deviation(s)*, of a result is the square root of the sum of the squares of individual deviations divided by $(n-1)$.

$$s = \sqrt{\frac{d_1{}^2 + d_2{}^2 + d_3{}^2 + d_4{}^2 + \cdots}{(n-1)}}$$

where d_1, d_2, d_3, d_4 etc., are individual deviations and 'n' is the number of individual deviations. Let us calculate the value of average and standard deviation for the following data :

Example 2($xxvi$)

%Ag	Individual deviation (d) $x - \bar{x} = d$	d^2
(x_1) 22·64	$(x_1 - \bar{x})$; $(22\cdot64 - 22\cdot58) = +0\cdot06$	0·0036
(x_2) 22·54	$(x_2 - \bar{x})$; $(22\cdot54 - 22\cdot58) = -0\cdot04$	0·0016
(x_3) 22·61	$(x_3 - \bar{x})$; $(22\cdot61 - 22\cdot58) = +0\cdot03$	0·0009
(x_4) 22·53	$(x_4 - \bar{x})$; $(22\cdot53 - 22\cdot58) = -0\cdot05$	0·0025

the sum is, 90·32   the sum is, 0·18   0·0086 (sum)

$$\text{Average} = \frac{90\cdot32}{4}\;;\qquad \text{(disregarding +ve and} \qquad s = \sqrt{\frac{0\cdot0086}{4-1}}$$
$$\text{—ve sign).}$$

$\bar{x} = 22\cdot58$;   Average deviation $s = 0\cdot05$

$$= \frac{0\cdot18}{4}\;;$$

$$\bar{d} = 0\cdot04$$

The square of standard deviation is called *variance* and coefficient of variation (C.V.) is defined as :

$$C.V. = \frac{s \times 100}{\bar{x}}$$

In example 2(*xxvi*), standard deviation is 0·05, hence the variance will be $(0·05)^2 = 0·0025$ and the coefficient of variation will be :

$$\frac{0·05}{22·58} \times 100 = 0·22\%.$$

Coefficient of variation is also known as relative standard deviation.

2·6·1. Physical Significance of Standard Deviation

Though it is easier to calculate mean deviation than to calculate standard deviation, but the latter is a better measure of the overall deviation. From the curve showing normal distribution of random errors or deviations in a large number of determinations of the same quantity (Fig. 2·1), it is concluded that small deviations are more frequent than large deviations. It has been shown that 68 per cent of the individual deviations are less than the standard deviation,

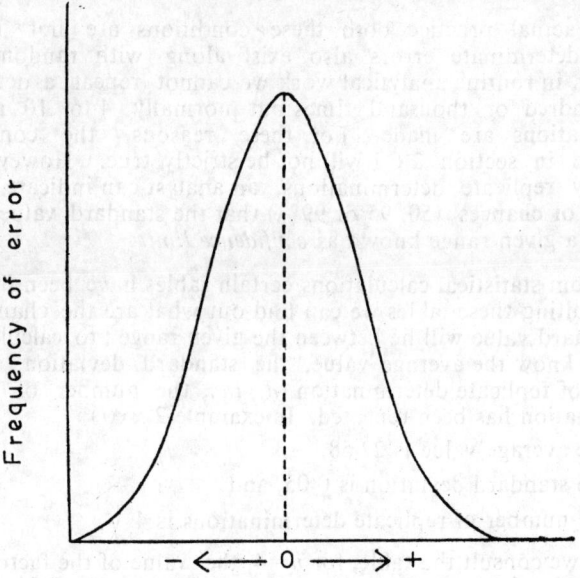

Magnitude of error

Fig. 2·1.   Normal or Gaussion distribution of errors.

95 per cent are less than twice the standard deviation and 99 per cent are less than 2·5 times the standard deviation. In other words 68 per cent of the observed values will be in the range ($\bar{x} \pm s$), 95 per cent in the range ($\bar{x} \pm 2s$) and 99 per cent within the range ($\bar{x} \pm 2·5s$) ; $\bar{x}$ is the average value and 's' is the standard deviation.

In example 2(xxvi), the average value is 22·58 and the standard deviation is 0·05. If a large number of determinations are made—

(a) 68% of the observed values will be between (22·58 ±0·05), i.e., between 22·53 and 22·63 ;

(b) 95% of the observed values will be between (22·58±0·1), i.e., between 22·48 and 22·68 ; and

(c) 99% of the observed values will be between (22·58±0·13), i.e., between 22·45 and 22·71.

2·6·2. Confidence Limit and Probability

The above conclusions have been derived by making two assumptions :

(i) determinations involve only random errors, and

(ii) a very large number of replicate determinations are made.

In actual practice both these conditions are not fulfilled. Firstly, determinate errors also exist along with random errors. Secondly, in routine analytical work we cannot repeat a determination hundred or thousand times but normally 4 to 10 replicate determinations are made. For these reasons, the conclusions described in section 2·6·1 will not be strictly true. However, even with few replicate determinations, an analyst can indicate the *probability* or chances (50, 95 or 99%) that the standard value will lie between a given range known as *confidence limit*.

From statistical calculations certain tables have been prepared. By consulting these tables we can find out what are the chances that the standard value will lie between the given range ; to calculate this, we must know the average value, the standard deviation and the number of replicate determination (n), i.e., the number of times a determination has been repeated. In example 2(xxvi) :

the average value is 22·58,

the standard deviation is 0·05, and

the number of replicate determinations is 4.

If we consult the table, for $n=4$, the value of the factor, f_{50}, is 0·38. Now, $(0·38 \times 0·05)=0·02$. it means that there is 50% probability that the true or standard value will lie between (22·58±0·02), i.e., 22·56 to 22·60. For $n=4$, $f_{99}=2·9$. Now, $(2·9 \times 0·05)=0·15$. It means that there is 99% probability that the standard value will lie between (22·58±0·15), *i.e.*, 22·43 and 22·73. In other words the analyst can confidently say that there are 99% chances that the correct answer is within 22·43 and 22·73. But this will be correct only when he has eliminated or atleast minimised the determinate error.

2·6·3. Rejection of an Observation

Sometimes one of the values obtained in a series of results of replicate determinations is found to be quite different from other values.

Example 2(*xxvii*)

Suppose the series of results, when the same quantity is measured four times is :

 (*a*) 22·64

 (*b*) 22·54

 (*c*) 22·22

 (*d*) 22·69

The third value is obviously out of line, showing a large error. This can be due to some reason which may be known. For example, some of the precipitate may be lost during a step of gravimetric analysis. In such a case the further analysis should be stopped. If the reason for the deviation is not known, statistical tests are applied to know whether to reject such an observation.

Let us apply the test to find out whether the third value (22·22) in example 2(*xxvii*), should be considered or rejected. First, considering all the four readings, find out the difference (R_1), for the highest and lowest value ; this will be $(22·69-22·22)=0·47$. Now, leave the doubtful value, *i.e.*, 22·22 and again find out the difference (R_2) between the highest and lowest value ; this time it will be $(22·69-22.54)=0·15$. Calculate the value of the ratio R_1/R_2 and use the following table to know whether to retain or reject the doubtful value, *i.e.*, 22·22.

Table 2·1. Factors for Retaining or Rejecting an Observation

n	Value of R_1/R_2 at 99% probability level
4	9·0
6	3·3
10	2·1
n=number of readings	

In our example, the value of $R_1/R_2=0·47/0·15$ or 3:1. For four determinations, the value of this ratio from the above table is

9·0. Because the value in the table is more than that calculated, hence the value 22·22 should not be rejected. If the value of R_1/R_2 comes out to be greater than that given in the table, the doubtful value is rejected. This is also known as Q test.

2·6·4. Student's t Test

Suppose a sample is analysed for a particular constituent by two different methods. Several replicate determinations are made and average value calculated in both the cases. Now, it is not possible to say which one is correct, but by statistical considerations we can tell whether the two average values are significantly different or should be considered as similar. This question can be answered by applying a test known as t test which was suggested by an English chemist writing under the pen name Student. The quantity t is defined as :

$$t = \frac{\bar{x} - \bar{y}}{s} \sqrt{\frac{n \times m}{n + m}}$$

where $\bar{x}$ is the average of n values obtained by first method and $\bar{y}$ is the average of m values obtained by the second method. The standard deviation in both the method has the same value s.

Example 2(xxviii)

A given sample containing chloride ion was analysed volumetrically. Four determinations ($n=4$) were made and their average ($\bar{x}$) was found to be 22·54% for chloride ion. Four gravimetric determinations ($m=4$) were also done for chloride ion in the same sample and the average came out to be 22·44% ($\bar{y}$). In both the procedures the standard deviation was calculated to be 0·08. Now, the question is whether the average values, i.e., 22·54 and 22·44% should be treated as almost similar or they should be regarded as significantly different. (Note that although the two values are different but we must not forget that even if the same quantity is measured two times, the two values will not be identical but will differ from each other). This can be known with the help of t test. In the above example, the t value is calculated as :

$$t = \frac{\bar{x} - \bar{y}}{s} \sqrt{\frac{n \times m}{n + m}} \ ;$$

$$t = \frac{22·54 - 22·44}{0·08} \sqrt{\frac{4 \times 4}{4 + 4}} = 1·77$$

The table for t values is then consulted.

Table 2·2.   t Values for Comparing Averages

D.F.	t value at 99% probability level
2	63·7
4	4·6
6	3·7
8	3·4
10	3·2

D.F. means degree of freedom $= m+n-2$.

In example $2(xxviii)$, the value of t comes out to be 1·7 for D.F. value $(4+4-2)=6$. From Table 2·2., at 99% probability level, the value of t, for D.F. equal to 6, is 3·7, which is higher than the observed t value of 1·7. Hence, statistically the two average values, $i.e.$, 22·54 and 22·44% cannot be regarded as significantly different. In this example both the procedures had the same value for standard deviation, $i.e.$, 0·08. If the values of standard deviation in the two methods used is different, the calculation of t value becomes more complicated.

2·6·5. F Test

If the values of standard deviations s_1 and s_2 for the first and second method respectively differ, there is a test called F test to know whether this difference is significant. The value of F is calculated as :

$$F = \frac{s_1{}^2}{s_2{}^2}$$

The larger value of standard deviation s is always kept in the numerator so that the value of F is always greater than unity. The value of F so calculated is compared with those theoretically calculated (these are given in tables). If the F value in the table is less than the observed F value, then the two standard deviations are significantly different. If the observed value of F is smaller than that given in the table, the two standard deviations s_1 and s_2 are not significantly different.

2·6·6. Chi Square Test

This test is used to find out whether the observed data differs significantly from the one obtained from theoretical distribution.

2·7. THE IMPORTANCE OF STATISTICAL TREATMENT

We have seen that in quantitative chemical analysis we are mainly interested in finding out the amount of a particular constituent present in a given sample. Obviously, if only one determination is made, the value obtained cannot be confidently taken to be correct. Hence, the same determination is repeated a number of times (normally 6 to 10 times). The different values obtained in these different determinations are not similar but usually differ from each other. Now the question is how to get a value that will be quite near to the standard value. This problem is solved by statistically treating the observed data. The average value, average deviation and standard deviation etc., are calculated for a given set of readings. Then by statistical considerations, we can calculate the probability that the standard value will be between $(\bar{x} \pm f s)$, where $\bar{x}$ is the average value, s is the standard deviation and f is a factor whose value is theoretically found.

3

Stoichiometric Calculations

3.1. USE OF CHEMICAL REACTIONS IN CHEMICAL ANALYSES

Most of the analytical procedures make use of some or the other chemical reaction. For example, gravimetric determination of silver (in a given soln. of $AgNO_3$) as silver chloride is based on the reaction of silver nitrate and hydrochloric acid ; titrimetric determination of oxalic acid is based on its reaction with potassium permanganate. But every chemical reaction cannot be employed for developing an analytical method. There are two important conditions which a chemical reaction must fulfil in order that it may act as a basis of an analytical procedure. Firstly, the reaction should be rapid and secondly it must go to completion. The second condition may or may not be important in qualitative analysis but it is absolutely necessary if the reaction is being used in quantitative analysis.

3.1.1. Advantages of Rapid Reactions

As mentioned above, a chemical reaction can be used in chemical analysis only when the time taken by the reaction is much smaller than the time required during the analytical operation.

Example 3(i)

Suppose a substance X forms a coloured compound when a solution of substance Y is added to it. Hence, the solution of substance Y can be used as a reagent for recognising or identifying the substance X. Here, the important requirement is that the reaction between X and Y should be quick so that we immediately see the colour change. If the reaction between them takes place slowly, the colour will appear after sometime. Moreover, it will be faint and will gradually develop. Thus, this will not be a good test.

Example 3(*ii*)

Suppose we are titrating solution A (known as titrand) with solution B (known as titrant). If the two substances present in these solutions react slowly, the titration between them will be both inconvenient and inaccurate. After each addition of the titrant, we will have to wait for some time so that the reaction between solution A and added solution B is complete. Thus a very long time will be required for completing the titration. Furthermore, due to slow reaction, there will be difficulty in judging the end point also, hence the titration will be inaccurate.

From the above two examples, it is evident that only those reactions can be successfully used in analytical chemistry which proceed more rapidly than the time required for performing an analytical operation. In example 3(*ii*), we add small amount of titrant to the titrand, shake the solution and then add little more titrant. Suppose in between these successive additions, there is a time gap of 30 seconds, then the reaction between the titrand and the added titrant must be complete in less than 30 seconds.

If the chemical reaction under consideration is not rapid, some steps should be taken to make it rapid before it can be used as a basis of an analytical method.

Example 3(*iii*)

When oxalic acid is titrated with potassium permanganate at room temperature, the pink colour of the added permanganate disappears gradually due to slow reaction between oxalic acid and permanganate. Hence, oxalic acid solution is heated to about 70°C before being titrated with permanganate.

Apart from heating, other steps can also be taken to speed up a reaction ; these will be discussed in detail in Chapter 4.

3·1·2. Completeness of Chemical Reaction

Theoretically speaking, a chemical reaction is never complete but if it proceeds to about 99·8% or more, it is supposed to be practically complete or quantitative and can be used as a basis of a quantitative method. Apart from being quantitative, the reaction should be fast also, so that equilibrium is rapidly attained.

Example 3(*iv*)

Hydrochloric acid reacts rapidly and quantitatively with sodium hydroxide according to the equation :

$$HCl \quad + \quad NaOH \quad = \quad NaCl \quad + \quad H_2O$$
$$\underset{36·5\,g}{(1+35·5)\,g} \quad \underset{40·0\,g}{(23+16+1)\,g} \quad \underset{58·5\,g}{(23+35·5)\,g} \quad \underset{18·0\,g}{(2+16)\,g}$$

The above equation tells us that 36·5 g of hydrochloric acid (acid) react with 40·0 g of sodium hydroxide (alkali) to produce 58·5 g of sodium chloride (salt) and 18·0 g water. Even if we add 100·0 g of alkali to 36·5 g acid, the acid will react only with 40·0 g of alkali. We can take any other unit for weight also. Such as, 36·5 kg of the acid would react with 40·0 kg of the alkali to form 58·5 kg of the salt and 18·0 kg of water. Further, the different quantities involved can be divided or multiplied by a common factor such as, $(36·5 \times 2) = 73$ mg of the acid would react with $(40·0 \times 2) = 80·0$ mg of the alkali to form $(58·5 \times 2) = 117·0$ mg of the salt and $(18·0 \times 2) = 36·0$ mg of water ; or, $(36·5/10) = 3·65$ tons of the acid will react with $(40·0/10) = 4·0$ tons of the alkali to give $(58·5/10) = 5·85$ tons of the salt and $(18·0/10) = 1·8$ tons of water.

In this example, we have calculated the quantities of the reactants (acid and alkali) which combine and those of the products (salt and water) formed, with the help of the chemical equation representing the reaction. The branch of chemistry which deals with the weight relations between reactants and products in chemical reactions is called *stoichiometry*. If we say that the reaction between hydrochloric acid and sodium hydroxide is stoichiometric, it is understood that 36·5 parts by weight of the acid will react with 40·0 parts by weight of alkali to produce 58·5 parts by weight of the salt and 18·0 parts by weight of water. In quantitative analysis only those reactions can be used which have known stoichiometry, *i.e.*, in which there is a fixed ratio between the quantities of the different reactants and products.

3·1·3. Stoichiometric Calculation

In methods of quantitative analysis, some quantity such as weight or volume is measured and from this measurement, the amount of a particular substance present in a sample solution is calculated. Suppose we are given a hydrochloric acid solution (called sample solution) and we have to find out the weight of the acid in given volume of the sample solution. To do this, first of all, we will have to prepare a known solution (called standard solution) of alkali say of sodium hydroxide. A known volume of the sample solution is then titrated with standard alkali solution using a suitable indicator, to know that what volume of standard alkali is chemically equivalent to the volume of acid taken for the titration. Knowing the strength of alkali, volumes of the acid and alkali used in the titration and from the known stoichiometry of the reaction between hydrochloric acid and sodium hydroxide, the quantity of hydrochloric acid in known volume of acid sample can be calculated. Such calculations are known as *stoichiometric calculations*.

Example 3(v)

We are given 25·0 ml of hydrochloric acid solution and we have to find out the weight of acid present in this solution. To do this, we require a known or standard solution of alkali. Suppose we have an alkali solution containing 40·00 g of sodium hydroxide in 1000 ml of solution. On carrying out the titration we find out that for 25·0 ml of acid, 20·0 ml of alkali solution is required. Now, we have to calculate the weight of acid present in 25·0 ml of sample solution. First of all, calculate the amount of sodium hydroxide present in 20·0 ml of alkali solution.

1000 ml alkali solution contains 40·00 g NaOH.

$$\therefore 20\text{·}0 \text{ ml alkali solution contains} \frac{20\text{·}0}{1000} \times 40\text{·}00 = 0\text{·}80 \text{ g NaOH}$$

Now, from stoichiometry of the reaction between hydrochloric acid and sodium hydroxide, we know that 40·00 g of alkali reacts with 36·50 g of the acid [see example 3(iv)]. With the help of this stoichiometric relation, we can calculate the amount of hydrochloric acid which must have reacted with 0·80 g of sodium hydroxide.

40·00 g NaOH reacts with 36·50 g HCl.

$$\therefore \quad 0\text{·}80 \text{ g NaOH reacts with } \frac{0\text{·}80}{40\text{·}00} \times 36\text{·}50 = 0\text{·}73 \text{ g of HCl.}$$

Thus, we can say that 25·0 ml of acid sample solution contains 0·73 g of hydrochloric acid.

Example 3(vi)

25·0 ml of given solution of barium chloride was treated with an excess of sulphuric acid. The precipitate of barium sulphate so obtained was washed, dried and weighed. If the weight of barium sulphate has been found to be 0·3298 g, calculate the weight of $BaCl_2.2H_2O$ or $BaCl_2$ or Ba in the given solution.

Barium chloride and sulphuric acid react to form barium sulphate according to the equation :

$$BaCl_2 + H_2SO_4 = BaSO_4 + 2HCl$$

Molecular weight of

$BaCl_2$ = at. wt. of barium $= 137\text{·}34$
$+2 \times$ at. wt. of chlorine $= (2 \times 35\text{·}45) = 70\text{·}90$

$\overline{\qquad\qquad}$
$208\text{·}24$

$BaCl_2.2H_2O = 208\text{·}24 + 2(2+16) = 208\text{·}24 + 36\text{·}00 = 244\text{·}24.$
$BaSO_4 = 137\text{·}34 + 32\text{·}06 + (4 \times 16\text{·}00)$
$\qquad = 137\text{·}34 + 32\text{·}06 + 64\text{·}00 = 233\text{·}40.$

From the stoichiometry, it is known that 208·24 g of barium chloride (or 244·24 g of $BaCl_2.2H_2O$) on reaction with an excess of sulphuric acid will produce 233·40 g of barium sulphate. With the help of this stoichiometric relationship, we can calculate the weight of barium chloride bihydrate ($BaCl_2.2H_2O$) or barium chloride or of barium present in the sample solution (which produced 0.3298 g of barium sulphate).

233.40 g $BaSO_4$ is obtained from 244.24 g $BaCl_2.2H_2O$.

∴   0.3298 g $BaSO_4$ is obtained from $\dfrac{0.3298}{233.40} \times 244.24$

$$= 0.3451 \text{ g } BaCl_2.2H_2O.$$

233.40 g of $BaSO_4$ is obtained from 208.24 g $BaCl_2$

∴   0.3298 g of $BaSO_4$ is obtained from $\dfrac{0.3298}{233.40} \times 208.24$

$$= 0.2942 \text{ g of } BaCl_2.$$

233.40 g of $BaSO_4$ is obtained from 137.34 g Ba.

∴   0.3298 g of $BaSO_4$ is obtained from

$$\frac{0.3298}{233.40} \times 137.34 = 0.1941 \text{ g of Ba.}$$

Thus, 25.0 ml of given solution contains 0.3451 g of barium chloride bihydrate or 0.2942 g of barium chloride or 0.1941 g of barium.

3.1.4. Incomplete Reactions

There are many reactions which do not go to completion. Such reactions generally do not have any fixed stoichiometry and, therefore, cannot act as a basis of a quantitative analytical method.

Example 3(*vii*)

Acetic acid reacts with ethyl alcohol according to the equation :

$$CH_3COOH + C_2H_5OH \rightleftharpoons CH_3COOC_2H_5 + H_2O$$

If this reaction is stoichiometric, 1 g mole of acid should combine with 1 g mole of alcohol to produce 1 g mole of ethyl acetate (ester) and 1 g mole of water. But this is not so. The reaction does not go to completion, and forms only 0.666 g mole of ester and 0.666 g mole of water, *i.e.*, the reaction goes only up to 66.6 per cent. Thus the ratio in g mole between the amount of reactant taken and the amount of product formed is 1 : 0.66. Even if this ratio remains fixed, the reaction can be used in developing a quantitative analytical method. But on increasing the amount of acid or alcohol, this ratio is changed, because now the reaction proceeds beyond 66.6 per cent. Thus the stoichiometry of this reaction is not fixed and hence we cannot calculate how much product would be formed. So, the above reaction cannot act as a basis of a quantitative method of analysis. Note that in the reaction between hydrochloric acid and sodium hydroxide the ratio of amounts of acid and base reacting with each other is always fixed (36.5 : 40.0) no matter what amounts of alkali and acid are mixed with each other. Similarly a definite amount of barium chloride will always give a definite amount of barium sulphate even if sulphuric acid is added in larger amounts than required theoretically according to the chemical equation. Hence, these two reactions can be successfully used in developing quantitative method of analysis.

3·1·5. Test for Completeness of a Reaction

It has been seen that only those reactions are used in quantitative analysis which go to virtual completion. Hence, if we wish to make use of a chemical reaction as a basis of a quantitative analytical procedure, we must find out whether it goes to completion. This can be known by calculating the value of equilibrium constant (K) for the reaction under consideration.

Consider a simple reversible reaction at constant temperature :

$$A+B \rightleftharpoons C+D$$

It can be shown that the equilibrium constant, represented by K, is given by

$$K = \frac{[C] \times [D]}{[A] \times [B]}$$

where [A], [B], [C] and [D] are concentrations of A, B, C and D respectively when the reaction has reached equilibrium. The condition for equilibrium is that the concentrations of reactants, *i.e.*, [A] and [B] and those of the products, *i.e.*, [C] and [D] remain constant and do not change with time.

Example 3(*viii*)

We have solution (1) containing 1 g mole of substance A and solution (2) containing 1 g mole of substance B. The two solutions are mixed and suppose the total volume of the reaction mixture is 1 litre. Further, at a fixed temperature, say T°C, the reaction proceeds to 80 per cent and then reaches equilibrium. Then, 0·8 g mole of C and 0·8 g mole of D will be formed and 0·2 g mole of A and 0·2 g mole of B will remain unreacted. Thus,

[A]=0·2 g mole/litre

[B]=0·2 g mole/litre

[C]=0·8 g mole/litre

[D]=0·8 g mole/litre

([A], [B], [C] and [D] are concentrations of A, B, C and D respectively at equilibrium.)

The value of equilibrium constant K will be

$$K = \frac{[C] \times [D]}{[A] \times [B]} = \frac{0·8 \times 0·8}{0·2 \times 0·2} = 16 \text{ at } T°C.$$

If the reaction is 99·9% complete at a particular temperature (T_1°C), only 0·1 per cent of reactant will remain at equilibrium. Thus, 0·999 g mole each of C and D will be formed and 0·001 g mole each of A and B will remain unreacted, *i.e.*,

[A]=0·001 g mole/litre.

[B]=0·001 g mole/litre.

[C]=0·999 g mole/litre.

[D]=0·999 g mole/litre.

The value of equilibrium constant K at T_1°C will be :

$$K = \frac{0·999 \times 0·999}{0·001 \times 0·001} = 998001.$$

It is seen from the above example that when the reaction goes to virtual completion say 99·9 per cent, the value of equilibrium constant is very high. If we wish to use a chemical reaction as a basis of a quantitative analytical method, we must find out the value for its equilibrium constant, K.   From the value of K we can have an idea about the percentage completion of the reaction. Greater the value of K, greater is the percentage completion of the reaction.

3·2. THE CONCEPT OF MOLE

In chemical studies we frequently deal with number of parti- cles such as molecules, atoms or ions that are involved in chemical processes. It is not possible to count these particles. What we can measure is the weight of different reactants and products taking part in a chemical reaction. However, from these weights we can theoretically find out the number of different particles involved in a reaction on the basis of the following considerations.

It is known that one *gram atom* (a g atom) of an element contains $6·023 \times 10^{23}$ atoms ; this number is called *Avogadro's number* and is represented by N. As per definition, Avogadro's number is equal to the number of carbon atoms present in exactly 12 g of C^{12} (a particular isotope of carbon). By one g atom of an element, we mean its atomic weight expressed in g. For example, the atomic weight of sodium is 23, hence one g atom of sodium means 23 g of sodium and this would contain $6·023 \times 10^{23}$ sodium atoms, or 0·1 g atom, *i.e.*, $23/10 = 2·3$ g. of sodium would contain $6·023 \times 10^{23}/10$ $= 6·023 \times 10^{22}$ sodium atoms. The number of g atoms of an element present in a given sample is calculated by :

$$\text{No. of g atom} = \frac{\text{Wt. of the element in g}}{\text{atomic weight of the element}}$$

It is also known that one gram molecular weight of any sub- stance   contains $6·023 \times 10^{23}$ molecules of that substance.   By gram molecular weight of a substance is meant its molecular weight expressed in g. *Gram molecular weight* is also written as *g mole* or *simply mole*. The molecular weight of water is 18, hence a mole of water means 18 g of water and this would contain $6·023 \times 10^{23}$ water molecules.

The following reaction :

$$N_2 + 3H_2 \longrightarrow 2NH_3$$

tells us that a mole $(1 \times 28 = 28$ g) of nitrogen will react with three moles $(3 \times 2 = 6$ g) of hydrogen to produce 2 moles $(2 \times 17 = 34$ g) of ammonia. We can also say that $6·023 \times 10^{23}$ nitrogen molecules will react with $3 \times 6·023 \times 10^{23}$ hydrogen molecules to produce $2 \times 6·023 \times 10^{23}$ molecules of ammonia.

The number of moles in a given system is calculated as :

$$\text{No. of moles} = \frac{\text{wt. of the substance in g}}{\text{mol. wt. of the substance}}$$

Suppose in a given volume of alkali solution, 4 g of NaOH is present, then the number of moles of NaOH in the solution will be $4/40 = 0·1$ mole, where 40 is the molecular weight of NaOH.

The term mole, strictly speaking, refers to a fixed number that is $6·023 \times 10^{23}$. It does not refer to any fixed amount of weight of a substance. For example, the correct use of the term mole is, one mole of hydrogen *atoms* and not one mole of hydrogen. However, ordinarily we say a mole of hydrogen meaning 2 g of hydrogen (2 is the molecular weight of hydrogen). Thus, mole is a general term related to the number $6·023 \times 10^{23}$. For example, one mole of electrons means $6·023 \times 10^{23}$ electrons.

3·2·1. Gram Formula Weight

The *gram-formula weight* or *formula weight* of a substance is obtained by adding atomic weights of all atoms shown in the chemical formula of that substance. Generally formula weight is the same as the molecular weight. But sometimes it is preferred to use the term formula weight rather than molecular weight because, in some cases, it is not appropriate to talk about molecules, such as in ionic compounds. For example, NaCl even in the solid state does not contain molecules but has Na^+ and Cl^- ions, hence it is not proper to use the term molecular weight in this case. However, the formula weight and the molecular weight of NaCl are similar, *i.e.*, $23 + 35·5 = 58·5$. Thus, 58·5 g of NaCl, which is the formula weight of NaCl, will contain a mole of Na^+ $(6·023 \times 10^{23}$ $Na^+)$ and a mole of Cl^- $(6·023 \times 10^{23}$ $Cl^-)$ ions.

One *gram ion weight* is the formula weight of the ion expressed in g. For example, the formula weight of SO_4^{2-} ion is $32 + 64 = 96$, hence one g ion of SO_4^{2-} means 96 g of sulphate ions. A gram ion weight is also written briefly as a *g ion*.

3·2·2. Molar and Formal Solutions

If one g mole of a substance is present in a litre of solution it is called a *molar solution*. If a litre of solution contains 40 ,g of NaOH, *i.e.*, one g mole of NaOH, the solution is called a molar solution or the molarity of solution will be unity.

$$\text{Molarity of a solution} = \frac{\text{No. of g mole}}{\text{Volume of solution in litres}}$$

If 2 g mole of a substance are present in 10 litres of its solution, the molarity of the solution will be 2/10=0˙2 or the solution will said to be 0˙2 molar or 0˙2 M.

If the formula weight of the substance is considered then the term formality is used. For example, the formula weight of NaCl is 58˙5, hence if 58˙5 g NaCl is present in a litre of solution, it will be called a *formal solution*.   If 58˙5 g NaCl is present in 10 litres of solution, the formality of the solution will be 1/10=0˙1.   Thus,

$$\text{Formality of a solution} = \frac{\text{No. of g formula weight}}{\text{Volume of solution in litres}}$$

(See Appendix II for formula weight of some common substances).

4

Some Theoretical Principles Underlying Analytical Operations

A method of qualitative or quantitative analysis may involve one or more steps. These steps are generally based on some theoretical consideration. It is, therefore, necessary to study theoretical principles which are frequently used in various analytical steps or operations. (These principles will be only briefly discussed here, for a detailed and more complete treatment one should consult a text book of physical chemistry). This study should enable us to know why a particular operation is necessary, *i.e.*, we should not only know what we are doing but must also know why are we performing a particular operation.

4·1. THE LAW OF MASS ACTION

Most of the methods of chemical analysis make use of some chemical reactions. Normally those reactions are preferred which are fast and proceed to virtual completion. Such information can be obtained by the application of law of mass action.

Many of the reactions used in analytical chemistry are *reversible, i.e.*, they proceed simultaneously in two opposite directions. According to *law of mass action*, the rate of a chemical reaction is proportional to the product of the active masses of the reacting substances ; the active mass may be taken as equal to concentration in g mole per litre. Consider the following homogeneous and reversible reaction taking place at a fixed temperature, T° C :

$$A+B \rightleftharpoons C+D$$

A homogeneous reaction is one in which all the reactants and products are in the same phase, such as all of them may be in gaseous state or in the form of aqueous solution. In the above equation the sign of equality is replaced by the double arrow ($\rightleftharpoons$) representing reversibility.

Suppose a solution containing one g mole of substance A and another solution containing one g mole of B are mixed and total volume of the reaction mixture is one litre. As time proceeds, the reaction will also proceed in the forward direction so that the concentrations of A and B, represented by (A) and (B) respectively will go on decreasing. At the same time the concentrations of C and D, i.e., (C) and (D) will go on increasing. Now, as per law of mass action, the rate of forward reaction, r_1, will be proportional to the product (A) $\times$ (B) and the rate of backward reaction, r_2, will be proportional to (C) $\times$ (D). Note that for the backward reaction C and D are reactants. Thus,

$$r_1 \propto (A) \times (B) \text{ or, } r_1 = k_1 (A) \times (B)$$
$$\text{and, } r_2 \propto (C) \times (D) \text{ or, } r_2 = k_2 (C) \times (D)$$

where k_1 and k_2 are proportionality constant ; k_1 is called the forward velocity constant and k_2, the backward velocity constant.

Now, as time increases :

more and more of A and B will react,

concentrations of A and B, i.e., (A) and (B), will go on decreasing,

∴ the value of the product (A) $\times$ (B) will go on decreasing,

∴ the value of r_1 will go on decreasing.

On the other hand with increase in time :

more and more of C and D will be formed,

∴ concentrations of C and D, i.e., (C) and (D), will go on increasing,

∴ the value of the product (C) $\times$ (D) will go on increasing,

∴ the value of r_2 will go on increasing.

In this way, a stage will be reached when the decreasing value of r_1 will become equal to the increasing value of r_2 as shown in Fig. 4·1. At time t, the forward and backward reaction rates will be equal, i.e., the reaction will reach or attain *equilibrium*. At this stage, the forward and the backward reactions do not stop but the extent of the forward reaction is equal to that of the backward reaction, i.e., the amounts of reactants consumed in the forward reaction will be equal to the amounts formed by the backward reaction. This is the principle of *dynamic equilibrium*.

Thus the important condition of equilibrium is that the amounts of the reactants and the products remain constant and do not change with time although both the forward and backward reactions are still going on.

If at *equilibrium*, the concentratians of A, B, C and D are [A], [B], [C] and [D] respectively, then

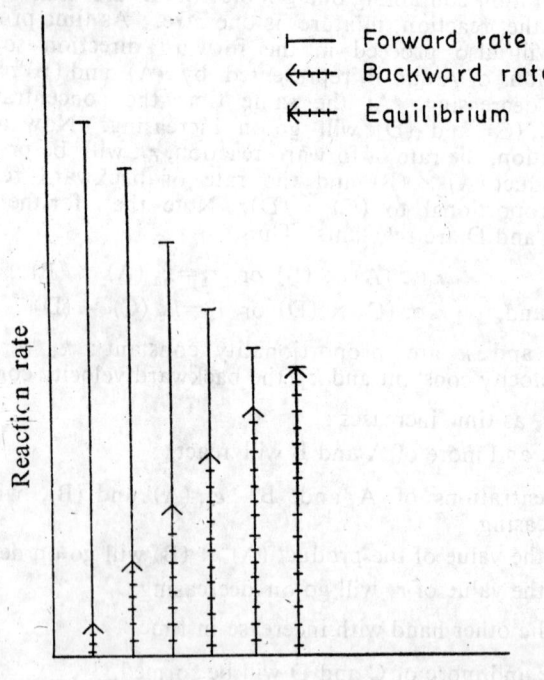

Fig. 4·1. Increase of backward and decrease of forward reaction rate with time.

$$r_1 = k_1 [A] \times [B] \quad \text{and} \quad r_2 = k_2 [C] \times [D]$$

At equilibrium, $r_1 = r_2$, therefore,

$$k_1[A] \times [B] = k_2[C] \times [D]$$

or

$$K = \frac{k_1}{k_2} = \frac{[C] \times [D]}{[A] \times [B]}$$

where K is the ratio of the forward and backward velocity constants and is called the equilibrium constant of the reaction at T° C.

Consider the following reaction :

$$aA + bB \rightleftharpoons cC + dD$$

where a g mole of substance A react with b g mole of substance B to produce c g mole of C and d g mole of substance D. The value of equilibrium constant K for this reaction will be given as :

$$K = \frac{[C]^c \times [D]^d}{[A]^a \times [B]^b}$$

It should be noted that equilibrium constant is more correctly given as :

$$K = \frac{a_C{}^c \times a_D{}^d}{a_A{}^a \times a_B{}^b}$$

where a_A, a_B, a_C and a_D are *activities* of substances A, B, C and D respectively at equilibrium. The activity and concentration are related by the equation :

$$a_i = c_i \times f_i$$

where a_i is activity, c_i is concentration and f_i is activity coefficient of any species i. Now, when concentrations are low, as in dilute solutions of A, B, C and D, the value of activity coefficient is unity and hence activity is equal to concentration. Thus for all practical purposes the term activity can be replaced by concentration, provided the solutions involved are dilute. The equilibrium constant can, therefore, be expressed as :

$$K = \frac{[C]^c \times [D]^d}{[A]^a \times [B]^b}$$

4·1·1. Application of Law of Mass Action to Analytical Chemistry

It has already been seen that only those reactions can act as a basis of analytical procedures which are fast and proceed to completion. It has also been shown that those reactions proceed to completion whose equilibrium constant has a very large value. For example, the value of equilibrium constant for the reaction between ferrous sulphate and potassium permanganate is 3×10^{63} at ordinary temperature hence, this reaction will proceed to completion. For the reaction between ferrous chloride and chlorine, again the value of equilibrium constant is quite large, $(K = 4 \cdot 7 \times 10^{23})$ hence this reaction would also go to virtual completion.

If the value of equilibrium constant for a reaction is small it will not go to completion and hence would be unsuitable for use in a quantitative analytical method. In such cases, conditions should be created which will favour the forward reaction. These conditions are derived by applying the law of mass action. If a reaction is incomplete, following three steps can be taken to increase its speed and push it in the forward direction.

(i) *By increasing the concentration of reactants.* The value of equilibrium constant is given as :

$$K = \frac{[C] \times [D]}{[A] \times [B]}$$

If concentration of A or B or of both is increased, the value of [A]×[B] will also increase and consequently the value of K will decrease. But K must remain constant so long as the temperature remains constant. Hence, to maintain K constant, the value of the product [C]×[D] also must increase, *i.e.*, the concentration terms [C] and [D] must increase which means that the formation of products will be in greater amounts, *i.e.*, the reaction would move in the forward direction.

Example 4(i)

The reaction between acetic acid, potassium iodide and potassium iodate takes place according to the equation :

$$6CH_3COOH + KIO_3 + 5KI = 6CH_3COOK + 3H_2O + 3I_2$$

It follows from the above equation that 6 g mole of acetic acid would liberate 3 g mole of iodine provided the iodate and iodide are added in excess. Molecular weight of acetic acid is 60 and that of iodine is 254. From the stoichiometry, we know that (6×60) =360 g of acetic acid will liberate $(3 \times 254) = 762$ g iodine.

If a given acetic acid solution contains 0˙360 g acid, on adding excess of iodide and iodate it must produce 0˙762 g iodine. It would then mean that the reaction is complete and can be used for the determination of acetic acid. But it has been found that the reaction is slow and does not go to completion, when a small excess of iodate-iodide reagent solution is added. Now, if to the sample acid solution, a very large excess of iodide and iodate (3 g each of KI and KIO_3) is added, the reaction becomes fast and is complete in 3-5 minutes. Thus, by increasing the concentration of the reactants KI and KIO_3, the reaction has been made fast and pushed forward to completion. Under these experimental condi-tions this reaction can be used for the quantitative determination of acetic acid.

In many qualitative and quantitative analytical procedures it is recommended that an excess of the reagent should be added, the object is to make the reaction fast and quantitative. But in adding a very large excess of reagent, one should check that this would not produce an adverse effect on the result of determination. From preliminary experiments one can find out the suitable excess of reagent that must be added to obtain accurate results.

(*ii*) *By decreasing the concentration of products.* Remember that equilibrium constant K is given by :

$$K = \frac{[C] \times [D]}{[A] \times [B]}$$

If value of [C] or [D] is made small, the value of K will also decrease. To maintain the value of K constant, the value of [A] and [B] must also decrease, that is, A and B will react further to produce C and D, *i.e.*, the reaction would be pushed in the forward direction.

Example 4(*ii*)

We have seen in example 4(*i*), that the reaction between acetic acid, potassium iodate and iodide is slow and incomplete hence, cannot be used for determining acetic acid. In this reaction, one of the products is iodine which readily reacts with sodium thiosulphate ; this fact is used for decreasing the concentration of iodine.

To a known volume of given acetic acid solution, a known excess of thiosulphate solution is first added and then an excess of iodate-iodide reagent. As soon as iodine is formed it immediately reacts with thiosulphate and to maintain the value of equilibrium constant, the reaction moves in the forward direction. The reaction is thus speeded up and is practically complete in about 15-30 min. The unreacted thiosulphate is then titrated with standard iodine solution and knowing the quantity of thiosulphate consumed, the amount of iodine liberated or the amount of acetic acid present in the given solution can be calculated using the relationship :

$$6CH_3COOH \equiv 3I_2 \equiv 6Na_2S_2O_3$$

(*iii*) *By increasing the temperature of reaction mixture.* On increasing the temperature, the value of equilibrium constant (K) increases. It means that the value of numerater increases and that of the denominator decreases, *i.e.*, more products are formed and less of reactants remain unreacted $\left[\text{Remember } K = \frac{[C] \times [D]}{[A] \times [B]} \right]$.The effect is that reaction moves in the forward direction.

Example 4(*iii*)

We have seen that the reaction between acetic acid, iodate and iodide can be accelerated either by adding greater amounts of iodide and iodate to the acid sample solution or by removing the iodine from the sphere of action, as soon as it is formed, by adding thiosulphate. The third approach to increase the rate of reaction is to heat the reaction mixture. Because iodine is volatile, the reaction mixture should be heated in a closed pressure bottle. On increasing the temperature, the value of K increases. This is possible only when the product [C]×[D] increases and the product [A]×[B] decreases, *i.e.*, concentrations of products increase and those of reactants decrease. It means the reaction moves in the forward direction. Thus by heating the reaction mixture, there is stoichiometric liberation of iodine which can be titrated with thiosulphate. Knowing the amount of iodine produced the quantity of acetic acid present in the sample can be calculated from the stoichiometry of the reaction.

4·2. LE CHATELIER AND BRAUN PRINCIPLE

According to this principle, if a reaction in equilibrium is subjected to a change, the reaction tends to move in such a direction that the effect of the change would be neutralised.

Consider the reaction :

$$6CH_3COOH + 5KI + KIO_3 \rightleftharpoons 6CH_3COOK + 3H_2O + 3I_2$$

At equilibrium, the concentrations of acetic acid, iodide, iodate, potassium acetate, water and iodine are fixed. If we add a small amount of one of the reactants say, iodate then its concentration will increase and the equilibrium will be disturbed. The reaction will, therefore, move in a direction that would cause decrease of iodate concentration. This is possible if the iodate reacts with acetic acid and iodide to produce acetate, water and iodine, *i.e.*, the reaction moves in the forward direction. *In general, a reaction can be pushed forward by increasing the concentration of reactants.*

If one of the products say iodine is removed from the reaction mixture by some means, say by adding sodium thiosulphate, the concentration of iodine would decrease and again the equilibrium of the reaction will be disturbed. The reaction would oppose the decrease in the concentration of iodine by producing more iodine. This is possible if the reaction moves in the forward direction forming more iodine. *In general a reaction can be made to proceed in the forward direction by decreasing the concentration of products.*

In. this way, by the application of Le Chatelier and Braun principle also we come to the same conclusion that in order to speed up a reaction and to push it in forward direction we should either increase the concentration of reactants or decrease the concentration of products.

4·3. VAN'T HOFF REACTION ISOTHERM

Consider the following reaction in which *a* g mole of substance A reacts with *b* g mole of substance B to form *c* g mole of product C and *d* g mole of D :

$$aA + bB \rightleftharpoons cC + dD$$

For this reaction, the equilibrium constant K is written as :

$$K = \frac{a_C{}^c \times a_D{}^d}{a_A{}^a \times b_B{}^b}$$

where a_A, a_B, a_C and a_D are activities of substances A, B, C and D respectively at equilibrium. In dilute solutions activity can be considered to be practically equal to concentration of these substances, hence we can write :

$$K = \frac{[C]^c \times [D]^d}{[A]^a \times [B]^b}$$

Now, according to the reaction isotherm first derived by J.H. van't Hoff :

$$\triangle F_{T.P} = -RT \; ln \; \frac{[C]^c \times [D]^d}{[A]^a \times [B]^b} + RT \; ln \frac{(C)^c \times (D)^d}{(A)^a \times (B)^b}$$

where :

$\triangle F_{T.P}$ = free energy change for the reaction at temperature T and pressure P ;

R = gas constant ; [A], [B], [C] and [D] are concentrations of A, B, C and D respectively at equilibrium ; (A), (B), (C) and (D) are any arbitrary concentrations of A, B, C and D respectively (not necessarily at equilibrium).

The reaction isotherm can also be written in the following form :

$$\triangle F_{T.P} = -RT \; ln \; K + RT \; ln \; J_a$$

where

$$J_a = \frac{(C)^c \times (D)^d}{(A)^a \times (B)^b}$$

According to reaction isotherm, a reaction moves in forward direction only when $\triangle F_{T.P}$ is negative ; this is possible if the value of K is greater than that of J_a. Hence, to make a reaction proceed in the forward direction those conditions should be used which will decrease the value of J_a or increase the value of K. The value of J_a can obviously be decreased by decreasing the concentration of the products C and D or by increasing the concentration of the reactants A and B. The value of K can be increased by increasing the temperature of the reaction mixture.

It is thus seen that we come to the same conclusion that a reaction can be pushed forward by increasing the concentration of reactants or by decreasing the concentration of products or by increasing the temperature of the reaction mixture.

4·4. THE DISSOCIATION THEORY

The reactions used in analytical methods may involve heating of solid sample material with solid reagent or interaction between sample and reagent in the form of their solutions, these are known as *dry* and *wet* methods respectively. An example of a dry method is that when a cobalt salt is heated with borax powder, a blue bead (glassy material) is formed ; this is a dry test for cobalt. In analytical chemistry we mostly deal with the reactions between substances in solutions. The solvent generally used is water.

4·4·1.   Electrolytes and Nonelectrolytes

Solutions of certain substances do not contain charged particles (or ions) and hence cannot conduct electricity. Such substances are called *non-electrolytes*. Glucose, urea, cane sugar are non-electrolytes. There are certain other types of substances which when dissolved in water (or in any other suitable solvent) produce free ions and their solutions can conduct electricity. Such ubstances are known as *electrolytes*. Sodium chloride, sodium hydroxide, potassium acetate are examples of electrolytes.

4·4·2.   Degree of Dissociation : Strong and Weak Electrolyte

When an electrolyte, AB, is dissolved in water, it is dissociated into positively and negatively charged particles called positive and negative ions respectively. Thus,

$$AB \rightleftharpoons A^+ + B^-$$

Atoms or group of atoms carrying electrical charge are called ions. Positively charged ions are called cations and negatively charged ions are called anions. Now, it is not necessary that all the molecules of the electrolyte AB will break away into ions. If only 60 per cent molecules dissociate, we will say that the dissociation is 60 per cent or the *degree of dissociation*, α, is 60/100, *i.e.*, 0·6. In other words, if one g mole of AB is dissolved in water and if only 0·6 g mole dissociates and 0·4 g mole remains undissociated, the degree of dissociation, *i.e.*, the fraction of the g mole undergoing dissociation would be 0·6. The degree of dissociation of electrolytes is of great importance in analytical chemistry because the chemical activity of electrolytes depend on it. The degree of dissociation, α, depends on the nature of the substance, nature of the solvent, concentration of the solution and temperature.

The value of α varies from zero to unity. Those substances which dissociate to a greater extent have high value for α ; these are called *strong electrolytes*. On the other hand, when the value of α is small, the substance is said to be a *weak electrolyte*. For example, in a dilute solution of sodium chloride practically all the molecules give ions that are free to move in the solution. Sodium chloride is, therefore, known as a strong electrolyte. If we consider a solution of acetic acid of the same concentration, a few molecules will dissociate to produce hydrogen and acetate ions, hence acetic acid is called a weak electrolyte or a weak acid. (It should be noted that the properties of ions differ from those of the corresponding atoms. Thus sodium ions do not decompose water but sodium atoms decompose water to form sodium hydroxide and hydrogen.) The charge carried by an ion is equal to its valency.

4·4·3. Classification of Acids, Bases and Salts According to Their Degree of Dissociation

Solution of $HClO_4$, HCl, HNO_3, H_2SO_4, HI, HBr are almost completely dissociated these are, therefore, called strong acids. Most of the organic acids such as CH_3COOH, C_2H_5COOH, C_3H_7COOH etc., and acids like H_2CO_3 and H_3BO_3 are poorly dissociated in aqueous solution hence, these are called weak acids. When for an acid, the value of α is neither high nor low, it is said to be an acid of intermediate strength, e.g., monochloroacetic acid. (see Appendix IV).

Sodium hydroxide and potassium hydroxide are strong bases because in water solution they almost completely dissociate giving a very large number of hydroxyl ions. In ammonium hydroxide solution of the same concentration, the number of hydroxyl ions is much smaller hence it is a weak base.

Most salts are strong electrolytes. Salts like NaCl, KNO_3, K_2SO_4, CH_3COONa, CH_3COONH_4 are strong electrolytes. There are, however, salts like $HgCl_2$, $Hg(CN)_2$ which are poorly dissociated, hence are weak electrolytes.

4·4·4. Dissociation of Acids and Dissociation Constant

According to the theory of electrolytic dissociation, an acid is a substance which in aqueous solution gives hydrogen ions.

Monobasic acids are those whose molecules contain only one replaceable hydrogen ; these dissociate in one stage. For example :

$$HCl \rightleftharpoons H^+ + Cl^- \quad \text{and} \quad CH_3COOH \rightleftharpoons H^+ + CH_3COO^-$$

Diabasic acids are those whose molecules contain two replaceable hydrogen, such as H_2CO_3, H_2SO_3, H_2SO_4, $H_2C_2O_4$ etc. These acids dissociate in two stages :

First stage $\quad H_2SO_4 \rightleftharpoons H^+ + HSO_4^-$ (hydrogensulphate ion)
Second stage $\quad HSO_4^- \rightleftharpoons H^+ + SO_4^{2-}$ (sulphate ion)

In the first stage the dissociation is to a much greater extent as compared to that in the second. Note that a solution of sulphuric acid contains three types of ions, H^+, HSO_4^- and SO_4^{2-}.

In a *tribasic acid* there are three replaceable hydrogen in the acid molecule and it dissociates in three stages.

First stage $H_3PO_4 \rightleftharpoons H^+ + H_2PO_4^-$ (dihydrogenphosphate ion)

Second stage $H_2PO_4^- \rightleftharpoons H^+ + HPO_4^{2-}$ (hydrogenphosphate ion)

Third stage $HPO_4^{2-} \rightleftharpoons H^+ + PO_4^{3-}$ (phosphate ion)

Thus, in an aqueous solution of phosphoric acid there will be four types of ions, H^+, $H_2PO_4^-$, HPO_4^{2-} and PO_4^{3-}. There is maximum dissociation in the first stage therefore concentration of $H_2PO_4^-$ ions will be much larger than that of HPO_4^{2-} ions. The second dissociation is greater than that in the third stage hence, the concentration of HPO_4^{2-} ion would be greater than that of PO_4^{3-} ion. It has been found that for 0·1 M phosphoric acid solution, the first dissociation is 26 per cent, second is 0·11 per cent and the third is only 0·001 per cent.

The dissociation of a molecule into ions is a reversible process. Let us apply the law of mass action to the following equilibrium :

$$CH_3COOH \rightleftharpoons CH_3COO^- + H^+$$

Suppose at equilibrium, the concentrations of acetic acid, hydrogen ion and acetate ion are represented as $[CH_3COOH]$, $[H^+]$ and $[CH_3COO^-]$ respectively. Then the value of the equilibrium constant (K_a) is given as :

$$K_a = \frac{[H^+] \times [CH_3COO^-]}{[CH_3COOH]}$$

K_a is called the dissociation constant of acetic acid. The quantity K_a is the measure of the tendency of an acid to split up into ions. The greater the value of K_a, higher must be the ionic concentrations, i.e., greater is the dissociation of the acid.

For example,

Boric acid : $H_3BO_3 \rightleftharpoons H^+ + H_2BO_3^-$; $K_a = 6·4 \times 10^{-10}$

Acetic acid : $CH_3COOH \rightleftharpoons H^+ + CH_3COO^-$; $K_a = 1·75 \times 10^{-5}$

Sulphamic acid : $NH_2SO_3H \rightleftharpoons H^+ + NH_2SO_3^-$; $K_a = 1·0 \times 10^{-1}$
(at room temperature)

From the values of K we can say that boric acid is a very weak acid, acetic acid is a weak acid and sulphamic acid is relatively a strong acid.

For phosphoric acid the values of primary, secondary and tertiary dissociation constants $(K_1, K_2$ and K_3 respectively) are :

$$H_3PO_4 \rightleftharpoons H^+ + H_2PO_4^- \; ; \; K_1 = 7·5 \times 10^{-3}$$
$$H_2PO_4^- \rightleftharpoons H^+ + HPO_4^{2-} \; ; \; K_2 = 6·2 \times 10^{-8}$$
$$HPO_4^{2-} \rightleftharpoons H^+ + PO_4^{3-} \; ; \; K_3 = 4·8 \times 10^{-13}$$

The primary dissociation constant is greater than the secondary dissociation constant which is greater than the third $(K_1 > K_2 > K_3)$.

From known values of K, it is easy to calculate the degree of dissociation and ionic concentrations in solution of a weak electrolyte.

Example 4(iv)

To calculate the concentrations of HS^- and S^{2-} ions in a saturated solution of hydrogen sulphide.

A saturated solution of H_2S in water at room temperature is about 0.1 M, i.e., $[H_2S]=0.1$. The solution behaves like a weak dibasic acid for which the primary and secondary dissociation constants are given by :

First stage : $\quad\quad H_2S \rightleftharpoons H^+ + HS^-$

Second stage : $\quad\quad HS^- \rightleftharpoons H^+ + S^{2-}$

$$K_1 = \frac{[H^+] \times [HS^-]}{[H_2S]} = 9.1 \times 10^{-8} \quad\quad ...(4.1)$$

and

$$K_2 = \frac{[H^+] \times [S^{2-}]}{[HS^-]} = 1.2 \times 10^{-15} \quad\quad ...(4.2)$$

The value of K_2 is very much smaller than that of K_1, hence, the concentration of S^{2-} ions, which are formed in the second stage, is extremely small and can be neglected. The primary dissociation is, therefore, is of importance which gives equal concentrations of H^+ and HS^- ions. Thus,

$$[H^+]=[HS^-] \text{ and } [H_2S]=0.1$$

Substituting these values in equation (4.1) :

$$\frac{[HS^-]^2}{0.1} = 9.1 \times 10^{-8}$$

$$[HS^-] = \sqrt{9.1 \times 10^{-8} \times 0.1} = 9.5 \times 10^{-5}$$

$$[H^+] = 9.5 \times 10^{-5} \quad (\text{note that } [H^+]=[HS^-]=9.5 \times 10^{-5})$$

Substituting the value of $[HS^-]$ and $[H^+]$ in equation (4.2) :

$$\frac{9.5 \times 10^{-5} \times [S^{2-}]}{9.5 \times 10^{-5}} = 1.2 \times 10^{-15}$$

or

$$[S^{2-}] = 1.2 \times 10^{-15} \text{ g ion/litre.}$$

4.4.5. Dissociation of Bases

According to the theory of electrolytic dissociation, a base is a substance which in aqueous solution gives hydroxyl ions, (OH^-), for example :

$$NaOH \rightleftharpoons Na^+ + OH^-$$

$$Ba(OH)_2 \rightleftharpoons Ba^{2+} + 2OH^-$$

$$Al(OH)_3 \rightleftharpoons Al^{3+} + 3OH^-$$

In general,

$$MOH \rightleftharpoons M^+ + OH^-$$

The equilibrium constant for this equilibrium is given by

$$K_b = \frac{[M^+] \times [OH^-]}{[MOH]}$$

= dissociation constant of the base.

Smaller the value of K, weaker will be the base. For example, K_b for ammonium hydroxide at room temperature is 1.8×10^{-5}, hence it is a weak base.

4·4·6.   Dissociation of Salts

Neutral salts on dissolving in water give metallic ions and acid radical ion :

$$KNO_3 \rightleftharpoons K^+ + NO_3^-$$
$$K_2SO_4 \rightleftharpoons 2K^+ + SO_4^{2-}$$
$$Al_2(SO_4)_3 \rightleftharpoons 2Al^{3+} + 3SO_4^{2-}$$

Dissociation of acid salts proceeds in two stages. For example :

First stage : $KHSO_4 \rightleftharpoons K^+ + HSO_4^-$
Second stage : $HSO_4^- \rightleftharpoons H^+ + SO_4^{2-}$

A basic salt contains one or more hydroxyl groups, such a salt dissociates in two or more stages. For example :

First stage : $Mg(OH)Cl \rightleftharpoons Mg(OH)^+ + Cl^-$
Second stage : $Mg(OH)^+ \rightleftharpoons Mg^{2+} + OH^-$

A basic salt thus contains metal ions, hydroxyl ions and acid radical ions.

If hydrogen atoms of a polybasic acid are replaced by two different metals, a double salt is formed. For example, Rochelle salt (sodium potassium tartrate) ; this will dissociate as follows :

$$NaKC_4H_4O_6 \rightleftharpoons Na^+ + K^+ + C_4H_4O_6^{2-}$$

We can also have complex salts, such as potassium ferrocyanide, $[K_4Fe(CN)_6]$; this will dissociate as follows :

$$K_4[Fe(CN)_6] \rightleftharpoons 4K^+ + [Fe(CN)_6]^{4-}$$

It should be noted that the solution does not contain Fe^{2+} and CN^- ions but K^+ and a complex ion $[Fe(CN)_6]^{4-}$.

4·5.   COMMON ION EFFECT

A weak electrolyte AB when dissolved in water will dissociate to a small extent into A^+ and B^- ions. If to this solution, we add a strong electrolyte CB, it will dissociate into C^+ and B^- ions. Note that both the electrolytes will give B^- which is called the *common ion*. The two dissociations are represented as follows : -

$$AB \rightleftharpoons A^+ + B^- \quad \text{(Poorly dissociated)} \qquad ...(4\cdot3)$$

$$CB \rightleftharpoons C^+ + B^- \quad \text{(Strongly dissociated)} \qquad ...(4\cdot4)$$

Common ion

The effect of addition of CB to solution of AB will thus increase the concentration of the common ion, B^-. This would push equilibrium (4·3) in the backward direction (shown by bold arrow) as per law of mass action so that the poor dissociation of AB will further decrease. Thus, when to a solution of a weak electrolyte, a strong electrolyte with common ion is added, the dissociation of the weak electrolyte is suppressed ; this is known as the *common ion effect*.

Example 4(v)

If H_2S gas is passed through water containing HCl, the following dissociation equilibria exist :

$$H_2S \rightleftharpoons H^+ + HS^- \qquad ...(4\cdot5)$$

$$HS^- \rightleftharpoons H^+ + S^{2-} \qquad ...(4\cdot6)$$

$$HCl \rightleftharpoons H^+ + Cl^- \qquad ...(4\cdot7)$$

Hydrochloric acid dissociates strongly giving high concentration of H^+ hence dissociation (4·5) and (4·6) will be suppressed so that the concentrations of HS^- and S^{2-} ions will be less as compared to their concentrations in absence of hydochloric acid.

In inorganic qualitative analysis, to the filtrate from first group, HCl is added and then H_2S gas is passed. In presence of HCl, due to common ion effect, the dissociation of H_2S is suppressed hence sulphide ion concentration, (S^{2-}), is also decreased. This decreased sulphide ion concentration is sufficient only to precipitate sulphides of Cu, Hg, Bi, Cd, As, Tin and Sb hence, only these are precipitated. The sulphide ion concentration becomes so small in presence of HCl that it cannot precipitate sulphides of Fe, Al, Cr, Ni, Co, Zn, Mn, Ba, Sr, Ca and Mg, hence they remain in solution. Thus metal ions placed in the second group of qualitative analysis can be separated from those kept in higher groups.

4·6. SOLUBILITY PRODUCT

Silver chloride is poorly (or sparingly) soluble in water. Consider a saturated solution of AgCl in water at a fixed temperature. The dissolved salt will dissociate into Ag^+ and Cl^-, at the same time these ions due to opposite charge are attracted towards each other to form AgCl. As a result of these opposite processes, the following equilibrium is established :

$$AgCl \text{ (solid)} \rightleftharpoons AgCl \text{ (solution)} \rightleftharpoons Ag^+ + Cl^- \qquad ...(4.8)$$

At equilibrium the concentration of AgCl, Ag^+ and Cl^- are fixed and these do not change with time so long as temperature remains constant. By applying the law of mass action to equilibrium (4.8), the equilibrium constant is given by :

$$K = \frac{a_{Ag^+} \times a_{Cl^-}}{a_{AgCl}}$$

The activity of solid AgCl, a_{AgCl} , is taken to be unity by convention, hence :

$$K_{ap} = a_{Ag^+} \times a_{Cl^-} = \text{constant} \quad \left| \begin{array}{l} a_{Ag^+} \text{ and } a_{Cl^-} \text{ are activities of } Ag^+ \text{ and } Cl^- \text{ respectively.} \end{array} \right.$$

The constant K_{ap} is called the *thermodynamic activity product*. Thus, the product of activities of Ag^+ and Cl^- is constant at constant temperature. The solubility of AgCl is small hence, the concentrations of Ag^+ and Cl^- are also small, therefore, activity can be replaced by concentration terms (remember that $a = c \times f$ and in dilute solution $f = 1$). Thus,

$$[Ag^+] \times [Cl^-] = K_{sp} \text{ (or } S_{AgCl})$$

where $[Ag^+]$ and $[Cl^-]$ are concentrations of Ag^+ and Cl^- respectively in a saturated solution of AgCl, *i.e.* AgCl in equilibrium with its ions Ag^+ and Cl^-. The constant K_{sp} is called the *solubility product* of silver chloride at a given temperature, this can also be represented as S_{AgCl}.

(See Appendix III for solubility product constants).

Intrinsic Solubility. Consider the following equilibrium (saturated soln of AgCl in water in contact with solid AgCl) :

$$AgCl \text{ (s)} \rightleftharpoons AgCl \text{ (aq)}$$

The equilibrium constant S° for the above equilibrium is given as :,' ·

$$\frac{a_{AgCl} \text{ (aq)}}{a_{AgCl} \text{ (s)}} = S°$$

where, a_{AgCl} (aq) = activity of AgCl in aqueous soln and

a_{AgCl} (s) = activity of solid AgCl

.As per convention a_{AgCl} (s) is unity, so :

$$a_{AgCl}\ (aq) = S°$$

$S°$ is also known as the *intrinsic solubility* of AgCl in water at a parti‐cular temperature.

The solubility product of some other substances can be expressed in the following manner.

For a saturated solution of $BaSO_4$ in water at a given temperature :

$$BaSO_4 \rightleftharpoons Ba^{2+} + SO_4{}^{2-}$$

The solubility product of $BaSO_4$, S_{BaSO_4}, is given as :

$$S_{BaSO_4} = [Ba^{2+}] \times [SO_4{}^{2-}]$$

In a saturated solution of silver chromate, (Ag_2CrO_4) :

$$Ag_2CrO_4 \rightleftharpoons 2Ag^+ + CrO_4{}^{2-}$$
$$S_{Ag_2CrO_4} = [Ag^+]^2 \times [CrO_4{}^{2-}]$$

In a saturated solution of arsenic trisulphide (As_2S_3) :

$$As_2S_3 \rightleftharpoons 2As^{3+} + 3S^{2-}$$
$$S_{As_2S_3} = [As^{3+}]^2 \times [S^{2-}]^3$$

In general, for a substance A_xB_y, dissociating as follows :

$$A_xB_y \rightleftharpoons xA^{y+} + yB^{a-}$$
$$S_{A_xB_y} = [A^{y+}]^x \times [B^{a-}]^y$$

If the value of solubility product of a substance is known we can calculate its solubility.

Example 4(vi)

The solubility product of AgCl at 25°C is 2.8×10^{-10}, calculate its solubility at the same temperature.

$$[Ag^+] \times [Cl^-] = 2.8 \times 10^{-10} \qquad \qquad ...(4.9)$$

Each mole (g mole) of AgCl will give a mole of Ag^+ and a mole of Cl^-, *i.e.*, the concentration in g ion per litre of Ag^+ and Cl^- will be equal.

$$[Ag^+] = [Cl^-]$$

Substituting in equation (4.9),

$$[Ag^+] \times [Cl^-] = [Ag^+]^2 = 2.8 \times 10^{-10}$$
$$\therefore \quad [Ag^+] = 1.7 \times 10^{-5} \text{ g ion per litre}$$

Now, because each AgCl molecule produces one Ag^+, hence $[Ag^+]$ will be equal to the solubility of AgCl in g mole per litre. Thus, solubility of AgCl at 25° will be 1.7×10^{-5} g mole per litre.

The molecular weight of AgCl is $(108+35\cdot5)=143\cdot5$. Hence, solubility of AgCl in g/litre will be :

$$1\cdot7\times10^{-5}\times143\cdot5=2\cdot44\times10^{-3} \text{ g/litre}$$

(solublity in g/litre=solubility in g mole/litre×molecular weight).

Example 4(*vi*) is quite simple because each molecule of AgCl on dissociation gives one Ag^+ and one Cl^- ion, *i.e.*, the number of Ag^+ and Cl^- ions obtained is equal. The solubility calculations are a bit complicated if a molecule dissociates to give unequal numbers of positive and negative ions as is the case in the following example.

Example 4(*vii*)

The solubility product of iron (III) hydroxide in water at room temperature is 4×10^{-38}, calculate its solubility in water at room temperature.

Ferric hydroxide dissociates as shown by the equation :

$$Fe(OH)_3 \rightleftharpoons Fe^{3+}+3OH^-$$

It is given that :

$$S_{Fe(OH)_3} =[Fe^{3+}]\times[OH^-]^3=4\times10^{-38} \qquad ...(4\cdot10)$$

Suppose the solubility of $Fe(OH)_3$ is S g mole per litre.

Now, one molecule of $Fe(OH)_3$ dissociates to give one Fe^{3+}, hence, the solubility of $Fe(OH)_3$ in g mole/litre will be equal to the concentration of Fe^{3+} in g ion/litre, so :

$$S=[Fe^{3+}]$$

Also, one molecule of $Fe(OH)_3$ gives three OH^- ions, hence the concentration of OH^- will be three time the solubility of $Fe(OH)_3$, so :

$$3S=[OH^-]$$

Substituting these results in equation (4·10), we get :

$$(S)\times(3S)^3=4\times10^{-38}$$

or, $$S\times27S^3=27S^4=4\times10^{-38}$$

$$S=2\times10^{-10} \text{ g mole per litre.}$$

Thus the solubility of $Fe(OH)_3$ in water at room temperature comes out to-be 2×10^{-10} g mole per litre.

It is also possible to calculate the solubility product if the solubility of a sparingly soluble electrolyte is given.

4·6·1. Condition for Precipitation

Consider a solid electrolyte AB which is sparingly soluble in water. Suppose we take some water in a beaker, add a very small amount of AB and stir. The added electrolyte will dissolve giving A^+ and B^- ions. If the concentrations of these ions are (A^+) and (B^-) respectively, the product $(A^+) \times (B^-)$ is called the *ionic product*. If little more of AB is added which dissolves on stirring, the values of (A^+) and (B^-) will increase and so the value of the ionic product will also increase. As we go on adding the salt, the value of the ionic product goes on increasing. After sometime, a stage will come when on further adding the salt, it will not go into solution but will settle down at the bottom of the beaker. Thus, we will obtain a saturated solution of AB in water at room temperature. In this saturated solution, there will be an equilibrium between AB and its ions A^+ and B^-. Suppose $[A^+]$ and $[B^-]$ represent the concentrations of A^+ and B^- at *equilibrium*, then the product $[A^+] \times [B^-]$ is the *solubility product* of AB. It should be noted that as we go on adding AB it goes on dissolving and the ionic product also goes on increasing but the moment the value of ionic product becomes equal to the solubility product, the precipitation starts. Thus, the condition for precipitation is that the ionic product must exceed the solubility product. Remember that so long as the ionic product is smaller than the solubility product, AB remains in solution. Hence the condition for precipitation is :

$$(A^+) \times (B^-) > [A^+] \times [B^-]$$

(ionic product is greater than the solubility product).

Example 4(*viii*)

The reaction between cadmium chloride solution and hydrogen suphide gas is given by the equation :

$$CdCl_2 + H_2S \rightarrow CdS + 2HCl$$

The solubility product of CdS in water at room temperature is 1.4×10^{-28}. Suppose a little H_2S gas is passed through an aqueous solution of $CdCl_2$. the yellow precipitate of CdS will not be formed if the value of the ionic product, *i.e.*, $(Cd^{2+}) \times (S^{2-})$, is smaller than 1.4×10^{-28}. On passing more H_2S gas, the value of the ionic product will increase and as soon as it becomes equal to 1.4×10^{-28} the yellow precipitate of CdS will appear.

4.6.2. Order of Precipitation

Sometimes a reagent forms sparingly soluble precipitates with more than one ions present in a solution. For example, in the second group of inorganic qualitative analysis, S^{2-} ions from H_2S gas passed, form precipitates with Hg^{2+}, Pb^{2+}, Cu^{2+}, Cd^{2+} etc. Now in such a case we want to know that which precipitate will appear first ? This question can be answered if we know the values of the solubility products of the different precipitates formed. The precipitate which has the smallest value of the solubility product will be first to be formed because the ionic product will exceed its solubility product first.

Example 4(ix)

We have a mixture of $HgCl_2$ and $CdCl_2$ solutions. The solubility products of HgS (black) and CdS (yellow) are 4×10^{-54} and 1.4×10^{-28} respectively. If H_2S gas is passed through the solution of the mixture, a black precipitate will appear which is of HgS, i.e., HgS will be precipitated first and not CdS. The reason is that as H_2S gas is being passed, the S^{2-} ion concentration goes on increasing, so also the ionic products $(Hg^{2+}) \times (S^{2-})$ and $(Cd^{2+}) \times (S^{2-})$. Because the solubility product of HgS has a smaller value, i.e., 4×10^{-54}, hence, this is first exceeded that is why HgS is precipitated first. The value for the solubility product of CdS is greater so it will be exceeded later and hence it will be precipitated after HgS.

4.6.3. Condition for Solution

It is known that AgCl is insoluble in HNO_3 but dissolves readily in NH_4OH solution. From the concept of solubility product we can explain why AgCl dissolves in NH_4OH.

Suppose we have a precipitate of AgCl in contact with its saturated solution in water. Because solid AgCl is present, it means that the ionic product $(Ag^+) \times (Cl^-)$ must be equal to the solubility product $[Ag^+] \times [Cl^-]$. If by some means we can decrease the value of the ionic product below the solubility product value, condition for precipitation will not exist hence, AgCl will start dissolving. On adding NH_4OH solution, Ag^+ reacts to form a complex according to the equation :

$$Ag^+ + 2NH_3 \rightarrow [Ag(NH_3)_2]^+$$

Thus, the concentration of Ag^+ decreases and hence also the value of the product $(Ag^+) \times (Cl^-)$ and as soon as it becomes smaller than the solubility product value, AgCl starts dissolving. Thus the condition for solution is :

$$(Ag^+) \times (Cl^-) < [Ag^+] \times [Cl^-]$$
ionic product < solubility product.

4.7. DIVERSE ION EFFECT

So far we have considered the solubility of a substance in pure water. In several analytical procedures, the formation or dissolution of a precipitate takes place in presence of a large concentration of ions which are not common to the ions of the precipitate, such ions are known as *foreign ions*. For example, if AgCl is being precipitated from a solution which contains a large amount of KNO_3, potassium nitrate will be called a foreign electrolyte ; this on dissociation produces K^+ and NO_3^- ions which are not common to AgCl ; these are called foreign ions.

We have already studied the common ion effect. Now, let us study the effect of foreign ions on the solubility of a precipitate : This effect is called *diverse ion effect, uncommon ion effect, neutral salt effect or activity effect*. It has been observed that if we go on adding KNO_3 solution to a precipitate of AgCl or $BaSO_4$, the solubility of these precipitates goes on increasing with increasing concentrations of K^+ and NO_3^- ions which are not common to AgCl or $BaSO_4$. The increase in the solubilities of these precipitates can be explained by the following considerations. We have seen that in a saturated solution of AgCl in water at a fixed temperature :

$$a_{Ag^+} \times a_{Cl^-} = K_{ap}$$

where a_{Ag^+} and a_{Cl^-} are activities of Ag^+ and Cl^- ions respectively and K_{ap} is the activity product of AgCl at a given temperature. It is known that the terms activity and concentration are related by :

$$a_i = c_i \times f_i$$

where f_i is the activity coefficient of ion i ; this becomes unity when ionic concentration is small so that, $a_i = c_i$ in dilute solutions. For example, if we have a saturated solution of AgCl in pure water, due to poor solubility of AgCl there will be a very small concentration of Ag^+ and Cl^- ions in the solution. In this way, though the solution is saturated yet it will be very dilute. Hence, in such a solution the values of activity coefficients of Ag^+ and Cl^-, *i.e.*, f_{Ag^+} and f_{Cl^-} can be taken to be unity so that $a_{Ag^+} = [Ag^+]$ and $a_{Cl^-} = [Cl^-]$, and we can write that solubility product of AgCl $= ([Ag^+] \times [Cl^-])$ is constant at a given temperature. But if a large amount of KNO_3 solution is added to the precipitate of AgCl, there will be now a large number of ions of different kinds present in the solution (Ag^+, Cl^-, K^+, NO_3^- H^+, OH^-) hence the ionic strength of the medium will be quite high. (Note that in calculating the ionic strength of a solution all types of ions present in the solution are considered). In such a solution of high ionic strength, the values of f_{Ag^+} and f_{Cl^-} will not be unity but will be smaller than 1, suppose these become 0.8. Then,

$$a_{Ag^+} = [Ag^+] \times 0.8 \qquad \qquad f_{Ag^+} = 0.8$$
$$\text{and} \quad a_{Cl^-} = [Cl^-] \times 0.8 \qquad \qquad f_{Cl^-} = 0.8$$
$$\text{and} \qquad a_i = c_i \times f_i$$

The activities of Ag^+ and Cl^-, *i.e.*, a_{Ag^+} and a_{Cl^-} will thus decrease and to maintain activity product constant more AgCl will dissolve. This explains why the solubility of a precipitate increases in presence of large amounts of foreign salts.

4·8. IONISATION OF WATER

Mostly the reactions used in analytical chemistry take place in aqueous solution. It has been found that even highly purified water possesses a small conductivity. The conduction of electricity requires presence of ions hence, water must be ionising to produce H^+ and OH^- ions. Thus water possesses properties of an acid (because it gives H^+) and also properties of a base (as it gives OH^-). The conducting power of water is poor which shows that there are very few H^+ and OH^- ions present in water, *i.e.* all the water molecules do not ionise. It means that water is a very weak electrolyte which very slightly ionises as follows :

$$H_2O \rightleftharpoons H^+ + OH^-$$

The degree of ionisation of water has been determined from conductivity measurements. It has been observed that out of 1 g mole of water only $1/10,000,000$ g mole (10^{-7} g mole) of water ionises, rest of the water remains in the form of molecules.

A molecule of water on ionisation produces one ion each of H^+ and OH^- ion hence, in water the concentrations of these ions are equal. Thus,

$$[H^+] = [OH^-] = 10^{-7} \text{ g ion per litre at } 22°C.$$

$$\therefore \quad [H^+] \times [OH^-] = 10^{-7} \times 10^{-7} = 10^{-14} = K_w$$

where K_w is known as the *ionic product of water*. Its value depends on temperature and at room temperature its value can be taken to be 10^{-14}.

Strictly speaking H^+ ion does not remain as such but takes up water molecule to form H_3O^+, known as *hydroxonium* or *hydronium* ion. The ionisation of water should, therefore, be represented as :

$$2H_2O \rightleftharpoons H_3O^+ + OH^-.$$

4·8·1. pH Value

In pure water there is a poor ionisation producing small but equal concentrations of H^+ and OH^-.

$$[H^+] = [OH^-] = 10^{-7} \text{ g ion per litre.}$$

Because the two concentrations are equal, pure water is neither acidic nor basic but is neutral. If in a solution, $[H^+] > [OH^-]$, the solution will be acidic or if $[OH^-] > [H^+]$, the solution will be basic. In general we can say that if in a solution :

$[H^+]$ is smaller than 10^{-7} g ion/litre, it will be basic

$[H^+]$ is equal to 10^{-7} g ion/litre, it will be neutral

$[H^+]$ is greater than 10^{-7} g ion/litre, it will be acidic

Thus, the acidity or alkalinity of a solution can be expressed in terms of 10^{-x}, where x is hydrogen ion concentration in g ion per litre ; if x is less than 7, the solution is acidic and if it is more than 7, the solution is basic (note the negative sign of x). But this method of representing the acidity or alkalinity of a solution is cumbersome. A simple and convenient method was proposed by S.P.L. Sorensen. In pure water, $[H^+]=10^{-7}$ g ion per litre. Hence,

Remember

$$\log [H^+] = \log [10^{-7}] = -7$$

$$\log 10^x = x$$

or

or, $\quad -\log [H^+] = -\log [10^{-7}] = -(-7) = 7$

$$\log 10^{-x} = -x$$
(See Appendix X)

Now, $-\log$ is denoted by p, so we can write :

$$-\log [H^+] = pH = 7.$$

It means that pH value of pure water is 7. Suppose in a solution, $[H^+]$ is 10^{-8} g ion/litre, *i.e.*, smaller than 10^{-7} g ion/litre, so that the solution will be basic. The pH of this solution will be :

$$pH = -\log [H^+] = -\log 10^{-8} = -(-8) = 8.$$

Thus, when the pH of a solution is more than 7, it is basic.

In another solution, $[H^+]$ is 10^{-4} g ion/litre, *i.e.*, more than 10^{-7} g ion/litre, hence the solution will be acidic and its pH will be :

$$pH = -\log [H^+] = -\log 10^{-4} = -(-4) = 4.$$

It means that when pH of a solution is less than 7, it is acidic.

The pH value of a solution is thus defined as the negative logarithm of its hydrogen ion concentration in g ion per litre.

Remember

$$pH = -\log [H^+] = \log \frac{1}{[H^+]}$$

$$-\log x = \frac{1}{\log x}$$

Example 4(x)

In a solution the hydrogen ion concentration is 0·01 g ion per litre, calculate its pH.

(0·01 means 10^{-2} g ion per litre).

$$pH = -\log [H^+] = -\log 10^{-2} = -(-2) = 2$$

or $\qquad pH = \log \dfrac{1}{[H^+]} = \log \dfrac{1}{10^{-2}} = \log 10^2 = 2.$

4·8·2. pOH Value

pOH value of a solution can be calculated by the same method that is used for finding out pH. Suppose in a solution the concentration of OH^- is 10^{-5} g ion per litre, then its pOH value will be :

$$pOH = -\log [OH^-] = -\log 10^{-5} = -(-5) = 5.$$

4·8·3.   Relation Between pH and pOH

We have seen that the value of ionic product of water, K_w, is 10^{-14} at room temperature, hence pK_w will be given as :

$$pK_w = -\log K_w = -\log 10^{-14} = -(-14) = 14$$

$$K_w = [H^+] \times [OH^-] = 10^{-14} \qquad \qquad ...(4·11)$$

$$\therefore \quad \log K_w = \log [H^+] \times \log [OH^-] = \log 10^{-14}$$

or, $\quad \log K_w = \log [H^+] + \log [OH^-] = \log 10^{-14} \qquad ...(4·12)$

(Remember that $\log a \times \log b = \log a + \log b$)

Multiplying equation (4·12) throughout by -1,

$$-\log K_w = -\log [H^+] - \log [OH^-] = -\log 10^{-14}$$

or, $\quad pK_w = pH + pOH = -(-14) = 14$

Thus, $pH + pOH = 14 \qquad \qquad ...(4·13)$

It should be noted that relation (4·13) is applicable to all dilute solutions at room temperature. With the help of this relationship, if pH value of a solution is known, the value of pOH of that solution can be calculated and vice versa. Thus,

$$pH = 14 - pOH$$

and, $\qquad pOH = 14 - pH.$

Example 4(xi)

In an aqueous solution, $[H^+] = 10^{-3}$ g ion per litre, calculate the pH and pOH value of the solution.

$$[H^+] = 10^{-3} \text{ g ion per litre}$$

$$pH = -\log [H^+] = -\log 10^{-3} = 3$$

[or $\qquad pH = \log \dfrac{1}{[H^+]} = \log \dfrac{1}{10^{-3}} = \log 10^3 = 3$]

The pH of the solution will be 3, the pOH value can be calcuted as follows :

$$[H^+] \times [OH^-] = 10^{-14}$$

$$\therefore \quad [OH^-] = \frac{10^{-14}}{[H^+]} = \frac{10^{-14}}{10^{-3}} = 10^{-14} \times 10^{+3} = 10^{-11}$$

$$pOH = -\log [OH^-] = -\log 10^{-11} = 11$$

The pOH value of the solution will be 11.

Note that $pH + pOH = 3 + 11 = 14.$

4·8·4. pH Scale

A normal HCl solution means a solution containing 1 g ion of H^+ per litre, *i.e.* $[H^+]=1$, hence pH of this solution will be

Remember

$$pH=-\log[H^+]=-\log 1=0 \qquad \log 1=0$$

(In the above calculation it has been assumed that HCl is completely dissociated into H^+ and Cl^- ; normal HCl soln means that 1 g mole of HCl/l, this would give 1 g ion of H^+ ions/l).

In N/10 (or 0·1 N or 10^{-1} N) HCl solution, the concentration of H^+, $[H^+]$, is 0·1 or 10^{-1} g ion per litre, hence its pH will be :

$$pH=-\log[H^+]=-\log[10^{-1}]=-(-1)=1.$$

In N/100 (or 0·01 N or 10^{-2} N) HCl solution, $[H^+]=0·01$ or 10^{-2} g ion per litre, hence pH is :

$$pH=-\log 10^{-2}=-(-2)=2.$$

Similarly it can be shown that pH of :

N/1000 or 0·001 N HCl is 3

N/10,000 or 0·0001 N HCl is 4

N/100,000 or 0·00001 N HCl is 5 and so on.

From the above discussion it is clear that if N HCl is diluted 10 times (N to N/10) its pH increases by 1 unit (0 to 1). If N/10 HCl is further 10 times diluted (N/10 to N/100), again pH value increases by 1 unit (1 to 2) and so on. It should be noted that if we go on diluting the acid solution, its pH will keep on increasing but it will never exceed 7, because if pH becomes greater than 7 it means that the solution has become basic. But we cannot obtain a base simply by diluting an acid solution. The reason is that for dilution we use water which itself contains 10^{-7} g ions per litre of H^+ ions hence, the concentration of H^+ can never become smaller than 10^{-7} g ion per litre, *i.e.*, pH will never become greater than 7 when an acid is diluted with pure water.

Now consider a normal solution of NaOH. In this solution the concentration of OH^- will be 1 g ion per litre if NaOH is supposed to be completely dissociated. In this solution :

$$[H^+]\times[OH^-]=10^{-14}$$

substituting the value $[OH^-]$,

$$[H^+]\times 1=10^{-14}$$

or

$$[H^+]=\frac{10^{-14}}{1}=10^{-14} \text{ g ion per litre}$$

$$pH=-\log 10^{-14}=14.$$

and, $pOH = -\log [OH^-] = -\log 1 = 0$

Remember
$[OH^-] = 1$
and
$\log 1 = 0$

[It should be noted that even in alkaline solution, H^+ ions are present but their concentration is smaller than that of OH^- ion concentration, that is why the solution shows alkaline property. It is wrong to think that an alkaline solution will contain only OH^- ions and no H^+ ions will be present]. Thus, for a normal solution of NaOH, pH is 14 and pOH is zero.

In N/10 (or 0·1 N or 10^{-1} N) NaOH solution, $[OH^-]$ is 0·1 or 10^{-1} g ion per litre. Using the relation,

$$[H^+] \times [OH^-] = 10^{-14}$$

and substituting 10^{-1} for $[OH^-]$ we get :

$$[H^+] \times 10^{-1} = 10^{-14}$$

or $[H^+] = \dfrac{10^{-14}}{10^{-1}} = 10^{-14} \times 10^{+1} = 10^{-13}$ g ion/litre

$\therefore$ $pH = -\log [H^+] = -\log 10^{-13} = 13$

and $pOH = -\log [OH^-] = -\log 10^{-1} = 1.$

The pH of N/10 NaOH solution will be 13 and its pOH will be 1. Thus, by diluting N NaOH ten times the pH decreases by 1 unit. Hence, we can write that for :

	pH	pOH	pH+pOH
N —NaOH solution	14	0	14
N/10 or 0·1 N NaOH	13	1	14
N/100 or 0·01 N NaOH	12	2	14
N/1000 or 0·001 N NaOH	11	3	14
N/10,000 or 0·0001 N NaOH	10	4 and so on	

These observations have been summarised in Table 4·1.

Example 4(*xii*)

The hydrogen ion concentration of a solution is $5·0 \times 10^{-7}$ g ion per litre, calculate its pH and pOH.

$pH = -\log [H^+] = -\log [5·0 \times 10^{-7}]$
$pH = -[\log 5·0 + \log 10^{-7}]$
$pH = -[0·6990 + (-7·0000)]$
$pH = -[0·6990 - 7·0000]$
$pH = -[-6·3010] = +6·3010$
$pOH = 14 - pH$
$pOH = 14 - 6·3010 = 7·6990$

Remember
$\log a \times b = \log a + \log b$
$\log 10^{-7} = -7·0000$ or
$\bar{7}·0000$
$\log 5·0 = 0·6990$
(from log table)

Table 4·1. The pH Scale.

$[H^+] > [OH^-]$ Acidic Range

Normality of HCl (g eq./litre)	[H+] in g ion/litre	pH	[OH−] in g ion/litre	pOH
1 or N or 1N	1 or 1	0	10^{-14}	14
0·1 N/10 10^{-1} N	0·1 10^{-1}	1	10^{-13}	13
0·01 N/100 10^{-2} N	0·01 10^{-2}	2	10^{-12}	12
0·001 N/1000 10^{-3} N	0·001 10^{-3}	3	10^{-11}	11
0·0001 N/10,000 10^{-4} N	0·0001 10^{-4}	4	10^{-10}	10

$[H^+]=[OH^-]=10^{-7}$: Neutral Solution : pH $=7$

$[OH^-] > [H^+]$ Alkaline Range

Normality of NaOH (g eq./litre)	[OH−] in g ion per litre	pOH	[H+] in g ion per litre	pH
0·0001 N/10,000 10^{-4} N	0·0001 10^{-4}	4	10^{-10}	10
0·001 N/1000 10^{-3} N	0·001 10^{-3}	3	10^{-11}	11
0·01 N/100 10^{-2} N	0·01 10^{-2}	2	10^{-12}	12
0·1 N/10 10^{-1} N	0·1 10^{-1}	1	10^{-13}	13
or N or 1	1 or 1	0	10^{-14}	14

The pH of the solution will be 6·3010 and its pOH will be 7·6990.

Example 4(xiii)

Calculate the pH of 0·01 N HCl and 0·01 N CH_3COOH. (The percentage dissociation of CH_3COOH is 12·5%).

In 0·01 N HCl, $[H^+]=10^{-2}$ g ion/litre

$pH=-\log 10^{-2}=2$.

In 0·01 N HCl solution, 0·01 g eq of HCl is present in a litre of solution. Since HCl is a strong acid, it is completely dissociated. Hence, 0·01 g eq of HCl will dissociate to give 0·01 or 10^{-2} g ion of H^+ and 10^{-2} g ion of Cl^- ion. But CH_3COOH is a weak acid which in 0·01 N solution is only 12·5% dissociated. It means that only 12·5% molecules will dissociate to give H^+ and rest 87·5% will remain undissociated. The degree of dissociation, α, of CH_3COOH in 0·01 N solution will be 12·5/100=0·125. Thus only 12·5% of replaceable hydrogen (present in COOH group) will be in the form of H^+. Therefore, hydrogen ion concentration in the solution will not be 0·01 (equal to that of CH_3COOH) but only (0·01 × 0·125) g ion per litre.

$pH=-\log[0·01 \times 0·125]$ $\log 0·01 = \bar{2}·0000$

$pH=-[\log 0·01+\log 0·125]$ $\log 0·125=\bar{1}·0969$

$pH=-[\bar{2}·0000+\bar{1}·0969]$ $=\bar{3}·0969$

$pH=-[\bar{3}·0969]=-[-3·0000+0·0969]*$

$pH=-[-2·9031]=2·9031$

The pH of 0·01 N HCl is 2 but that of 0·01 N CH_3COOH will be 2·9031.

Example 4(xiv)

The pH of a solution is 10·70, calculate the hydrogen ion concentration in the solution.

---

*Logarithms are divided into two parts, characteristic which comes at the left of the decimal point and mantissa which appears after the decimal point. For example, in $\bar{3}·0969$, $\bar{3}$ (pronounced three bar) is characteristic and 0·0969 is mantissa. Here, characteristic is negative (as shown by bar at the top) and mantissa is positive, i.e., a part of the quantity is positive and another part is negative. But the quantity should be either completely positive or completely negative. This can be done by writing $\bar{3}·0969$ as $-3·0000+0·0969$ $=-2·9031$ (when minus sign is written before characteristic, characteristic and mantissa both are negative).

$$pH = 10.70 = -\log [H^+]$$
$$\therefore \quad \log [H^+] = -10.70 = 0.30 - 11.0$$
$$[H^+] = \text{antilog } 0.30 \times \text{antilog } (-11.0)$$
$$[H^+] = 2.0 \times 10^{-11}.$$

4.9. SALT HYDROLYSIS

When salts are dissolved in water, the solution is not always neutral but may be acidic or basic depending upon the nature of the salt ; this is due to salt hydrolysis which means interaction between ions of a salt and ions of water. For a convenient study of this interaction, salts have been divided into four categories.

A. Salts of strong acids and strong bases, such as, NaCl, K_2SO_4 etc.

B. Salts of weak acids and strong bases, such as HCOOK, CH_3COONa etc.

C. Salts of strong acids and weak bases, such as NH_4Cl, $(NH_4)_2SO_4$ etc.

D. Salts of weak acids and weak bases, such as, CH_3COONH_4, $(CH_3COO)_3Al$ etc.

A.   Salts of strong acids and strong bases

Let us take the example of NaCl which is dissolved in water. In this solution the following two equilibria will exist :

$$NaCl \rightleftharpoons Na^+ + Cl^- \text{ (Strongly dissociated)} \qquad ...(4.14)$$
$$H_2O \rightleftharpoons OH^- + H^+ \text{ (Poorly dissociated)} \qquad ...(4.15)$$

Now, Na^+ ions do not have any tendency to combine with OH^- to form NaOH, similarly Cl^- ions do not combine with H^+ to form HCl because NaOH and HCl are strong electrolytes which are completely dissociated in solution. Thus, ions of the salt, i.e., Na^+ and Cl^- do not disturb the equilibrium (4.15), so that the solution remains neutral with pH equal to 7, the same that of pure water. *It is concluded that the salts of strong acids and strong bases are not hydrolysed.*

B.   Salts of weak acids and strong bases

An example of this type of salt is CH_3COONa which is a salt of a , weak acid, CH_3COOH, and a strong base, NaOH. Salts are completely dissociated hence, CH_3COONa will be completely dissociated in aqueous solution :

$$CH_3COONa \rightleftharpoons CH_3COO^- + Na^+$$

Water being a weak electrolyte will be poorly dissociated giving a very small concentration of H^+ and OH^- ions. Acetate ions combine with H^+ ions to form poorly dissociated acetic acid hence water will further dissociate to give more H^+ and OH^- ions. Because CH_3COOH is a weak acid it will slightly dissociate to give a small concentration of H^+ ions. On the other hand, Na^+ ions do not combine with OH^- as NaOH is completely dissociated, so that OH^- ion concentration in the solution will be much larger than that of H^+ ions. The solution therefore will be basic.

$$CH_3COONa \rightleftharpoons \boxed{CH_3COO^- \quad + \quad Na^+} \ldots (\text{strongly dissociated})$$
$$H_2O \rightleftharpoons \boxed{H^+ \quad + \quad OH^-} \ldots (\text{poorly dissociated}).$$

$$\downarrow \qquad\qquad\qquad \downarrow$$

$$CH_3COOH \qquad NaOH$$

weak acid   strong base
poorly   strongly
dissociated   dissociated

$$\therefore \text{ [H}^+\text{] is small} \qquad \therefore \text{ [OH}^-\text{] is larger}$$

Thus, due to interaction between ions of sodium acetate and water, a weak acid and a strong base is produced so the resultant solution is alkaline and the salt is said to be hydrolysed.

C. Salts of strong acids and weak bases

Ammonium chloride, for example, is a salt of a strong acid HCl and a weak base NH_4OH. In an aqueous solution NH_4Cl will completely dissociate :

$$NH_4Cl \rightleftharpoons \boxed{Cl^- \quad + \quad NH_4^+}$$
$$H_2O \rightleftharpoons \boxed{H^+ \quad + \quad OH^-}$$

$$\downarrow \qquad\qquad\qquad \downarrow$$

$$HCl \qquad\qquad NH_4OH$$

strong acid   weak acid
completely dissociated   poorly dissociated

$$\therefore \text{ [H}^+\text{] is large} \qquad \therefore \text{ [OH}^-\text{] is small}$$

Thus, it can be shown that a salt of a strong acid and a weak base will interact with water to produce a weak base so that its solution is acidic.

D. Salts of weak acids and weak bases

Ammonium acetate is a salt of a weak acid (CH_3COOH) and a weak base (NH_4OH). In aqueous solution, this salt will be completely dissociated into NH_4^+ and CH_3COO^- ions which will interact with H^+ and OH^- ions obtained by the weak dissociation of water.

$$CH_3COONH_4 \rightleftharpoons \quad CH_3COO^- \quad + \quad NH_4^+ \quad \text{(completely dissociated)}$$

$$H_2O \rightleftharpoons \quad H^+ \quad + \quad OH^- \quad \text{(poorly dissociated)}$$

$$\downarrow \qquad\qquad \downarrow$$

$$CH_3COOH \qquad NH_4OH$$
weak acid   weak base
poorly dissociated   poorly dissociated

The question, now, is whether the salt solution will be neutral or acidic or basic ? This will depend upon the relative strengths of the weak acid and weak base, formed as a result of hydrolysis. If K_a and K_b represent dissociation constant of weak acid and weak base respectively then :

if $K_a = K_b$, solution will be neutral,

if $K_a > K_b$, solution will be acidic and

if $K_b > K_a$, solution will be basic.

After considering these four types of salts, we can give a general definition of hydrolysis ; this is defined as the interaction between ions of salts and ions of water to produce either a weak acid or a weak base or both. If a weak acid or a weak base is not formed the salt will not be hydrolysed such as, NaCl, KCl or $NaNO_3$ are not hydrolysed because when they react with water a strong acid and a strong base is formed. Thus, for salt hydrolysis, the formation of a weak acid or weak base is a must.

4·9·1. Degree of Hydrolysis and Hydrolysis Constant

Case I. Salt of a weak acid and a strong base.

Suppose such a salt is represented by MA, which in its aqueous solution completely dissociates into M^+ and A^- ions. The anion, combines with H^+, from water, to form a weak acid HA. Thus :

$$MA \rightleftharpoons M^+ + A^- \text{ (completely dissociated)}$$

$$H_2O \rightleftharpoons H^+ + OH^- \text{ (poorly dissociated)}$$

The ions of the salt MA will then react with water :

$$M^+ + A^- + H_2O \rightleftharpoons HA + M^+ + OH^- \qquad ...(4·16)$$

As HA is a weak acid it will poorly dissociate to give very small concentration of H^+ and A^- ions and most of it will be in the form of HA molecules. This is the reason that in equation (4·16) it is written as HA and not as H^+ and A^-. Similarly water is a weak electrolyte therefore, it is written as H_2O and not as H^+ and OH^-. On the other hand, because MOH is a strong base which completely dissociates in solution, it is not written in the molecular form MOH.

but in terms of ions as M^+ and OH^-. In equation (4·16), M^+ ion is common on both the sides hence, it cancels out and we can write :

$$A^- + H_2O \rightleftharpoons HA + OH^- \qquad ...(4·17)$$

As there is formation of a weak acid HA, the salt is said to be hydrolysed. In the hydrolysed salt solution, there is a greater concentration of free OH^- ions than that of H^+ ions hence, the salt solution will be basic.

By applying law of mass action to equilibrium (4·17), we get :

$$\frac{a_{HA} \times a_{OH^-}}{a_{A^-} \times a_{H_2O}} = \text{constant} = K_h \text{ (hydrolysis constant)}$$

Now, activity of water is taken as unity.

$$K_h = \frac{a_{HA} \times a_{OH^-}}{a_{A^-}}$$

$$K_h = \frac{[HA] \times [OH^-]}{[A]^-} \times \frac{f_{HA} \times f_{OH^-}}{f_{A^-}}$$

Remember
$a = c \times f$ and $f = 1$
in dilute solutions

The terms in brackets represent concentration and f_{HA}, f_{OH^-} and f_{A^-} are activity coefficients of HA, OH^- and A^- respectively. In dilute solution activity coefficients become unity so that :

$$K_h = \frac{[HA] \times [OH^-]}{[A^-]} \qquad ...(4·18)$$

The equilibrium constant in this case is called *hydrolysis constant* and is represented by K_h.

Suppose one g mole of a salt is dissolved in water, out of which x g mole is hydrolysed then, x will be called the *degree of hydrolysis.* The hydrolysis of a salt of a weak acid and a strong base is given as :

$$A^- + H_2O \rightleftharpoons HA + OH^- \qquad ...(4·19)$$

If one g mole of the salt is present in V litres of solution and x is the degree of hydrolysis, then the concentration of the unhydrolysed salt $[A^-] = 1 - x/V$ g mole/litre and that of HA and OH^- will be x/V each. [Each molecule of MA dissociates to give one M^+ ion and one A^- ion so that one g mole of MA on dissociation will give 1 g ion of M^+ and 1 g ion of A^-. Hence, if concentration of salt (unhydrolysed) is $1 - x/V$ g mole, the concentration of M^+ or A^- ion will also be $1 - x/V$ g ion per litres.]

By substituting these values in (4·18), we get :

$$K_h = \frac{x/V \times x/V}{(1-x)/V}$$

$$K_h = \frac{x^2}{V^2} \times \frac{V}{(1-x)} = \frac{x^2}{(1-x)/V} \qquad \ldots(4\cdot20)$$

With the help of the above relationship, K_h can be calculated if x is known and *vice versa*.

In an aqueous solution of such a salt, the following equilibria exist :

$$H_2O \rightleftharpoons H^+ + OH^- \text{ (poorly dissociated)}$$
$$HA \rightleftharpoons H^+ + A^- \quad \text{(poorly dissociated)}$$

and
$$A^- + H_2O \rightleftharpoons HA + OH^-$$

Now, it is known that :

$$[H^+] \times [OH^-] = K_w \text{ (ionic product of water)}$$

$$\frac{[H^+] \times [A^-]}{[HA]} = K_a \text{ (dissociation constant of weak acid HA)}$$

and,
$$\frac{[HA] \times [OH^-]}{[A^-]} = K_h \text{ (hydrolysis constant)}$$

$$\therefore \quad \frac{K_w}{K_a} = \frac{[H^+] \times [OH^-] \times [HA]}{[H^+] \times [A^-]}$$

$$= \frac{[OH^-] \times [HA]}{[A^-]} = K_h$$

Thus for a salt of a weak acid and a strong base :

$$\boxed{\frac{K_w}{K_a} = K_h}$$

or, $$\log K_w - \log K_a = \log K_h$$
or, $$-\log K_w + \log K_a = -\log K_h$$
or, $$pK_w - pK_a = pK_h$$

The pH of a solution of a hydrolysed salt can be calculated in the following manner. From equation (4·19) it is evident that as a result of hydrolysis, one molecule of HA and one OH^- ion is formed, *i.e.*, $[HA] = [OH^-]$ so that :

$$\frac{[HA] \times [OH^-]}{[A^-]} = \frac{[OH^-]^2}{[A^-]} = K_h = \frac{K_w}{K_a} \bigg| \text{ putting } [HA] = [OH^-]$$

If concentration of the salt is c g mole per litre and it is assumed that very little of the salt is hydrolysed (x is small) then, c can be taken as approximately equal to the concentration of the unhydrolysed salt, *i.e.*, $[A^-]$. Substituting c for $[A^-]$:

$$\frac{[OH^-]^2}{c} = K_h = \frac{K_w}{K_a}$$

or, $$[OH^-]^2 = \frac{K_w \times c}{K_a}$$

$$[OH^-] = \sqrt{\frac{K_w \times c}{K_a}} = \frac{K_w^{1/2} \times c^{1/2}}{K_a^{1/2}}$$

or, $[OH^-] = K_w^{1/2} \times c^{1/2} \times K_a^{-1/2}$

$$[H^+] = \frac{K_w}{[OH^-]} = \frac{K_w}{K_w^{1/2} \times c^{1/2} \times K_a^{-1/2}}$$

$$[H^+] = \frac{K_w^{1/2}}{c^{1/2} \times K_a^{-1/2}} = K_w^{1/2} \times K_a^{1/2} \times c^{-1/2}$$

$\log [H^+] = \log K_w^{1/2} + \log K_a^{1/2} + \log c^{-1/2}$

$\log [H^+] = \frac{1}{2} \log K_w + \frac{1}{2} \log K_a - \frac{1}{2}\log c$

$-\log [H^+] = -\frac{1}{2} \log K_w - \frac{1}{2} \log K_a + \frac{1}{2} \log c$

$pH = \frac{1}{2} pK_w + \frac{1}{2}pK_a + \frac{1}{2}\log c$ ...(4.21)

Remember

$\sqrt{x} = x^{1/2}$

$1/x^{1/2} = x^{-1/2}$

$[H^+] \times [OH^-] = K_w$

$\therefore [H^+] = \dfrac{K_w}{[OH^-]}$

$K_w = K_w^{1/2} \times K_w^{1/2}$

$\log a^x = x \log a$ and $\log a \times b = \log a + \log b$

(multiplying both sides by -1)

($-\log$ written as p)

Equation (4.21) can be used to calculate pH of a solution of a salt of a weak acid and a strong base provided the concentration of the salt, c and the value of the dissociation constant of the weak acid, K_a, is known.

$[K_w = 10^{-14}$; $\log K_w = -14$; $-\log K_w = 14$ or $pK_w = 14$; $\frac{1}{2} pK_w = 7]$

Example 4(xv)

Calculate pH of 0.05 M solution of sodium acetate. (The dissociation constant of acetic acid is 1.8×10^{-5}).

$pH = \frac{1}{2} pK_w + \frac{1}{2} pK_a + \frac{1}{2} \log c$

$\log K_a = \log [1.8 \times 10^{-5}]$

$\log K_a = [\log 1.8 + \log 10^{-5}]$

$\log K_a = -4.7447$

$-\log K_a = +4.7447$

$pK_a = 4.7447$

$\frac{1}{2} pK_a = 2.3724$

$\frac{1}{2} pK_w = 7.0000$

$\frac{1}{2} \log c = -0.6505$

$pH = 7.0000 + 2.3724 - 0.6505$

$= 8.72$

Remember

$\log a \times b = \log a + \log b$

$\log 10^{-5} = \bar{5}.0000$
$\log 1.8 = 0.2553$
_____
$\bar{5}.2553$

or $(-5.0000 + 0.2553)$
$= -4.7447$

$c = 0.05$ g mole/litre

$\log 0.05 = \bar{2}.6990$

$\frac{1}{2} \log 0.05 = \bar{1}.3495$

$= (-1.0000 + 0.3495)$

$= -0.6505$

Thus, the pH of 0·05 M sodium acetate would be 8·72.

Case II. Salt of a strong acid and a weak base

Suppose MA is a salt of a strong acid and a weak base which hydrolyses to give a weak base (MOH) and a strong acid (HA). If one g mole of the salt is present in V litres of solution and x is the degree of hydrolysis, the concentration of unhydrolysed salt will be $1-x/V$ and that of MOH and HA will be x/V each. The hydrolysis of the salt is represented as :

$$M^+ + A^- + H_2O \rightleftharpoons MOH + H^+ + A^-$$

or,
$$M^+ \mid + H_2O \rightleftharpoons MOH + \mid H^+ \qquad ...(4·22)$$

$\dfrac{1-x}{V}$ g ion per litre $\quad \dfrac{x}{V}$ g mole per litre $\quad \dfrac{x}{V}$ g ion per litre

The hydrolysis constant will be given as :

$$K_h = \frac{[MOH] \times [H^+]}{[M^+]}$$

$$= \frac{x/V \times x/V}{(1-x)/V} = \frac{x^2}{(1-x)V}$$

The weak base MOH poorly dissociates as

$$MOH \rightleftharpoons M^+ + OH^-$$

and its dissociation constant K_b is given as :

$$K_b = \frac{[M^+] \times [OH^-]}{[MOH]} \qquad ...(4·23)$$

Relation between K_h, K_w and K_b ·

$$\frac{K_w}{K_b} = \frac{[H^+] \times [OH^-] \times [MOH]}{[M^+] \times [OH^-]}$$

$$= \frac{[MOH] \times [H^+]}{[M^+]} = K_h$$

Thus for a salt of a strong acid and a weak base :

$$\boxed{K_h = \frac{K_w}{K_b}} \qquad ...(4·24)$$

Calculation of pH of a hydrolysed salt solution

$$K_h = \frac{[MOH] \times [H^+]}{[M^+]} \qquad (\because \ [MOH] = [H^+])$$

$$\therefore \quad K_h = \frac{[H^+]^2}{c} = \frac{K_w}{K_b} \qquad (\because \ [M^+] = c, \text{ assuming } x \text{ to be small})$$

or, $$[H^+] = \sqrt{\frac{K_w \times c}{K_b}} = K_w^{1/2} \times K_b^{-1/2} \times c^{1/2}$$

or, $$\log [H^+] = \tfrac{1}{2} \log K_w - \tfrac{1}{2} \log K_b + \tfrac{1}{2} \log c$$

$$-\log [H^+] = -\tfrac{1}{2} \log K_w + \tfrac{1}{2} \log K_b - \tfrac{1}{2} \log c$$

$$pH = \tfrac{1}{2} pK_w - \tfrac{1}{2} pK_b - \tfrac{1}{2} \log c \qquad \ldots(4\cdot25)$$

Example 4(xvi)

The dissociation constant of NH_4OH is $1\cdot85 \times 10^{-5}$, calculate the pH of $0\cdot02$ N solution of NH_4Cl.

$$pH = \tfrac{1}{2} pK_w - \tfrac{1}{2} pK_b - \tfrac{1}{2} \log c \qquad \qquad \tfrac{1}{2} pK_w = 7\cdot00$$

$$pH = 7 - 2\cdot37 - \tfrac{1}{2} (-2\cdot00 + 0\cdot30) \qquad \qquad pK_b = 4\cdot74$$

$$pH = 7 - 2\cdot37 - \tfrac{1}{2} (-1\cdot7) = 4\cdot63 + 0\cdot85 = 5\cdot48 \qquad \log 0\cdot02 = \overline{2}\cdot30$$

Case III. Salt of a weak acid and a weak base

The hydrolysis of a salt, MA, of a weak acid and a weak base can be represented as :

$$M^+ + A^- + H_2O \rightleftharpoons MOH + HA$$

If 1 g mole of salt is present in V litres of solution and x is degree of hydrolysis :

$$[M^+] = [A^-] = \frac{1-x}{V} \text{ g ion per litre and}$$

$$[MOH] = [HA] = \frac{x}{V} \text{ g mole per litre.}$$

The hydrolysis constant will be given by :

$$K_h = \frac{[MOH] \times [HA]}{[M^+] \times [A^-]}$$

$$= \frac{x/V \times x/V}{\dfrac{(1-x)}{V} \times \dfrac{(1-x)}{V}} = \frac{x^2}{(1-x)^2} \qquad \ldots(4\cdot26)$$

Relation between K_h, K_w, K_a and K_b

$$\frac{K_w}{K_a \times K_b} = [H^+] \times [OH^-] \times \frac{[HA]}{[H^+] \times [A^-]} \times \frac{[MOH]}{[M^+] \times [OH^-]}$$

$$= \frac{[HA] \times [MOH]}{[M^+] \times [A^-]} = K_h \qquad ...(4.27)$$

Thus, for a salt of a weak acid and a weak base

$$\boxed{K_h = \frac{K_w}{K_a \times K_b}}$$

or, $\log K_h = \log K_w - \log K_a - \log K_b$

or, $-\log K_h = -\log K_w + \log K_a + \log K_b$

$pK_h = pK_w - pK_a - pK_b$

| $-\log$ is denoted as p ; $+\log$ can be denoted by $-p$.

Calculation of pH of a hydrolysed salt solution

The dissociation constant of a weak acid is given as :

Remember

$[HA] = x/V$ and $[A^-] = 1 - x/V$

$$K_a = \frac{[H^+] \times [A^-]}{[HA]}$$

$$\therefore \quad \frac{[HA]}{[A^-]} = \frac{x}{V} \times \frac{V}{1-x} = \frac{x}{1-x}$$

$$\therefore \quad [H^+] = K_a \times \frac{[HA]}{[A^-]}$$

$$\frac{x^2}{(1-x)^2} = K_h \text{ [see equn. (4.26)]}$$

$$[H^+] = K_a \times \frac{x}{1-x}$$

$$[H^+] = K_a \times \sqrt{K_h}$$

$$\therefore \quad \frac{x}{(1-x)} = \sqrt{K_h}$$

$$[H^+] = K_a \times \sqrt{\frac{K_w}{K_a \times K_b}}$$

$$K_h = \frac{K_w}{K_a \times K_b}$$

$$[H^+] = \frac{K_a \times K_w^{1/2}}{K_a^{1/2} \times K_b^{1/2}}$$

$$\sqrt{x} = x^{1/2}$$

$$[H^+] = K_w^{1/2} \times K_a^{1/2} \times K_b^{-1/2}$$

$$\frac{1}{K_b^{1/2}} = K_b^{-1/2}$$

$$\log [H^+] = \tfrac{1}{2} \log K_w + \tfrac{1}{2} \log K_a - \tfrac{1}{2} \log K_b$$

or, $$pH = \tfrac{1}{2} pK_w + \tfrac{1}{2} pK_a - \tfrac{1}{2} pK_b \qquad ...(4.28)$$

Example 4(*xvii*)

Calculate the pH of a solution of ammonium formate. The dissociation constant of formic acid is $1·77 \times 10^{-4}$ and that of ammonium hydroxide is $1·85 \times 10^{-5}$.

Dissociation constant of the acid, $K_a = 1·77 \times 10^{-4}$

$$pK_a = -\log K_a = -\log [1·77 \times 10^{-4}]$$

$$pK_a = -[\log 1·77 + \log 10^{-4}] = -[0·2480 + (-4·0000)]$$

$$pK_a = -[-3·7520] = +3·7520$$

$$\tfrac{1}{2} pK_a = \frac{3·7520}{2} = 1·88$$

Dissociation constant of the base, $K_b = 1·85 \times 10^{-5}$

$$pK_b = -\log [1·85 \times 10^{-5}] = -[0·2672 - 5·0000]$$

$$pK_b = -[-4·7328] = 4·7328$$

$$\tfrac{1}{2} pK_b = 2·37$$

$$pH = \tfrac{1}{2} pK_w + \tfrac{1}{2} pK_a - \tfrac{1}{2} pK_b \text{ [see equn. } 4·28]$$

$$= 7·0 + 1·88 - 2·37 = 6·51.$$

The pH of ammonium formate solution will be 6·51, *i.e.*, it will be slightly acidic.

4·10. BUFFER SOLUTION OR BUFFER SYSTEMS

We have seen that the pH of water is 7. Now, if to a litre of water, 1 ml of N-HCl is added, the acid will be diluted 1000 times hence, the normality of the resultant acid solution will be N/1000 and its pH will be 3. Thus, the addition of 1 ml of N-HCl to a litre of water will cause a pH change from 7 to 3, *i.e.*, by 4 pH units. Likewise, it can be shown that if 1 ml of N-NaOH is added to a litre of water, the pH will rise from 7 to 11.

It has been seen in 4·9 that salts of strong acids and strong bases do not hydrolyse so their aqueous solutions remain neutral. For example, aqueous solutions of KCl, NaCl, KNO_3 etc., have pH equal to 7. Hence, if 1 ml of N-HCl is added to a litre of N-NaCl solution, the pH will decrease from 7 to 3 as was observed in the case of water. Similarly, the addition of 1 ml of N-NaOH to a litre of N-NaCl will increase the pH of the solution from 7 to 11. Thus, there is a great change in pH of water or NaCl solution on the addition of even small amounts of acid or alkali. On the other hand, if 1 ml of N-HCl is added to a litre of N-ammonium acetate solution (whose pH is 7), there would be a very small change in pH.

Solutions which resist the change in pH when a small amount of acid or alkali is added to them, are called *buffer solutions* and this resistance to change in pH, upon the addition of small amounts of acid or alkali is called *Buffer action.*

In many analytical procedures, it is sometimes necessary to carry out some analytical operation at a fixed pH. In such cases, a buffer solution of desired pH is used to control the pH of the system under consideration.

Buffer solutions can be obtained by mixing a solution of a weak acid with a solution of its salt. For example, a mixture containing solutions of acetic acid and sodium acetate will form a buffer system. The pH of this buffer system will depend upon the value of the dissociation constant of acetic acid and the relative amounts of acetic acid and sodium acetate. A buffer solution can also be obtained by mixing a solution of a weak base and a solution of its salt. For example, a solution containing NH_4OH (a weak base) and its salt NH_4Cl will form a buffer solution. The pH of a buffer solution depends upon the nature of the weak acid or base taken and the relative amounts of the acid or base and its salt. Thus, we can prepare a buffer system of desired pH by selecting a suitable weak acid or base and mixing it with its salt in a particular ratio.

4'10'1. Buffer Action

To understand buffer action, consider a mixture containing acetic acid and sodium acetate. Sodium acetate is a strong electrolyte hence, it will completely dissociate whereas acetic acid being a weak electrolyte will only slightly dissociate in aqueous solution :

$$CH_3COONa \rightleftharpoons CH_3COO^- + Na^+ \text{ (strongly dissociated)} \quad ...(4'29)$$

$$CH_3COOH \rightleftharpoons CH_3COO^- + H^+ \text{ (poorly dissociated)} \quad ...(4'30)$$

Let us now consider what will happen if a small amount of HCl is added to this buffer system. The added acid will give H^+ ions but equilibrium (4'30) permits only a small concentration of H^+ ions as acetic acid is weakly dissociated. Hence, H^+ ions provided by HCl will combine with CH_3COO^- ions of the salt to form undissociated CH_3COOH. In this way there is a regulation of H^+ ion concentration which is not permitted to increase so, there is practically no change in pH when a small amount of HCl is added to acetic acid-acetate mixture.

$$
\begin{array}{ll}
HCl \rightleftharpoons & \boxed{\begin{array}{c} H^+ \\ CH_3COO^- \end{array}} \begin{array}{l} +Cl^- \\ +Na^+ \end{array} \\
CH_3COONa \rightleftharpoons &
\end{array}
$$

$$\downarrow$$

$$CH_3COOH \text{ (poorly dissociated)}$$

If to the above system, a small amount of NaOH is added, the concentration of OH^- ions will increase, consequently the pH of the system must also change. But OH^- ions at once combine with H^+ ions from acetic acid. The H^+ ions used up in this reaction are replaced by the dissociation of CH_3COOH. Thus, again the H^+ ion concentration in the system remains unchanged.

$$NaOH \rightleftharpoons Na^+ \quad + \boxed{\begin{array}{c} OH^- \\ \\ H^+ \end{array}}$$

$$CH_3COOH \rightleftharpoons CH_3COO^- +$$

$$\downarrow$$
$$H_2O \text{ (poorly dissociated)}$$

Thus, on addition of NaOH to acetic acid-acetate buffer system its pH remains practically unchanged.

Buffer solutions can also be prepared by mixing different acid salts such as, NaH_2PO_4 and Na_2HPO_4 or $NaHCO_3$ and Na_2CO_3. A mixture of a weak base and its salt can also act as a buffer.. For example, a mixture of NH_4OH and NH_4Cl. If to such a mixture a small amount of HCl is added, OH^- ion from NH_4OH will combine with H^+ ions from HCl so that H^+ ion concentration of the system will remain the same.

$$HCl \rightleftharpoons \boxed{\begin{array}{c} H^+ \\ \\ OH^- \end{array}} + Cl^-$$

$$NH_4OH \rightleftharpoons \qquad\quad + NH_4^+$$

$$\downarrow$$
$$H_2O \text{ (poorly dissociated)}$$

If a small amount of NaOH is added to NH_4Cl-NH_4OH buffer, OH^- ions from NaOH will combine with NH_4^+ ions from NH_4Cl so that the pH of the solution will not change.

$$NaOH \rightleftharpoons Na^+ + \boxed{\begin{array}{c} OH^- \\ \\ NH_4^+ \end{array}}$$

$$NH_4Cl \rightleftharpoons Cl^- +$$

$$\downarrow$$
$$NH_4OH \text{ (poorly dissociated)}$$

- It is thus seen that a mixture of a weak acid and its salt or a weak base and its salt has the property to regulate H^+ ion concentration and it has the capacity to reduce the influence of any factors which tend to change the pH of the solution ; this capacity is known as *buffer capacity*.

4·10·2. Calculation of pH of a Buffer Solution

Consider a buffer solution obtained by mixing a weak acid HA and its salt MA. The dissociation of HA is given as :

$$HA \rightleftharpoons H^+ + A^- \qquad \text{...(poorly dissociated)}$$

The extent of dissociation will depend on the value of the dissociation constant, K_a (greater the magnitude of K_a, greater is the dissociation of HA into H^+ and A^- ions) :

$$K_a = \frac{[H^+] \times [A^-]}{[HA]}$$

Making the approximation that in dilute solution, activity is equal to concentration.

$$\therefore \quad [H^+] = K_a \times \frac{[HA]}{[A^-]} \quad \text{...(4·31)}$$

This relationship exists in the mixture of HA and MA.

Suppose the concentration of the acid is c_a and that of the salt is c_s. The concentration of the undissociated acid will be :

$$c_a - [H^+], \; i.e., \; [HA] = c_a - [H^+].$$

In this buffer solution, A^- ions will be produced from the dissociation of MA and also from that of HA. The salt MA is a strong electrolyte and so it completely dissociates. Each molecule of MA gives one M^+ and one A^- ion, and because the concentration of MA is c_s, the concentration of A^- ions will also be c_s. A molecule of HA on dissociation gives a H^+ ion and a A^- ion, hence $[A^-]$ will be equal to $[H^+]$. Thus the total concentration of A^- in the solution will be $c_s + [H^+]$. Substituting the values of $[HA]$ and $[A^-]$ in equation (4·31), we get :

$$[H^+] = K_a \times \frac{c_a - [H^+]}{c_s + [H^+]} \qquad \text{...(4·32)}$$

Now, in the buffer solution the following equilibria exist :

$$MA \rightleftharpoons M^+ + \boxed{A^-} \quad \text{(strongly dissociated)}$$

$$HA \rightleftharpoons H^+ + \boxed{A^-} \quad \text{(poorly dissociated)}$$

common ion

Due to common ion effect, the dissociation of weak acid HA will be further decreased hence, the concentration of H^+ ion, *i.e.*, $[H^+]$ will be small and can be neglected in comparison to c_s and c_a so equation (4·32) can be written as :

$$[H^+] = K_a \times \frac{c_a}{c_s}$$

or, $$[H^+] = K_a \times \frac{[Acid]}{[Salt]}$$

$$\log [H^+] = \log \left[K_a \times \frac{[Acid]}{[Salt]} \right]$$

$$\log [H^+] = \log K_a + \log \frac{[Acid]}{[Salt]}$$

$$-\log [H^+] = -\log K_a - \log \frac{[Acid]}{[Salt]}$$

$$pH = pK_a + \log \frac{[Salt]}{[Acid]} \quad \ldots(4\cdot33)$$

Remember
$-\log$ is written as p.
$\log\frac{a}{b} = -\log\frac{b}{a}$

Similarly, for a buffer solution containing a weak base and its salt, it can be shown that :

$$pOH = pK_b + \log \frac{[Salt]}{[Base]} \quad \ldots(4\cdot34)$$

where K_b is the dissociation constant of the weak base.

If in a buffer solution the concentrations of a weak acid is equal to that of its salt, i.e., [Salt]=[Acid], then equation (4·33) reduces to :

$$pH = pK_a + \log 1$$
or, $$pH = pK_a \quad \ldots(4\cdot35) \quad [\log 1 = zero]$$

For example, the dissociation constant of acetic acid is $1\cdot82 \times 10^{-5}$ (pK$_a$=4·74) ; if 10 ml of 0·1 M, CH_3COOH and 10 ml of 0·1 M, CH_3COONa are mixed, the pH of the resultant buffer solution will be equal to pK$_a$, i.e., 4·74.

4·10·3. pH Range of a Buffer

Suppose we mix 10 ml of 0·1 M, CH_3COOH and 1 ml of 0·1 M, CH_3COONa, then the pH of resultant buffer system will be given by :

$$pH = pK_a + \log \frac{[Salt]}{[Acid]}$$
$$pH = 4\cdot74 + \log \frac{1}{10}$$
$$pH = 4\cdot74 - 1 = 3\cdot74$$

Remember
[Acid]=10 [salt]
$\log \frac{1}{10} = \log 10^{-1}$, and
$\log 10^{-1} = -1$

If 1 ml of 0·1 M, CH_3COOH and 10 ml of 0·1 M, CH_3COONa are mixed, the pH of the buffer will be :

$$pH = 4·74 + \log \frac{10}{1}$$ $\qquad$ [Salt] = 10 [Acid]

$$pH = 4·74 + \log 10$$ $\qquad$ log 10 = 1

$$pH = 4·74 + 1 = 5·74$$

It is thus seen that when the salt-acid ratio changes from 1 : 10 to 10 : 1, the pH of a weak acid buffer changes from pK_a—1 to pK_a+1, thus the approximate pH range of such a buffer is

$$pH = pK_a \pm 1 \qquad\qquad ...(4·36)$$

For a buffer solution containing a weak base and its salt, the pOH of the solution is given as :

$$pOH = pK_b + \log \frac{[Salt]}{[Base]}$$

Now, $\qquad\qquad pH = 14 - pOH$ $\qquad\qquad$ (see section 4·8·3)

∴ $\qquad\qquad pH = 14 - pK_b - \log \frac{[Salt]}{[Base]} \qquad ...(4·37)$

The dissociation constant of $NH_4OH(K_b)$ is $1·85 \times 10^{-5}$ so that pK_b is 4·74. Suppose we mix 10 ml of 0·1 M, NH_4OH and 10 ml of 0·1 M, NH_4Cl, then the pH of the mixture will be :

$$pH = 14 - 4·74 - \log 1$$ $\qquad$ ∵ [Salt] = [Base]

$$pH = 14 - 4·74 = 9·26$$ $\qquad$ ∴ $\log \dfrac{[Salt]}{[Base]} = \log 1 = 0$

The following points should be remembered about buffer solutions.

It has been seen that a buffer solution maintains practically constant pH even if acid or alkali is added to it. But it should be noted that the amount of acid or alkali added should be small. If too much acid or alkali is added, the pH of the buffer solution will change. The components of a buffer react with H^+ or OH^- ions of the acid or alkali added. If the amount of acid or alkali added is large, the buffer components are not sufficient to combine with H^+ or OH^- ions, hence the buffer will not be able to regulate H^+ ion concentration and so cannot maintain constant pH. However, if concentrations of the components of a buffer are higher it will have higher buffer capacity. For example, a mixture of 1 N, NH_4OH and NH_4Cl will be more effective in maintaining constant pH as compared to a buffer mixture of 0·1 N, NH_4OH and NH_4Cl.

4·10·4. Preparation of a Buffer Solution of Desired pH

Certain analytical procedures are carried out at a particular fixed pH. For this purpose, buffer solutions of desired pH are used. A buffer solution of desired pH can be prepared by properly selecting buffer components and mixing them in a particular proportion. For example, pK_a of acetic acid is 4·75 ; buffer solutions of pH in the range 3·75 to 5·75 ($pK_a \pm 1$) can be prepared by mixing acetic acid and sodium acetate solutions in different proportions as shown in Table 4·2.

Table 4·2. pH of Acetic Acid-Sodium Acetate Buffer Mixtures

ml of 0·2 M Acetic Acid	ml of 0·2 M Sodium Acetate	pH of the buffer Mixture (18°C)
9·5	0·5	3·42
9·0	1·0	3·72
8·0	2·0	4·05
7·0	3·0	4·27
6·0	4·0	4·45
5·0	5·0	4·63
4·0	6·0	4·80
3·0	7·0	4·99
2·0	8·0	5·23
1·0	9·0	5·57
0·5	9·5	5·89

Suppose we have to prepare a buffer solution in the alkaline range, then we should use a weak base and its salt. If the pH of the buffer to be prepared is in the pH range 8-10, a weak base whose pK_b is about $(14-9)=5$, should be used.

Example 4(xviii)

Calculate the pH of a buffer mixture containing 7·5 ml of 0·1 M, NH_4Cl and 2·5 ml of 0·1 M, NH_4OH. The dissociation constant of NH_4OH is $1·79 \times 10^{-5}$.

$$pK_b = -\log 1·79 \times 10^{-5} = -[\log 1·79 + \log 10^{-5}]$$
$$pK_b = -[0·25 + (-5·00)] = -[0·25 - 5·00]$$
$$pK_b = -[-4·75] = +4·75$$

$$pH = 14 - pK_b - \log \frac{[Salt]}{[Base]} \quad [(\text{see equation } 4\cdot34)]$$

$$pH = 14 - 4\cdot75 - \log \frac{7\cdot5}{2\cdot5}$$

$$pH = 14 - 4\cdot75 - \log 3 = 9\cdot25 - 0\cdot48$$

$$pH = 8\cdot77.$$

4·11. COMPLETENESS OF A CHEMICAL REACTION

It has been noted that only those chemical reactions are employed in quantitative analysis which are fast and proceed to virtual completion. Whether or not a chemical reaction will be complete can be known by finding out the value of the equilibrium constant of that reaction ; if the value is quite large the reaction would go to completion. It was mentioned in section 4·1·1 that an incomplete reaction can be pushed in forward direction by :

(i) Increasing the concentration of the reactant,

(ii) Increasing the temperature of the reaction mixture, and

(iii) Decreasing the concentrations of the products of the reaction.

Apart from the above steps there are certain other means by which a reaction can be accelerated and made to proceed to completion in a reasonable period of time.

EFFECT OF CATALYSTS. Some reactions are slow and hence are not complete in a reasonable period of time. In such cases, suitable catalysts, can be added which helps the reaction to attain equilibrium in a much shorter time. For example, the oxidation of mannitol by alkaline potassium permanganate (in presence of barium chloride) is a slow process which can be accelerated by adding a small amount of nickel salt. Here, it should be remembered that a catalyst cannot alter the value of equilibrium constant, it can only diminish the time required for the attainment of equilibrium.

EFFECT OF LIGHT. There are some reactions which in the absence of light are not complete in a reasonable period of time hence, are of no practical value in quantitative chemical analysis. Such reactions on exposure to light of a suitable wavelength can proceed to completion in much shorter time. For example, reaction between mercuric chloride and potassium oxalate is slow but if the mixture is exposed to sun light in presence of ferric chloride the reaction is quantitative in about half an hour and can then be used in the photochemical determination of mercuric chloride.

EFFECT OF SOLVENT. A change in solvent in some reaction gives important effects. For example, quantitative oxidation of sodium oxalate by iodine dissolved in aqueous potassium iodide requires about 6 hrs. heating at $100°C$ but if iodine solution in carbon tetrachloride is used the reaction period is considerably reduced.

EFFECT OF pH. In a number of reactions the equilibrium is pH dependent and the reaction can be controlled by maintaining a particular pH. For example, the reaction of sodium formate and mercuric chloride does not proceed to completion. However, if sodium acetate is added to the reaction mixture, the reaction becomes quantitative. Here, sodium acetate produces buffer action and controls the pH of the reaction mixture.

PART II
QUALITATIVE INORGANIC ANALYSIS

5

Qualitative Inorganic Analysis

There are analytical schemes by means of which cations and anions present in a mixture can be identified. The students of undergraduate classes are familiar with such analytical tables and use them in their practical work for qualitative inorganic analysis. The purpose of this chapter is not to simply describe such a scheme in detail but discuss how theoretical principles have been employed for framing a scheme for the qualitative analysis of inorganic mixtures.

The purpose of analytical chemistry is to provide theoretical basis for methods of chemical analysis. Chemical analysis is of two type ; qualitative and quantitative. The aim of qualitative analysis is to detect or identify individual elements or ions present in a sample. Once these are known, their amounts can be determined by means of methods of quantitative analysis.

5'1. IMPORTANCE OF QUALITATIVE ANALYSIS

Qualitative analysis is of great scientific and practical importance. In chemical studies it is used to characterise different substances and the changes that they undergo during chemical reactions. It is also important to other branches of science such as geology, physiology, microbiology, medicine, agriculture etc. The properties of materials depend on their composition hence, in order to control the properties of a substance it is important to analyse it qualitatively. It should be remembered that if we are required to determine a component of a given sample, the other components of the sample must also be known then only we can select a suitable method for determining the particular component. For example, suppose we have to determine the amount of Ag in a given sample whose composition is not known. Suppose we add an excess of HCl to precipitate AgCl and thus determine Ag gravimetrically. Now, if the sample contains some other ion such as, Hg_2^{2+} which also gives an insoluble chloride, the gravimetric determination of Ag as AgCl will not be correct and some other method for determining Ag has to be used in which Hg_2^{2+} ions do not interfere. Thus, if a particular component of a mixture is to be determined it is very necessary to know the other components present in the mixture, *i.e.*, it is necessary to analyse the mixture qualitatively.

5·2. TYPES OF METHODS OF QUALITATIVE ANALYSIS

Different types of methods are employed for qualitative analysis. In physical methods, analysis depends on relationship between chemical composition and some physical property. For example, let us consider a physical method such as spectro-chemical analysis. It is known that when spectrum of an element is produced, it contains particular lines having fixed wavelengths which are characteristic of the element producing them ; this relationship can act as a basis for identifying various elements. Suppose we want to identify different elements in a mixture. The spectrum of the mixture should be excited and wavelengths of different spectral lines should be measured. A table showing wavelengths of various elements is then consulted and from comparison it is possible to know different elements present in the mixture. Polarographic and radiochemical techniques are also useful in the identification of elements.

Besides these physical or instrumental methods, chemical methods are also used in chemical analysis ; these continue to play leading role and constitute an important part of analytical chemistry. In chemical methods, qualitative analysis is carried out in two ways ; by *dry method* in which dry sample is used and by *wet method* in which substance under examination is dissolved and the resultant solution is analysed. Wet method is much more important in a systematic qualitative analysis however, some dry tests too are quite useful for a rapid identification of certain elements. Some of the dry tests are given below.

1. **Flame test.** In this test the material under examination, with the help of a platinum wire, is introduced into a non-luminous flame. From the colour of the flame the element present in the material can be recognisted. This test is applied for identifying the following metals whose salts give the flame colours shown against their names.

Sodium salt	—	Yellow
Potassium salt	—	Lilac
Strontiam salt	—	Crimson red
Barium salt	—	Yellowish green
Calcium salt	—	Dull red.

2. **Bead test.** A loop is made at the end of a platinum wire which is heated on a flame. Some borax ($Na_2B_4O_7 . 10H_2O$) is put on the loop and it is again heated when a transparent glassy material is formed ; this is called bead. The substance under test is touched with this bead and it is again heated. Different coloured oxides impart characteristic colours to the borax bead. For example, cobalt gives blue, nickel gives yellowish brown and chromium gives green bead.

3. **Charcoal test.** A little of the substance to be tested is mixed with Na_2CO_3 and is heated in a charcoal cavity with the help of a blow pipe. First carbonates of metals are formed which then decompose to oxides, thus coloured or white deposits are observed. For example, lead gives a yellow deposit and arsenic, a white deposit. On adding a drop of cobalt nitrate and again heating, coloured deposits are seen in the cavity. Aluminium gives blue, zinc shows a green and magnesium forms a pink deposit.

The above tests which involve heating solid test material with solid reagents constitute *pyrochemical methods*.

The wet methods which are most often used in chemical analysis are based on reaction between solution of test substance with that of a suitable reagent. These methods will therefore be discussed in greater detail.

5·3. WET METHOD OF QUALITATIVE INORGANIC ANALYSIS

In qualitative inorganic analysis the cations (called basic radicals) and anions (called acid radicals) are separately analysed. The basic radicals which we are generally required to identify are Ag^+, Pb^{2+}, Hg_2^{2+}, Hg^{2+}, Bi^{3+}, Cu^{2+}, Cd^{2+}, Sb^{3+}, As^{3+}, Tin, Iron, Al^{3+}, Cr^{3+}, Co^{2+}, Ni^{2+}, Zn^{2+}, Mn^{2+}, Ba^{2+}, Sr^{2+}, Ca^{2+}, Mg^{2+}, Na^+, K^+ and NH_4^+. A given test material may contain one or more of these 24 ions. Now, if we have 24 separate specific tests for each of these ions and each such test is applicable to an individual ion even in presence of others, then we can apply them one by one and can thus recognise different basic radicals present in the given mixture. But it is not possible to have such tests which will be applicable only to individual ions and will not be interferred by other ions. Hence, for the sake of convenience and rapid analysis, the above mentioned ions have been divided into the following groups :

Group	Cations	Group Reagent
I	Ag^+, Pb^{2+}, Hg_2^{2+}	Dilute HCl
II (A)	Hg^{2+}, (Pb^{2+}), Bi^{3+}, Cu^{2+}, Cd^{2+}	H_2S in dilute HCl medium
II (B)	Sb^{3+}, As^{3+}, tin	
III	Al^{3+}, Fe^{3+}, (Fe^{2+}), Cr^{3+}	NH_4OH in presence of NH_4Cl
IV	Co^{2+}, Ni^{2+}, Zn^{2+}, Mn^{2+}	H_2S in presence of NH_4OH
V	Ba^{2+}, Sr^{2+}, Ca^{2+}	$(NH_4)_2CO_3$
VI	Mg^{2+}, Na^+, K^+, NH_4^+	

This division is based on the principle of solubility product which has already been discussed in section 4·6. If we consider the chlorides of different metals placed in these six groups it will be found that the values of solubility product of AgCl, $PbCl_2$ and Hg_2Cl_2, i.e., chlorides of metals kept in the first group, are extremely small as compared to those for the chlorides of remaining metals. In other words, the solubility of AgCl, $PbCl_2$ and Hg_2Cl_2 is very small hence, if we add dilute HCl to a solution containing these metal ions, only chlorides of Ag, Pb and Hg (I) will be precipitated and can be separated from other metal ions by filtration. It should be noted that the solubility product values of remaining metal chlorides are quite high therefore, on adding dilute HCl their ionic products will not be able to exceed their solubility products, so other metal chlorides will not be precipitated and these will be collected in the filtrate.

Consider a solution which contains 24 basic radicals already mentioned. On adding dilute HCl, a white ppt containing AgCl, $PbCl_2$ and Hg_2Cl_2 will be obtained. The precipitate is filtered and further examined, the filtrate contains the remaining radicals.

After eliminating Ag^+, Pb^{2+} and Hg_2^{2+} ions we have to examine the filtrate from Gr. I for only 21 basic radicals. If we consider the values of solubility product for metal sulphides it is found that these are very small for HgS, PbS, Bi_2S_3, CuS, CdS, As_2S_3, Sb_2S_3 and tin sulphides. Hence, if H_2S gas is passed through the filtrate from Gr. I only these sulphides will be precipitated. But the solubility product values of CoS, NiS, ZnS and MnS are not very high so these will also be precipitated on passing H_2S making the further examination of the sulphides very complicated. The advantage here is taken of the common ion effect discussed in section 4·5. If the filtrate from Gr. I is made acidic by adding HCl and then H_2S gas is passed, the poor dissociation of H_2S is further decreased due to common ion effect so that the sulphide ion concentration $[S^{2-}]$, in the solution is very small. This decreased $[S^{2-}]$ is sufficient only to precipitate HgS, PbS, As_2S_3, Sb_2S_3. tin, sulphide, Bi_2S_3, CuS and CdS which can be separated by filtration. The $[S^{2-}]$ in acidic medium is so low that ionic products of CoS, NiS, ZnS and MnS never exceed their solubility products hence, they are not precipitated. In this way by passing H_2S gas through acidified filtrate from Gr. I, Hg^{2+}, Pb^{2+}, Bi^{3+}, Cu^{2+}, Cd^{2+}, Sb^{3+}. As^{3+} and tin can be separated leaving only 14 basic radicals in the filtrate from Gr. II. (It will be noted that although Pb^{2+} is kept in Gr. I, it has also been included in Gr. II. The reason for this is that $PbCl_2$ has some solubility in cold water therefore, some of it will come into filtrate from Gr. I and Pb^{2+} will form a precipitate of PbS on passing H_2S. That is why if Pb^{2+} ions are present they will give $PbCl_2$ precipitate in Gr. I and also form PbS in Gr. II).

In Gr. II are precipitated eight sulphides namely HgS, PbS, Bi_2S_3, CuS, CdS, Sb_2S_3, As_2S_3 and tin sulphide ; this is fairly a large number making the subsequent individual identification difficult. Hence Gr. II was divided into two sections Gr. II(A) and Gr. II(B). It was known that HgS, PbS, Bi_2S_3. CuS and CdS do not dissolve in NaOH solution whereas Sb_2S_3, As_2S_3 and tin sulphide are soluble. Thus the precipitate obtained in Gr. II is warmed with NaOH solution and filtered. The precipitate contains Gr. II(A) precipitates,. i.e., HgS, PbS, Bi_2S_3, CuS and CdS whereas the filtrate will contain Sb^{3+}, As^{3+} and tin [Gr. II(B) radicals]. These can be then further analysed for identifying individual ions.

The filtrate from Gr. II may contain as many as 14 basic radicals If solubility product data of remaining metal hydroxides, are examined, it is found that for $Al(OH)_3$, $Cr(OH)_3$ and $Fe(OH)_3$, the solubility product values are very small, i.e., these are highly insoluble. If NH_4OH solution is added to filtrate from Gr. II (after boiling off the dissolved H_2S from the filtrate), Al^{3+}, Cr^{3+} and Fe^{3+} ions will precipitate out in the form of their hydroxides. But the solubility product values of $Zn(OH)_2$, $Mn(OH)_2$, $Co(OH)_2$ are not very high consequently they will also be precipitated. Again, advantage is taken of the principle of common ion-effect. Filtrate from Gr. II is boiled until all the dissolved H_2S gas is driven out, solution is cooled, little HNO_3 is added and it is again boiled (to convert any Fe^{2+} to Fe^{3+} ions). The filtrate is cooled and first NH_4Cl and then NH_4OH solution is added. Due to the common ion, i.e., NH_4^+, the dissociation of NH_4OH is suppressed consequently there is a very small concentration of OH^- which is enough to precipitate only $Al(OH)_3$, $Cr(OH)_3$ and $Fe(OH)_3$ but not $Mn(OH)_2$, $Zn(OH)_2$ etc. By filteration precipitate is separated which is further examined for identifying individual radical.

To the filtrate from Gr. III which can contain 11 basic radicals, little NH_4OH solution is added and H_2S gas is passed. Both H_2S and NH_4OH are weak electrolytes which poorly dissociate as follows :

$$H_2S \rightleftharpoons \boxed{2H^+} + S^{2-} \qquad \ldots(5\cdot1)$$

$$NH_4OH \rightleftharpoons \boxed{OH^-} + NH_4^+ \qquad \ldots(5\cdot2)$$

$$\downarrow$$
water

The H^+ ions from H_2S combine with OH^- ions from NH_4OH to form water and to maintain the equilibrium (5·1), more H_2S must dissociate. Thus the dissociation of H_2S is increased in presence of NH_4OH consequently, the $[S^{2-}]$ in the solution increases. This increased $[S^{2-}]$ is sufficient to precipitate CoS, NiS, ZnS and MnS which could not be precipitated in Gr. II. (Remember, in Gr. II, H_2S was passed in acidic solution so that due to common ion effect the dissociation of H_2S was suppressed resulting in small $[S^{2-}]$ which was not enough to precipitate CoS, NiS, ZnS and MnS). Thus in Gr. IV, Co^{2+}, Ni^{2+}, Zn^{2+} and Mn^{2+} ions are separated as their sulphides.

The filtrate from Gr. IV can have only 7 basic radicals. Out of these Ba^{2+}, Sr^{2+} and Ca^{2+} form insoluble carbonates. The filtrate from Gr. IV is boiled to drive out dissolved H_2S gas, then cooled and NH_4OH and $(NH_4)_2CO_3$ are added. This causes precipitation of $BaCO_3$, $SrCO_3$ and $CaCO_3$ which can be filtered out.

The filtrate from Gr. V can contain Na^+, K^+, NH_4^+ and Mg^{2+}. There is no group reagent for this Group called the sixth group ; these are individually tested.

The purpose of the above discussion is to bring about the fact that the division of basic radicals into different groups is not empirical based on trial and error but is based on sound theoretical considerations making use of principles of solubility product and common ion effect.

5·4. ANALYSIS OF CATIONS OF GR. I

Cations of Gr. I : Ag^+, Pb^{2+}, Hg_2^{2+}

Group reagent : Dilute HCl.

Reaction between these cations and Cl^- ions from HCl can be written as :

$$Ag^+ + Cl^- \longrightarrow AgCl$$
$$Pb^{2+} + 2Cl^- \longrightarrow PbCl_2$$
$$Hg_2^{2+} + 2Cl^- \longrightarrow Hg_2Cl_2$$

[white precipitates]

For example, if nitrates of metals are present, the reactions in the molecular form can be written as :

$$AgNO_3 + HCl \longrightarrow AgCl + HNO_3$$
$$Pb(NO_3)_2 + 2HCl \longrightarrow PbCl_2 + 2HNO_3$$
$$Hg_2(NO_3)_2 + 2HCl \longrightarrow Hg_2Cl_2 + 2HNO_3$$

On adding dilute HCl to a solution (soln) of mixture, if no precipitate is observed, it shows that Gr. I is absent, *i.e.*, Ag^+, Pb^{2+} and Hg_2^{2+} are not present in the given mixture. If white precipitate (ppt) is obtained any one or any two or all the three from Ag^+, Pb^{2+} and Hg_2^{2+} ions may be present. The ppt is boiled with water and filtered.

Lead chloride is soluble in hot water but AgCl and Hg_2Cl_2 do not dissolve. If all the ppt dissolves it means that only Pb^{2+} ions are present and Ag^+ and Hg_2^{2+} ions are absent. If some ppt remains it means that Ag^+ or Hg_2^{2+} or both may also be present. On filtering (step 5·4A), filtrate will contain $PbCl_2$ while the ppt will contain either AgCl or Hg_2Cl_2 or both. The filtrate is divided into three parts and the following tests are performed to confirm the presence of Pb^{2+} ions.

(a) First part, cooled when white crystals of $PbCl_2$ are observed.

(b) Second part + potassium chromate soln when yellow ppt of lead chromate is formed.

$$PbCl_2 + K_2CrO_4 \longrightarrow PbCrO_4 + 2HCl$$
or,
$$Pb^{2+} + CrO_4^{2-} \longrightarrow PbCrO_4 \text{ (yellow ppt)}$$

(c) **Third** part + potassium iodide soln when yellow ppt of lead iodide is formed.

$$PbCl_2 + 2KI \longrightarrow PbI_2 + 2KCl$$
or,
$$Pb^{2+} + 2I^- \longrightarrow PbI_2 \text{ (yellow ppt)}$$

If tests (a), (b) and (c) are positive, it confirms the presence of Pb^{2+} ions in the given mixture.

The remaining precipitate from step 5·4A is shaken with NH_4OH soln and filtered (step 5·4 B). If all the ppt dissolves, Ag^+ ions are present and Hg_2^{2+} ions are absent. But if some ppt remains and turns black on adding NH_4OH, Hg_2^{2+} ions are also present along with Ag^+ ions. The ppt of AgCl dissolves in NH_4OH because Ag^+ ions form complex with ammonia :

$$AgCl + 2NH_4OH \longrightarrow [Ag(NH_3)_2]Cl + 2H_2O$$

or, $$Ag^+ + 2NH_4OH \longrightarrow [Ag(NH_3)_2]^+ + 2H_2O$$

The remaining black ppt (from step 5·4B) is dissolved in aqua-regia.

$$Hg_2Cl_2 + 2NH_4OH \longrightarrow \underset{\text{(black ppt)}}{Hg(NH_2)Cl} + Hg + NH_4Cl + 2H_2O$$

(Mercurous chloride turns black when NH_4OH is poured on it, the blackened ppt dissolves in aqua-regia).

$$\underset{\text{(aqua-regia)}}{3HCl + HNO_3} \longrightarrow NOCl + Cl_2 + 2H_2O$$

$$2Hg(NH_2)Cl + 3Cl_2 \longrightarrow 2HgCl_2 + 4HCl + N_2$$

The solution is divided into two parts :

(a) First part + stannous chloride soln when white ppt is obtained.

$$2HgCl_2 + SnCl_2 \longrightarrow \underset{\text{(white ppt)}}{Hg_2Cl_2} + SnCl_4$$

(b) To the second part, a copper foil is added. After sometime a shining deposit of mercury on the copper foil is observed.

5·5. ANALYSIS OF CATIONS OF GR. II

Cations of Gr. II : Hg^{2+}, (Pb^{2+}), Bi^{3+}, Cu^{2+}, Cd^{2+} (Gr. II A.) Sb^{3+}, As^{3+}, tin (Gr. II B)

Group reagent : H_2S gas in presence of dilute (dil) HCl.

Reaction between cations of Gr. II and sulphide ions from H_2S can be written as :

$$Hg^{2+} + S^{2-} \longrightarrow HgS \text{ (mercuric sulphide ; black ppt)}$$

$$Pb^{2+} + S^{2-} \longrightarrow PbS \text{ (lead sulphide ; black ppt)}$$

$$2Bi^{3+} + 3S^{2-} \longrightarrow Bi_2S_3 \text{ (bismuth sulphide ; brownish black ppt)}$$

$$Cu^{2+} + S^{2-} \longrightarrow CuS \text{ (copper sulphide ; black ppt)}$$

$$Cd^{2+} + S^{2-} \longrightarrow CdS \text{ (cadmium sulphide ; yellow ppt)}$$

$$2Sb^{3+} + 3S^{2-} \longrightarrow Sb_2S_3 \text{ (antimony sulphide ; orange ppt)}$$

$$2As^{3+} + 3S^{2-} \longrightarrow As_2S_3 \text{ (arsenic sulphide ; yellow ppt)}$$

$$Sn^{2+} + S^{2-} \longrightarrow SnS \text{ (stannous sulphide ; brown ppt)}$$

$$Sn^{4+} + 2S^{2-} \longrightarrow SnS_2 \text{ (stannic sulphide ; yellowish brown ppt)}$$

A small portion of the filtrate from Gr. I is taken, acidified with dil HCl, warmed and H_2S gas is passed through it. If no ppt is observed it means that Gr. II radicals are absent and so one can proceed for the detection of Gr. III radicals in the remaining portion of the filtrate. If a ppt is obtained it shows the presence of one or more cations of Gr. II. [If H_2S gas is passed through warm solution, bigger particles of metal sulphides are formed which cannot pass through filter paper. On passing H_2S through cold solution very fine particles of ppt will be formed which can pass through the pores of an ordinary filter paper into the filtrate and will then interfere in the examination of radicals of later groups]. On filtering (step 5·5 A), the second group sulphides remain on the filter paper while radicals of subsequent groups come down in the filtrate. The filtrate is diluted, warmed and H_2S is again passed through it. If a ppt appears, it is filtered and H_2S is again passed through the filtrate. This process is repeated until there is no appearance of ppt. The purpose of this process is to completely precipitate out all the second group cations in the form of their sulphides. If the precipitation is incomplete, Gr. II cations will pass into the filtrate and will then interfere with the detection of radicals of higher group. In general a large excess of a group reagent should be added so that the reacting cations are completely precipitated and thus totally separated from radicals of higher group. It should be noted that H_2S gas is passed through diluted filtrate. The reason for diluting the filtrate is that if acid (HCl) concentration in the filtrate is high, it will suppress the dissociation of H_2S due to common ion effect. This decreased $[S^{2-}]$ will not be sufficient to completely precipitate out cadmium sulphide because its solubility product value is relatively higher ($S_{CdS}=3·6\times10^{-29}$) as compared to those of sulphides of other cations of Gr. II (for example $S_{HgS}=4\times10^{-53}$). When filtrate is diluted, the concentration of acid also decreases hence, suppression of dissociation of H_2S is to a smaller extent. Under these conditions the $[S^{2-}]$ is sufficient to completely precipitate out cadmium sulphide. (Remember that if too much HCl is present CdS will not be precipitated at all and we will miss the cadmium ion).

5·5·1.   Analysis of Cations of Gr. II.A

The ppt obtained from step 5·5 A is shaken with yellow ammonium sulphide (or warmed with sodium hydroxide solution) and filtered (step 5·5 B). The ppt contains sulphides of metals of Gr. II.A while Gr. II.B radicals are collected in the filtrate. The ppt is washed with warm water and then boiled with 33% nitric acid solution and filtered (step 5·5 C), the ppt contains HgS while Pb^{2+}, Cu^{2+}, Bi^{3+} and Cd^{2+} ions pass into filtrate. The black ppt of HgS is dissolved in aqua-regia and the resultant solution divided into two parts :

(a) First part+$SnCl_2$ soln—a white ppt is observed.

(b) Second part+a copper piece—a shining deposit of mercury on copper is observed.

To a small portion of the filtrate obtained in step 5·5°C, dilute H_2SO_4 and alcohol is added, if a white ppt is not seen then it means that lead is absent, if white ppt is obtained then dilute H_2SO_4 and alcohol is added to the entire filtrate when all the lead is precipitated as $PbSO_4$. ($PbSO_4$ dissolves in a concentrated soln of ammonium acetate. The resultant soln.+acetic acid+potassium chromate soln gives a yellow ppt of $PbCrO_4$). On filtering (step 5·5°D), the ppt contains $PbSO_4$ and filtrate contains Bi^{3+}, Cu^{2+} and Cd^{2+} ions. This filtrate is boiled to drive out alcohol and an excess of NH_4OH is added. (NH_4OH solution is gradually added. After each addition, soln is shaken and smelt. When a clear smell of NH_3 is given out, it means that the soln is alkaline).

If Bi^{3+} is present, it will be precipitated as $Bi(OH)_3$ which can be separated by filtration (step 5·5°E). The ppt of $Bi(OH)_3$ is dissolved in a small quantity of concentrated HCl.

$$Bi(OH)_3 + 3HCl \longrightarrow BiCl_3 + 3H_2O$$

A few drops of this soln are added to a large volume of water which turns milky due to formation of bismuth oxychloride.

$$BiCl_3 + H_2O \longrightarrow BiOCl + 2HCl$$

If the filtrate from step 5·5°E is colourless Cu^{2+} will be absent but if the filtrate is blue in colour Cu^{2+} or Cu^{2+} and—Cd^{2+} both may be present. This filtrate is divided into two parts.

(a) First part+acetic acid soln gradually added until the blue colour disappears+potassium ferrocyanide soln—a brown ppt shows presence of Cu^{2+}.

(b) Second part+excess of concentrated HCl and pass H_2S gas—a black ppt of CuS is obtained which is filtered. Filtrate is diluted and on passing H_2S, a yellow ppt of CdS is obtained. (Note that in presence of large quantity of HCl, due to common ion effect, a very small $[S^{2-}]$ is available which can precipitate out only CuS which has a small value for solubility product, the Cd^{2+} ions goes to the filtrate. On diluting the filtrate, acid concentration decreases, common ion effect is less so $[S^{2-}]$ increases and now it is sufficient to precipitate out CdS which has a higher value for solubility product. This is the reason why in presence of higher acid concentration only CuS is observed and yellow ppt of CdS is seen only when filtrate is diluted and H_2S passed through it).

5·5·2. Analysis of Cations of Gr. II.B.

The filtrate from step 5·5°B which contains As^{3+}, Sb^{3+} and tin is acidified with dilute HCl and filtered. The filtrate is rejected and the ppt which contains sulphides of arsenic, antimony and tin is boiled with concentrated HCl and filtered (step 5'5°F). Arsenic sulphide being insoluble remains on the filter paper whereas antimony and tin pass into filtrate. The yellow ppt of As_2S_3 is dissolved in hot concentrated HNO_3 and ammonium molybdate soln is added, a yellow ppt indicates the presence of As^{3+}.

The filtrate from step 5'5°F is boiled to drive out H_2S, it is then cooled and made alkaline with NH_4OH. To this soln, 5 g oxalic acid is added, it is boiled and H_2S gas is passed through it. On filtering Sb_2S_3 is found as orange coloured ppt and tin goes to the filtrate. The filtrate is made first alkaline by adding NH_4OH and then just acidic with acetic acid. The solution is boiled and H_2S gas is passed through it, a brownish yellow ppt shows the presence of tin. It should be noted that tin ions form a complex with oxalic acid. This is the reason that on passing H_2S, although Sb^{3+} ions form an orange ppt of Sb_2S_3 but because tin ions are bound in the complex, they cannot form a ppt of tin sulphide. The Sb_2S_3 can be separated by filtration. The soluble complex present in the filtrate is decomposed by the addition of NH_4OH so that tin ions now become free and give a yellowish brown ppt of tin sulphide on passing H_2S.

5'6. ANALYSIS OF CATIONS OF GR. III

Cations of Gr. III : Fe^{3+}, Al^{3+}, Cr^{3+}.

Group reagent : NH_4OH in presence of NH_4Cl.

Reaction between cations of Gr. III and OH^- ions from NH_4OH can be written as :

$$Fe^{3+} + 3OH^- \longrightarrow Fe(OH)_3 \text{ (reddish brown ppt)}$$
$$Al^{3+} + 3OH^- \longrightarrow Al(OH)_3 \text{ (gelatinous white ppt)}$$
$$Cr^{3+} + 3OH^- \longrightarrow Cr(OH)_3 \text{ (green ppt)}$$

Filtrate from Gr. II, obtained in step 5'5°A, is boiled to completely remove the dissolved H_2S gas from it. About 1 ml of concentrated HNO_3 is added and it is again boiled. The purpose of addition of HNO_3 is to oxidise Fe^{2+} ions to Fe^{3+} because in Gr. III we want to precipitate iron as $Fe(OH)_3$ and not as $Fe(OH)_2$. The solubility product of $Fe(OH)_3$ is smaller than that of $Fe(OH)_2$ so iron can be completely separated if it is precipitated in the form of $Fe(OH)_3$. (At this stage if phosphate is present it must be removed before testing for Gr. III radicals). After boiling with HNO_3, the soln is cooled and, first NH_4Cl and then NH_4OH is added and filtered (step 5'6°A). The ppt contains hydroxides of iron, aluminium and chromium. Due to the presence of common ion, NH_4^+, the dissociation of NH_4OH is suppressed resulting in a small (OH^-). The values of solubility product for $Fe(OH)_3$, $Al(OH)_3$ and

$Cr(OH)_3$ are small hence, even the decreased $[OH^-]$ is enough to precipitate them completely. But the solubility product values of hydroxides of higher group metals (and also that of $Fe(OH)_2$) are higher so the decreased $[OH^-]$ is not sufficient to precipitate them hence they pass into solution. Thus, Fe^{3+}, Al^{3+} and Cr^{3+} can be separated from Ni^{2+}, Co^{2+}, Zn^{2+}, Mn^{2+}, Ba^{2+}, Sr^{2+}, Ca^{2+}, Mg^{2+}, K^+, Na^+ and NH_4^+. The ppt obtained in step $5\cdot6°A$ is washed and boiled with NaOH and bromine water and filtered (step $5\cdot6°B$). The ppt is of $Fe(OH)_3$ which is dissolved in dilute HCl and soln divided into two parts :

(a) First part $+ K_4Fe(CN)_6$ soln—deep blue colour is given

$$4FeCl_3 + 3K_4Fe(CN)_6 \longrightarrow Fe_4[Fe(CN)_6]_3 + 12 \text{ KCl}$$
$$\downarrow$$
ferric ferrocyanide
or prussian blue

(b) Second part $+$ KCNS soln—a red colour is observed.

$$FeCl_3 + 3KCNS \longrightarrow [Fe(CNS)]^{2+} + 2CNS^- + 3KCl$$
$$\downarrow$$
red colour complex

If the above tests are given, the presence of iron is confirmed.

The filtrate from step $5\cdot6°B$ contains soluble chromate and aluminate. This filtrate is boiled to drive out excess of bromine and is divided into two parts :

(a) First part $+$ Acetic acid $+$ lead acetate solution a yellow ppt shows presence of chromium.

$$Na_2CrO_4 + Pb(CH_3COO)_2 \longrightarrow \underset{\text{yellow ppt}}{PbCrO_4} + 2CH_3COONa$$

or, $$CrO_4^{2-} + Pb^{2+} \longrightarrow PbCrO_4.$$

(b) Second part $+$ NH_4Cl and boil—a white ppt of $Al(OH)_3$ is obtained in which the presence of aluminium is confirmed by charcoal cavity test.

5·7. ANALYSIS OF CATIONS OF GR. IV

Cations of Gr. IV : Ni^{2+}, Co^{2+}, Mn^{2+}, Zn^{2+}.

Group reagent : H_2S gas in presence of NH_4OH.

Reactions between cations of Gr. IV and S^{2-} ions from H_2S can be written as :

$$Ni^{2+} + S^{2-} \longrightarrow NiS \text{ (black ppt)}$$
$$Co^{2+} + S^{2-} \longrightarrow CoS \text{ (black ppt)}$$
$$Mn^{2+} + S^{2-} \longrightarrow MnS \text{ (light brown ppt)}$$
$$Zn^{2+} + S^{2-} \longrightarrow ZnS \text{ (dirty white ppt)}$$

To the filtrate from step 5·6°A, NH₄OH is added, H₂S gas is passed and filtered (step 5·7°A). The values of solubility product of NiS, CoS, MnS and ZnS are higher hence they could not be precipitated in Gr. II when the $[S^{2-}]$ was small. In presence of NH₄OH, the dissociation of H₂S is increased giving high concentration of S^{2-} ions which is enough to precipitate NiS, CoS, MnS and ZnS. The filtrate contains Ba^{2+}, Sr^{2+}, Ca^{2+}, Mg^{2+}, Na^+, K^+ and NH₄⁺ ions. The ppt obtained from step 5·7°A is shaken with dilute HCl and filtered (step 5·7°B). The ppts of NiS and CoS are insoluble hence, remain on the filter paper whereas Zn^{2+} and Mn^{2+} ions go into the filtrate. The separation of cobalt and nickel is based on the fact that cobalt forms a complex with sodium bicarbonate while nickel does not. The ppt obtained from step 5·7°B is dissolved in aqua regia, cooled and a strong solution of sodium bicarbonate is added when cobalt forms a stable soluble complex but nickel does not form any complex. Now, bromine water is added, if soln has a green colour—it shows the presence of cobalt. The green solution is then boiled, if a black ppt appears both cobalt and nickel are present. (Black ppt containing nickel can be separated by filtration). If the green soln does not turn black on heating, only cobalt is present and nickel is absent. If there is no green colour in cold but a black ppt appears on boiling, nickel is present but cobalt is absent. After separation, nickel and cobalt can be tested by borax bead test ; cobalt gives a blue bead while nickel forms a brown bead. Nickel, even in extremely small amounts, forms a red ppt with dimethylglyoxime.

The filtrate from step 5·7°B, which contains Zn^{2+} and Mn^{2+} ions, is boiled to drive out the dissolved H₂S from it. (If we want to separate two ions, a simple way is to select a reagent which forms an insoluble product with one ion and a soluble product with the other. On filtration, the ion giving insoluble product remains on the filter paper in the form of a ppt while the other ion forming a soluble product goes into the filtrate). To the filtrate containing Zn^{2+} and Mn^{2+} ions, an excess of NaOH soln is added when insoluble manganese hydroxide and soluble sodium zincate is formed.

$$MnCl_2 + 2NaOH \longrightarrow \underset{\text{(insoluble)}}{Mn(OH)_2} + 2NaCl$$

$$ZnCl_2 + 2NaOH \longrightarrow Zn(OH)_2 + 2NaCl$$

$$Zn(OH)_2 + 2NaOH \longrightarrow \underset{\text{(soluble)}}{Zn(ONa)_2} + 2H_2O$$

The ppt of Mn(OH)₂ is separated by filtration (step 5·7°C) and is fused with KNO₃ and Na₂CO₃—formation of a green mass shows the presence of manganese. Through the filtrate obtained from step 5·7°C, H₂S gas is passed when a white ppt of ZnS is obtained which indicates the presence of zinc. By applying charcoal cavity test to this ppt with cobalt nitrate—a bright green deposit is observed.

5·8. ANALYSIS OF CATIONS OF GR. V

Cations of Gr. V : Ba^{2+}, Sr^{2+}, Ca^{2+}.

Group reagent : $(NH_4)_2CO_3$ in presence of NH_4OH.

Reaction between cations of Gr. V and CO_3^{2-} ions from $(NH_4)_2CO_3$ can be written as :

$$Ba^{2+} + CO_3^{2-} \longrightarrow BaCO_3 \text{ (white ppt)}$$
$$Sr^{2+} + CO_3^{2-} \longrightarrow SrCO_3 \text{ (white ppt)}$$
$$Ca^{2+} + CO_3^{2-} \longrightarrow CaCO_3 \text{ (white ppt)}$$

The filtrate from Gr. IV obtained from the step 5·7°A is boiled to completely remove H_2S and is concentrated to a smaller volume. (While testing for different radicals from Gr. I to Gr. IV, several reagents are added hence the solution of the given mixture becomes very dilute so that the concentrations of Ba^{2+}, Sr^{2+}, Ca^{2+} and Mg^{2+} become very small. On adding the group reagent these ions form a very small amount of ppt which is not sufficient for performing further tests. This is the reason why the filtrate from Gr. IV is boiled for sometime so that its volume is reduced to about 25-30 ml). After cooling, ammonium hydroxide and then a slight excess of ammonium carbonate is added and filtered (step 5·8°A). The values of solubility product of carbonates of barium, strontium and calcium are smaller than that of magnesium carbonate hence, $BaCO_3$, $SrCO_3$ and $CaCO_3$ are precipitated but Mg^{2+} ions pass into the filtrate. (The medium is alkaline, if it is acidic the carbonates of barium, strontium and calcium will dissolve that is why these are precipitated in presence of NH_4OH).

The ppt obtained from step 5·8°A is dissolved in dilute acetic acid and to the resultant soln (Soln A), an excess of potassium chromate solution is added (when all the barium is precipitated as barium chromate) and filtered (step 5·8°B).

$$Ba^{2+} + CrO_4^{2-} \longrightarrow BaCrO_4$$
$$\text{(yellow ppt)}$$

The filtrate from step 5·8°B contains Sr^{2+} and Ca^{2+} ions. To this filtrate, an excess of ammonium sulphate soln is added (when all the strontium is precipitated as strontium sulphate) and filtered (step 5·8°C).

$$Sr^{2+} + SO_4^{2-} \longrightarrow SrSO_4$$
$$\text{(white ppt)}$$

The filtrate from step 5·8°C contains Ca^{2+} ions. Ammonium oxalate soln is added to this filtrate when a white ppt of calcium oxalate is formed.

$$Ca^{2+} + C_2O_4^{2-} \rightarrow CaC_2O_4$$
white ppt

The above paragraph describes a scheme for the separation of Ba^{2+}, Sr^{2+} and Ca^{2+} when all of them are present in a mixture. This separation scheme is based on the following consideration.

The first point to be noted is that the ppt of barium, strontium and calcium carbonate are dissolved in dilute acetic acid and not in dilute HCl. If dilute HCl is used for dissolving these carbonates, there will be difficulty in testing Ba^{2+} and Ca^{2+} ions because $BaCrO_4$ and CaC_2O_4 are soluble in HCl hence, they will not be precipitated. This is the reason why acetic acid is used for dissolving carbonates of metals of Gr. V.

Another point to be noted is the order in which Ba^{2+}, Sr^{2+} and Ca^{2+} ions are tested. It has already been mentioned that if two or more ions present in a mixture are to be separated, such a reagent should be added which will form an insoluble product with one of the ions and the others must remain in the soln so that they can be separated by filtration. The carbonates of barium, strontium and calcium are dissolved in dilute acetic acid and to the soln first we add K_2CrO_4 soln. Potassium chromate reagent is selected because it forms insoluble $BaCrO_4$ with Ba^{2+} ions while Sr^{2+} and Ca^{2+} ions remain in soln hence, separated by filtration. (Note that the solubility product value for barium chromate is smaller than those for strontium and calcium chromates hence, only barium chromate is precipitated). The filtrate containing Sr^{2+} and Ca^{2+} is treated with $(NH_4)_2SO_4$ soln ; the reason for selecting this reagent is that it forms insoluble $SrSO_4$ and because $CaSO_4$ has a high value for solubility product hence, Ca^{2+} ions pass into the filtrate. This filtrate has Ca^{2+} ion which can be tested by adding $(NH_4)_2C_2O_4$ soln when a white ppt of CaC_2O_4 is obtained.

It is necessary that barium should be tested first then strontium and then calcium. If this order is changed it will not be possible to separate Ba^{2+}, Sr^2 and Ca^{2+} ions. For example, suppose to a soln containing Ba^{2+}, Sr^{2+} and Ca^{2+} ions, $(NH_4)_2SO_4$ is added first in place of K_2CrO_4, then $BaSO_4$ and $SrSO_4$ both will be precipitated hence the separation of Ba^{2+} and Sr^{2+} will not be possible. If $(NH_4)_2C_2O_4$ soln is added first, then Sr^{2+} and Ca^{2+} will be precipitated and their separation will not be possible. It is, therefore, necessary that K_2CrO_4 should be added first so that only Ba^{2+} will be precipitated and not Sr^{2+} and Ca^{2+} ions. Then, to the filtrate containing Sr^{2+} and Ca^{2+}, $(NH_4)_2SO_4$ soln should be added when only Sr^{2+} is precipitated and not Ca^{2+} ions. Thus, these three ions can be successfully separated.

5·9. ANALYSIS OF CATIONS OF GR. VI

To the filtrate from Gr. V obtained in step 5·8°A, ammonium chloride, ammonium hydroxide and sodium phosphate soln is added when a white ppt of magnesium ammonium phosphate is obtained.

$$MgCl_2 + Na_2HPO_4 + NH_4OH \longrightarrow Mg(NH_4)PO_4 + 2NaCl + H_2O$$

Although sodium, potassium and ammonium are kept in Gr. VI, they are not tested in the filtrate from Gr. V but are tested in the original mixture. The reason is that while testing for cations of Gr. I to Gr. V, reagents containing NH_4^+ and Na^+ ions (NH_4Cl, NH_4OH, NaOH etc.) have already been added.

Test for K^+

In neutral or acetic acid soln, potassium ions form a yellow crystalline ppt with sodium cobaltinitrite. The reagent cannot be used in alkaline or strongly acidic medium because then the complex is decomposed. Further, NH_4^+ ions interfere with this test as they also form a similar complex.

Potassium can also be detected by flame test. It gives a violet flame. If sodium is also present its yellow flame masks the violet colour. Hence, then the flame should be seen through a cobalt glass when yellow colour due to sodium is cut off.

Test for Na^+

Zinc uranyl acetate in neutral or acetic acid soln forms a greenish yellow ppt with sodium ions. Sodium can also be recognised by its golden yellow flame which is not visible when viewed through cobalt glass.

Test for NH_4^+

For testing NH_4^+ ions, the original mixture is heated with sodium hydroxide soln when smell of ammonia gas shows the presence of ammonium radical in the mixture. Another test for NH_4^+ ions is by using Nessler's reagent. This reagent is obtained by adding excess of KI to $HgCl_2$ soln until a colourless soln is obtained. A mixture of this soln and KOH gives a yellowish brown ppt or colour with NH_4^+ ions.

5·10. INTERFERING RADICALS

There are certain acid radicals, such as phosphate, oxalate, fluoride and—borate, which interfere with the systematic group separation of different cations : these are called *interfering radicals*. These do not cause any disturbance so long as the medium is acidic, *i.e.*, up to Gr. II but as soon as the medium is made alkaline in Gr. III, their interference begins. Due to the presence of these radicals, we not only get hydroxides of Gr. III metals but also oxalates, phosphates and fluorides of members of higher group metals such as Zn, Ca, Mg etc. (It should be noted that these are soluble in acidic medium hence interfering radicals do not present any problem up to Gr. II when the medium is acidic).

5'10'1. Detection of Interfering Radicals

Oxalate. A small amount of mixture is heated with concentrated H_2SO_4 when CO gas is evolved which burns with blue flame.

Borate. A small amount of mixture is heated with concentrated H_2SO_4 and little of C_2H_5OH. A volatile compound ethyl borate is formed which burns with a green flame. Presence of copper salt interferes with this test.

Fluoride. A small amount of mixture is taken in a dry test tube and heated with a little SiO_2 and a few drops of concentrated H_2SO_4. A drop of water in a wire loop is taken inside the tube. The water in the drop becomes turbid due to the formation of silicic acid.

Phosphate. A small amount of mixture is heated with nitric acid and ammonium molybdate soln when a yellow ppt is formed. The presence of arsenic interferes with this test.

5'10'2. Removal of Interfering Radicals

It has been seen in 5'10, that if borate, fluoride, phosphate or oxalate radical is present in the mixture, it interferes with the normal procedure of detection of the basic radicals after Gr. II. Even if Gr. III radicals are absent, on adding NH_4OH, phosphates, borates, fluorides and oxalates of Gr. IV and V metals and of magnesium will be precipitated causing confusion. (Note that these are soluble in acid hence were not precipitated up to Gr. II when the medium was acidic). It is therefore obvious that the interfering radicals must be removed from test soln after Gr. II.

The filtrate from Gr. II is boiled until the dissolved H_2S is completely driven out. A few drops of nitric acid are then added and soln again boiled to convert Fe^{2+} ions, which might be present, into Fe^{3+} ions. After cooling, NH_4Cl and NH_4OH are added when hydroxides of only Gr. III metals are precipitated if no interfering radical is present. If an interfering radical is present, the metals of higher group will also be precipitated along with Gr. III metals, and steps will have to be taken to remove the interfering radicals present.

Removal of fluoride and borate. The ppt obtained in Gr. III is taken in a procelain dish, about 2 ml of concentrated HCl is added and the mixture evaporated to dryness. Again 2 ml of concentrated HCl is added and the process repeated. By doing this three or four times, all the borate and fluoride is decomposed leaving behind the metal. The ppt is finally dissolved in dilute HCl, NH_4Cl and an excess of NH_4OH are then added and if ppt is obtained it is tested for Fe^{3+}, Al^{3+} and Cr^{3+}. The filtrate is mixed with the original filtrate obtained from Gr. II.

Removal of oxalate. The ppt obtained in Gr. III is taken on a procelain piece and ignited for about 20 min when the oxalate is decomposed to carbonate or oxide. The ignited mass is dissolved in dilute HCl. To the resultant soln, NH_4Cl and NH_4OH are added. The ppt obtained is examined for Gr. III radicals while the filtrate is mixed with the filtrate obtained after Gr. II.

Removal of phosphate. The filtrate from Gr. II is boiled to remove the dissolved H_2S, little HNO_3 is added and soln again boiled to convert any Fe^{2+} ions which might be present into Fe^{3+} ions. The soln is cooled and to a small portion of it potassium ferrocyanide soln is added, if iron is present a deep blue ppt is observed. To the rest of the soln, NH_4Cl and then an excess of NH_4OH is added. The ppt thus obtained contains hydroxides and phosphates of the metals of Gr. III along with phosphates of metals of higher groups. To this ppt sodium acetate soln and an excess of acetic acid is added. If the whole ppt dissolves, Gr. III radicals are absent. If a portion of ppt remains undissolved it is filtered out and tested for iron, aluminium and chromium. The filtrate is collected and from it phosphate is removed by the following procedure. (Note that in the presence of acetate-acetic acid buffer, only phosphates of iron, aluminium and chromium are precipitated whereas the phosphates of metals of higher group remain in soln and are collected in the filtrate from which phosphate is removed).

To the filtrate, first sodium acetate and then neutral ferric chloride soln is gradually added dropwise with constant shaking tlll the soln becomes raddish brown. The soln is then boiled for 5 min and filtered. The ppt is rejected. To the filtrate an excess of NH_4OH is added when the excess of Fe^{3+} ions are precipitated and can be filtered out. The filtrate contains cations of Gr. IV, V and VI free from phosphate. (Note that ferric phosphate is insoluble in acetic acid-acetate buffer medium. Hence, on adding neutral $FeCl_3$, all the phosphate is precipitated in the form of ferric phosphate and can be filtered out. Phosphates of higher group metals are soluble hence are not precipitated in the buffered medium and thus cations of higher group free from phosphate ions are collected in the filtrate).

5'11. DETECTION OF ACID RADICALS

These radicals are negetively charged hence they are also known as anions. There is no generally accepted analytical classification of anions, however, for the sake of convenience the anions can also be divided into groups. The acid radicals include carbonate, sulphite, sulphide, nitrite, chloride, bromide, iodide, sulphate, thiosulphate, nitrate, phosphate, oxalate, fluoride, borate, acetate, thiocyanate, ferrocyanide, ferricyanide, arsenate, arsenite, etc. We already know the chemical tests used to identify these radicals hence these will not be discussed here. However, we shall consider some analysis schemes for analysing certain groups of anions in order to understand how chemical reactions are utilized to detect these anions in presence of each other.

5'11'1. Preparation of Sodium Carbonate Extract

About 1 g of the given mixture is heated with about 5 g of sodium carbonate and 50 ml of distilled water for about 15 min and filtered. The filtrate is called sodium carbonate extract which is used for testing acid radicals.

5'11'2. Carbonate and Sulphite Present Together

A mixture containing both CO_3^{2-} and SO_3^{2-}, on treatment with dilute HCl produces CO_2 and SO_2 gases. We can smell SO_2 in presence of CO_2. But the lime water test for CO_2 will fail in presence of SO_2 because SO_2 can also turn lime water milky. It is therefore necessary to remove SO_2 in such a manner that CO_2 remains unaffected. To achieve this, the given mixture is heated with $K_2Cr_2O_7$ and dilute H_2SO_4 in a test tube ; SO_2 evolved reacts with acidic $K_2Cr_2O_7$ whereas CO_2 does not. Hence now only CO_2 will come out of the test tube which can be tested with lime water.

5'11'3. Sulphide and Sulphite Present Together

A mixture containing S^{2-} and SO_3^{2-} on treatment with dilute HCl will produce H_2S and SO_2 ; these cannot be recognised by smell in presence of each other. Hence, the following tests are performed.

(a) To a small amount of sodium carbonate extract, NH_4OH and then a fresh soln of sodium nitroprusside is added, a violet colour indicates sulphide. The presence of SO_3^{2-}, SO_4^{2-} and $S_2O_3^{2-}$ ions do not interfere with this test.

(b) To another small portion of sodium carbonate extract, acetic acid is added till it is acidic and then $BaCl_2$ soln is added, a white ppt soluble in dil HCl shows the presence of SO_3^{2-} ion. (It should be noted that such reactions are searched that in one case only one component will react while the other would not In a second test the second component will undergo change while the first will remain unaffected).

5'11'4. Carbonate and Oxalate Present Together

On adding dilute HCl to a mixture containing CO_3^{2-} and $C_2O_4^{2-}$, oxalate remains unaffected but CO_3^{2-} decomposes to give CO_2 which can be tested with lime water. Thus carbonate can be tested in the presence of oxalate. In order to test for oxalate, the mixture is heated with concentrated H_2SO_4 when oxalate decomposes to give CO gas. Normally oxalate is recognised by the fact that CO burns with blue flame. But when carbonate is present CO_2 is also produced and blue flame of burning CO is not observed. Under such condition the following test can be used.

A small amount of mixture is heated with an excess of dil H_2SO_4 till all the carbonate is decomposed and evolution of CO_2 stops. Then a small quantity of MnO_2 is added when again CO_2 starts coming out. Manganese dioxide oxidises oxalate in presence of acid and the product of oxidation is CO_2. This is why there is evolution of CO_2 on adding MnO_2.

5'11'5. Sulphate, Sulphite and Sulphide Present Together

Sodium carbonate extract of the mixture is prepared, acidified with dilute HCl and $BaCl_2$ soln is added to it, a while ppt (of $BaSO_4$) shows the presence of SO_4^{2-} ions. The ppt is filtered out and to the filtrate bromine water is added and it is boiled, a white ppt (of $BaSO_4$) shows the presence of SO_3^{2-} ions. The ppt is filtered out and to the filtrate a few drops of con. HNO_3 are added and it is boiled, a white ppt shows the presence of S^{2-} ions.

The sodium carbonate extract contains SO_4^{2-}, SO_3^{2-} and S^{2-} ions. On adding $BaCl_2$ soln to the acidified extract SO_4^{2-} ions form a white ppt of $BaSO_4$ which is insoluble in acids. Barium sulphite and barium sulphide are soluble in acidic medium and hence are not precipitated. On filtering, the filtrate contains SO_3^{2-} and S^{2-} ions. When the filtrate is boiled with bromine water, SO_3^{2-} ions are oxidised to SO_4^{2-} ions hence a white ppt of $BaSO_4$ again appears. Note that S^{2-} ions remain unaffected. After removing $BaSO_4$ by filtration, the filtrate contains only S^{2-} ions which by HNO_3 are oxidised to SO_4^{2-} ions which again form a white ppt of $BaSO_4$. This test illustrates clever use of redox reactions in identifying SO_3^{2-} in presence of S^{2-} ions. The selection of bromine as oxidant is such that it converts SO_3^{2-} to SO_4^{2-} but cannot oxidise S^{2-} ions which in the later stage are oxidised by HNO_3 to SO_4^{2-} ions.

5·11·6.   Chloride, Bromide and Iodide Present Together

Chloride can be detected in presence of bromide and iodide by chromyl chloride test, because Br^- and I^- do not interfere in the test. For recognising Br^- and I^-, the following test can be performed.

A small volume (about 2 ml) of sodium carbonate extract is acidified with dilute HNO_3. A few drops of $CHCl_3$ and chlorine water are then added and soln shaken when $CHCl_3$ layer becomes violet showing the presence of iodide. On adding more chlorine water and shaking $CHCl_3$ layer becomes colourless and then brown showing the presence of bromide.

The extract contains Cl^-, Br^- and I^-. On adding chlorine water I^- ions are oxidised to iodine which dissolves in $CHCl_3$ to give it a violet colour. (Iodide is more easily oxidised than bromide). On adding more chlorine water iodine is further oxidised to a colourless product, i.e., iodic acid. When no iodide ions are left, chlorine water oxidises bromide ions to bromine which dissolves in chloroform to give it a brown colour.

Many other acid radical combinations can also be analysed by using various types of chemical reactions. A few examples given above simply demonstrate how chemical reactions are cleverly chosen so that in one case only one species reacts and the other remains unaffected. In a second test, reaction selected is such that the second species reacts and can be tested while the first remains unchanged.

PART III

CLASSICAL METHODS OF QUANTITATIVE ANALYSIS

6

Methods of Gravimetric Analysis

6`1. GRAVIMETRIC ANALYSIS

Gravimetric, volumetric, radiant energy and electrical methods are the four major techniques of quantitative analysis. Of these the gravimetric technique is the oldest and quite accurate though it is tedious and time-consuming ; the final step (or the measurement step) in this case is weighing hence, the name gravimetric analysis. In this type of quantitative analysis, the constituent to be determined is separated from all other components of the sample in the form of an insoluble ppt by adding a suitable reagent. By filtration and drying, the solvent is also removed leaving only dried ppt of a definite chemical composition which is weighed in the final or the measurement step. From the atomic and formula weight, the weight of the constituent sought is calculated.

A soluble chloride, such as sodium chloride, when treated with a soluble silver salt, such as silver nitrate, gives a white ppt of silver chloride according to the equation :

$$\underset{(58\cdot448)}{NaCl} + \underset{(169\cdot888)}{AgNO_3} \longrightarrow \underset{(84\cdot999)}{NaNO_3} + \underset{(143\cdot337)}{AgCl}$$

The formula weights of the different substances involved are shown in parantheses. The reaction will always take place according to these weights or weights proportional to them. The equation shows that 143·337 parts by weight of AgCl are always produced by 58·448 parts by weight of NaCl when an excess of AgNO₃ is added to NaCl soln.

Example 6(*i*)

A given soln of NaCl on treatment with excess AgNO₃ soln gave a ppt of AgCl which was washed, dried and on weighing was found to be 0·2987 g. Calculate the weight of NaCl in the given soln.

143·337 g of AgCl is produced by 58·448 g of NaCl

$$\therefore \quad 0·2987 \quad ,, \quad ,, \quad \frac{0·2987}{143·337} \times 58·448$$

$$=0·1218 \text{ g of NaCl}$$

Thus, wt. of NaCl=wt. of AgCl$\times \dfrac{\text{Formula wt of NaCl}}{\text{Formula wt of AgCl}}$

In general, wt. of substance sought

$$\text{wt. of ppt} \times \frac{\text{Formula wt. of substance (a), sought}}{\text{Formula wt. of substance (b), weighed}}$$

If we calculate the value of the factor a/b, we can directly calculate the weight of NaCl from known weight of AgCl. The value of such a chemical factor a/b for **AgCl to NaC** conversion is :

$$\frac{a}{b}=\frac{58·448}{143·337}=0·4077.$$

If the weight of AgCl is 0·2987 g, the weight of NaCl in the sample solution will be :

$$0·2987 \times 0·4077 = 0·1218 \text{ g}$$

Example 6(ii)

Calculate the weight of $BaCl_2$ required to produce 0·3000 g of AgCl.

$$\mathbf{BaCl_2} + 2AgNO_3 \longrightarrow 2AgCl + Ba(NO_3)_2$$

$$BaCl_2 \equiv 2AgCl$$

$$(208·27) \quad (2 \times 143·34 = 286·68).$$

Now, 286·68 g AgCl is produced by 208·27 g of $BaCl_2$

$$\therefore \quad 0·3000 \text{ g AgCl is produced by } \frac{0·3000}{286·68} \times 208·27$$

$$=0·2179 \text{ g } BaCl_2$$

6·2. GRAVIMETRIC FACTORS

These are used for simplifying gravimetric calculations. In example 6 (i), we have seen that the factor for conversion of AgCl to NaCl is 0·4077. Hence, if we know the weight of AgCl, by multiplying it with 0·4077, we can easily calculate the weight of NaCl which produced the given weight of AgCl. Similar factors can be calculated for other cases.

Table 6·1   Chemical Factors for some Metals

Metal	Form in which precipitated	Gravimetric factor
Pb	$PbSO_4$	0·6838
Ag	AgCl	0·7526
Hg	HgS	0·8622
Cu	$Cu_2(CNS)_2$	0·5226
Al	Al_2O_3	0·5291
Fe	Fe_2O_3	0·6994
Zn	$Zn(NH_4)PO_4$	0·3665
Ca	$CaC_2O_4.H_2O$	0·2743
Ca	C_2CO_3	0·4004
Ca	CaO	0·7147
Ba	$BaSO_4$	0·5885
Mg	$Mg_2P_2O_7$	0·2185

Example 6(iii)

In a gravimetric method for determining iron the weight of ppt of Fe_2O_3 was found to be 0·3158 g. Calculate the weight of iron in the sample solution.

The chemical factor for the conversion Fe_2O_3 to Fe is 0·6994.

∴   weight of iron will be $= 0·3158 \times 0·6994 = 0·2209$ g.

Example 6(iv)

A sample containing 0·2000 g chloride gave 0·1250 g ppt of AgCl. Calculate the per cent chlorine in the sample.

$$\underset{(35·46)}{Cl^-} \equiv \underset{(143·34)}{AgCl}$$

Chemical factor for the conversion AgCl to Cl^- is calculated

as : $\dfrac{\text{Formula weight of } Cl^-}{\text{Formula weight of AgCl}} = \dfrac{35·46}{143·34} = 0·2474$

Weight of chlorine in 0·1250 g AgCl is

$$0·1250 \times 0·2474 = 0·0309 \text{ g}$$

Now, 0·2000 g sample contains 0·0309 g chlorine

∴   100 g sample contains $\dfrac{100 \times 0·0309}{0·2000} = 15·45$ g.

Thus the per cent chlorine in the given sample of chloride is 15·45%.

6·3. GENERAL PRINCIPLE OF GRAVIMETRIC ANALYSIS

It has already been seen that gravimetric determinations are based on the measurement of weights. Generally two weight determinations are involved ; first being the weight of the sample taken for analysis and second the weight of the pure ppt containing the constituent of the sample that is to be determined. In example 6(iv), we weigh the given chloride sample (0·2000 g) and then the resultant AgCl (0·1250 g). From these two weight measurements we can calculate the amount of chloride or chlorine in a known amount of the given chloride sample.

A gravimetric determination is based on a chemical reaction such as :

$$aA + rR \longrightarrow A_a R_r$$

Here, 'a' molecules of analyte (substance A which is to be analysed) react completely with 'r' molecules of another substance R (called reagent) to produce a highly insoluble substance of formula $A_a R_r$ (called precipitate). This ppt sometime can be weighed as such after drying. For example, silver from a soln of $AgNO_3$ can be precipitated as AgCl which can be weighed after washing and drying because AgCl does not change its composition on heating. Knowing the weight of AgCl, the quantity of silver in a given amount of $AgNO_3$ can be calculated.

Sometimes, on heating the composition of a ppt may change. For example, if a ppt of $Fe(OH)_3$ is dried by heating, its composition will change depending upon temperature and period of heating. The ppt of $Fe(OH)_3$, therefore, cannot be weighed as such after drying. The procedure in this case would be to ignite the ppt of $Fe(OH)_3$ for sufficient period of time so that all the hydroxide is converted into stable Fe_2O_3 of fixed composition.

6·3·1. Requirements of Quantitative Separation

In gravimetric analysis, an element or a definite compound is separated from a weighed portion of the sample material. This is done by converting the element or radical to be determined, into a pure, stable and insoluble compound of definite composition that is suitable for weighing.

Example 6(v)

Gravimetric determination of calcium in a sample containing calcium and magnesium :

A weighed portion of the sample containing calcium and magnesium is dissolved in HCl and ammonium oxalate soln (reagent) is added in a neutral medium when calcium precipitates out as a white ppt of calcium oxalate monohydrate ($CaC_2O_4.H_2O$) leaving

Mg^{2+} ions in the soln. The ppt of calcium oxalate is filtered, washed, dried at 110° for about half an hour and then weighed. From the known weight of calcium oxalate, the quantity of calcium in the given amount of sample can be calculated.

In the above example, the reaction between Ca^{2+} and oxalate ion has been used for the quantitative separation of calcium from magnesium and other components of the sample. In selecting a chemical reaction for quantitative separation the following requirements must be fulfilled.

(*i*) *The desired constituent must be precipitated quantitatively.* In example 6(*v*), on adding $(NH_4)_2C_2O_4$ soln, calcium is virtually completely precipitated as $CaC_2O_4.H_2O$ leaving negligible quantity of calcium in soln. If the reaction is, say only, 95% complete, an error of -5% will be observed because our calculations are based on 100% reaction. (The solubility of the ppt must be negligibly small).

(*ii*) *The ppt must be pure.* The ppt obtained must be pure so that it has a known composition. If the ppt contains other substances they must be removed by washing or heating or by some other means.

(*iii*) *The ppt must be in a suitable physical form.* The particles of the ppt should not be very fine otherwise they will pass through filtering medium. Furthermore, the ppt should not change its composition during the drying process, it must not be hygroscopic or volatile in nature.

The precipitation should be so planned that the above conditions are fulfilled. In such a plan, several factors are to be controlled; these are choice of compound to be precipitated, selection of precipitating reagent, concentration of reagent, use of proper solvent, rate of addition of reagent, pH and temperature of soln etc.

6·4. THE PROCESS OF PRECIPITATION

Precipitation is the most important step in gravimetric analysis. The formation of a ppt involves both a physical process and a chemical process. The physical process consists of two stages, (*a*) formation of nuclei (nucleation) and (*b*) crystal growth; these will be discussed in some detail in the following paragraphs.

6·4·1.   Saturated and Supersaturated Solution

If to a given amount of a solvent at a fixed temperature, we go on gradually adding a solute and stir the solution after each addition, a stage will come when the added solute will not dissolve any more but settle down at the bottom of the container. This solution is known as a *saturated solution*. (If 100 g of solvent is taken the amount in g of solute that has dissolved will be called the solubility of the substance in that particular solvent at given temperature). In a saturated soln, the dissolved substance is in equilibrium with the undissolved substance present at the bottom of the vessel.

Sometimes a soln contains greater amount of dissolved substance as compared to that present in a saturated soln—such a soln is referred to as a *supersaturated soln*. This state of supersaturation is generally unstable and exists only for a short period of time.

6·4·2. Nucleation (Formation of Nuclei)

Theoretically it is possible that in a supersaturated soln ions will join together to form a nucleus—this is known as *spontaneous nucleation*. Also, if a small crystal of the solute or any other substance is added (called seeding the soln), it acts as nucleus for growth of a crystal of the solute—this is called *induced nucleation*. The impurities present in the reagent or walls of the container can also act as sites for growth. Stirring a supersaturated soln also helps the nucleation process. It has been found that the larger the extent of supersaturation, the smaller is the size of the individual particle of the ppt.

6·4·3. Crystal Growth

Once a nucleus is formed, crystal growth on it consists of two steps, the diffusion of ions to the surface of the growing crystal and deposition of these on the crystal surface. The diffusion rate depends on nature of ions, their concentration, rate of stirring, and the temperature of the solution. The rate of deposition depends on concentration, impurities present and nature of the crystal.

6·4·4. Conditions of Precipitation

In gravimetric analysis precipitation is carried out under such experimental conditions that it is rapid and complete moreover, the particles of the ppt are large enough so that they do not pass through filtering medium (filter paper, sintered glass or gooch crucible).

According to von Weimern, the rate of precipitation is proportional to $Q-S/S$; where, Q is the actual concentration of solute, *i.e.*, concentration of solute in supersaturated soln and S is the equilibrium concentration, *i.e.*, concentration of solute in its saturated solution. It should be noted that this equation is applicable only when Q is large as compared to S. It was shown by von Weimern that for the production of an easily filtrable crystalline ppt the value of the factor $Q-S/S$ should be as small as possible. In order to decrease the value of $Q-S/S$, the value of Q should be decreased. This can be done by increasing the dilution of the sample and reagent soln but then we will have to handle a very large volume which is tedious and time consuming. Furthermore, in a very dilute soln, due to small value of Q−S/S, the rate of precipitation will be very poor and it will take a long time for complete precipitation. Owing to these practical difficulties the value of Q−S/S cannot be very much decreased simply by decreasing Q. Another approach to reduce the value of Q−S/S is to increase the value of S. This can be done by raising the temperature of the sample soln during precipitation and also by using such medium in which the ppt will have a greater solubility. For example, the solubility of $BaSO_4$ is greater in acid medium than in neutral medium hence, the precipitation is done in presence of HCl. When the precipitation is nearly complete the mother liquor is partially neutralised so that there is no solubility loss (in neutral medium the solubility of $BaSO_4$ will decrease).

6·4·5. Completeness of Precipitation

In order that the desired constituent is completely precipitated, we must add the precipitating reagent in excess. Because the amount of the constituent is unknown it is not possible to know that how much reagent should be added. The procedure is that some amount of reagent is added, the ppt is allowed to settle and then a few drops of the reagent are added slowly through a rod to the upper clear liquid (supernatant liquid). If there is ppt formation in the upper clear liquid it means that more reagent should be added, if ppt formation is not observed it shows that the precipitation is complete and there is no need to add more reagent.

Another consideration that influences the completeness of precipitation is the solubility of the ppt at the time of filtration. For example, if the solubility of a ppt just before filtration is $0·2\%$, then the weight of the ppt obtained will be only $99·8\%$ of the theoretically calculated value.

In the example given in 6·4·4, we have seen that the precipitation of $BaSO_4$ is done in acidic medium when the solubility of $BaSO_4$ is greater. This was necessary to decrease the value of Q−S/S in order to obtain a crystalline ppt of $BaSO_4$. If filtration is done at this stage the amount of ppt of $BaSO_4$ will be smaller due to higher solubility of $BaSO_4$ in acidic medium. Hence, before filtration most of the acid present is neutralised so that the solubility of $BaSO_4$ decreases and the solubility loss is minimum.

6·4·6. Factors Influencing Solubility

The solubility of a ppt is influenced by several factors. One of the most important factors is the common-ion effect. In gravimetric procedures an excess of reagent is added to achieve complete precipitation. On doing so, due to common-ion effect, the solubility of the ppt decreases hence the solubility loss also decreases.

Example 6(vi)

If an excess of Na_2SO_4 is added to $BaCl_2$ soln, the reaction is :

$$BaCl_2 + Na_2SO_4 \longrightarrow BaSO_4 + 2NaCl$$

Now, $BaSO_4$ is poorly dissociated while Na_2SO_4 is strongly dissociated

$$BaSO_4 \rightleftharpoons Ba^{2+} + SO_4^{2-} \text{ (Poorly dissociated)}$$
$$Na_2SO_4 \rightleftharpoons 2Na^+ + SO_4^{2-} \text{ (Strongly dissociated)}$$

Due to the common ion (SO_4^{2-}) the poor dissociation of $BaSO_4$ is further decreased, the i.e., solubility of $BaSO_4$ decreases. It has been found that the solubility of $BaSO_4$ is more in distilled water as compared to that in presence of Na_2SO_4 or $BaCl_2$ (substances that contain common ion).

It should be noted that in some cases excess reagent forms a complex with the ppt. In such cases, too much of the reagent should not be added otherwise some of the ppt would dissolve due to complex formation. For example, the solubility of AgCl increases in presence of high Cl^- ion concentration due to the formation of $AgCl_2^-$ and $AgCl_3^{2-}$ species.

Another factor influencing the solubility of a ppt is the diverse ion effect (see 4.7). The presence of any ions not in common with the ppt tends to increase its solubility.

Temperature increases the solubility of a ppt. The nature of the solvent also influences the solubility of a ppt. Most of the ppts are inorganic solids and are more soluble in a polar solvent like water and less soluble in non-polar solvents like carbon tetrachloride. However, it should be remembered that if a non polar solvent is used for decreasing the solubility of a ppt, the solubilities of various impurities may also be diminished hence the ppt will be less pure.

6.4.7. Purity of a Precipitate

One of the advantages of gravimetric analysis is that the ppt after final weighing can be analysed to find out the amount of impurities and then necessary correction in the result can be made.

In spite of all precautions sometimes, the desired ppt contains one or more substances because these substances are not sufficiently soluble in the medium used.

The contamination of the ppt by substances which are normally soluble in the mother liquor is called *co-precipitation* ; this can be of two type. The first is concerned with the adsorption on the surface of the ppt and the second involves *occlusion* of foreign substances during the growth of the ppt. Another term that is used is called *post-precipitation* which means deposition of another substance on the ppt after its formation. It occurs with sparingly soluble substances which usually have an ion in common with the ppt.

6'4'8.   Adsorption of Ions on Precipitates

Let us consider the process of precipitation of a salt, say, $BaSO_4$. Suppose we have a soln of $BaCl_2$ to which we add a very small amount of Na_2SO_4. The soln will contain Ba^{2+}, Cl^-, Na^+ and SO_4^{2-} ions and also H^+ and OH^- ions. (The diameter of these ions is of the order of 10^{-8} cm.) The concentration of SO_4^{2-} ions is very small, the solubility product (S_{BaSO_4}) of $BaSO_4$ is not exceeded hence, its precipitation will not take place. If we go on adding Na_2SO_4 a stage will be reached when the ionic product for $BaSO_4$ will exceed S_{BaSO_4} and Ba^{2+} and SO_4^{2-} ions will join together to form a small particle of $BaSO_4$. Now it has been found that only those particles settle at the bottom whose diameter is greater than 10^{-4} cm. The particles of $BaSO_4$ initially formed are smaller hence do not settle. Gradually particles grow and when their diameters become greater than 10^{-4} cm, the particles under the influence of gravity settle at the bottom of the container. It is obvious that during the growth process a particle of the ppt passes through the colloidal range **(particle of diameter** $10^{-7}-10^{-4}$ cm**)**. The precipitation process can be represented as

$$\begin{array}{ccccc} \text{ions in soln} & \longrightarrow & \text{colloidal particles} & \longrightarrow & \text{ppt} \\ \left[\begin{array}{l}\text{particle } 10^{-8}\text{ cm} \\ \text{size}\end{array}\right. & & 10^{-7}-10^{-4}\text{ cm} & & \begin{array}{l}\text{greater} \\ \text{than } 10^{-4}\text{ cm}\end{array} \end{array}$$

The colloidal particles are electrically charged so they repel each other and are not able to come close to each other to form bigger particles. Thus, one of the main reasons for the stability of colloids is the charge on their particles. This electrical charge on the particles is due to the adsorption of ions from the mother liquor on to the surface of the colloid particles. Colloid particles which are very small in size have a very high surface to mass ratio.

Example 6(*vii*)

Suppose we have a 1 cm cube of a substance then its total area will be 6 sq cm. If this cube is subdivided into 10^{18} cubes the total area of these very small cubes will be about 6,000,000 sq cm. Thus the surface to mass ratio increases from 6 : 1 to 6,000,000 : 1.

Colloid particles are very small in size hence their surface to mass ratio would be very high ; surface effects are very important in colloid chemistry. In colloid particles there exists several localised positive and negative charge centres on which adsorption of ions from the mother liquor takes place. For example, if a drop of

$AgNO_3$ soln is added to a NaCl soln and if the solubility product value of AgCl is exceeded the white particles of AgCl will appear. In the beginning these particles are of colloidal size and have a large number of Ag^+ and Cl^- ions (centres of localised positive and negative charge) on the surface. In the solution (mother liquor), there are Na^+, Cl^- and NO_3^- ions. The Ag^+ ions on the particle surface attract negative ions, i e., NO_3^- and Cl^- ions present in the mother liquor. The surface Cl^- ions attract Na^+ ions. Now, according to Paneth-Fajans-Hahn rule, when two or more types of ions are available for adsorption, that ion which forms the least soluble salt with one of the ions of the particle (called lattice ions) will be adsorbed in preference to the other ion (this is called preferential adsorption). In the above example, Ag^+ and Cl^- are the lattice ions and NO_3^- and Cl^- ions are available for adsorption. Because AgCl is less soluble than $AgNO_3$, it is the Cl^- ion which will be preferentially adsorbed. Thus there will be a layer of Cl^- ions on the particle of AgCl hence the particle will become negatively charged. The Cl^- ions are said to form a *primary layer*. These Cl^- ions now attract positively charged sodium ions thus forming a *secondary layer*. These primary and secondary layers constitute what is known as an *electrical double layer*, which is mainly responsible for the stability of colloids (see Fig. 6·1).

The adsorption of an ion on a particle depends on the concentration of the ion present in the soln. Further, a multicharged ion is more readily adsorbed than a singly charged ion. Size of the ion also influences the adsorption process.

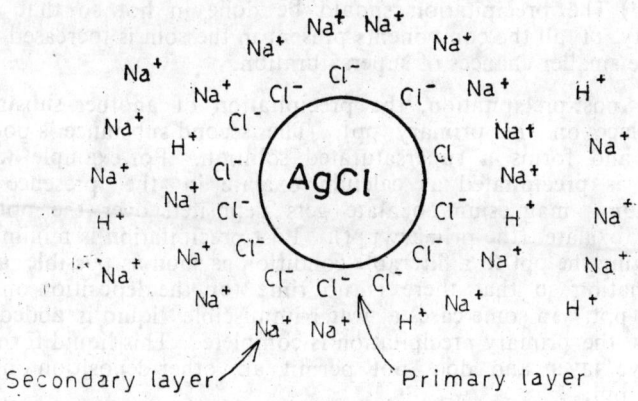

Fig. 6 1.   Electrical double layer on a colloid particle.

6·4·9. Coprecipitation, Occlusion and Post-Precipitation

When a substance is precipitated from a soln it is not perfectly pure but contains various impurities depending on the nature of the ppt and conditions of precipitation. The contamination of a ppt by substances normally soluble in the mother liquor is called *precipitation*. The main reason for coprecipitation is adsorption of ions on the particles of the ppt.

Example 6(*viii*)

To determine Cl^- ions in a given soln of NaCl, an excess of $AgNO_3$ soln is added to it and the resultant ppt of AgCl is washed, dried and weighed. In the mother liquor there are Ag^+, Na^+ and NO_3^- ions, Silver ions are the only ions that are common to those of AgCl (Ag^+ and Cl^- ions) hence, Ag^+ ions will be preferentially absorbed on the particle surface forming the primary layer, the nitrate ions will form the secondary layer. Thus $AgNO_3$ which is ordinarily a soluble salt is coprecipitated with AgCl.

Another type of coprecipitation can be understood by considering the process of growth of crystals of the ppt. If the rate of growth is rapid, some impurities are enclosed inside the growing crystals ; this is known as *occlusion*.

Following steps are taken to minimise coprecipitation :

(*i*) The soln from which precipitation is made should be dilute so that the concentration of foreign ions which may be adsorbed or occluded is small.

(*ii*) Stir the soln during precipitation so that larger crystals are formed, this will keep adsorption and occlusion at a minimum.

(*iii*) The precipitation should be done in hot so that the solubility of all the components present in the soln is increased and there are smaller chances of supersaturation.

In post-precipitation, the precipitation of another substance takes place on the primary ppt. The second substance is poorly soluble and forms a supersaturated solution. For example, when calcium is precipitated as calcium oxalate in the presence of magnesium, magnesium oxalate gets deposited over the ppt of calcium oxalate (the primary ppt). Post-precipitation is minimised by bringing the ppt to a filterable condition as soon as possible after its formation so that there is no time for the deposition on the primary ppt. In some cases a water-immiscible liquid is added as soon as the primary precipitation is complete. This liquid forms a protective layer and does not permit any other deposition on the primary ppt.

6·5. DIGESTION OF PRECIPITATES

It has been seen that by properly choosing the precipitating agent and by carying out precipitation in dilute and and hot solution with constant stirring, coprecipitation can be kept at a minimum.

But even after such steps a ppt may contain impurities and digestion may be necessary. Digestion is carried out by allowing the ppt to stand for 12-24 hours at room temperature or warming the ppt for some time in contact with the soln from which it was precipitated. On doing so there is complete precipitation and bigger particles of the ppt are formed which can be readily filtered. During the process smaller particles of the ppt goes into soln and then are redeposited on the larger particles that are easy to filter. Furthermore, co-precipitation is greater on smaller particles and since during digestion small particles form larger particles, coprecipitation is minimised. Thus the effect of digestion is to reduce coprecipitation and to increase the size of the particles which are easier to filter.

6·6. WASHING OF PRECIPITATES

After filtration it is necessary to wash the ppt so as to remove the ions adsorbed on it. Pure water is generally not used for washing precipitates because during repeated washing some of the ppt can go into solution due to *peptisation*. It is known that when an electrolyte is added to a colloidal soln, the colloid particles join together to form bigger particles that settle down at the bottom of the container ; this phenomenon is called *coagulation*. The reverse of this is peptisation in which coagulated particles pass back into colloidal state. It has been found that if a ppt is washed repeatedly with pure water, a stage comes when wash water contains colloidal particles of the ppt. Thus pure water cannot be used as a wash liquid for precipitates.

The composition of the wash soln depends upon the solubility and chemical properties of the ppt. Usually a very dilute soln of an electrolyte is used as a wash soln. The electrolyte selected is such that it contains an ion common to the ions of the ppt. The presence of the electrolyte in the wash soln has two advantages : (a) it helps in the formation of bigger particles of the ppt which can be easily filtered (note that the presence of electrolytes helps coagulation) ; and (b) the common ion present in the electrolyte prevents solubility loses of the ppt [see example, 6(vi)]. For example, the ppt of CaC_2O_4 is washed with 0·1 to 0·2% $(NH_4)_2C_2O_4$ soln. If the ppt is a salt of a weak acid or weak base it will have a tendency to hydrolyse ; this can be prevented by using dilute acid or basic soln as a wash liquid. For example, $Mg(NH_4)PO_4$ undergoes hydrolysis hence this ppt is washed with dilute soln of ammonia. The ions present in the wash liquid should be such that it can be easily volatalised during drying or igniting the ppt. Sometimes a non-aqueous solvent (or a mixture of water and non-aqueous solvent) is used as a wash liquid. The property of the wash liquid should be such that the impurities should have greater solubility in it but the solubility of the ppt should be negligible. Furthermore, the solvent should be volatile so that it is easily removed during drying or ignition of the ppt.

If too much wash soln is used there may be considerable solubility losses. The correct procedure is to use a small volume (about 10 ml) of wash liquid each time for washing. It is advantageous to do washing several times, each time using a small volume of wash liquid rather than using a large volume and doing fewer washings.

6.7. DRYING AND IGNITION OF PRECIPITATES

The washed ppt may contain occluded and adsorbed water. Also, water of crystallisation may be present in certain cases. Apart from water the electrolyte added to wash water may also be present.

Some precipitates are dried at ordinary temperature. For example, $MgNH_4PO_4.6H_2O$ is dried by washing it with a mixture of alcohol and ether and drawing air through the ppt for a few minutes. This procedure of drying is normally not recommended because some water which is occluded is rather difficult to remove by this method.

In some cases, on heating the ppt to 100-110°C for 30-60 minutes, water is driven out and the dried ppt can be weighed in the form in which it was precipitated. For example, by heating the ppt of AgCl in an oven at about 100-120°C it becomes dry and can be weighed as AgCl. (The drying is continued until two successive weights of the ppt are equal).

There are certain precipitates which decompose when heated and hence their composition changes during the drying process carried out to drive out occluded water. In such cases the ppt is heated at a suitable temperature for certain period of time so that all the water is removed and the ppt is completely converted to some other compound of definite chemical composition. For example, when the ppt of aluminium hydroxide is heated to drive out water, it partly decomposes into its oxide making the composition of the ppt uncertain. This problem is solved by heating the ppt to a sufficiently high temperature for about half an hour. The ppt is then cooled in a desiccator and weighed. The ppt is again heated for some time then cooled and weighed. This process is repeated until two weight readings are almost equal. This ensures that all the hydroxide has been converted into oxide which has a fixed chemical composition.

6.7.1. Thermal Decomposition of Precipitates

In thermogravimetric analysis the temperature of a substance is gradually increased and its weight is recorded at different temperatures. From such a study it is possible to know that at what temperature the ppt is decomposing. For example, when the ppt of calcium oxalate is heated to about 475°C its weight rapidly decreases because it starts decomposing into $CaCO_3$. At about 500°C, if ppt is heated for a sufficient period all of it is converted into $CaCO_3$. The weight then remains constant in the temperature range 510-520°C, but as the temperature is increased beyond 530°C, the weight again starts decreasing showing that $CaCO_3$ is being decomposed into CaO. Hence, if in the gravimetric determination we choose $CaCO_3$ as the weighing form, the crucible should be heated to 500-510°C for a sufficient period so that all the oxalate is converted into carbonate and because the temperature is controlled, the decomposition of $CaCO_3$ to CaO does not take place. Hence, the substance that is weighed has a definite chemical composition, *i.e.*, it is $CaCO_3$ alone.

6·8. LABORATORY EXERCISES

In this section some gravimetric procedures are described. The purpose of this description is not only to provide methods for determining certain substances but also to demonstrate various operations that are performed during a gravimetric determination.

Experiment 6·1

Gravimetric Determination of Chloride as Silver Chloride

Apparatus and Chemicals required

Two sintered-glass crucibles, analytical balance (weighing up to 0·2 or 0·1 mg), oven, desiccator, watch-glasses, weighing bottles, crucible-tongs, beakers, glass rods, washing bottle, filtration assembly and suction pump.

The chemicals needed are silver nitrate, nitric acid and distilled water.

Procedure

This determination involves the following steps :

(*i*) *Determining the constant weights of the sintered crucibles.* Two sintered crucibles should be cleaned, thoroughly rinsed with distilled water and kept over a watch-glass in an oven at 120°C. After approximately one hour, hte crucibles should be taken out of the oven with the help of crucible tongs (crucibles should not be touched with hand or a piece of cloth or paper), placed on a clean watch-glass and thus cooled in air for about 2 to 3 minutes. (Hot crucibles should not be directly transferred to a desiccator). The crucibles are then transferred to a desiccator with the aid of crucible tongs (see Fig. 6.2). After about 30 minutes the crucibles are

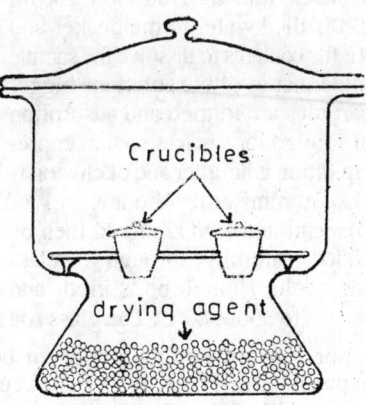

Fig. 6 2. Desiccator.

weighed. The heating and cooling steps should be repeated until the two weight readings for a particular crucible are within 0·2 mg. For example, suppose the different weight readings for a particular crucible are : 20·8258 ; 20·8089; 20·8078 ; 20·8074 and 20·8072 g then 20·8072 g should be regarded as the constant weight of that crucible. Similarly the constant weight of the other crucible should be determined.

(ii) *Preparation of the sample solutions.* In order to have reliable results at least two determinations should be carried out. Sufficient amount of sample containing Cl^- ion should be taken in a watch-glass (from which two portions can be weighed) and dried in an oven at 120°C for one hour (to remove any moisture present in the sample), cooled in air for 2 to 3 minutes and then in a desic-cator for about 30 minutes. The dried and cooled sample should be transferred to a clean and dry weighing bottle of known weight and the bottle should be weighed again. The difference in the two weight readings will give the weight of the sample. In this way two weighed sample should be taken. The weight of each portion should be such that it will form 0·4 to 0·7 g of AgCl. (Note that 35·46 g of Cl^- ions produces 143·34 g of AgCl). If the weight of AgCl formed is small, say 0·1 g, the weighing error will be greater. However, the final veight of AgCl should not be too much otherwise there will be ifficulty in handling the large quantity of the ppt during filtering and washing.

The weighed sample is then completely transferred from a weigh-ing bottle to a clean 400 ml beaker with the help of a washing bottle (see Fig. 6.3).

(iii) *Precipitation of chloride as silver chloride.* Add about 100 ml of distilled water to the beaker and stir the contents to dissolve the sample (note that in dilute solutions bigger particles are formed and adsorption of foreign ions is less so that copre-cipitation is smaller and occlusion is also minimised). About 1 ml of concentrated HNO_3 should then be added carefully through a glass rod, soln should be stirred and heated to about 80°C. The glass rod

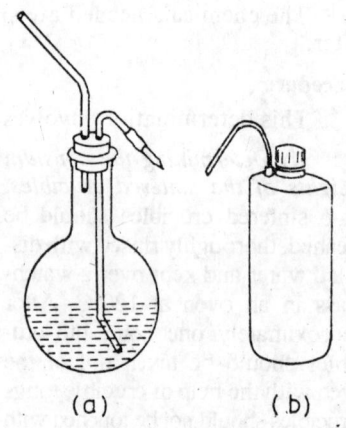

(a)   (b)

Fig. 6·3. Wash bottles:
(a) glass, (b) polyethylene.

dipped into the soln should not be taken out from it throughout the experiment. If it is to be taken out, it must be thoroughly washed with distilled water and then removed from the soln. For separate solutions separate rods should be used. A 5 per cent $AgNO_3$ soln in water should be gradually added in slight excess with the help of the glass rod to the hot soln and then it should be stirred thoroughly (gradual addition, stirring and hot soln helps in the formation of bigger crystals of AgCl ; in hot condition adsorption of foreign ions on the ppt is minimum). Some authors recommend precipitation in cold and then heating at about 80°C for half an hour.

(iv) Digestion of the precepitate. After the addition of AgNO$_3$ soln the mixture should be kept at about 80°C (on a hot water bath) for about 30 minutes or overnight at room temperature. The process of digestion brings about coagulation, i.e., formation of bigger particles. In the upper clear liquid, called supernatant soln, 2 or 3 drops of AgNO$_3$ soln should be added through the glass rod, if no ppt appears it means that all the chloride ions have been precipitated as AgCl. If ppt appears in the supernatant liquid, it indicates that the precipitation is not complete and more AgNO$_3$ soln should be added. Silver chloride on exposing to direct light especially sun light) undergoes decomposition hence exposure of the ppt to light should be avoided.

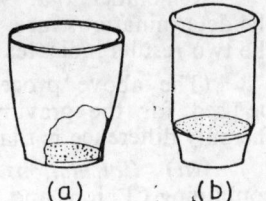

(a)   (b)

Fig. 6·4. Filter crucibles :
(a) porous porcelain,
(b) sintered glass.

(v) Filtration and washing of the precipitate. A suction flask and trap for filtration is arranged, the weighed sintered crucible (see Fig. 6.4) is inserted into a crucible holder on the suction flask and a mild suction is applied to the filtration assembly (see Fig. 6.5). Filtration should be started by pouring the supernatant liquid through the glass rod on to the crucible. The beaker should be so

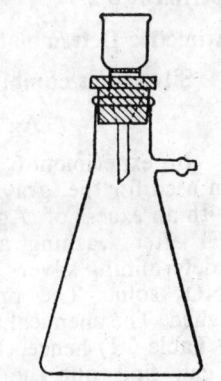

Fig. 6·5. Suction filtration with filter crucible.

held that the ppt remains at the bottom of the beaker. The water level in the crucible should not be allowed to rise above two-thirds of the height of the crucible otherwise there is a danger of some ppt moving out of the crucible. After transferring almost all the upper clear liquid, about 20 ml of dilute HNO$_3$ (2 ml of concentrated HNO$_3$ added to 500 ml of water) should be added to the ppt and the mixture should be thoroughly stirred (pure water causes peptisation of ppt). The ppt should be allowed to settle and the supernatant liquid should be poured into the crucible through the glass rod. This process of washing should be repeated about four times. The purpose of washing the ppt is to remove Ag$^+$ and other ions adsorbed on it. After each washing the filtrate should be collected and a few drops of dilute HCl added to it—if a white ppt of AgCl appears it means Ag$^+$ ions are still present and the ppt needs more washing.

(vi) Drying and weighing of the precipitate. The crucible along with the washed ppt should be kept in an oven at 120° C for one hour. After heating, the crucible should be cooled in air for 2 to 3 minutes and then in a desiccator for about 30 minutes. The crucible is then weighed. The heating, cooling and weighing opera-

tions are repeated until the weight of the crucible and the ppt is constant, *i.e.*, two successive weights do not differ by more than 0·2 mg.

Remember that we had taken two weighed samples. Both the determinations are simultaneously carried out. Agreement in the two results indicates the reliability of the result.

(The above procedure for the determination of Cl^- ions can be used for the gravimetric standardisation of hydrochloric acid the only difference is that the addition of nitric acid is not required.)

(*vii*) *Calculations.* Suppose we have taken '*a*' g of the sample containing Cl^- ions and the weight of AgCl formed is '*b*' g. Now, it has been seen in example 6. (*iv*) that the chemical factor for the conversion AgCl to Cl^- ion is 0·2474. Hence '*a*' g of the sample will contain ($b \times 0·2474$) g Cl^- ions.

Experiment 6·2.

Gravimetric Determination of Silver as Silver Chloride

Silver ions combine with Cl^- ions to form insoluble AgCl :

$$Ag^+ + Cl^- \longrightarrow AgCl \text{ (white ppt)}$$

In experiment 6·1. we have seen that this ionic reaction has been used for the gravimetric determination of Cl^- ions by treating it with an excess of $AgNO_3$ soln and weighing the resultant ppt of AgCl after washing and drying. The same reaction can be used for determining silver by adding an excess of dilute HCl to given $AgNO_3$ soln. The ppt of AgCl obtained is washed, dried and weighed. The chemical factor for the conversion AgCl to Ag is 0·7526 (see Table 6·1) hence, by multiplying the weight of AgCl by 0·7526 we can find out the weight of silver in the given volume of the sample.

Notes :

1 In the determination of Ag^+ as AgCl, the precipitant is dilute HCl which gives H^+ ions ; these serve the same function as HNO_3 in a chloride determination. Silver salts of weak acids are soluble in HCl so they remain in soln and their precipitation is prevented (in neutral medium some silver salts such as silver acetate will not dissolve but will be collected along with AgCl ; thus the composition of the ppt will not be definite). Hydrochloric acid soln contains H^+ and Cl^- ions which help in the coagulation of colloidal AgCl (remember that the addition of electrolytes causes coagulation of colloid particles.) Furthermore, these ions prevent the peptisation of the ppt of AgCl during its washing. Because in silver[1] determination, HCl is used as a precipitant and because it performs all the functions of HNO_3, hence it is not necessary to add HNO_3 before precipitation as is done in the gravimetric determination of chlorides.

2. A slight excess of HCl is added so that Ag^+ ions are completely precipitated. The presence of excess HCl decreases the solubility of AgCl so that the solubility losses are minimum. However, a large excess of HCl should be avoided because then the

solubility of AgCl increases due to the formation of soluble chloro. complexes of silver : $AgCl + Cl^- \rightarrow AgCl_2^- (AgCl_3^{2-}$ etc.)

Experiment 6'3.

Gravimetric Determination of Barium as Barium Sulphate

The gravimetric determination of barium as barium sulphate is based on the reaction :

$$Ba^{2+} + SO_4^{2-} \longrightarrow BaSO_4 \text{ (white ppt)}$$

The procedure involves the following steps.

(*i*) By repeatedly heating (500-600° C), cooling and weighing, the constant weight of a porcelain or a silica crucible is found out as described in experiment 6.1.

(*ii*) If barium is to be determined in a given soln, its definite volume is taken in a beaker. In case a solid sample is given, it should be dried, an accurately weighed portion of the sample transferred to a beaker and dissolved in distilled water.

(*iii*) About 5 ml of dilute HCl is added (presence of electrolyte helps in coagulation and impurities which are soluble in acid are not precipitated).

(*iv*) To the sample soln, about 150 ml of water is added (in dilute soln bigger particles are formed and coprecipitation is also minimised).

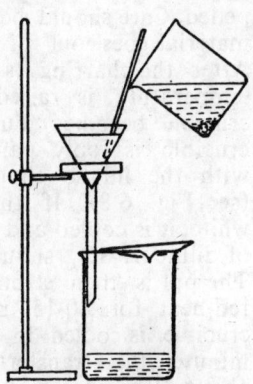

Fig. 6·6. Filtration using a filter paper.

(*v*) The soln is heated to about 80°C, an axcess of hot dilute H_2SO_4 is gradually added through a glass rod and the mixture is stirred thoroughly for 2 to 3 minutes (at high temperature, colloidal particles coagulate to form bigger particles which can be easily filtered).

(*vi*) A few drops of dilute H_2SO_4 are added to the supernatant soln to test for complete precipitation.

(*vii*) A filter paper (Whatman no. 40) is properly fitted in a funnel, the supernatant liquid is poured through it and the filtrate is collected in a clean beaker (see Fig. 6.6). The ppt is washed first with hot water containing a few drops of dilute H_2SO_4 and then with distilled water alone until the acid is removed. When the filtrate does not give any ppt or turbidity with $AgNO_3$, the ppt

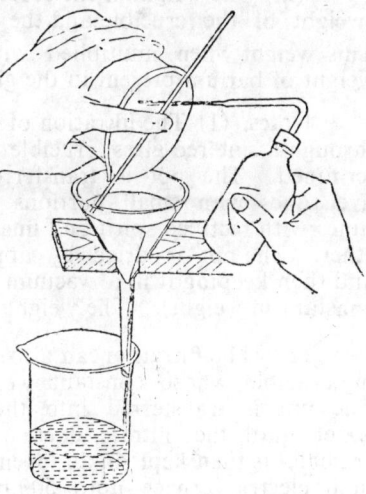

Fig. 6·7. Transfer of a precipitate from a beaker to the filter assembly with the help of a polyethylene wash bottle.

is completely transferred to the filter paper with the help of a jet of hot water from the wash bottle (see Fig. 6·7). If some ppt is sticking to the walls of the beaker or to the stirring rod, it should be removed by means of rubber-tipped glass rod called "policeman".

(*viii*) After all the ppt has been transferred on to the filter paper, it is folded and placed in a procelain or a silica crucible whose constant weight has already been determined. The crucible is loosely covered and slowly heated when the filter paper chars (turns black) and volatile mater is expelled. Care should be taken that no material goes out of the crucible. After the charring is complete the temperature is raised so that the crucible becomes dull red. The crucible is only partially covered with the lid so that air can enter (see Fig. 6·8). If the ppt is not white, it is cooled and a drop or two of dilute H_2SO_4 should be added. The ppt is then strongly heated to red-heat for 10-15 minutes. The crucible is cooled in air for 2 to 3 minutes, then transferred to a desiccator in which it is cooled for about 10 to 15 minutes and is weighed. The heating and cooling is continued until two successive weights of the crucible do not differ by more than 0·2 mg.

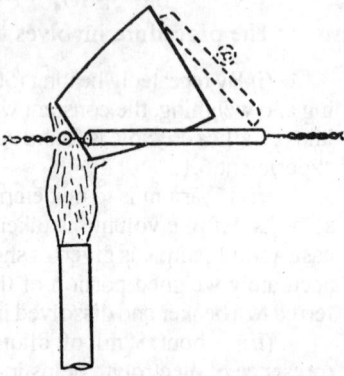

Fig. 6·8. Ignition of a precipitate.

(*ix*) The weight of the crucible is subtracted from the combined weight of the crucible and the ppt to obtain the weight of $BaSO_4$. This weight when multiplied with 0·5885 (see Table 6·1) gives the weight of barium present in the given amount of the sample material.

Notes. (1) The filtration of the ppt of $BaSO_4$ can also be done through a sintered-glass crucible whose constant weight is predetermined. The ppt is transferred to the crucibile, washed about five times with small portions of hot distilled water then five times with rectified spirit and finally five to six times with anhydrous ether. The ppt is dried by applying suction through the crucible and then keeping it in a vacuum desiccator for 10 minutes (or until constant in weight). The weight of the crucible is then taken.

(2) The filtration can also be done through a procelain filtering crucible whose constant weight has already been determined. The ppt is transferred into the crucible and washed with warm water until the filtrate does not gives test for Cl^- ions. The cruicble is then kept in an oven for drying after which it is heated in an electric furnace upto 500-600° C until constant weight of the crucible is recorded.

(3) **Precipitation from homogeneous solution**

In this technique precipitant is not added from outside but is generated by a homogeneous chemical reaction in the soln. In the gravimetric determination of Ba^{2+} ions as $BaSO_4$, the precipitant added is dilute H_2SO_4. Another method of precipitation is to add sulphamic acid to the given soln containing Ba^{2+} ions. Sulphamic acid produces SO_4^{2-} ions on boiling :

$$NH_2SO_3H + H_2O \longrightarrow NH_4^+ + SO_4^{2-} + H^+$$

The SO_4^{2-} ions are gradually produced during the above reaction and they combine with Ba^{2+} ions present in the sample soln to form $BaSO_4$. When the ppt of $BaSO_4$ appears, the boiling is continued for another 30 minutes. Filtration is done through a weighed porcelain filter crucible, ppt is washed with warm water and crucible is heated to 900°C until constant weight. (This technique is known as the precipitation from homogeneous soln. The advantage of this technique is that it gives rise to bigger particles and co-precipitation is also at a minimum).

Experiment 6.4.

Gravimetric Determination of Sulphate as Barium Sulphate

An accurately weighed portion of the given sample (the amount should contain 0.05 to 0.06 g sulphur) is taken in a 400 ml beaker. About 25 ml water and 0.5 ml of concentrated HCl are added to dissolve the solid. This soln is diluted to about 200 ml and heated to boiling. Through a burette 10 to 15 ml of 5 per cent barium chloride soln (5 g $BaCl_2.2H_2O$ in 100 ml of water) is gradually added with thorough stirring. The ppt is allowed to settle and test for complete precipitation is done in the supernatant liquid with the help of $BaCl_2$ soln. The beaker is kept hot by keeping it on a steam bath for an hour. The ppt of $BaSO_4$ is then filtered, washed, dried and weighed as in the case of determination of Ba^{2+} ions described in experiment 6.3.

The formula weight of $BaSO_4$ is equal to $137.36 + 32.06 + 64.00$ $= 233.42$ and that of SO_4^{-2} ion is $32.06 + 64.00 = 96.06$. The chemical factor for the conversion $BaSO_4$ to SO_4^{2-} ions will be $96.06/233.42 = 0.4115$. Hence, the weight of $BaSO_4 \times 0.4115$ will give the quantity of sulphate ions present in the given amount of the sample.

Example 6(ix)

Twenty five ml of a soln of barium chloride was treated with an excess of H_2SO_4. The resultant ppt of $BaSO_4$ was filtered, washed, dried and was found to weigh 0.3521 g. Calculate the weight of $BaCl_2.2H_2O$ present in the soln.

The formula weight of $BaSO_4$ is 233.42.

The formula weight of $BaCl_2.2H_2O$ is 244.32.

$$[137.36 + (2 \times 35.46) + (4 \times 1.01) + (2 \times 16.00) = 244.32]$$

The gravimetric factor for the conversion $BaSO_4$ to $BaCl_2$. $2H_2O$ is :

$$\frac{244\cdot32}{233\cdot42} = 1\cdot0467.$$

The weight of $BaCl_2.2H_2O$ in 25 ml of the given soln will be :
$$0\cdot3521 \times 1\cdot0467 = 0\cdot3685 \text{ g.}$$

Example 6(x)

A sample contains $0\cdot0500$ g of sulphur in the form of SO_4^{2-} ions. If the sample is treated with an excess of $BaCl_2$ soln, what weight of $BaSO_4$ will be obtained ?

$$\underset{(32\cdot06)}{S} \equiv \underset{(233\cdot42)}{BaSO_4}$$

$32\cdot06$ g sulphur forms $233\cdot42$ g $BaSO_4$

$\therefore$ $0\cdot0500$ g sulphur forms $\dfrac{0\cdot0500}{32\cdot06} \times 233\cdot42$

$$= 0\cdot3640 \text{ g of } BaSO_4.$$

or, the chemical factor for the conversion S to $BaSO_4$ is $233\cdot42/32\cdot06 = 7\cdot2807$, hence the weight of $BaSO_4$ will be—

$$0\cdot0500 \times 7\cdot2807 = 0\cdot3640 \text{ g of } BaSO_4.$$

Experiment 6·5.

Gravimetric Determination of Calcium as Calcium Oxalate

Discussion. The sample containing calcium is dissolved in hot HCl and ammonium oxalate is added. On adding NH_4OH slowly, calcium is precipitated as calcium oxalate monohydrate :

$$Ca^{2+} + C_2O_4^{2-} + H_2O \longrightarrow CaC_2O_4.H_2O$$

(It should be noted that CaC_2O_4 is soluble in HCl that is why it was not precipitated in acidic medium. On adding NH_4OH, acid is neutralised and ppt of CaC_2O_4 appears). The ppt is washed with a dilute soln of $(NH_4)_2C_2O_4$ (it contains a common ion hence, the solubility of CaC_2O_4 is less in its presence). The ppt can be weighed either as $CaC_2O_4.H_2O$ or $CaCO_3$ or CaO.

Procedure :

(i) Sufficient amount of sample that contains about $0\cdot2$ g of calcium is accurately weighed and transferred to a 500 ml beaker. The mixture is heated with HCl to dissolve the solid and soln is boiled for 5 to 10 minutes. About 200 ml of water and 2 drops of methyl red indicator are then added and sides of beakers are washed.

(ii) To the hot soln (about 80°C), 1 per cent hot soln of $(NH_4)_2C_2O_4$ (about 50 ml) is slowly added with stirring. Ammonia soln is then added dropwise with stirring until the mixture is neutral or slightly alkaline (as shown by the colour change from red to yellow). Test for complete precipitation should be made in the supernatant liquid.

(iii) After the precipitation either $CaC_2O_4.H_2O$ is weighed or it is converted into $CaCO_3$ or CaO which can be weighed.

(a) *Weighing as* $CaC_2O_4.H_2O$: The ppt is filtered through a weighed sintered glass crucible, washed with 0·1 to 0·2 per cent cold soln of $(NH_4)_2C_2O_4$ until the filtrate does not give test for Cl^- ions (5 ml of filtrate after each washing is acidified with HNO_3 and $AgNO_3$ soln is added to test for Cl^- ions). The ppt is then dried at 100 to 105°C for 1 to 2 hours and weighed. This method is not recommended because the oxalate is hygroscopic and coprecipitated ammonium oxalate is difficult to remove at this low temperature.

(b) *Weighing as* $CaCO_3$: The ppt is allowed to settle and the supernatent liquid is poured into a weighed porcelain filtering crucible. The ppt is washed with 0·1 to 0·2 per cent ammonium oxalate and completely transferred to the crucible. The ppt is further washed until the washing is free from Cl^- ions. The ppt is first dried in an oven at 100 to 120°C for 1 hour and then in an electric furnace at 500 to 525°C until the constant weight.

(c) *Weighing as* CaO : The ppt is allowed to settle and supernatant liquid is poured on a Whatman no. 40 filter paper fitted in a funnel. The ppt is washed with 0·1 to 0·2 per cent cold ammonium oxalate soln until the washings do not give test for Cl^- ions. The filter paper containing the washed ppt is folded and kept in a platinum crucible whose constant weight has already been determined. The crucible is heated first gently and then strongly over a bunsen flame for about 15 minutes. It is cooled first in air, then in a desiccator and it is weighed. The heating and cooling process is repeated until two successive weight readings do not differ by more than 0·2 mg. The weight of the crucible is subtracted from the weight of the crucible and ppt—this gives the weight of CaO which on multiplying with 0·7147 gives the weight of calcium in the sample soln (see Table 6·1).

Experiment 6·6.

Gravimetric Determination of Iron as Iron(III) oxide

Discussion. On adding aqueous ammonia soln to a salt soln containing Fe^{3+} ions, a reddish brown ppt of hydrated oxide of iron, $Fe_2O_3.XH_2O$, is obtained. This ppt has no definite composition as it contains variable amount of water hence, it cannot be weighed as such after drying. The ppt is neither curdy like $AgCl$ nor crystalline like $BaSO_4$ but is rather gelatinous. The precipitation is carried out using dilute soln at about 100°C, in presence of an electrolyte (HCl) by adding the precipitant (aqueous ammonia soln) gradually with constant stirring (all these steps help in the formating of bigger particles and coprecipitation is also minimum). One advantageous point is that ferric hydroxide is highly insoluble hence is completely precipitated and losses during washing are negligible. The ppt is washed with a dilute soln of ammonia (or ammonium nitrate) and ignited to give Fe_2O_3 which has a definite composition hence it is a suitable weighing form.

Procedure

(*i*) A weighed portion of the sample containing Fe^{3+} ions is transferred into a 400 ml beaker. The solid is dissolved in 50 ml of water and 10 ml of dilute HCl (1 : 1). (About 2 ml of concentrated HNO_3 should be added and soln boiled for about 5 minutes, if the sample contains Fe^{2+} ions, so that these are converted into Fe^{3+} ions).

(*ii*) About 150 ml of water is added, soln is thoroughly stirred, heated to boiling and 1 : 1 ammonia soln is slowly added with stirring until it is in excess (this is indicated by the smell of NH_3).

(*iii*) The soln is boiled for about 1 minute and ppt allowed to settle. (In some cases it is beneficial to redissolve the ppt in HCl and then again precipitate with ammonia soln ; most of the impurities are thus removed during first precipitation and filtration). The supernatant liquid is poured through a glass rod over a ashless filter paper fitted properly in a funnel. The beaker is so held that the ppt remains at the bottom of the beaker. The ppt is washed three or four times with hot 1 per cent soln of ammonium nitrate and it is completely transferred to the filter paper.

(*iv*) The ppt is then washed on the filter paper with hot 1 per cent NH_4NO_3 soln until no test for Cl^- ions is obtained in the washing.

(*v*) The constant weight of a porcelain, silica or a platinum crucible is determined. The filter paper containing the ppt is folded and placed in the crucible which is heated slowly in the beginning and then strongly The crucible is then cooled (using a desiccator) and weighed. The heating and cooling is repeated until two weight readings do not differ by more than 0.2 mg. Thus the weight of Fe_2O_3 is known from which the weight of iron in the given amount of the sample can be calculated.

wt. of iron present in the sample = wt. of $Fe_2O_3 \times 0.6994$.

Example 6(*xi*)

Twenty five ml of a soln of ammonium. iron(II) sulphate also called ferrous ammonium sulphate $[(NH_4)_2SO_4.FeSO_4.6H_2O]$ was boiled with HNO_3 and an excess of ammonia soln was added. The ppt of hydrated ferric oxide was obtained which was filtered, washed, dried and ignited. The weight of the resultant Fe_2O_3 was found to be 0.3145 g. Calculate the weights of :

(*a*) Ammonium iron (II) sulphate hexahydrate,

(*b*) Ferrous sulphate and

(*c*) Iron

in the given sample soln.

The formula weights of :

(*a*) $(NH_4)_2SO_4.FeSO_4.6H_2O = 392.14$

(*b*) $FeSO_4$ $\qquad = 151.91$

(b) The precipitation of nickel dimethylglyoxime (B) is done by adding the alcoholic soln of dimethylglyoxime to a hot (70 to 80°C), slightly acidic soln of the nickel compound and then adding a slight excess of ammonia soln. The reaction involved is

$$NiSO_4 + 2H.DMG \longrightarrow Ni(DMG)_2 + H_2SO_4$$

Since nickel dimethylglyoxime (B) is soluble in mineral acids, its bright red ppt appears only when the soln is made alkaline with ammonia soln. Note that during the precipitation, acid (H_2SO_4 in this case) is produced ; even this small amount of acid can dissolve the ppt.

(c) If the precipitation of nickel dimethylglyoxime is done in cold ammonical soln, the particles of the precipitate formed are very small. Hence, the precipitation is done in hot, slightly acidic soln and then ammonia soln in slight excess is added. Excessive amounts of ammonium hydroxide retard the precipitation.

(d) The precipitation of nickel dimethylglyoxime begins to dissolve if the soln contains more than 50 per cent of alcohol by volume. Hence, for the precipitation, only slight excess of the reagent soln should be used. If the reagent (dimethylglyoxime) soln in large excess is used, then some of it may be precipitated (due to its poor solubility in water) along with the ppt of nickel dimethylglyoxime. Furthermore, if too much reagent soln (which is prepared in alcohol) is added, the alcohol content of the medium will increase and some of the ppt of nickel dimethylglyoxime will dissolve.

(e) The ppt of nickel dimethylglyoxime is slightly soluble in hot water hence, it is washed with cold water and not with hot water.

(f) The ppt of nickel dimethylglyoxime, after washing with cold water, should be dried between 110−120°C to constant weight. The ppt whose composition is $Ni(C_4H_7O_2N_2)_2$ contains 20 32 per cent of nickel.

[Note. 1. The sodium salt of dimethylglyoxime $Na_2C_4H_6O_2N_2$.9 H_2O is soluble in wate and its 2-3 per cent aqueous soln can be used for the precipitation of nicket.

Note. 2. α-Furildioxime can also be used for the determination of nickel. This reagent also gives a red precipitate with nickel salts in ammonical soln. It has the advantage of being soluble in water. Its molecular weight is high hence, the ppt formed with nickel has

α-Furildioxime.

greater weight. This ppt is less soluble as compared to the ppt of nickel with dimethylglyoxime.]

Dimethylglyoxime can also be used for the determination of palladium (Pd).

To a soln containing about 0·1 g of Pd in 250 ml (if more than 0·1 g of Pd is present, the volume of the ppt formed would be large and present practical difficulties) add HCl or HNO₃ so th the normality of the soln in term of acid content is about 0·25 M. (The soln should be free from nickel and gold which interfere.) Add, at room temperature, a 1 per cent soln of dimethylglyoxime in 95 per cent alcohol. Use 2-5 ml of this soln for every 10 mg of Pd. A yellow ppt of palladium dimethylglyoxime $Pd(C_4H_7N_2O_2)_2$ is formed. Wash with hot water (ppt is insoluble in hot water but soluble in ammonia) and filter through a weighed filtering crucible (Gooch, sintered glass or porcelain). Dry at 110°C to constant weight and calculate the amount of Pd in the given solution.

Solutions of bismuth salts in the presence of EDTA give a yellow ppt $[B_2O_2(C_4H_6N_2O_2)]$ with dimethylglyoxime. The precipitation is quantitative at pH 11 0 to 11·5. The ppt is dried at 105—125°C and weighed. (This reaction provides a sensitive test for identifying small quantities of bismuth.)

[Note. Cyclohexane-1, 2-dione dioxime (nioxime) has also been used for the gravimetric determination of Pd using an empirical correction. 4-methylcy-clohexane-1, 2-dione dioxime (4-methyl-nioxime) is quite useful for determining Ni and Pd.]

(ii) 8-Hydroxyquinoline (Oxine)

This reagent (molecular farmula : C_9H_7ON) forms sparingly soluble compounds (called oxinates) with several metal ions hence, it can be used for determining many metals.

Metals	Coordination number	Formula of the oxinate formed
Mg, Zn, Cu, Cd, Pb, In	4	$M(C_9H_6ON)_2$
Al, Fe, Bi, Ga	6	$M(C_9H_6ON)_3$
Th, Zr	8	$M(C_9H_6ON)_4$

Compounds like $TiO(C_9H_6ON)_2$, $MnO_2(C_6H_9ON)_4$ and $UO_2(C_6H_9ON)_2$ are also formed.

8-hydroxyquiroline
or, 8-quinolinol
or, oxine

Cupric oxinate

Copper replaces the hydrogen of the hydroxyl group. Similarly it can be shown that Al^{3+} **will combine with three molecules of oxine.**

Although the oxinates are insoluble in water but are soluble in less polar solvents like chloroform or carbon tetrachloride. The oxinates can, therefore, be extracted with such solvents and the colour intensity measured with a colorimeter or a spectrophotometer. In this way these metals can be determined colorimetrically also.

The reagent oxine can be used in the titrimetric determination of metals. A known excess of the reagent is added to a given solution containing metal ions and ppt obtained is filtered. The unused reagent passes down into the filtrate ; its amount can be found out by a suitable titrimetric method. Thus the quantity of the reagent used up in the reaction becomes known hence, the amount of metal in the test soln can be calculated.

The advantage with oxine is that it can be used for determining several metal ions. But since many metal ions form insoluble complexes with oxine, the reagent loses its specificity. For example, Cu cannot be determined in presence of Mg, Al, Fe, Zn, Cd, Pb. Similarly, Zn cannot be determined in presence of Cd, Mg, Cu, Th, Zr, Al. However, with proper control of precipitation conditions, use of complex forming reagents to remove the interfering metal ion (or by some other method) it is possible to determine a metal in presence of some other metal. For example, Al can be separated from Be by carrying out precipitation in presence of ammonium acetate-acetic acid buffer.

While using 8-hydroxyquinoline (oxine) as a reagent for gravimetric determination, the following points should be remembered :

(a) Oxine is insoluble in water, hence its 2 per cent soln in methyl or ethyl alcohol is used. This soln is stable for about ten days provided it is protected from light. The alcoholic solution is used where precipitation is required to be carried out at a high pH. Another way to prepare the reagent soln is to dissolve 2 g of oxine in 100 ml of 2N-acetic acid. To this soln ammonia soln is gradually added until a turbidity appears. Acetic acid is then added in a dropwise manner so that the solution again becomes clear. The soln is fairly stable if protected from light and can be used when the precipitation is done at a low pH.

(b) The reagent soln is gradually added to metal salt soln until the supernatant liquid acquires a faint yellow colour ; this shows that the slight excess of the reagent has been added. The precipitation is done either in cold solution or at 50—60°C. The ppt is then heated to 70°C for a short period so that small particles coagulate to form bigger particles.

(c) The ppt is filtered through a sintered crucible. The filtrate should have a faint yellow colour indicating a slight excess of the reagent.

(d) The ppt is washed with hot water but if the oxinate of the metal being determined is soluble in hot water then cold water should be used for washing. Washing should be continued until the filtrate becomes colourless. The ppt can also be washed with alcohol provided the ppt is insoluble in alcohol.

(e) The washed ppt is dried at 105—110°C when hydrated oxinate is formed or at 130°—140°C to obtain anhydrous oxinate. If the ppt decomposes at 130—140°C then it is strongly heated to get metal oxide which can be weighed.

(iii) 1-Nitroso-2-napthol (α-Nitroso-β-napthol)

This reagent is a brown powder which is insoluble in water.

The reagent soln is prepared by dissolving 4 g of powder in 100 ml of glacial acetic acid and then adding 100 ml of hot distilled water. The soln is cooled, filtered and used immediately.

This reagent

quantitatively **precipitates**	Co, Iron (III), Pd and Zr	from slightly acidic soln
partially **precipitates**	Sn, Ag, Bi, Cr (III), Ti, tungsten (VI), Uranium (VI) and V (VI)	
does not **precipitate**	Pb, Cd, Hg, As, Sb, Be, Al, Ni, Mn, Zn, Ca and Mg	

This reagent is used mainly for separation of Co from large amounts of Ni from which iron has been previously removed.

On adding the reagent to a cobalt soln in presence of dilute HCl, a red-brown bulky ppt of $Co(C_{10}H_6O_2N)_3$ is formed. Since, the composition of the ppt is doubtful, it is ignited to obtain cobalt oxide which is then reduced to cobalt and weighed as metal provided the amount of cobalt is large.

1-nitroso-2-napthol

(*iv*) **Cupferron.** This reagent which is the ammonium salt of nitrosophenyl hydroxylamine, is soluble in water. Its 6 per cent aqueous soln is used but the soln used for precipitation should be freshly prepared. The reagent forms insoluble compounds with many metals both in weakly acidic and strongly acidic soln. In strongly acidic soln iron (III), vanadium (V), titanium (IV), zirconium (IV), cerium (IV), niobium (V), tantalum (V), tungsten (VI) and tin (IV) are precipitated with this reagent and can be separated from aluminium, beryllium, chromium, manganese, nickel cobalt, zinc, uranium (VI), calcium, strontium and barium.

This reagent is mainly used for separations such as iron and titanium from aluminium.

While precipitating metals with cupferron, the following points should be remembered :

(*a*) The solid reagent should be protected from light by storing it in a dark-coloured bottle.

(*b*) Since the reagent soln is not very stable, its 6 per cent soln should be prepared just before use.

(*c*) The precipitation should always be done in cold because cupferron decomposes at higher temperature. (Nitric acid or other oxidising agents should not be present during the precipitation since the reagent is easily oxidised).

(d) The precipitate formed should be filtered as soon as possible since the cupferron (which is present as excess) is not very stable in acid solution.

(e) The ppt cannot be weighed after drying but has to be ignited to the oxide which is weighed.

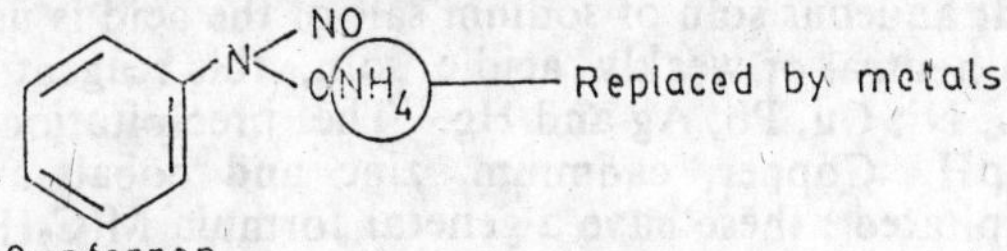

Cupferron

[Note. Neo-cupferron is ammonium salt of N-nitroso-N-2-napthyl-hydroxylamine. This reagent forms more insoluble and bulky ppt than cupferron].

(v) α-Benzoinoxime (cupron)

It is a white crystalline solid which is poorly soluble in water but fairly soluble in alcohol. A 2 per cent soln of the reagent in rectified spirit is used.

α-Benzoinoxime is a good reagent for copper with which it forms a green ppt in dilute ammonical soln. The ppt is dried at 110°C to constant weight. By adding tartrate, copper can be separated from Cd, Pb, Ni, Co and Al.

Molybdate and tungstate ions are quantitatively precipitated

from strong acidic soln by means of this reagent. Molybdate complex is ignited at $500-525°C$ to obtain MoO_3 which is then weighed. Chromate, vanadate and palladium (II) are partly precipitated.

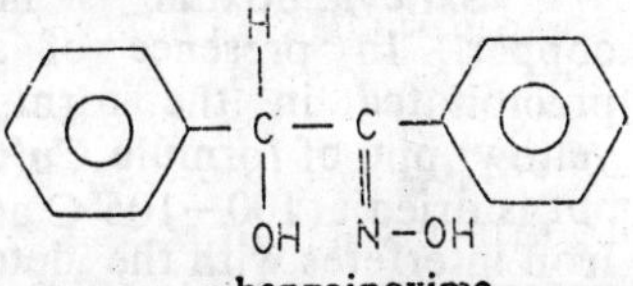

, α-benzoinoxime

(vi) Quinaldic acid

This is an expensive reagent. The reagent soln consists of a 2 % aqueous soln of the acid or its sodium salt.

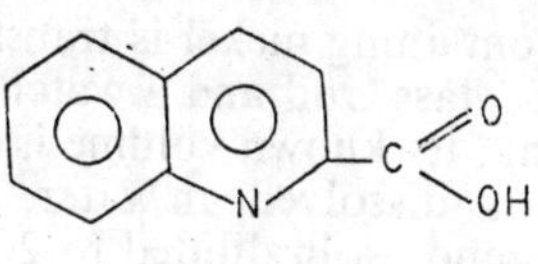

Quinaldic acid

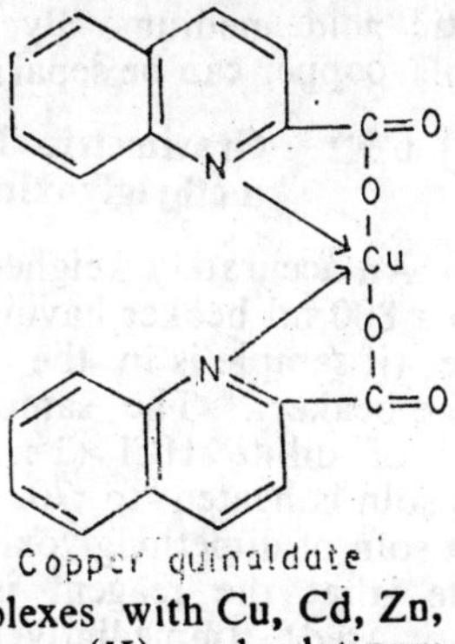

Copper quinaldate

This reagent gives insoluble complexes with Cu, Cd, Zn, Mn, Ag, Co, Ni, Pb, Hg, iron (II), palladium (II) and platinum (II). The precipitates so obtained are influenced by the pH of the solution. For example, cadmium and zinc complexes are soluble in acidic medium as compared to the copper quinaldinate. By properly controlling the pH of the solution copper can be precipitated while cadmium and zinc will remain in solution. Thus, copper can be separated from cadmium and zinc. Many other separations can be achieved by making proper use of complexing reagents.

Copper quinaldate after drying at 110—115°C has a composition represented by $(Cu(C_{10}H_6NO_2)_2 . H_2O$.

(vii) Anthranalic acid

A 3 per cent aqueous soln of sodium salt of the acid is used as reagent. In neutral or weakly acidic soln, this reagent precipitates Zn, Cd, Co, Ni, Cu, Pb, Ag and Hg. The precipitation is done at controlled pH. Copper, cadmium, zinc and cobalt are quantitatively precipitated ; these have a general formula $M(C_7H_6ON)_2$. The ppt. is dried at 105—110°C.

NH2

COO(H) ————Replaced by metals

Anthranilic acid

(viii) Salicylaldoxime

It is a white crystalline solid which is not much soluble in water. Hence, the reagent soln is prepared in water-alcohol mixture.

Copper quinaldate

This reagent reacts with Cu, Pb, Bi, Zn, Ni and Pd.

Salicylaldoxime is mainly used for the determination of copper. In presence of acetic acid (pH of soln 2·6) copper is precipitated in the form of a greenish yellow ppt of formula $Cu(C_7H_6O_2N)_2$. The ppt is dried at 100—105°C and then weighed. Iron interferes with the determination but Ag, Cd, Hg, As and Zn fhave no effect in acetic acid medium. By proper control of pH copper can be separated from nickel.

CH=NOH

OH

Salicyaldoxime

6·9·1. Gravimetric Determination of Nickel as Nickel Dimethylglyoxime

An accurately weighed sample containing nickel is transferred into a 800 ml beaker having a stirring glass rod and a watch-glass cover (if sample is in the form of soln, its known volume is taken in the beaker). The sample material is dissolved in water, about 5 ml of dilute HCl (1 : 1) is added and soln diluted to 200 ml. The soln is heated to 70 to 80° C and about 30 to 40 ml of 1 per cent soln of dimethylglyoxime (DMG) in rectified spirit is added (note that the reagent is insoluble in water hence its alcoholic soln is used). Immediately after this, a soln of ammonia in water is dropwise added with stirring until a red ppt appears (Ni-DMG is soluble in acid hence, its ppt did not appear in acidic medium) and then ammonia soln is added in slight excess. The beaker containing the ppt is kept over a steam bath for about 30 minutes so that the ppt settles down. Test for complete precipitation is done in the supernatant liquid. The ppt is allowed to stand for 1 hour when it cools down. The supernatant liquid is poured through a glass rod into a weighed sintered-glass crucible and the ppt in the beaker is washed with cold water. The ppt is then completely transferred to the crucible with the help of policeman and again washed with cold water until it is free from Cl^- ions. The crucible along with the ppt is kept in an electric oven at 100-120° C for about 1 hour, cooled in a desiccator and weighed. The drying process is repeated until constant weight is obtained. The weight of the ppt of nickel dimethylglyoxime $[Ni (C_4H_7O_2N_2)_2]$ thus becomes known and hence the weight of nickel in the given sample can be calculated.

(The weight of Ni-DMG $\times 0.2031 =$ wt of nickel).

Note. 1. The ppt of Ni-DMG is soluble in acids yet we add DMG to acidic soln of nickel salt and then bring about precipitation of Ni-DMG by neutralising the acid with amonia soln ; this helps in the formation of more easily filterable ppt than that obtained by direct precipitation from ammonical soln.

2. Only a slight excess of DMG should be added because it is not very soluble in water and, if present in large excess, may precipitate. Further, if alcohol is used to dissolve this excess DMG, some of the ppt of Ni-DMG may also dissolve.

6'10. ELECTROGRAVIMETRY

In electrogravimetric analysis, the given soln, containing ions of the element to be determined, is electrolysed. The element gets deposited on an electrode which has been previously weighed. This electrode is weighed again after the deposition is complete. From the difference in two weights, the amount of the element in the given soln can be found out. In fact ordinary gravimetric analysis and electrogravimetric analysis are quite similar. The only difference is that in the latter, in place of a crucible an electrode is used and no reagent is added as a precipitant but electric current deposits the element on a particular electrode. Here the advantage is that filtration is avoided and if the conditions of electrolysis are properly controlled, codeposition, i.e., deposition of other metals present in the soln, can also be avoided.

6'10'1. Electrodeposition of Metals

In electrogravimetry there are two important points that must be considered.

[A] The deposit of the metal on the electrode must be dense, smooth and should stick to the electrode surface so that no material is lost during the washing, drying and weighing of the electrode. The formation of such a deposit is favoured by the following conditions :

(i) The metal should be deposited from a soln in which it is present as a complex ion rather than as a simple ion. For example, if $AgNO_3$ soln is given, sufficient KCN should be added to it so that $[Ag(CN)_2]^-$ complex ions are formed and then electrolysis should be carried out.

(*ii*) The soln during electrolysis should be kept at about 70 to 80° C and should be constantly stirred.

(*iii*) The current strength used for electrolysis also influences the nature of deposit, hence, it should be suitably regulated.

[B] The electrolysis of a soln begins only when certain minimum exernal E.M.F. is applied—this is called *decomposition potential*. Hence, in order to bring about electrodeposition of a metal from a soln, the applied voltage must be greater than the decomposition voltage of the soln.

It has been found that the deposition of a particular metal starts at a particular value of cathode potential—this is called its deposition potential. Suppose we have a soln containing ions of two metals whose deposition potentials are different. If we gradually increase the applied voltage, as soon as the cathode potential exceeds the deposition potential of one of the metals—it will be deposited while the other will remain in the soln. In this way, by properly controlling the cathode potential, electroseperation of metals can be achieved.

6·10·2. Electrogravimetric Determination of Copper

To 100 ml of soln containing 0·2 to 0·3 g of Cu, 2 ml of concentrated H_2SO_4 and 1 ml of concentrated HNO_3 are added

A = Ammeter

B = Battery

Rh = Rheostat

K = Key

V = Voltmeter

P = Platinum electrodes

S = Electrolyte solution

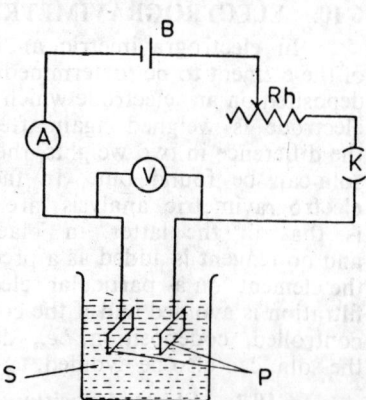

Fig. 6·9. Electrodeposition.

and soln is kept in an electrolysis vessel. Platinum electrodes are used for electrolysis. The platinum electrode which is to be made the cathode is cleaned with hot dilute HNO_3, washed thoroughly with distilled water, dried completely at 100-110° C and weighed. The circuit is arranged as shown in Fig. 6·9. A voltage of 3-4 volts is applied, current strength is adjusted to 2 to 4 amperes and soln is stirred. After about 30 minutes, a drop of the soln is taken out and tested with H_2S water. If no black ppt appears it means that all the copper has been deposited. The cathode is than carefully taken out, washed, dried and weighed. From the increase in the weight of the cathode, the amount of copper present in the soln is calculated.

7

Titrimetric Analysis

It has already been mentioned that the methods of quantitative analysis can be divided into two categories. The quantitative procedures which make use of instruments, such as a colorimeter, a conductivity bridge or a potentiometer etc., are classified under *instrumental* or *physicochemical* methods of analysis. Gravimetric and volumetric methods constitute what is known as the *classical chemical analysis.*

The final or the measurement step of a volumetric method is the measurement of volume. Volumetric methods can be divided into the following three types depending on whether the volume of a gas or that of a soln is measured.

(*i*) *Gas analysis.* Suppose we have a known volume (X ml) of a mixture containing CO_2 and H_2 gases. If this gas mixture is bubbled through NaOH soln, all the CO_2 is absorbed and the gas coming out of the soln will be H_2 whose volume can be measured. If the volume of H_2 gas is found to be Y ml, then the volume of CO_2 will be (X—Y) ml. Thus the gas mixture can be quantitatively analysed. This type of analysis is known as gas analysis.

(*ii*) *Gasometric analysis.* Suppose we have a definite amount of a sample containing a substance, which on treatment with another substance, is completely decomposed giving out a gas as one of the products. Now, if this decomposition takes place according to a chemical equation and if we measure the volume of the liberated gas, it is possible to calculate the amount of the substance present in the given amount of the sample. This type of method of quantitative analysis is called a gasometric method.

Example 7(*i*)

A sample (0˙1603 g) containing hydrazine was treated with lead dioxide. Hydrazine was completely decomposed into H_2O and

N_2 gas. The volume of N_2 gas at N.P.T. was found to be 89·6 ml. Calculate the percentage of hydrazine in the sample.

Hydrazine is oxidised by lead dioxide in accordance with the equation :

$$NH_2-NH_2+O_2(PbO_2) \rightarrow 2H_2O+N_2$$
$$(32·05 \text{ g}) \qquad\qquad\qquad (28·01 \text{ g})$$

32·05 g hydrazine$\equiv$28·01 g nitrogen or 1 g mole of N_2

$\equiv$22,400 ml of nitrogen at N.T.P.

22,400 ml of $N_2\equiv$32·05 g hydrazine

$$\therefore \quad 89·6 \text{ ml} \quad \cdots \quad \cdots \quad \frac{89·6}{22,400}\times 32·05 \text{ g}$$

$$=0·1282 \text{ g hydrazine}$$

Now, 0·1603 g sample contains 0·1282 g hydrazine

$$\therefore \quad 100 \text{ g} \quad \cdots \quad \cdots \quad \frac{100\times 0·1282}{0·1603}\%$$

$$=79·98\%.$$

(*iii*) *Titrimetric analysis.* Suppose we are given a soln of a substance (called analyte) and we have to find out its concentration. This can be done by gradually adding soln of another substance (called reagent) until the reaction between the analyte and the reagent is just complete. If we know :

(*a*) chemical equation representing the reaction between the analyte and the reagent,

(*b*) the volume of the sample soln taken,

(*c*) the concentration of the reagent soln, and

(*d*) the volume of the reagent soln required for complete reaction, then the concentration of the sample soln can be calculated. Such methods are known as *titrimetric methods*. These methods are simple and rapid as compared to gravimetric methods, hence titrimetric methods are extensively ueed for the determination of a large number of organic and inorganic compounds.

7·1. GENERAL PRINCIPLE OF TITRIMETRIC ANALYSIS

It has been mentioned above that a titrimetric method makes use of a chemical reaction between the substance to be determined (analyte) and another substance (reagent). This reaction should be fast, quantitative and should take place according to a chemical equation, such as :

$$aA+rR \rightarrow \text{products} \qquad\qquad \cdots(7·1)$$

The above equation tells us that '*a*' molecules of analyte 'A' react with '*r*' molecules of reagent 'R', *i.e.*, a given amount of the analyte will react with a definite amount of the reagent and this amount can be calculated with the help of equation (7·1) (see section 3·1·3).

The titrimetric determination of the analyte with the reagent involves the following steps :

(*i*) A known amount of the reagent is dissolved in a known volume of water so that the concentration of the reagent soln can be calculated. Such a soln is called a *standard soln*. A volumetric flask (see Fig. 7·1) is used to prepare a standard soln.

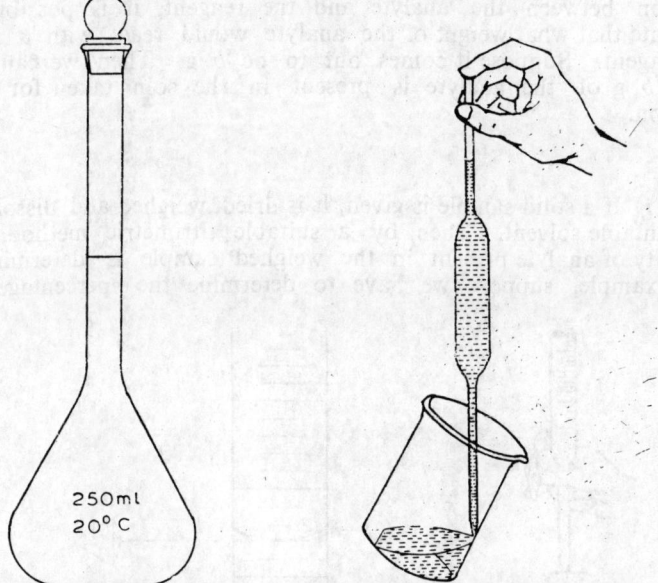

250 ml
20° C

Fig. 7·1. Volumetric or   Fig. 7·2. Adjusting liquid level
        measuring flask.   in a pipette.

(*ii*) With the help of a pipette (see Fig. 7·2), a known volume of the analyte soln is taken in a conical flask. (The analyte soln is also called sample soln, test soln or titrand soln).

. (*iii*) A few drops of an indicator soln are added to the titrand soln, taken in the conical flask. The function of the indicator is to show when the reaction between the analyte and the reagent is just complete. Indicator shows a colour change at the completion of the reaction.

(*iv*) The standard soln of the reagent, *i.e.*, the titrant soln is taken in a burette and gradually added to the analyte soln taken in the conical flask until the reaction between them is just complete as shown by the colour change of the indicator. This step is known as *titration* which is the most important operation of titrimetric analysis (see Fig. 7·3).

(*v*) The volume of the titrant needed for the complete reaction is recorded, suppose it is 'X' ml. (This is called titre value).

(*vi*) Because the concentration of the reagent soln is known, the quantity of the reagent present in X ml of the soln can be calculated. Suppose this comes out to be '*d*' g.

(*vii*) With the help of the chemical equation representing the reaction between the analyte and the reagent, it is possible to calculate that what weight of the analyte would react with '*d*' g of the reagent. Suppose it comes out to be '*b*' g. Then we can say that '*b*' g of the analyte is present in the soln taken for the titration.

Notes :

(*i*) If a solid sample is given, it is dried, weighed and dissolved in a suitable solvent. Then by a suitable titrimetric method, the quantity of analyte present in the weighed sample is determined. For example, suppose we have to determine the percentage of

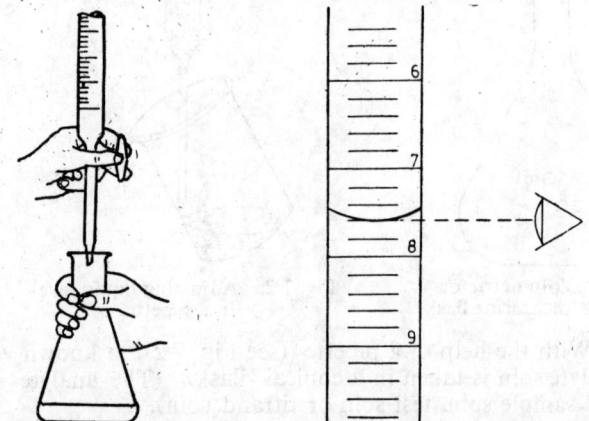

Fig. 7·3. Titration process.   Fig. 7·4.   Noting the burette reading.

manganese in a sample of its ore. A portion of the ore will be dried, weighed and dissolved in HCl. By a suitable titration the quantity of manganese in the weighed sample will then be determined. If '*a*' g of the ore-sample contains '*b*' g of manganese then 100 *b*/*a* will be the percentage of manganese in the ore.

(*ii*) Certain substances do not have a definite chemical composition or they are hygroscopic, hence it is not possible to prepare their standard soln by dissolving a weighed amount of the substance in a known volume of water. In such cases, an approximate soln of the reagent is prepared by weighing and this soln is then titrated with a standard soln of some other substance. In this way, the concentration of the reagent soln is determined ; this process is called *standardisation*.

(*iii*) It is not always necessary, to take analyte soln in a conical flask and titrant in a burette. For example, in titrating NaOH (titrand) with HCl (titrant) using methyl orange as indicator, HCl is taken in a burette because then the colour at the end point changes from yellow to red, which is easier to observe rather than that from red to yellow. But when phenolphthalein is used as indicator, a known volume of HCl is taken in a conical flask and titrated with NaOH soln taken in a burette because then the change is colourless to pink which is easier to note rather than that from pink to colourless. In a titration we want to know the volumes of titrand and titrant solutions when the reaction between them is just complete, it is immaterial which of them is taken in a conical flask or in a burette.

7·2. EQUIVALENCE POINT AND END POINT

During a titration, the point at which the reaction between a titrand and a titrant is just complete is called *equivalence point* or *theoretical end point* or *stoichiometric end point*. The point at which an indicator changes its colour is known as the *end point*. If the visible end point coincides with the theoretical end point, the titration is ideal. But in practice there is a very small difference between these two ; this is called the end point error. The volume of the titrant required in a titration is called *titre*.

7·3. FUNDAMENTAL REQUIREMENTS OF A TITRIMETRIC METHOD

In order to develop a titrimetric procedure the following conditions must be fulfilled :

(*i*) The reaction between the titrand and the titrant should take place only in one way, *i.e.*, a single reaction should take place between them. If a side reaction also occurs, it will not be possible to calculate how much titrant was consumed in the main reaction and how much in the side reaction.

(*ii*) The reaction must be well defined, *i.e.*, definite amounts of reactants must react to produce definite amounts of products. There should be a chemical equation representing the reaction so that it is possible to calculate that what amount of analyte must have reacted with a particular amount of the reagent.

(*iii*) The reaction must be rapid so that little time is needed for performing the titration. Most ionic reactions are quite rapid. If the reaction involved is slow it can be accelerated by adding a catalyst.

(*iv*) The reaction must be complete when equivalent amount of reactants are brought together, because titrimetric calculations are based on 100 per cent reaction between the reactants.

(*v*) It should be possible to prepare a standard soln of the reagent which will fulfil the above meationed four conditions.

(*vi*) An indicator must be available to show the completion of the reaction when the addition of the titrant to titrand soln can be stopped.

Example 7(*ii*)

Suppose we are given a soln of NaOH (analyte) whose concentration is to be found out. The first thing is to select a suitable substance (reagent) which will rapidly and stoichiometrically react with NaOH and there would be no side reactions. Benzoic acid (C_6H_5COOH) reacts rapidly and completely with NaOH according to the equation :

$$C_6H_5COOH + NaOH \rightarrow C_6H_5COONa + H_2O$$
$$\underset{122\cdot12\ g}{} \qquad \underset{40\cdot00\ g}{}$$

This equation tells us that $122\cdot12$ g of C_6H_5COOH will react with $40\cdot00$ g of NaOH. Benzoic acid is non-hygroscopic and has a fixed composition, hence its standard soln can be readily prepared by dissolving a known weight of the acid in a known volume of water. (The substances whose standard soln can be directly prepared by weighing are known as primary standards). Phenolphthalein is colourless when added to a soln of benzoic acid but gives a pink colour when the acid is neutralised and there is an extra drop of NaOH soln. In this way, all the conditions are fulfilled, hence benzoic acid can be used as a reagent in the titrimetric determination of NaOH.

The procedure is that a known volume (X ml) of benzoic acid soln is taken in a conical flask and 2 to 3 drops of phenolphthalein indicator are added. The given soln of NaOH is gradually added from a burette with constant shaking until the soln becomes just pink. The addition of alkali soln is then stopped and burette reading is taken. Suppose the volume of NaOH soln required for the complete reaction is Y ml. Because the concentration of benzoic acid soln is known, hence the weight of the acid present in its X ml of soln can be calculated—suppose this comes out to be '*a*' g. Now,

$$122\cdot12 \text{ g } C_6H_5COOH \equiv 40 \text{ g NaOH}$$

$$\therefore \quad 'a' \text{ g} \quad \cdots \quad \cdots \quad \frac{a \times 40}{122 \cdot 12} \text{ g}$$

Thus, $a \times 40/122 \cdot 12$ g of NaOH will be present in Y ml of alkali soln.

7·4. STANDARD SOLUTIONS

A soln whose concentration is accurately known is called a *standard solution*. There are two methods by which a standard soln may be prepared.

(A) **DIRECT METHOD.** An exactly weighed amount of the substance, of definite and known composition is dissolved and made up to known volume in a volumetric flask. From the known weight and volume, the concentration of the soln is calculated.

Standard soln, by direct method, can be prepared of only those substances which fulfil the following conditions :

(*i*) The substance must be either 100% pure or at least of known purity. For example, suppose 0·2000 g Na_2CO_3 is weighed whose purity is only 98·5% (rest 1·5% is NaCl) then the actual weight of Na_2CO_3 will be taken as

$$0 \cdot 2000 \times 98 \cdot 5/100 = 0 \cdot 1970 \text{ g.}$$

(*ii*) The impurity must not react with either analyte or reagent. In the above example, Na_2CO_3 contains NaCl as impurity. Because NaCl does not react with Na_2CO_3 or HCl, hence Na_2CO_3 can be used as a reagent for titrating HCl.

(*iii*) Tests should be available for knowing the impurities present in the substance.

(*iv*) Before weighing, the substance is dried to remove moisture. The substance should be stable during drying at the oven temperature.

(*v*) The substance should not absorb moisture or should not react with oxygen or carbon dioxide during weighing.

(*vi*) The reaction of the substance with the analyte should be single, rapid, complete and stoichiometric.

A substance which fulfils above condition is called a primary standard.

(B) **INDIRECT METHOD.** Many substances to be used as titrants are not primary standards, hence their standard solutions cannot be prepared directly by weighing. For example, in the case of sodium thiosulphate ($Na_2S_2O_3.5H_2O$) there is always some uncertainty about its water content, so its standard soln cannot be prepared by the direct method. A soln of approximate concentration of $Na_2S_2O_3$ is first prepared by weighing and then it is titrated with a standard soln of KIO_3, which is a primary standard. With the help of this titration, the exact concentration of thiosulphate soln can be calculated. This process is known as standardisation.

7·5. DETECTION OF END POINT

The end point of a titration is detected by a sudden change in some property of the reaction mixture. In most cases the end points are located either by visual observation of the change or by measurement of some electrical property of the reaction mixture.

[A] VISUAL METHODS

(i) *The titrant may act as a self-indicator.* In titrating a soln containing Fe^{2+} ions with that of $KMnO_4$ taken in a burette, $KMnO_4$ is reduced by Fe^{2+} ions to a colourless product. When all the Fe^{2+} ions are converted to Fe^{3+} ions, the next added drop of $KMnO_4$ soln imparts pink colour to the reaction mixture.

(ii) *A change of colour of the added indicator solution.* In titrating $K_2Cr_2O_7$ soln with iron (II) soln, ferroin is used as an indicator. This indicator has a greenish blue colour in $K_2Cr_2O_7$ soln. After the completion of the reaction, an extra drop of iron (II) soln turns the reaction mixture red.

(iii) *Formation of a soluble product.* A soln of $HgCl_2$ can be titrated with KI soln. First a red ppt of HgI_2 is formed which reacts with more KI to form a soluble colourless complex K_2HgI_4. The disappearance of the red ppt is the end point of the titration.

(iv) *Appearance of a precipitate.* Mercuric nitrate reacts with a chloride soln in accordance with the equation.

$$Hg(NO_3)_2 + 2KCl \longrightarrow HgCl_2 + 2KNO_3$$

Mercuric nitrate is a strong electrolyte, hence gives Hg^{2+} ions but $HgCl_2$ is a poor electrolyte. Now, sodium nitroprusside reacts with Hg^{2+} ions to form a white ppt. Hence, when $Hg(NO_3)_2$ soln is gradually added to a chloride soln containing little sodium nitroprusside, a white turbidity appears when all the chloride has reacted and a drop of $Hg(NO_3)_2$ soln is added in excess.

(v) *Formation of a soluble coloured product.* In the titration of silver with a soln of thiocyanate using ferric salt soln as indicator, Ag^+ ions are completely precipitated by thiocyanate ions :

$$Ag^+ + CNS^- \longrightarrow AgCNS \text{ (white ppt)}$$

The next drop of thiocyanate produces a red colour due to the reaction :

$$Fe^{3+} + CNS^- \longrightarrow Fe(CNS)^{2+} \text{ (red soln)}$$

The appearance of red colour thus indicates the end point of the titration.

(vi) *Formation of a coloured ppt.* Silver ions react with Cl^- ions to form a white ppt of AgCl and with CrO_4^{2-} ions to form a red ppt of Ag_2CrO_4. If a soln of $AgNO_3$ is gradually added to a chloride soln containing little K_2CrO_4, a red ppt of Ag_2CrO_4 will appear as soon as all the Cl^- ions have been precipitated and an extra drop of $AgNO_3$ soln is added. (The solubility of AgCl is smaller than that of Ag_2CrO_4, hence AgCl is precipitated first.)

(vii) *External indicators.* Potassium ferricyanide acts as an external indicator in the titration of iron(II) soln with $K_2Cr_2O_7$. Ferricyanide ion reacts with iron(II) to form a blue ppt. The titration of iron(II) is done by adding $K_2Cr_2O_7$ soln very gradually from a burette. At different stages of the titration, a drop of the reaction mixture is taken out and added to potassium ferricyanide soln. The point at which this soln ceases to turn blue is the end point of the titration (after the completion of the reaction there are no Fe^{2+} ions left, hence the indicator soln does not turn blue).

[B] **ELECTRICAL METHODS.** There are several titrations in which end point is located by measuring the change in some electrical properties of the titration mixture during the course of the titration. Later a graph is plotted between the magnitude of the electrical property and corresponding volumes of the titrant added. A sudden change in the graph gives the end point of the titration. Such titrations are known as electrometric titrations. These generally involve the measurement of potential (potentiometric), conductance (conductometric), current strength (amperometric) or quantity of electricity (coulometric titrations). These will be dealt in some detail in Chapter 14.

7·6. INDIRECT TITRATIONS

In a direct titration a known volume of an analyte is titrated with a standard soln of a reagent (taken in a burette) or, a known volume of the reagent soln can be titrated with the analyte soln (taken in a burette). For example, iodine soln can be titrated with a standard soln of thiosulphate or, HCl can be titrated with standard NaOH soln. In these titrations, at the equivalence point, neither the analyte nor the reagent is present in excess.

If the reaction between the analyte and the reagent is slow, the direct titration will take too much time for completion and is, therefore, not practicable. In such cases, those conditions are used which are helpful in accelerating the reaction rate, such as adding excess of reagent or heating the reaction mixture. To a known volume of the analyte soln, a known excess (100 to 200%) of the reagent is added. The reaction mixture is heated or kept for some time so that the reaction is complete. Then the unreacted reagent is determined by titration with another suitable reagent. Such titrations are known as indirect titrations. Knowing the amount of the reagent consumed, the quantity of the analyte is found out by stoichiometric calculations.

Example 7(iii)

A sample soln containing HCOOH was heated with an excess of $KMnO_4$ soln (containing 'a' g of $KMnO_4$). After the completion of the reaction, the unconsumed $KMnO_4$ was determined by titration with a standard soln of oxalic acid. Suppose, the amount of $KMnO_4$ left unreacted came out to be 'b' gm, then $(a-b)$ g is the quantity of $KMnO_4$ that has been consumed in the reaction. It is then possible to find out the quantity of HCOOH that has reacted with $(a-b)$ g of $KMnO_4$ by making use of chemical equation representing the reaction of HCOOH with $KMnO_4$.

7.7. MINIMISATION OF THE TITRATION ERROR

In performing a titration, the following points must be considered in order to keep the titration error at a minimum.

(i) The amount of sample weighed should not be too small otherwise weighing error will be considerable. For example, if there is a weighing error of 0.2 mg in 100 mg, the percentage error is 0.2. If the same error is in 2000 mg, the percentage error will be 0.01. A sample of at least 0.200 g must be taken.

(ii) The concentration of the titrant should be so chosen that the titre value is not too small. Suppose in a titration, the burette used can read up to 0.1 ml. If the titre value is 5.0 ml, error of 0.1 ml means 2% error in the titration. If the titre is about 50 ml the percentage error will be only 0.2. The volume of the titrant should not be more than 50 ml because then burette has to be refilled which is inconvenient. Furthermore, in the second addition, the volume measured may be small, consequently error percentage will be greater.

(iii) The sample taken should not be so large that burette has to be filled a second time. For example, suppose the titre value is 55.0 ml, then the second time we are reading only 5.0 ml. If in this volume the error is 0.1 ml, there will be an additional error on the total volume.

(iv) Indicator blank should be determined and this should be subtracted from the titre value. Suppose in a titration, the reaction is complete when 10.0 ml of titrant is added but the change in the colour of the indicator is observed only when the burette reading is 10.2 ml. Then the equivalence point and the end point of the titration would differ by 0.2 ml. This problem can be largely solved by using the similar titration for the standardisation of the reagent, as is used for the titration of the sample. For example, if we have to titrate a given soln of oxalic acid with NaOH, the alkali should be standardised by titration with a standard soln of oxalic acid (note that the titre values in the two titrations should be as close as possible). In some cases, distilled water is used in place of analyte soln and the volume of titrant required to produce the colour is noted this is known as *indicator blank*. The indicator blank is subtracted from the titre value in a titration.

(v) In order to have reliable result, a titration must be carried out a number of times until at least three values closely agree. The titration should also be repeated with varying amounts of sample.

7·8. TYPES OF REACTIONS IN TITRIMETRIC ANALYSIS

There are several reactions which meet all the fundamental requirements for acting as a basis of titrimetric methods. For the sake of convenience and in order to define equivalency, these reactions have been divided into four categories :

(i) Neutralisation or acid-base reactions.
(ii) Oxidation-reduction or redox reactions.
(iii) Precipitation reactions, and
(iv) Complex forming or complexation reactions.

The applications of these reactions to titrimetry (titrimetric analysis) will be considered in detail in Chapters 8, 9, 10 and 11.

7·9. CALCULATIONS IN TITRIMETRIC ANALYSIS

The purpose of a titrimetric method is to determine the concentration (N_1) of the given analyte soln. This is achieved by taking a known volume (V_1) of the analyte soln and adding to it a soln of a reagent of known concentration (N_2). The point at which the reaction between the analyte and the reagent is complete, the addition of reagent is stopped and its volume (V_2) is recorded. The value of N_1 is then calculated with the help of the following relationship.

$$V_1 \times N_1 = V_2 \times N_2$$

Because V_1, V_2 and N_2 are known, the value of N_1 can be calculated (for the derivation of the above relationship see Chapter 8).

Notes. (1) Sometimes a known volume (V_2) of the reagent of known concentration (N_2) is titrated with analyte soln whose concentration (N_1) is to be determined. By carrying out the titration, the volume of the analyte (V_1) which is chemically equivalent to the amount of the reagent taken is found out.

(2) At the equivalence point of a titration, the amount of the analyte is chemically equivalent to the amount of the reagent.

(3) The concentrations of the analyte and reagent (N_1 and N_2) are expressed in g equivalents present per litre. The concept of chemical equivalence and that of g equivalent are discussed in greater detail in Chapter 8.

8

Aqueous Acid-Base Titrimetry

An acid-base titration (or neutralisation titration) is based upon the chemical reaction between an acid and a base. Titrations involving acids and bases are extensively used in the analytical control of many commercial and industrial pruducts. The purpose of this chapter is to discuss the practical aspects as well as underlying theory of acid-base titrimetry in aqueous solutions.

8·1. CONCEPT OF ACIDITY AND BASICITY

According to the classical theory (Arrhenius theory) of dissociation, an acid is a substance which when dissolved in water gives H^+ ions, and a base is a substance which on dissolution in water furnishes OH^- ions (the modern concepts of acids and bases will be discussed in Chapter 9). For example,

HCl	$\rightleftharpoons H^+ + Cl^-$ (strongly dissociated)	...(8·1)
CH_3COOH	$\rightleftharpoons H^+ + CH_3COO^-$ (poorly dissociated)	...(8·2)
$NaOH$	$\rightleftharpoons Na^+ + OH^-$ (strongly dissociated)	...(8·3)
NH_4OH	$\rightleftharpoons NH_4^+ + OH^-$ (poorly dissociated)	...(8·4)

8·1·1. Strengths of Acids and Bases

A soln of HCl in water is strongly dissociated, i.e., its degree of dissociation, α, is quite high, hence it is called a strong acid. The value of α for CH_3COOH is small, hence it is a weak acid. Similarly in aqueous solutions, NaOH is a strong base while NH_4OH is a weak base (see 4·4·3).

8.2. ADVANTAGES OF ACID-BASE TITRATIONS

The neutralisation reaction between an acid and a base is quite fast—practically instantaneous. The common ionic reaction in all neutralisation processes is :

$$H^+ + OH^- \rightarrow H_2O \qquad\qquad ...(8.5)$$

Apart from being fast, neutralisation reactions are :

(i) single (free from side reactions),

(ii) proceed to completion, and

(iii) are stoichiometric (the amounts of the reactants and those of the products are as per chemical equation representing the reaction).

For the above-mentioned reasons, neutralisation or acid-base reactions are very suitable for titrimetric analysis.

8.3. THE CONCEPT OF EQUIVALENCE

Consider the reaction between HCl and NaOH :

$$\underset{(36.5)}{HCl} + \underset{(40.0)}{NaOH} \rightarrow \underset{(58.5)}{NaCl} + \underset{(18.0)}{H_2O} \qquad ...(8.6)$$

This reaction tells us that 36.5 parts by weight of HCl will combine with 40.0 parts by weight of NaOH to produce 58.5 parts by weight of NaCl and 18.0 parts by weight of H_2O (see 3.1.2).

In other words, we can say that 36.5 parts by weight of HCl are chemically equivalent (represented by $\equiv$) to 40.0 parts by weight of NaOH. Thus,

$$36.5 \text{ g HCl} \equiv 40.0 \text{ g NaOH}$$

or $\qquad\qquad 36.5 \text{ kg HCl} \equiv 40.0 \text{ kg NaOH}$

or $\qquad\qquad 36.5 \text{ mg HCl} \equiv 40.0 \text{ mg NaOH}$

If to 36.5 g HCl, 100.0 g NaOH is added, only 40.0 g alkali will react (which is chemically equivalent to 36.5 g HCl) and rest 60.0 g will remain unreacted. Likewise, if we add 100.0 g HCl to 40.0 g NaOH, only 36.5 g acid will react and the remainder (100—36.5) =63.5 g will remain unreacted. This is the principle of chemical equivalence.

8.4. EQUIVALENT WEIGHT

The equivalent weight (eq. wt.) of a substance is defined as the parts by weight of that substance which is chemically equivalent to 1.008 parts by weight of hydrogen (or 8 parts by weight of oxygen or 35.45 parts by weight of chlorine). Thus, in finding out eq wt of a substance, we find out how many g of that substance are directly or indirectly chemically equivalent to 1.008 g of hydrogen.

156   ANALYTICAL CHEMISTRY

Example 8(i)

On analysis it was found that 40·0 g of magnesium oxide (MgO) is produced by the combination of 24·0 g of Mg and 16·0 g of O_2. So,

$$16·0 \text{ g } O_2 \equiv 24·0 \text{ g Mg} \qquad \qquad ...(8\text{-}A)$$

Similarly, it was found that 18·0 g water is produced by the combination of 2·0 g of H_2 and 16·0 g of O_2. So,

$$16·0 \text{ g } O_2 \equiv 2·0 \text{ g } H_2 \qquad \qquad ...(8\text{-}B)$$

By combining (8-A) and (8-B), we get,

$$2·0 \text{ g } H_2 \equiv 16·0 \text{ g } O_2 \equiv 24·0 \text{ g Mg}$$
$$\therefore \qquad 1·0 \text{ g } H_2 \equiv 8·0 \text{ g } O_2 \equiv 12·0 \text{ g Mg}$$

or, in general,

1·0 parts by weight of H_2 $\equiv$ 8·0 parts by weight of O_2
$\equiv$ 12·0 parts by weight of Mg

Hence, the eq wt of O_2 will be 8·0 and that of Mg will be 12·0.

The eq wt of a substance is not a constant quantity but its value depends upon the reaction in which it is taking part.

8·4·1. Gram-Equivalent

The gram-equivalent (g eq) of a substance is the number of grams of the reagent which, in a given reaction, corresponds to a gram-atom or gram-ion (1·008 g) of hydrogen. In other words, a g eq of a substance is its eq wt expressed in g. The eq wt of HCl in acid-base reactions is 36·5, hence its one g eq means 36·5 g of HCl. The value of the g eq of the same substance can be different in different reactions.

8·4·2. Equivalent Weight in Acid-Base Reactions

The eq wt of an acid is that weight of it which contains one replaceable hydrogen, i.e. 1·008 g of hydrogen. For example 35·46 g HCl contains 1·008 g of replaceable hydrogen, hence eq wt of HCl will be 35·46, and a g eq of HCl means 35·46 g of HCl. It should be noted that mol wt of HCl is also 35·46. Thus for HCl, the mol wt and eq wt are equal.

An acid whose molecule contains only one replaceable (or ionisable) hydrogen is called a *monobasic acid* (or its basicity is said to be one). For example, HCl, HBr, HI, $HClO_4$ and HNO_3 are monobasic acids. For such an acid, the eq wt is equal to its mol wt. A molecule of acetic acid (CH_3COOH) contains four hydrogen atoms but only one of them, i.e., the one present in COOH group is ionisable, hence acetic acid also is a monobasic acid.

There are certain acids, such as, H_2SO_4 and H_2CO_3, whose molecules contain two replaceable hydrogens ; these are called *dibasic acids*. Now,

$$2H \equiv H_2SO_4$$

2·016 parts by wt $\equiv$ 98·082 parts by wt (mol wt)

∴ 1·008 parts by wt $\equiv$ 49·041 parts by wt (eq wt)

Thus for dibasic acids :

$$eq\ wt = \frac{mol\ wt}{2}$$

Similarly, it will be seen that for a tribasic acid like H_3PO_4 :

$$eq\ wt = \frac{mol\ wt}{3}$$

The *basicity* of an acid is defined as the number of ionisable hydrogen atoms present in a molecule of the acid. For example, the basicity of HCl is 1, that of H_2SO_4 is 2 and for H_3PO_4 it is 3. The eq wt of an acid is related to its mol wt by the following relationship :

$$eq\ wt = mol\ wt/basicity \qquad \qquad ...(8\text{-}C)$$

The eq wt of a base is that weight of it which contains 17·008 g ionisable hydroxyl group. The molecules of bases like NaOH, KOH, LiOH etc., have only one ionisable hydroxyl group, hence for them eq wt is equal to mol wt. In the case of $Ca(OH)_2$ or $Ba(OH)_2$, the eq wt will be half the mol wt (Although CH_3OH contains hydroxyl group but it does not ionise, hence CH_3OH cannot be regarded as a base).

8·5. EXPRESSING CONCENTRATION OF A SOLUTION

In titrimetric analysis a titration is performed between an analyte and a reagent soln. For titrimetric calculations the concentration of the reagent soln must be known. Now, the concentration of a solute can be expressed in a number of ways.

(i) *As weight per unit volume.* A standard soln of $AgNO_3$ reagent may be prepared by dissolving 10 g of solid $AgNO_3$ in water, diluting the soln to 1 litre and shaking the soln thoroughly. The concentration of the soln can be expressed by saying that it contains 10 g of $AgNO_3$ per litre (or 10 mg per ml). It can also be called a 1 per cent soln.

(ii) *By mentioning the weight of the solute and that of the solvent.* Such as, 20 g of KCl dissolved in 1000 g of water.

(iii) *In terms of molarity.* Gram-molecular weight or g mole or simply mole of a substance means its mol wt expressed in g. The mol wt of H_2SO_4 is 98·08, so, its one mole would mean 98·08 g of

H_2SO_4. A soln containing one mole of a substance per litre is known as its molar solution. A soln containing 98·08 g of H_2SO_4 per litre will be a molar soln of H_2SO_4 ; if this amount is 98·08/2, *i.e.*, 49·04 g per litre, then the soln will be M/2 or 0·5 molar (or molarity of the soln will be said to be 0·5). In general,

$$\frac{\text{wt of substance in g/litre}}{\text{mol wt}} = \text{molarity} \qquad ...(8\text{-}D)$$

In above example, weight of H_2SO_4 per litre is 49·04 g and mol wt of H_2SO_4 is 98·08. So

$$\text{molarity} = \frac{49·04}{98·08} = 0·5.$$

Molarity of a soln can also be calculated by finding out the number of moles of the substance present in 1 litre of its soln.

Example 8(*ii*)

We are given the following four solutions whose molarities are to be calculated :

    (*a*) 80 g NaOH in 1 litre soln,

    (*b*) 80 g NaOH in 5 litre soln,

    (*c*) 10 g NaOH in 1 litre soln, and

    (*d*) 10 g NaOH in 2 litre soln.

(The mol wt of NaOH is 40 ; so, its one mole means 40 g of NaOH).

Solution. (*a*). 40 g NaOH means 1 mole of NaOH

∴   80 g   ···   **2 moles** of NaOH

Thus, 2 moles of NaOH are present per litre of soln ; so, the molarity will also be 2.

The same result can be obtained by using relationship (8-D) ; weight of NaOH present per litre is 80 g and mol wt of NaOH is 40, so :

$$\text{Molarity} = \frac{\text{wt present per litre}}{\text{mol wt}} = \frac{80}{40} = 2.$$

(*b*) In 5 litre soln we have 80 g or 2 moles of NaOH.

∴   In 1 litre   ·   2/5 = 0·4 mole of NaOH

Because 0·4 mole of NaOH is present in a litre, the molarity will be 0·4. Or, weight present per litre = 80/5, *i.e.*, 16 g,

$$\text{molarity} = \frac{\text{wt present per litre}}{\text{mol wt}} = \frac{16}{40} = 0·4$$

(c) Ten g NaOH, *i.e.*, $10/40 = 0.25$ mole of NaOH is present in 1 litre, hence the molarity will be 0.25. (Note that, wt present per litre/mol wt, gives the number of moles present per litre of soln).

(d) Two litre soln has 10 g NaOH, so 1 litre will contain 5 g. Now,

$$\text{number of moles} = \frac{\text{wt present per litre}}{\text{mol wt}} = \frac{5}{40} = 0.125.$$

Thus, 0.125 mole is present in a litre of soln, hence, the molarity of the soln will be 0.125.

(iv) *In terms of normality.* A gram-equivalent (g eq) of a substance means its eq wt expressed in g. For example, the eq wt of HCl is 36.5, hence, its one g eq will contain 36.5 g of HCl. If a soln contains 1 g eq of a substance per litre, it is called a *normal solution* or its normality is said to be 1 ; such a soln is denoted as 1 N soln. If we have 1 g eq of HCl (36.5 g HCl) in 1 litre of a soln, it will be called a normal soln of HCl or the normality of the soln will said to be 1 ; such a soln is written as 1 N HCl soln. Now :

36.5 g HCl means 1 g eq of HCl

∴ 18.25 g HCl ··· 1/2 or 0.5 g eq of HCl

If we have 18.25 g HCl present in a litre of a soln, it will contain 0.5 g eq of HCl and normality of the soln will be 0.5. Thus normality is defined as the number of gram-equivalents present in a, litre of the given soln.

Table 8.1. Normalities of Different HCl Solutions

HCl (in g) present per litre	HCl (in g eq) present per litre	Normality	Soln denoted as
73.0	73/36.5 = 2	2	2N
36.5	36.5/36.5 = 1	1	1N (Normal)
18.25	18.25/36.5 = 0.5	0.5	0.5N (semi-normal)
3.65	3.65/36.5 = 0.1	0.1	0.1N (decinormal)
0.365	0.365/36.5 = 0.01	0.01	0.01N (centinormal)
	(eq wt of HCl = 36.5)		

We have already seen that HCl is a monobasic acid. The eq wt of HCl is, therefore, equal to its mol wt ; for a monobasic acid, the molar and normal solutions are identical. A soln of HCl which contains 36·5 g of the acid per litre will be a molar soln and also a normal soln of HCl. But for a polybasic acid (whose molecule contains more than one ionisable hydrogens) this is not true. For example, the basicity of H_2SO_4 is 2 and its mol wt is 98·08.

The eq wt of H_2SO_4 is given by :

$$\text{eq wt} = \frac{\text{mol wt}}{\text{basicity}} = \frac{98·08}{2} = 49·04$$

Thus, one g mole of H_2SO_4 means 98·08 g of the acid but its one g eq will be equal to only 49·04 g of H_2SO_4. If a soln of H_2SO_4 contains 98·08 g of the acid per litre, it will be called 1 M soln, but because it contains 2 g eq of the acid per litre, it will be 2N soln of H_2SO_4. The normality and molarity of an acid soln can be related through its basicity as is shown by the following relationship :

normality of an acid=molarity × basicity

Because, the basicity of H_2SO_4 is 2, hence its 0·1 M soln will be regarded as 0·2N H_2SO_4 soln. A soln 0·1 M in H_3PO_4 (basicity equal to 3) is the same as its 0·3N soln.

Similar considerations apply to solutions of bases. The normality of a 0·05M soln of NaOH will be the same, i.e., 0·05 because a molecule of NaOH contains only one ionisable hydroxyl group. But in a molecule of $Ca(OH)_2$, there are two ionisable hydroxyl groups, hence the normality of 0·05 M soln of $Ca(OH)_2$ will be 2×0·5, i.e., 0·1. (For formality and formal soln, see 3·2·2).

8·6. EXPRESSING CONCENTRATION OF SOLUTIONS IN TITRIMETRIC ANALYSIS IN TERM OF NORMALITY

In section 8·5, we have described the different ways of expressing concentration of a soln. The most convenient method, however, of expressing the concentrations of solutions in titrimetric work is with reference to eq wt, i.e., using the concept of normality. This point can be readily understood by considering the following example.

Example 8(iii)

Consider the reaction :

$$NaOH + HCl \rightarrow NaCl + H_2O$$

eq wt	40·0	36·5
g eq	40·0 g	36·5 g

Suppose, we have a soln which contains 40·0 g of NaOH (1 g eq of NaOH) and we gradually add to it a soln of HCl. As soon as the amount of the added HCl becomes 36·5 g (1 g eq of HCl), the reaction between NaOH and HCl will be just complete. Thus, exactly 1 g eq of HCl is needed to completely react with 1 g eq of NaOH. In general, at the end point, the number of g eq of the substance titrated is equal to the number of g eq of the reagent used for the titration. Now, the normality of a soln is defined as the number of g eq present per litre of the soln.

Hence, we may write :

$$\text{normality} = \frac{\text{number of gram-equivalents}}{\text{number of litres}}$$

[Note that :

1 g = 1000 milligram (mg)

1 litre = 1000 millilitre (ml)

1 g eq = 1000 milligram-equivalent (meq)]

We can also write :

$$\text{normality} = \frac{\text{number of milligram-equivalents (meq)}}{\text{number of millilitres (ml)}}$$

Hence, no of meq = normality × no. of ml.

Suppose, for the titration of V_A ml of substance A (analyte whose normality N_A is to be determined), V_B ml of the reagent soln of normality N_B are required. Then :

no. of meq of A = $N_A \times V_A$ and

no. of meq of B = $N_B \times V_B$

At the end point :

no. of meq of A = no. of meq of B

$$N_A \times V_A = N_B \times V_B \qquad \qquad \text{...(8-E)}$$

or,
$$N_A = \frac{N_B \times V_B}{V_A} \qquad \qquad \text{...(8-F)}$$

If volume and normality of the titrant soln and the volume of the analyte soln is known, the normality of the analyte soln can be easily calculated with the help of the relationship (8-F).

It has been seen that :

$$\text{normality of soln} = \frac{\text{no. of g eq present}}{\text{no. of litres of soln}} \qquad \text{...(8-G)}$$

Also,

$$\text{no. of g eq} = \frac{\text{wt in g}}{\text{eq wt}} \qquad \qquad \text{...(8-H)}$$

Substituting (8-H) in the relationship (8-G), we get :

$$normality = \frac{wt\ it\ g}{eq\ wt \times no.\ of\ litres}$$

or, $$normality \times eq\ wt = \frac{wt\ in\ g}{no.\ of\ litres}$$

or,   normality×eq wt=wt in g of the substance per litre of the soln.   ...(8-I)

The normality of the analyte soln is determined by means of (8-F) and then the weight of the analyte in g present per litre can be calculated with the help of the relationship (8-I).

From the above discussion it is evident that if equivalent system is followed, the titrimetric calculations become quite easy and simple. If we do not follow the equivalent system, the titrimetric calculations are lengthy and complicated as shown by the following example.

Example 8(*iv*)

Suppose a soln of NaOH is given and we have to find out the weight of NaOH present per litre. A standard soln of HCl is prepared which contains, say, 36·5 g HCl per litre (it is 1N). On titrating it is found that 25 ml of the alkali soln requires 20 ml of the acid soln. Now, two methods can be used for calculating the amount of NaOH present per litre.

(A) In the first method the following steps are involved :

(*i*) The quantity of HCl in 20 ml soln is calculated.

1000 ml contain 36·5 g HCl

∴   20 ml contain $\frac{20}{1000} \times 36 \cdot 5 = 0 \cdot 73$ g of HCl.

(*ii*) We know that 36·5 g HCl react with 40·0 g NaOH [see equation (8·6)].

36·5 g HCl react with 40·0 g NaOH,

∴   0·73 g HCl react with $\frac{0 \cdot 73}{36 \cdot 5} \times 40 \cdot 0 = 0 \cdot 8$ g of NaOH.

Thus, we know that 0·8 g of NaOH is present in 25 ml alkali soln.

(*iii*). 25 ml of alkali soln contain 0·8 g NaOH

∴   1000 ml of alkali soln contain $\frac{1000}{25} \times 0 \cdot 8$

=32·0 g of NaOH

Thus, is has been found out that 32·0 g of NaOH are present per litre.

(B)   In the second method, the use is made of normalities of solutions.

Volume of HCl (V_{HCl}) $=20.0$ ml.

normality of HCl(N_{HCl}) $=1.0$ N

volume of NaOH(N_{NaOH}) $=25.0$ ml

normality of NaOH(N_{NaOH}) is to be determined

$$N_{NaOH} \times V_{NaOH} = N_{HCl} \times V_{HCl}$$
$$N_{NaOH} \times 25.0 = 1 \times 20.0$$

$$N_{NaOH} = \frac{1 \times 20.0}{25.0} = 0.8 \text{ N}$$

wt present per litre $=$ normality $\times$ eq wt

wt of NaOH present per litre $=0.8 \times 40 = 32.0$ g

Both the methods give the same result, *i.e.*, 32.0 g NaOH per litre. But it can be easily seen that method B, which makes use of normalities of soln, is simple, rapid and more convenient.

8.7. PREPARATION OF STANDARD SOLUTIONS

In any titrimetric procedure there are two important steps on which the success of the method depends.

(*a*) Selecting a suitable reagent and preparing its standard soln.

(*b*) Choosing a suitable indicator to find out precisely the point at which the reaction between the analyte and reagent is just complete.

It has been seen (see 8.2) that a suitable reagent for a titration is one whose reaction with the analyte is single, fast, complete and stoichiometric. For example, benzoic acid reacts rapidly and completely with NaOH in accordance with a chemical equation, furthermore, no side reaction takes place. Hence, benzoic acid can be used as a reagent for the titrimetric determination of NaOH. The next step is to prepare a standard soln of the reagent. This can be done by weighing a portion of the dried reagent, dissolving it in water and then making up the volume in a measuring flask. But this is possible only when the reagent has a definite composition, is non-hygroscopic, does not decompose on drying at 100 to 120°C and does not react with CO_2 or O_2 of the atmosphere. A substance satisfying such conditions is called a *primary standard*.

8.7.1. Primary Standards in Acid-Base Titrimetry

The substances commonly used as primary standards in acid-base titrations are sodium carbonate (Na_2CO_3), borax ($Na_2B_4O_7$), succinic acid ($H_2.C_4H_4O_4$), benzoic acid ($H.C_7H_5O_2$), furoic acid ($H.C_5H_3O_3$) and adipic acid ($H_2C_6H_8O_4$).

If a substance contains water molecules, it is not a good primary standard. However, there are substances like borax ($Na_2B_4O_7.10H_2O$), oxalic acid ($H_2.C_2O_4.2H_2O$) and copper sulphate ($CuSO_4.5H_2O$) whose standard solutions can be prepared by weighing ; these are known as *secondary standards*.

8·7·2. Standardisation of Solutions·

When the reagent is not available in pure form or is unstable, its soln of approximate normality is prepared by weighing. This soln is then standardised by titration with a standard soln of some suitable reagent which is a primary standard (see expt. 8·1).

8·8. ACID-BASE OR NEUTRALISATION INDICATORS

The purpose of a titration is to find out the volume of the titrant which is chemically equivalent to the amount of the analyte. For example, when we titrate an acid soln with a standard soln of an alkali, the alkali soln is gradually added to the acid soln until the amount of the added alkali is chemically equivalent to that of the acid taken for the titration. At this point, the reaction between the acid and the alkali is just complete, hence the addition of the alkali soln is stopped and its volume is recorded ; this point is known as the equivalence point of the titration. The success of any titration depends upon the fact that how accurately the equivalence point is judged. *Indicators* are substances which at the equivalence point produce some change which can be readily seen. The point at which an indicator shows a colour change is called the end point of the titration. If the end point coincides with equivalence point, it in an ideal condition. But usually there is a small difference between the equivalence point and end point ; this difference is known as the *titration error* or end point error.

Acid-base or neutralisation indicators are those substances which possess different colours at different hydrogen ion concentrations (or pH ; see 4·8·1) of the soln. When a small amount of such an indicator is added to an acid soln it has a particular colour called *acid colour* and when added to an alkaline soln it has a different colour—*alkaline colour*. For example, for methyl red indicator, the acid colour is red while the alkaline colour is yellow. This colour change is not sudden but takes place gradually spread over a pH range of about 2 units. The pH range during which this colour change takes place is called *colour-change interval*. In the case of methyl red, the colour is clear red at pH 4·2 (or less) and distinct yellow at pH 6·3 (or more). In the pH range 4·2 to 6·3, the indicator colour is a mixture of red and yellow colour. Thus, the colour-change interval for methyl red is from pH 4·2 to 6·3 ; this range varies with the indicators.

8·8·1.   Theories of Indicator Action

Most of acid-base indicators are very weak organic acids or bases. W. Ostwald suggested the first theory to explain how an acid-base indicator works.

Let us consider an inidcator which is a weak organic acid represented as HIn. In aqueous soln it will dissociate :

$$HIn \rightleftharpoons H^+ + In^- \text{ (poorly dissociated)} \qquad ...(8·7)$$
Undissociated dissociated
colour   colour

The undissociated molecule HIn has one colour while the colour of In⁻ ion is different. If this indicator is placed in a soln of acid HA, then the following equilibria will exist :

$$HIn \overset{\leftarrow}{\rightleftharpoons} \boxed{H^+} + \text{ln}^- \text{ (dissociation decreased)}$$
$$HA \rightleftharpoons \boxed{H^+} + A^-$$
$$\downarrow$$
common ion

Due to common-ion effect, the dissociation of HIn which is already poor (because HIn is a weak acid) is further decreased as shown by the arrow at the top. Thus, in the presence of an acid the concentration of ln⁻ ion becomes very small and most of the indicator will be in the undissociated form, so, the colour shown will be that of HIn (undissociated colour). If the indicator is added to a soln of an alkali (MOH), the dissociation of HIn will increase as shown below :

$$HIn \overset{\rightarrow}{\rightleftharpoons} \boxed{H^+} + \text{ln}^- \text{ (dissociation increased)}$$
$$MOH \rightleftharpoons \boxed{OH^-} + M^+$$
$$\downarrow$$
$$H_2O$$

(MIn is a strong electrolyte, hence it will be in the form of M^+ and In⁻ ions).

The concentration of ln⁻ ions will be, therefore, greater than that of HIn, so, the colour exhibited will be that of ln⁻ ion, i.e., the dissociated colour.

For example, phenolphthalein, which we will represent as HPh is a weak acid. In the undissociated form it is colourless while Ph⁻ ion has a pink colour.

$$HPh \rightleftharpoons H^+ + Ph^- \quad \text{(poorly dissociated)}$$
$$\underset{\text{colourless}}{} \qquad \underset{\text{pink}}{}$$

In acid soln, due to common-ion effect, the dissociation of the indicator is suppressed, so most of it is present in the undissociated form consequently, the soln remains colourless. In alkaline medium, the OH$^-$ ions combine with H$^+$ ions from the indicator to form water ; this pushes the dissociation in the forward direction, the concentration of Ph$^-$ ion increases and hence the soln becomes pink.

Let us now consider an indicator that is a weak organic base which we shall represent as InOH. The indicator will dissociate as :

$$\underset{\substack{\text{undissociated} \\ \text{colour}}}{InOH} \rightleftharpoons \underset{\substack{\text{dissociated} \\ \text{colour}}}{In^+} + OH^- \quad \text{(poorly dissociated)} \quad ...(8\cdot8)$$

In alkaline soln, the concentration of the common-ion, OH$^-$, will be high, the already poor dissociation of InOH will be further decreased, so, most of the indicator will remain undissociated and the soln will have the undissociated colour. In acid soln, OH$^-$ ions from indicator will combine with H$^+$ ions from the acid ; this would push equilibrium (8·8) in the forward direction. The concentration of In$^+$ ion will, therefore, become greater than that of InOH so that the dissociated colour will be exhibited.

For example, methyl orange (shown as MeOH) is a weak organic base which dissociates as :

$$\underset{\substack{\text{undissociated} \\ \text{colour (yellow)}}}{MeOH} \rightleftharpoons \underset{\substack{\text{dissociated} \\ \text{colour (red)}}}{Me^+} + OH^- \quad \text{(poorly dissociated)} \quad ...(8\cdot9)$$

In presence of an alkali, MOH, the equilibria are :

$$MeOH \overset{\leftarrow}{\rightleftharpoons} Me^+ + \boxed{\begin{array}{c} OH^- \\ OH^- \end{array}} \quad \text{(dissociation decreased)}$$
$$MOH \rightleftharpoons M^+ +$$
$$\underset{\text{common ion}}{}$$

Due to common-ion effect, the dissociation of MeOH will be suppressed and the concentration of MeOH will be much greater than that of Me$^+$ ions. The colour in alkaline medium will be that of the undissociated form, MeOH, i.e., yellow. In acid medium, the H$^+$ ions from the acid (HA) will combine with OH$^-$ ions from the indicator as shown in following equation :

$$MeOH \overset{\rightarrow}{\rightleftharpoons} Me^+ + \left.\begin{array}{c} OH^- \\ \\ H^+ \end{array}\right| \text{(dissociation increases)}$$

$$HA \rightleftharpoons A^- +$$

$$\downarrow$$
$$H_2O$$

The dissociation of MeOH will be much greater, hence the concentration of Me^+ ions will be greater than that of MeOH so that the soln will turn red (dissociated colour).

Another theory which attempts to explain indicator action is the quinonoid theory. According to this theory the colour change is due to structural changes. The indicator exists in different structural forms in acidic and alkaline medium. Because these structural forms have different colours, therefore, indicator has one colour in acid soln and a different colour in alkaline soln.

8·9. INDICATOR CONSTANT

Consider an indicator which is a weak acid and is represented as HIn. In aqueous soln, it dissociates as shown by the equilibrium :

$$Hn \rightleftharpoons H^+ + In^- \text{ (poorly dissociated)} \qquad \dots(8·10)$$

By applying the law of mass action to equilibrium (8·10) we get:

$$K = \frac{a_{H^+} \times a_{In^-}}{a_{HIn}} \quad \left| \begin{array}{l} a_{H^+} = \text{activity of } H^+ \text{ ion} \\ \\ a_{In^-} = \text{activity of } In^- \text{ ion} \\ \\ a_{HIn} = \text{activity of HIn.} \end{array} \right.$$

The equilibrium constant K in this case is called *indicator constant* and is represented as K_{in}. If the soln is dilute, as an approximation, activity can be replaced by concentration. The simplified form so obtained is :

$$K_{in} = \frac{[H^+] \times [In^-]}{[HIn]} \quad \left| \begin{array}{l} \text{Remember} \\ \\ a = c \times f \text{ and in dil soln, } f = 1 \\ \\ \therefore \quad a = c \text{ (see 4·1)} \end{array} \right.$$

or, $\quad [H^+] = K_{in} \times \dfrac{[HIn]}{[In^-]}$

$$[H^+] = K_{in} \times \frac{[\text{unionised form}]}{[\text{ionised form}]}$$

Taking logarithms :

$$\log[H^+] = \log K_{in} + \log \frac{[HIn]}{[In^-]}$$

Multiplying by -1 :

$$-\log[H^+] = -\log K_{in} - \log \frac{[HIn]}{[In^-]}$$

$$pH = pK_{in} + \log \frac{[In^-]}{[HIn]} \qquad ...(8\cdot11)$$

$$\log a \times \frac{b}{c} = \log a + \log \frac{b}{c}$$

$-\log$ is written as p.

$$-\log \frac{a}{b} = \log \frac{b}{a}$$

From equation (8·11) it is obvious that the ratio $[In^-]/[HIn]$ is governed by the pH of the soln in which the indicator is placed. Now, if HIn and In^- both are present, our eye cannot detect their colours. However, if the pH of the soln is such that $[In^-] = 10[HIn]$, the colour of In^- ion will be clearly visible. Similarly, when $[HIn] = 10[In^-]$, the colour of HIn will be clearly seen.

Suppose $[In^-] = 10[HIn]$,

$$pH = pK_{in} + \log 10/1$$

$$= pK_{in} + \log 10$$

$$= pK_{in} + 1 \text{ (distinct colour of } In^- \text{ ion)}$$

if $[HIn] = 1$ then $[In^-] = 10$

see equation (8·11)

$\log 10 = 1$

If $[HIn] = 10[In^-]$

$$pH = K_{in} + \log \frac{1}{10}$$

$$= pK_{in} - \log 10$$

$$= pK_{in} - 1 \qquad \text{(distinct colour of HIn)}$$

if $[In^-] = 1$, $[HIn] = 10$

$$\log \frac{1}{10} = -\log \frac{10}{1} = -\log 10$$

$-\log 10 = -1$

From above calculations it is seen that when pH of the soln is equal to $pK_{in} + 1$, it has the colour of In^- ion and when $pH = pK_{in} - 1$ it will have the colour of HIn. Thus, a pH range of $pK_{in} \pm 1$ is known as the colour-change interval. For example, pK_{in} value for methyl red is 5·0. In all solutions whose pH is $(5-1) = 4$ (or less), the indicator will have a clear red colour. In case of solutions whose pH is $(5+1) = 6$ (or more), the colour will be distinctly yellow. Hence, for methyl red the colour-change interval is between pH 4 to 6. In this pH range the colour is neither yellow nor red but it is something between these two colours.

Table 8·2. Colour Changes and pH Range of Certain Indicators

Indicator	pH Range	Colour	
		Acid	Base
Cresol red	0·2—1·8	Red	Yellow
Methyl yellow	2·9—4·0	Red	Yellow
Methyl orange	3·1—4·4	Red	Yellow
Congo red	3·0—5·0	Blue	Red
Methyl red	4·2—6·3	Red	Yellow
Bromophenol red	5·2—6·8	Yellow	Red
Neutral red	6·8—8·0	Red	Orange
Thymol blue	8·0—9·6	Yellow	Blue
Phenolphthalein	8·3—10·0	Colourless	Red
Nitramine	10·8—13·0	Colourless	Orange

8·10. CHOICE OF INDICATOR

The most important condition that an indicator must satisfy is that its colour change must take place as close as possible, to the equivalence point of the titration. Suppose the reaction between an analyte and a reagent is just complete when 20·0 ml reagent soln is added. In other words, the equivalence point of the titration is reached when 20·0 ml reagent soln is added. If the indicator used for this titration shows a colour change when 20·1 ml reagent soln has been added, then there is a difference of 0·1 ml in the equivalence point (theoretical end point) and the actual end point ; this difference of 0·1 ml is called the indicator error. The most suitable indicator for this titration will be the one which will show a colour change when exactly 20·0 ml reagent soln has been added. The choice of a suitable indicator for an acid-base titration depends upon the nature of the acid and base involved.

8·11. TITRATION OF A STRONG ACID WITH A STRONG BASE

Consider, for example, the reaction between HCl and NaOH which can be represented as :

$$HCl + NaOH \rightarrow NaCl + H_2O$$

or

$$H^+ + OH^- \rightarrow H_2O$$

Suppose we take 50·0 ml of 0·1000 N NCl and gradually add to it 0·1000 N NaOH. As the reaction progresses, more and more H^+ ions from HCl will combine with OH^- ions from NaOH consequently, the concentration of H^+ ions (represented as $[H^+]$) will go on decreasing (but the pH will go on increasing ; see 4·8·4). When exactly 50·0 ml NaOH has been added, the neutralisation reaction between HCl and NaOH is just complete. At this stage the reaction mixture will be neither acidic nor basic but will be neutral whose pH will be 7. [It should be remembered that the salt NaCl formed during the reaction is a salt of a strong acid and strong base, hence it will not undergo hydrolysis and thus will not disturb the pH of the soln (which is 7)].

From the above consideration it appears that in the titration of HCl with NaOH, the indicator must show a colour change exactly at pH 7. But this is a hurriedly drawn conclusion which is not entirely correct. In order to know suitable indicators for this titration, we must find out that how pH changes during the titration.

8·11·1. Change in pH During the Titration of a Strong Acid with a Strong Base

Let us calculate pH at different stages of the titration of 50·0 ml of 0·1000 N HCl with 0·1000 N NaOH soln.

(i) *pH before any NaOH is added .*

In 0·1000 N HCl

$[H^+]=0\cdot1000$ g ion/litre $=1/10$ g ion/litre $=10^{-1}$ g ion/litre	Assuming that in the soln, HCl is completely dissociated
$\log[H^+]=\log 10^{-1}=-1$ $-\log[H^+]=-[-1]=1$ $pH=1$	$\log 10^{-X}=-X$ $-\log$ written as p

(ii) *pH after the addition of 10·0 ml NaOH.* 40·0 ml acid is left unreacted and total volume becomes 60·0 ml.

In this soln, the normality of HCl can be calculated by :

$$N_{HCl}\times60\cdot0=40\cdot0\times0\cdot1000$$

$$N_{HCl}=\frac{40\cdot0\times0\cdot1000}{60\cdot0}=0\cdot0667$$

It means that, now, 0·0667 g eq of HCl are present per litre or $[H^+]=0\cdot0667$ g ion per litre.

$$pH=-\log[H^+]=-[\log 0\cdot0667]$$

$$=-[\bar{2}\cdot8241]=-[-2\cdot0000+0\cdot8241]$$

$$= -[-1\cdot1759] = 1\cdot1759 \approx 1\cdot18$$
$$pH = 1\cdot18$$

Hence, when the titration is 20 per cent complete the pH rises from 1·00 to 1·18.

(iii) *pH after addition of 20·0 ml NaOH*

$[H^+]$ will be given as $\dfrac{0\cdot1000 \times 30\cdot0}{70\cdot0} = 0\cdot0428$ g ion per litre

$$pH = -[\log 0\cdot0428] = 1\cdot37$$

Thus, when the titration is 40 per cent complete the pH becomes 1·37.

(iv) *pH after the addition of 50·0 ml NaOH*. At this stage of the titration, the reaction is just complete, *i.e.*, equivalence point is reached. The titration mixture is now merely a soln of NaCl in water and because Na^+ or Cl^- ions do not hydrolyse, the soln is neutral with a pH of 7.

(v) *pH after the addition of 50·1 ml NaOH*. Out of 50·1 ml NaOH added, 50·0 ml is used in completely neutralising the acid and 0·1 ml is present in excess. The total volume of the reaction mixture is 100·1 ml or approximately 100·0 ml. In other words, 0·1 ml of 0·1000 N NaOH has been diluted to 100 ml. In this soln the normality of NaOH can be calculated :

$$N_{NaOH} \times 100 = 0\cdot1 \times 0\cdot1$$

or $\qquad N_{NaOH} = \dfrac{0\cdot1 \times 0\cdot1}{100} = \dfrac{10^{-1} \times 10^{-1}}{10^2} = 10^{-4}$ N

The normality of NaOH in the titration mixture is now 10^{-4}N, *i.e.*, 10^{-4} g eq of NaOH is present per litre of soln. Hence in this soln, the concentration of OH^- ion will be 10^{-4}g ion/litre ($\because NaOH \equiv OH^-$). Thus :

$$[OH^-] = 10^{-4}$$

Now, $\qquad [H^+] \times [OH^-] = 10^{-14}$

$$[H^+] = \dfrac{10^{-14}}{[OH^-]} = \dfrac{10^{-14}}{10^{-4}} = 10^{-14} \times 10^4$$

$$= 10^{-10} \text{ g ion/litre}$$

The $[H^+]$ in the soln is 10^{-10}, hence the pH of the soln will be 10.

In this way, the pH of the soln during the different stages of the titration and also after the completion of the titration can be calculated for different amounts of NaOH added. Table 8·3 gives the pH values of the titration soln for the different volumes of NaOH soln added.

Table 8·3. Titration of 50·0 ml of 0·1000 N HCl with 0·1000 N NaOH

NaOH added (ml)	HCl unreacted (ml)	% reaction	Total volume of soln (ml)	pH	Change in pH per ml of NaOH added
0·0	50·0	0·0	50·0	1·00	0·018
10·0	40·0	20·0	60·0	1·18	0·019
20·0	30·0	40·0	70·0	1·37	0·023
30·0	20·0	60·0	80·0	1·60	0·036
40·0	10·0	80·0	90·0	1·96	0·062
45·0	5·0	90·0	95·0	2·27	0·183
49·0	1·0	98·0	99·0	3·00	1·111
49·9	0·1	99·8	99·9	4·00	30·000
50·0	0·0	100·0	100·0	7·00	30·000
Excess NaOH (ml)					
50·1	0·1		100·10	10·00	30·000
51·0	1·0		101·0	11·00	1·111
55·0	5·0		105·0	11·68	0·170
60·0	10·0		110·0	11·96	0·056

The results given in Table 8·3, show that in the initial stages of the titration, pH increases very gradually even when large volumes of the titrant soln are added. But in the vicinity of the equivalence point, the addition of even small amount of NaOH causes relatively much greater rise in pH. For example, when the volume of NaOH is increased from 0·0 to 49·9 ml, the increase in pH is from 1·0 to 4·0 i.e., by 3 pH units. But when the volume is further increased from 49·9, to 50·0 ml, the pH jumps from 4·0 to 7·0, i.e., again by 3 units. Thus, the increase in pH caused by the addition of 49·9 ml of NaOH soln is equal to the rise in pH caused by adding only 0·1 ml NaOH in the vicinity of the equivalence point.

One more point is obvious from the results of Table 8·3. It is seen that after the addition of 49·9 ml NaOH, the pH of the titration mixture is 4 and 99·8 per cent reaction is complete. Now, if some indicator shows a colour change at this pH, the titration error will be only 0·2 per cent. Similarly if we use an indicator which shows a colour change at pH 10, the titre value will be 50·1 instead of the correct value 50·0, i.e., the error will be 0·2 per cent. Thus, although the pH at the equivalence point of the titration is 7, but it is not essential that the indicator used should necessarily show a colour change at pH 7. Any indicator which shows a colour change anywhere between pH 4 to 10 can be used because, the error introduced will not be greater than ±0·2%. For example, methyl orange, bromocresol green, methyl red, bromophenol red, bromothymol blue, phenol red and phenolphthalein can be used as indicators in this titration because their colour change interval falls within the pH limit 4 to 10.

The results recorded in Table 8·3 can be graphically represented as shown in Fig. 8·1. The curve obtained is called pH-

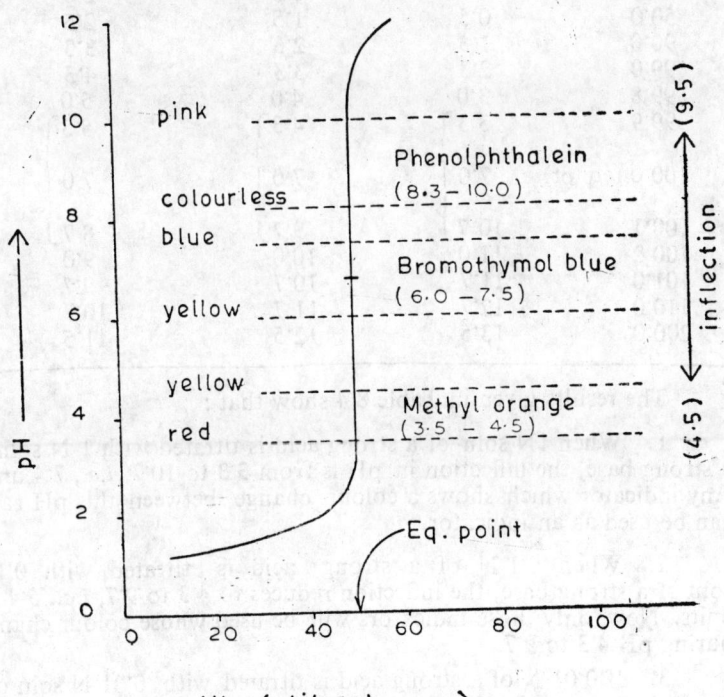

Fig. 8·1. pH-neutralisation curve for the titration of 0·1 N HCl with 0·1 N NaOH.

neutralisation curve. There are two turning points or points of inflection. The pH interval between these two points is called *inflection*. Inthe titration of 0.1 N HCl with 0.1 N NaOH, the inflection on the pH-neutralisation curve is from pH 4.5 to 9.5.

8.11.2. Effect of Concentration

The inflection on the pH-neutralisation curve depends upon the concentration of titrand and titrant soln, as shown by the results given in Table 8.4.

Table 8.4. pH Change During Titration of 1N, 0.1N and 0.01N HCl with 1N, 0.1N and 0.01N NaOH
- (Volume of acid taken = 100.0 ml)

NaOH added (ml)	pH		
	N soln	0.1 N soln	0.01 N soln
0.0	0.0	1.0	2.0
50.0	0.5	1.5	2.5
90.0	1.3	2.3	3.3
99.0	2.3	3.3	4.3
99.8	3.0	4.0	5.0
99.9	3.3 ⎤	4.3 ⎤	5.3 ⎤
100.0 (eq pt)	7.0	7.0	7.0
100.1	10.7 ⎦	9.7 ⎦	8.7 ⎦
100.2	11.0	10.0	9.0
101.0	11.7	10.7	9.7
110.0	12.7	11.7	10.7
200.0	13.5	12.5	11.5

The results given in Table 8.4 show that :

1. When 1N soln of a strong acid is titrated with 1 N soln of a strong base, the inflection in pH is from 3.3 to 10.7, *i.e.*, 7.4 units. Any indicator which shows a colour change between this pH range can be used as an indicator.

2. When 0.1 N of a strong acid is titrated with 0.1 N soln of a strong base, the inflection reduces to 4.3 to 9.7, *i.e.*, 5.4 pH units. Now, only those indicators will be used whose colour changes during pH 4.3 to 9.7.

3. If 0.01 N of a strong acid is titrated with 0.01 N soln of a strong base, the inflection further reduces to pH 5.3 to 8.7, *i.e.*, only 3.4 pH units. The choice of indicator will become limited. For example, now methyl orange cannot be used.

It is thus seen that as the concentration of acid and alkali soln is reduced, the inflection on the pH-neutralisation curve becomes smaller and smaller. This fact must be taken into consideration while selecting an indicator for the titration. Fig. 8·2 shows neutralisation curves for titration of HCl with NaOH at different concentration levels.

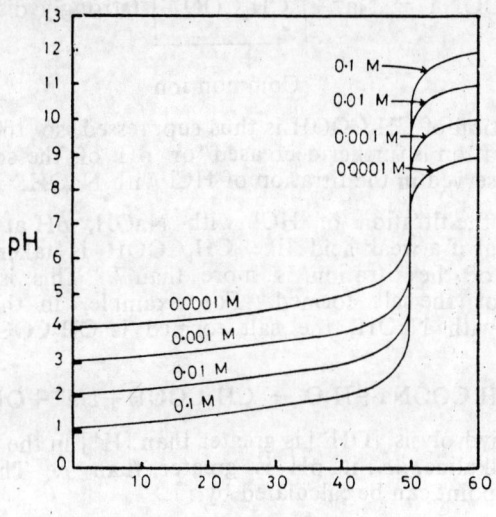

ml of NaOH

Fig. 8·2.   Effect of concentration on titration curves
of strong acids with strong bases.

8·12. TITRATION OF A WEAK ACID WITH A STRONG BASE

This type of titration may be represented by the general equation :

$$HA + OH^- \rightarrow H_2O + A^-$$

Here, HA represents a weak acid that is why it is written in the undissociated form. There are three important differences between this titration and that between a strong acid and a strong base :

1. The $[H^+]$ is small at the start of the titration (but pH will be greater). Note that in 0·1 N HCl, $[H^+]=0·1$ and pH$=1·0$, whereas in 0·1 N CH_3COOH, $[H^+]=1·34\times10^{-3}$ and pH$=2·87$. [Because CH_3COOH is a weak acid, it is poorly dissociated, hence it gives smaller concentration of H^+ ions.]

2. As alkali soln is added to the weak acid, the salt formed produces common-ion effect so that the dissociation of the weak

acid is suppressed. For example, when NaOH is added to CH_3COOH, there is formation of the salt CH_3COONa and the following equilibria exist :

$$CH_3COOH \; \underset{\leftarrow}{\rightleftharpoons} \; H^+ + \boxed{CH_3COO^-} \;\; \text{(poorly dissociated)}$$

$$CH_3COONa \rightleftharpoons Na^+ + \boxed{CH_3COO^-} \;\; \text{(strongly dissociated)}$$

$$\downarrow$$
$$\text{Common ion}$$

The dissociation of CH_3COOH is thus suppressed so the hydrogen-ion concentration is further decreased or pH of the soln is greater than that observed in the titration of HCl with NaOH.

3. In the titration of HCl with NaOH, pH at equivalence point is 7, but if a weak acid like CH_3COOH is taken, pH at the completion of the titration is more than 7. This is due to the hydrolysis of the salt formed. For example, in the titration of CH_3COOH with NaOH, the salt formed is CH_3COONa which is hydrolysed :

$$CH_3COONa + H_2O \rightarrow CH_3COOH + Na^+ + OH^-$$

Due to the hydrolysis, $[OH^-]$ is greater than $[H^+]$ in the soln, hence the soln is alkaline, *i.e.*, its pH is greater than 7. The pH at the equivalence point can be calculated by :

$$pH = \frac{1}{2} \, p \, K_w + \frac{1}{2} \, p \, K_a + \frac{1}{2} \log C \qquad \text{...(8-J)}$$

$$\text{(see equation 4·21)}$$

If 50·0 ml, 0·1 N NaOH is added to 50·0 ml, 0·1 N CH_3COOH, the total volume will become 100·0 ml and so the concentration of sodium acetate formed will be 0·05 M. Thus :

$$K_w = 10^{-14} \; ; \; \log K_w = -14\cdot00 \; ; \; pK_w = 14\cdot00$$

$$K_a = 1\cdot8 \times 10^{-5} \; ; \; pK_a = 4\cdot74$$

$$c = 0\cdot05 \; ; \; \log c = \log 0\cdot05 = \bar{2}\cdot70$$

$$\frac{1}{2} \, pK_w = 7\cdot00 \; ; \; \frac{1}{2} \, pK_a = 2\cdot37 \; ; \; \text{and}$$

$$\log c = \bar{2}\cdot70 = [0\cdot70 - 2\cdot00] = -1\cdot30$$

Substituting these values in equation (8-J) :

$$pH = 7\cdot0 + 2\cdot37 - \frac{1\cdot30}{2}$$

$$= 9\cdot37 - 0\cdot65 = 8\cdot72$$

It is thus seen that when 0.1 N CH_3COOH is titrated with 0.1 N NaOH, the pH at the equivalence point is 8.72 and not 7.00 as was observed in the case of titration of HCl with NaOH.

The above discussion can be summarised by stating that the titration of CH_3COOH with NaOH differs from the titration of HCl with NaOH in the following three important respects ; in the case of CH_3COOH :

(a) The initial pH is higher.

(b) The rate of increase of pH during the titration is greater.

(c) The pH at the equivalence point is higher.

These points can be clearly seen in the results of Table 8.5 which gives the change in pH during the titration of HCl and CH_3COOH with NaOH.

Table 8·5. Titration of 50.0 ml of 0.1000 N HCl/CH_3COOH with 0.1000 N NaOH solution

NaOH added (ml)	Unreacted acid (ml)	% reaction	Total vol (ml)	pH	
				HCl	CH₃COOH
0·0	50·0	0·0	50·0	1·00	2·87
10·0	40·0	20·0	60·0	1·18	4·14
20·0	30·0	40·0	70·0	1·37	4·57
30·0	20·0	60·0	80·0	1 60	4·92
40·0	10·0	80·0	90·0	1·96	5·35
45·0	5·0	90·0	95·0	2·27	5·70
49·0	1·0	98·0	99·0	3·00	6·43
49·9	0·1	99·8	99·9	4·00	7·44
50·0 (Eq pt)	0·0	100·0	100·0	7·00	8·72
	Excess NaOH (ml)				
50·1	0·1		100·1	10·0	10·00
51·0	1·0		101·0	11·0	11·00
55·0	5·0		105·0	11·68	11·68
60·0	10·0		110·0	11·96	11·96

The inflection range for the titration of 0.1 N CH_3COOH with 0.1 N NaOH is from pH 7.8 to 9.7 (see Fig. 8.3). In this titration, indicators like methyl orange or methyl red cannot be used. The pH at the equivalence point is 8·7, hence those indicators which show a colour change on the slightly alkaline side, such as phenolphtalein, thymolphthalein or thymol blue are suitable for the titration.

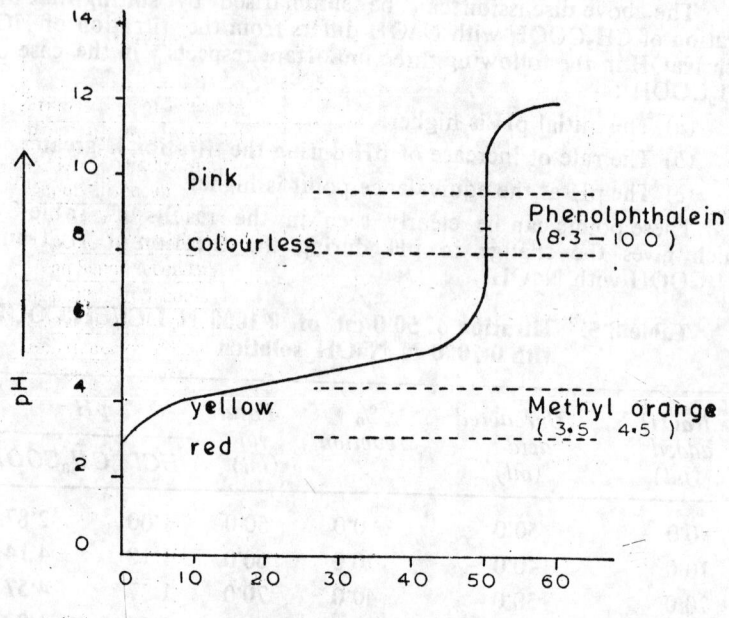

Fig. 8·3. pH-neutralisation curve for the titration of 0·1 N CH_3COOH with 0·1 N NaOH.

8·13. TITRATION OF A WEAK BASE WITH A STRONG ACID

As an example of such type of titrations, we shall consider the titration of 0·1 M (same as 0·1 N) aqueous ammonia soln with 0·1M HCl (same as 0·1 N), soln. The reaction involved is :

$$NH_4OH + HCl \longrightarrow NH_4Cl + H_2O$$

The salt NH_4Cl then hydrolyses :

$$NH_4 + H_2O \rightarrow NH_4OH + H^+$$

Due to formation of H^+ ions, the pH at the equivalence point will be slightly on the acidic side as shown by the following calculations. Suppose, we titrate 50 ml of 0·1 M NH_4OH with 0·1 M HCl. Then at the equivalence point :

$$pH = \tfrac{1}{2} pK_w - \tfrac{1}{2} pK_b - \tfrac{1}{2} \log c \qquad \text{(see eqn. 4·25)}$$

Now $\frac{1}{2}pK_w = 7\cdot00$; $pK_b = 4\cdot74$; $\frac{1}{2}pK_b = 2\cdot37$

where K_b=dissociation const. of NH_4OH.   At equivalence point the concentration, c, of the salt will be $0\cdot05$ M, so,

$$\log c = \log 0\cdot05 = \overline{2}\cdot70 = -1\cdot30$$

$$\frac{1}{2}\log c = -0\cdot65$$

$\therefore$ $pH = 7\cdot00 - 2\cdot37 - (-0\cdot65)$

$$= 7\cdot00 - 2\cdot37 + 0\cdot65 = 5\cdot28$$

The pH-neutralisation curve (Fig. 8·4) shows that the inflection is from pH 3 to 6·5. Hence, indicators such as methyl orange (3·1—4·4), methyl red (4·2—6·3), bromophenol blue (3·0—4·6) or bromocresol green (3·8—5·4) can be used in this titration. But indicators like phenolphthalein (8·3—10·0) or thymolphthalein (8·3—10·5) should not be used.

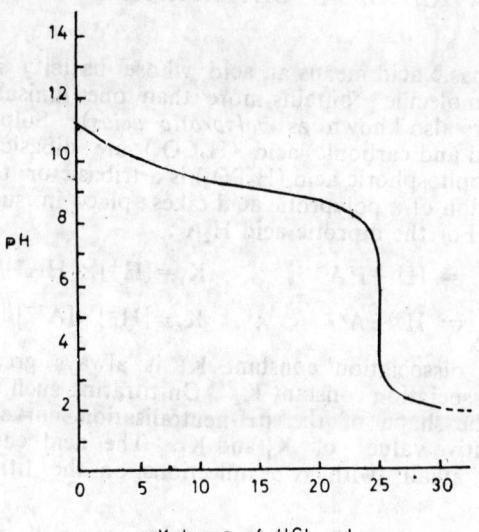

Volume of HCl, ml

Fig. 8·4.   pH-neutralisation curve for the titration of 0·1 N ammonia with 0·1 N HCl.

8·14.   TITRATION OF A WEAK ACID WITH A WEAK BASE

Let us consider the titration of 0·1 M CH_3COOH with 0·1 M NH_4OH :

$$CH_3COOH + NH_4OH \rightarrow CH_3COONH_4 + H_2O$$

The salt formed, CH_3COONH_4, undergoes hydrolysis :

$$CH_3COONH_4 + H_2O \rightarrow CH_3OOOH + NH_4OH$$

The disadvantage in such titrations is that the inflection on the pH-neutralisation curve is very small near the equivalence point. For example, in the titration of 0.1 N CH_3COOH with 0.1N NH_4OH, the pH near the equivalence point slowly rises from 6 to 8. With more dilute soln, the rise in pH is smaller. It should be noted that if the pH rise at the equivalence point is smaller than 2 pH units, it is very difficult to judge the colour change at the equivalence point and accurate results cannot be obtained.

The pH at the equivalence depends on the relative values of K_a (dissociation constant of acid) and K_b (dissociation constant of base). If $K_a = K_b$, it is 7, if $K_a > K_b$, it is less than 7 and if $K_b > K_a$, the pH at the equivalence point will be more than 7. From a study of the pH-neutralisation curve, the inflection can be found out and then suitable indicator can be selected.

8·15. TITRATION OF A POLYBASIC ACID WITH A STRONG BASE

A polybasic acid means an acid whose basicity is more than one, i.e., its molecule contains more than one ionisable hydrogen (such acids are also known as *polyprotic acids*). Sulphurous acid, sulphuric acid and carbonic acid (H_2CO_3) are dibasic or diprotic acids. Orthophosphoric acid (H_3PO_4) is a tribasic or triprotic acid. The dissociation of a polyprotic acid takes place in successive steps (see 4·4·4). For the diprotic acid H_2A :

$$H_2A \rightleftharpoons H^+ + HA^- \quad ; \quad K_1 = [H^+] \times [HA^-]/[H_2A]$$

$$HA^- \rightleftharpoons H^+ + A^{2-} \quad ; \quad K_2 = [H^+] \times [A^{2-}]/[HA^-]$$

The primary dissociation constant K_1 is always greater than the secondary dissociation constant K_2. On titrating such an acid with alkali soln, the shape of the pH-neutralisation curve will depend upon the relative values of K_1 and K_2. The acid can be titrated stepwise with alkali (with two inflections on the titration curve) provided :

'   (a) The values of K_1 and K_2 are not very small, and

(b) The ratio K_1/K_2 is more than 10,000.

The acid will then behave like a mixture of two acids with dissociation constants K_1 and K_2.

Let us consider, for example, sulphurous acid which dissociates in two steps :

$$H_2SO_3 \rightleftharpoons H^+ + HSO_3^- \quad ; \quad K_1 = 1.2 \times 10^{-2} \quad ; \quad pK_1 = 1.92$$

$$HSO_3^- \rightleftharpoons H^+ + SO_3^{2-} \quad ; \quad K_2 = 5.6 \times 10^{-8} \quad ; \quad pK_2 = 7.25$$

The titration of this acid with alkali can be done in stepwise manner with good separation because K_1/K_2 is more than 10,000 $(K_1/K_2 = 2.1 \times 10^5)$. At the first end-point, the pH is given by :

$$pH = 1/2\ (pK_1 + pK_2) = 1/2(1.92 + 7.25) = 4.58$$

For the first end point methyl orange, congo red or bromocresol green can be used as indicators. The colour change at the second end point in not sharp because the value of K_3 is not large enough. The pH at the second end point is 10.13 provided 0.2 M acid is used for titration. Thymolphthalein, however, can be employed for observing the second end point.

8.15.1. Titration of Phosphoric acid

Phosphoric acid dissociates in three steps :

$$H_3PO_4 \rightleftharpoons H^+ + H_2PO_4^- \quad ; \quad K_1 = 7.5 \times 10^{-3} \quad ; \quad pK_1 = 2.12$$
$$H_2PO_4^- \rightleftharpoons H^+ + HPO_4^{2-} \quad ; \quad K_2 = 6.2 \times 10^{-8} \quad ; \quad pK_2 = 7.21$$
$$HPO_4^{2-} \rightleftharpoons H^+ + PO_4^{3-} \quad ; \quad K_3 = 1 \times 10^{-12} \quad ; \quad pK_3 = 12.0$$

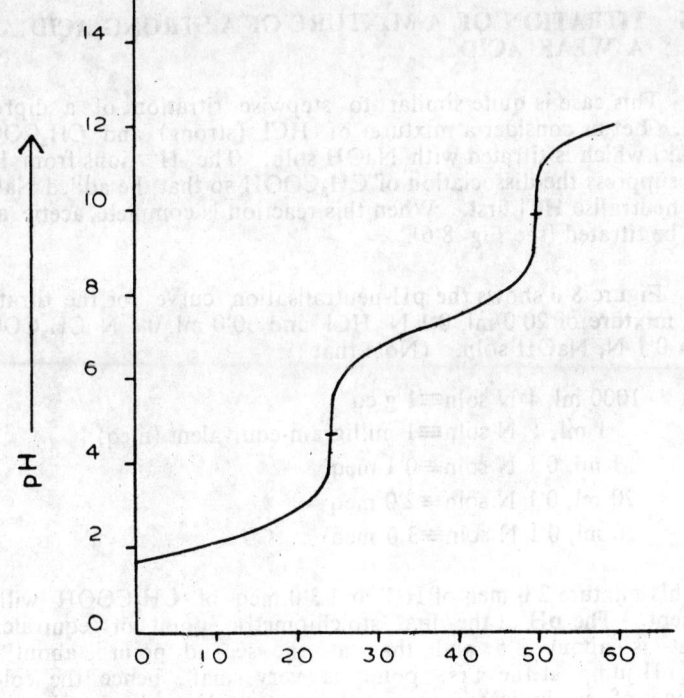

Fig. 8.5. pH neutralisation curve for the titration of 0.1 M phosphoric acid with 0.1 M (=0.1 N) NaOH.

Because $K_1/K_2 = 1.2 \times 10^5$ (more than 10,000) stepwise titration of the acid with alkali is possible. The pH at the first end point will be $\frac{1}{2}(2.12 + 7.21) = 4.67$; methyl orange or bromocresol green can be used as indicator to locate the first end point. The second end point is not very sharp because the value of K_2 is small and soln is buffered by HPO_4^{2-} ions present. The pH at the second end point is $1/2(7.21 + 12.0) = 9.6$; phenolphthalein or thymolphthalein can be used as an indicator. The third end point cannot be detected because the value of K_3 is very small. The two step titration of phosphoric acid has been graphically shown in Fig. 8.5. (Note that 25.0 ml 0.1 M H_3PO_4 soln is taken for titration. Because it is a tribasic acid, its 0.1 M soln means its 0.3N soln [see 8.5 and also relation (8-C)]. Thus :

$$25 \text{ ml, } 0.1 \text{ M } H_3PO_4 \equiv 25 \text{ ml, } 0.3 \text{ N } H_3PO_4$$

$$\equiv 75 \text{ ml, } 0.1 \text{ N } H_3PO_4$$

$$\equiv 75 \text{ ml, } 0.1 \text{ N NaOH.}$$

8.16. TITRATION OF A MIXTURE OF A STRONG ACID AND A WEAK ACID

This case is quite similar to stepwise titration of a diprotic acid. Let us consider a mixture of HCl (strong) and CH_3COOH (weak) which is titrated with NaOH soln. The H^+ ions from HCl will suppress the dissociation of CH_3COOH so that the added NaOH will neutralise HCl first. When this reaction is complete, acetic acid will be titrated (see Fig 8.6).

Figure 8.6 shows the pH-neutralisation curve for the titration of a mixture of 20.0 ml, 0.1 N HCl and 30.0 ml, 0.1 N CH_3COOH with 0.1 N, NaOH soln. (Note that :

1000 ml, 1 N soln $\equiv$ 1 g eq
1 ml, 1 N soln $\equiv$ 1 milligram-equivalent (meq)
1 ml, 0.1 N soln $\equiv$ 0.1 meq
20 ml, 0.1 N soln $\equiv$ 2.0 meq
30 ml, 0.1 N soln $\equiv$ 3.0 meq)

In this mixture 2.0 meq of HCl and 3.0 meq of CH_3COOH will be present. The pH at the first stoichiometric point or equivalence point is about 3.5 and that at the second point is about 8.5. The pH jump at the first point is very small, hence the colour change of an indicator cannot be accurately judged. However, it can be detected by potential measurement (by potentiometric titration).

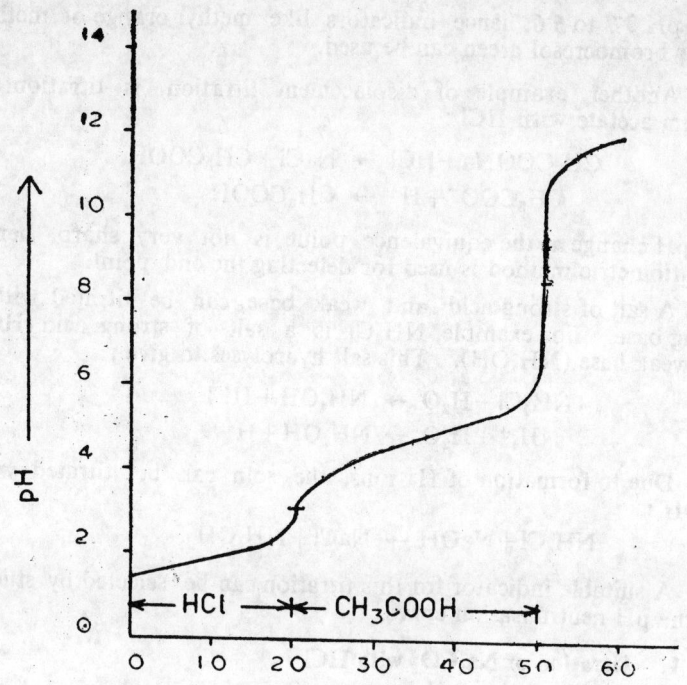

Fig. 8·6.   pH-neutralisation curve for the titration of a mixture
of 20 ml 0·1 N HCl and 30 ml 0 1 N CH₃COOH with
0·1 N NaOH.

8·17.   TITRATION OF A MIXTURE OF A STRONG BASE AND A WEAK BASE

The stepwise acidimetric titration (titration with a standard acid soln) of a mixture containing a strong base such as NaOH and a weak base like ammonia involves the same principles as those given in 8·16, for titrating a mixture of strong acid and weak acid.

8·18.   DISPLACEMENT TITRATION

Boric acid acts as a very weak monoprotic acid (dissociation constant is $6·4 \times 10^{-10}$). The reaction of borate ion with HCl is given by :

$$B_4O_7^{2-} + 2H^+ + 5H_2O \rightarrow 4H_3BO_3$$

On titrating 0·2 M sodium borate with 0·2 M HCl, the pH at the equivalence point is 5·1 The titration curve shows an inflection from pH 3·7 to 5·6, hence indicators like methyl orange or methyl red or bromocresol green can be used.

Another example of displacement titration is titration of sodium acetate with HCl :

$$CH_3COONa + HCl \rightarrow NaCl + CH_3COOH$$

or
$$CH_3COO^- + H^+ \rightarrow CH_3COOH$$

The pH change at the equivalence point is not very sharp, hence potentiometric method is used for detecting the end point.

A salt of strong acid and weak base can be titrated with a strong base. For example, NH_4Cl is a salt of strong acid (HCl) and weak base (NH_4OH). This salt hydrolyses to give :

$$NH_4Cl + H_2O \rightarrow NH_4OH + HCl$$
or
$$NH_4^+ + H_2O \rightarrow NH_4OH + H^+$$

Due to formation of H^+ ions, the soln can be titrated with NaOH :

$$NH_4Cl + NaOH \rightarrow NaCl + NH_4OH$$

A suitable indicator for this titration can be selected by studying the pH-neutralisation curve.

8·18·1. Titration of Na_2CO_3 with HCl

Sodium carbonate is sodium salt of carbonic solid (H_2CO_3), a dibasic acid, which dissociates in two steps :

$$H_2CO_3 \rightleftharpoons H^+ + HCO_3^- \quad : \quad K_1 = 4·2 \times 10^{-7} \quad ; \quad pK_1 = 6·38$$
$$HCO_3^- \rightleftharpoons H^+ + CO_3^{2-} \quad ; \quad K_2 = 4·8 \times 10^{-11} \quad ; \quad pK_2 = 10·32$$

In aqueous soln, Na_2CO_3 hydrolyses as shown by :

$$Na_2CO_3 + 2H_2O \rightarrow 2NaOH + H_2CO_3$$
or
$$(CO_3^{2-} + 2H_2O \rightarrow H_2CO_3 + 2OH^-)$$

The OH^- ions formed during hydrolysis can be titrated with HCl. Suppose 50·0 ml of 0·1000 M, Na_2CO_3 soln is titrated with 0·100 M of HCl (same as 0·100 N because HCl is a monobasic acid). The titration takes place in 2 steps :

(A) $$Na_2CO_3 + HCl \rightarrow NaCl + NaHCO_3 \qquad ...(8·12)$$
or $$(CO_3^{2-} + H^+ \rightarrow HCO_3^-)$$

(B) $$NaHCO_3 + HCl \rightarrow NaCl + H_2CO_3 \qquad ...(8·13)$$
or $$(HCO_3^- + H^+ \rightarrow H_2CO_3)$$

Sodium carbonate soln is alkaline due to hydrolysis and pH of its 0·100 M soln can be given by :

$$pH = 1/2\, pK_w + 1/2\, pK_a + 1/2 \log c \qquad \text{[see (4·21)]}$$

$$pK_w = 14.00 \qquad K_w = 1 \times 10^{-14} \therefore pK_w = 14.00$$

$$pK_a = 10.32 \qquad K_a = \text{dissociation constant of } H_2CO_3$$
$$= 4.8 \times 10^{-11}$$

$$\log c = \log 10^{-1} \qquad \therefore pK_a = 10.32$$

$$= -1.00 \qquad c = \text{concentration of sodium acetate}$$

$$= 0.100 = 10^{-1} \text{ g mole/litre}$$

$$pH = 7.00 + 5.16 - 0.5 = 11.56$$

When 50.0 ml of 0.100 N HCl has been added reaction (8.12) is complete. The pH at this point is $1/2(pK_1 + pK_2) = 1/2 (6.38 + 10.32) = 8.35$. The first end point can be detected with the help of phenolphthalein or thymolphthalein. The pH at the completion of the reaction (8.13) can be shown to be 3.93, hence the second end point will appear at pH 3.9 ; methyl orange can be used to detect the second point.

8.19. FLOURESCENT INDICATORS

Certain substances absorb radiant energy and then emit it in the form of light. These substances are called *fluorescent substances* and the phenomenon is known as *fluorescence*. The intensity and colour of many substances depend upon pH of the soln, hence these can be used as pH indicators and also in acid-base titrations. The advantage of these indicators is that they can be used when analyte soln is coloured or turbid so that the colour change of the usual indicators cannot be seen. The titrations are done using ultraviolet light and in a silica flask (a flask made of glass will not permit ultraviolet light to enter).

Table 8.6. Some Fluorescent Indicators

Name	pH range	Colour in	
		Acid	Base
Rosin	0.0—3.0	Colourless	Green
Chromotropic acid	3.0—4.5	Colourless	Blue
α-naphthylamine	3.4—4.8	Colourless	Blue
Fluorescein	4.0—6.0	Colourless	Green
Umbelliferone	6.5—8.0	Faint blue	Bright blue
β-naphthol	8.0—9.0	Colourless	Blue
Quinine sulphate	9.5—10.0	Violet	Colourless

8·20. NEUTRALIMETRY

Neutralimetry which includes all acid-base or neutralisation titrations, can be divided into two types :

(1) The determination of the amount of an acid in a sample, by titration with a standard alkali, called *alkalimetry.*

(2) The determination of the amount of a base in a sample by titration with standard acid soln, known as *acidimetry.*

8·20·1. Alkaline Primary Standards

For alkalimetry, the following substances can be used as primary standards.

(*i*) *Sodium carbonate*, Na_2CO_3 (mol wt=106·00). It is dried and then its known amount is dissolved in water and made up to known volume. Its soln is suitable only in the titration of strong acids, it is slightly hygroscopic and it has a low eq wt. The advantage is that it is available in pure form. The usual impurity is a small amount of $NaHCO_3$ which can be removed by heating :

$$2NaHCO_3 \rightarrow H_2O + CO_2 + Na_2CO_3$$

Sodium carbonate hydrolyses in aqueous soln as given by :

$$Na_2CO_3 + 2H_2O \rightarrow 2NaOH + H_2CO_3$$

$$Na_2CO_3 \equiv 2NaOH \equiv 2HCl$$

or
$$1/2\ Na_2CO_3 \equiv OH^- \equiv H^+$$

eq wt of Na_2CO_3 = 1/2 of its mol wt

$$= 53·0.$$

(*ii*) *Potassium acid carbonate.* $KHCO_3$ (mol wt=100·12 ; eq wt=100·12) is non-hygroscopic and its eq wt is greater than that of Na_2CO_3.

$$KHCO_3 + H_2O \rightarrow KOH + H_2CO_3$$

$$KHCO_3 \equiv KOH \equiv OH^- \equiv H^+$$

Eq wt of $KHCO_3$ is equal to its mol wt.

(*iii*) Thallous carbonate, Tl_2CO_3 (mol wt 468·80) is non-hygroscopic and its eq wt is quite high (234·40).

(*iv*) *Sodium tetraborate decahydrate*, borax $Na_2B_4O_7.10\ H_2O$ (mol wt—381·44) is available in pure form or it can be purified by crystallisation. Its eq wt is quite high (190·72). The reaction of borax with an acid is given as :

$$B_4O_7^{2-} + 2H^+ + 5H_2O \rightarrow 4H_3BO_3$$

$$Na_2B_4O_7.10H_2O \equiv 2H^+$$

$$1/2 \ Na_2B_4O_7.10H_2O \equiv H^+$$

$$\therefore \quad eq \ wt \ of \ Na_2B_4O_7.10H_2O = \frac{381\cdot44}{2} = 190\cdot72$$

(v) *Potassium iodate*, KIO_3 (mol wt$=214\cdot01$). This reagent is available in a high degree of purity. The soln of KIO_3 is very stable and can be kept for years without any change in the concentration of the soln. In presence of iodide ion it reacts with an acid according to the equation :

$$IO_3^- + 6H^+ + 5I^- \rightarrow 3H_2O + I_2$$
$$KIO_3 \equiv IO_3^- \equiv 6H^+$$
$$1/6 \ KIO_3 \equiv H^+$$

eq wt of $KIO_3 = 1/6$ of its mol wt
$$= 214\cdot01/6$$
$$= 35\cdot67.$$

The disadvantage with this reagent is its small eq wt so that we have to weigh a smaller amount and weighing error can be larger. This can be avoided by preparing a large volume of soln (say 1 litre) so that the amount weighed is not very small. Because the soln is highly stable it will not go waste.

(vi) *Gravimetric standardisation of acids.* Hydrochloric acid can be standardised by precipitation with $AgNO_3$ and weighing of the resultant AgCl after washing and drying (see expt. $6\cdot1$). Similarly, H_2SO_4 can be standardised by precipitation with $BaCl_2$ and weighing the ppt of $BaSO_4$ after washing and drying (see expt. $6\cdot4$).

8·20·2. Acidic Primary Standards

The following substances are generally used in acidimetry.

(i) Potassium acid phtahalate, $KHC_8H_4O_4$ (mol wt$=204\cdot22$). It is available in very pure form. It is dried at 125°C ; the dried substance is non-hygroscopic. Its reaction with a base is given as :

$$HC_8H_4O_4^- + OH^- \rightarrow C_8H_4O_4^{2-} + H_2O$$

The eq wt in this case is equal to mol wt.

(ii) *Oxalic acid dihydrate.* $H_2C_2O_4.2H_2O$ (mol wt$=126\cdot07$; eq wt$=63\cdot034$). It is a diprotic acid which can be used for the standardisation of alkali soln (also $KMnO_4$ soln) using phenolphthalein as indicator. The drawback of this reagent is that there is some occluded water present in the dihydrate crystals. By drying at about 100°C and then cooling in an atmosphere of about 60 per cent relative humidity, the dihydrate of exact composition is formed.

(iii) *Benzoic acid*, C_6H_5COOH or $HC_7H_5O_2$ (mol wt$=$eq wt$=122\cdot12$). It is available in pure form but is fluffy, hence difficult to handle during weighing. It should be molten in a platinum crucible and the resultant cake should be powdered and then weighed. Another disadvantage is poor solubility of the acid in water, hence alcohol-water mixture has to be used for the preparation of a fairly concentrated soln.

(*iv*) *Sulphamic acid*, [NH_2SO_3H] (mol wt 97·10), is a crystalline solid readily soluble in water and can be titrated with a strong base.

Potassium acid iodate ($KH(IO_3)_2$), HCl in the form of its constant boiling mixture, succinic acid, furoic acid, hydrazine sulphate etc., have also been used as primary standards for titrating a soln of a base.

8·21. LABORATORY EXERCISES

Experiment 8·1

Preparation of a 0·1000 M (the same as 0·1000 N) soln of NaOH.

The molecule of NaOH contains only one ionisable OH^- group, hence, for NaOH :

(*a*) Eq wt = mol wt = 40·00

(*b*) 1 g eq = 1 mole = 40·00 g

(*c*) 0·1 molar soln = 0·1 normal soln.

In order to prepare 0·1000 M soln we must have 0·1000 mole, *i.e.*, 40 g × 0·1000 = 4·0000 g NaOH in 1 litre soln. Now, because NaOH absorbs moisture during weighing, we cannot exactly weigh 4·0000 g so that its standard soln cannot be prepared directly by weighing, dissolving in water and then making up with distilled water to a known volume. In such a case, an indirect method is used which involves the following steps :

1. **Preparation of an approximate soln of NaOH.** Weigh out approximately 5 g of NaOH on a rough balance (the amount weighed should be more than the theoretically calculated amount, *i.e.*, 4·0000 g) and dissolve it in distilled water from which the dissolved CO_2 gas has been removed ; this gives NaOH soln that is free from carbonate. (In order to drive out CO_2, water is boiled for about 1 hour cooled and then used for dissolving NaOH). Make up the volume of the soln to 1 litre and shake thoroughly.

2. **Preparation of a standard acid solution.** [To find out the exact concentration of NaOH soln prepared in step 1, it is necessary to titrate it with a standard soln of an acid ; this process is called standardisation. A standard acid soln can be prepared by taking any acid which is a primary standard, such as furoric acid, sulphamic acid, succinic acid or oxalic acid. Suppose we are using oxalic acid. Now, its mol wt is 126·07 and because it is diprotic, its

eq wt is $126\cdot07/2 = 63\cdot04$.   To prepare $0\cdot1$ N soln, $63\cdot04/10 = 6\cdot304$ g oxalic acid should be present per litre soln ; if 250 ml soln is prepared, the amount of oxalic acid would be $6\cdot304/4 = 1\cdot576$ g]. Weigh out exactly $1\cdot576$ g of oxalic acid, dissolve in water, make up the volume to 250 ml in a volumetric flask and shake the soln thoroughly.

3.   Standardisation of NaOH soln. Take a known volume, say $25\cdot0$ ml, of oxalic acid soln by means of a pipette into a conical flask. Add 2 to 3 drops of phenolphthalein indicator soln and titrate with NaOH soln taken in a burette. Swirl the flask during the titration and stop the addition of alkali soln as soon as the titration soln becomes just pink. Note the volume of the alkali soln added by taking the burette reading ; suppose it is $20\cdot0$ ml (note that because NaOH soln is stronger than $0\cdot1$ N, hence its volume will be smaller than the volume of the acid taken, *i.e.*, $25\cdot0$ ml).

4.   Calculation of normality of NaOH solution. The normality of NaOH soln can be calculated by using the relation :

$$N_{NaOH} \times V_{NaOH} = N_{ox} \times V_{ox} \quad \text{(see 8-E)}$$

$$N_{NaOH} \times 20\cdot0 = 0\cdot1 \times 25\cdot0$$

$$N_{NaOH} = \frac{0\cdot1 \times 25\cdot0}{20\cdot0} = 0\cdot1250 \text{ N}$$

5.   Preparation of exact $0\cdot1000$ N NaOH. We want 1 litre soln of NaOH of normality $0\cdot1000$ but we have a soln whose normality is $0\cdot1250$. By calculation we can find out that what volume of $0\cdot1250$ N soln will be equivalent to $1000\cdot0$ ml of $0\cdot1000$ N NaOH soln.

$$0\cdot1250 \times V = 0\cdot1000 \times 1000\cdot0$$

$$V = \frac{0\cdot1000 \times 1000\cdot0}{0\cdot1250} = 800\cdot0 \text{ ml}$$

It means that if $800\cdot0$ ml of $0\cdot1250$ N NaOH is diluted to $1000\cdot0$ ml and thoroughly shaken, $0\cdot1000$ N soln of NaOH will be obtained.

Note. It is not necessary to prepare exactly $0\cdot1000$ N oxalic acid soln. All that we need is an oxalic acid soln of known concentration. However, preparation of exact $0\cdot1000$ or $0\cdot0100$ N soln simplifies titrimetric calculations considerably.

Experiment 8·2

Preparation of a $0\cdot1000$ M (the same as $0\cdot1000$ N) soln of HCl.

1.   Take about 10 ml of concentrated HCl, dilute it to 1000 ml and shake the soln. [Concentrated HCl is approximately 12 N.

If 1 ml of this soln is ten times diluted (to 10 ml), the normality of the diluted soln will be $12/10=1\cdot2$. If this soln is ten times further diluted so that the final volume is 100 ml, the normality will become $1\cdot2/10=0\cdot12$ that is slightly more than the desired value, *i.e.*, $0\cdot1000$. Thus, if 10 ml of concentrated HCl are diluted to 1000 ml, *i.e.*, dilution is hundred times, the normality of the resultant soln will be about $12/100=0\cdot12\cdot1$

2. Take a known volume ($25\cdot0$ ml) of the acid soln prepared in step 1 and titrate with $0\cdot1000$ N NaOH prepared by the method described in expt. 8·1. Suppose, the volume of NaOH required for the titration is $27\cdot8$ ml (note that the normality of HCl is greater than $0\cdot1$, hence the volume of alkali required will be more than $25\cdot0$ ml).

3. The normality of HCl can be calculated by :

$$N_{HCl} = \frac{N_{NaOH} \times V_{NaOH}}{V_{HCl}}$$

$$= \frac{0\cdot1 \times 27\cdot8}{25\cdot0} = 0\cdot1112$$

4. We have $0\cdot1112$ N HCl whereas we want to prepare $1000\cdot0$ ml of $0\cdot1000$ N HCl soln. We have to find out what volume of $0\cdot1112$ N HCl will be equivalent to $1000\cdot0$ ml of $0\cdot1000$ N HCl.

$$V \times 0\cdot1112 = 1000\cdot0 \times 0\cdot1000$$

$$V = \frac{1000\cdot0 \times 0\cdot1000}{0\cdot1112} = 899\cdot3 \text{ ml}$$

Thus an exact $0\cdot1000$ N HCl soln can be obtained if we take $899\cdot3$ ml of the acid soln prepared in step 1, dilute it to $1000\cdot0$ ml and shake the soln well.

Note. In step 2, the approximate soln of HCl prepared in step 1 has been standardised by titration with $0\cdot1$ N NaOH. This standardisation can also be done by titration with a substance which is a primary standard, like sodium carbonate, potassium hydrogen carbonate or borax.

Experiment 8·3

Determination of the normality of the given acid soln by alkalimetry.

1. Prepare a standard soln of a suitable alkali. The concentration of this alkali soln should not be very much different from that of the acid soln otherwise very small or very large titre value will be obtained.

2. Select a suitable indicator after studying the pH-neutralisation curve for the acid and alkali selected and also the colour change interval of the indicator.

3. Titrate a known volume of the acid soln with standard alkali soln.

Note. If the colour change of the indicator is better judged when the change is from basic to acidic form, a known volume of alkali is titrated with the given acid soln taken in a burette. For example, with methyl orange the colour change judgement is better when the medium changes from alkaline to acidic side, *i.e.*, colour changes from yellow to red. In this case a known volume of alkali is titrated with acid soln. If the colour change from acidic to alkaline side is easily seen (as in the case of phenolphthalein), a known volume of acid is titrated with alkali soln.

Experiment 8·4

Titration of 0·005 M acetic acid iodometrically with a standard thiosulphate soln.

Discussion

In acid-base titrimetry, the inflection on pH-neutralisation curve is smaller for a weak acid as compared to that for a strong acid (see 8·11 and 8·12). For example, in the titration of 0·1 M, HCl with 0·1 M, NaOH, the inflection is from pH 4·5 to 9·5 (5 pH unit), but on titrating 0·1 M, CH_3COOH with 0·1 M, NaOH the inflection is much smaller ; it is from pH 7·8 to 9·7 (only about 2 pH units). On increasing the dilution of acid and alkali solution, the inflection further decreases making the judgement of the colour change very difficult (see 8·11·1). When the inflection is less than 2 pH units, the end point cannot be located. It has been found that if the concentration of CH_3COOH is 0·01 M, it can be titrated with 0·01 M, NaOH, but when the concentration further decreases, the titration does not give satisfactory results. (Even with 0·01 M solutions, acetic acid has to be heated to remove dissolved CO_2 which interferes in the titration.) It follows that when the concentration of a weak acid is smaller than 0·01 M, titration with alkali does not give accurate results. In such cases an iodometric method can be successfully used, which makes use of the reaction :

$$IO_3^- + 5I^- + 6H^+ \longrightarrow 3H_2O + 3I_2$$

The liberated iodine is titrated with a standard thiosulphate soln and then the amount of acid present can be calculated.

Procedure

Take a known volume of the given acetic acid soln in a glass-stoppered conical flask (called iodine flask). Add about 1 g of KIO_3

and about 2 g of KI. Swirl the flask for 2 to 3 min and then titrate the liberated iodine with standard thiosulphate soln (0·01 M) using starch as indicator. The reactions involved are :

$$6CH_3COOH + 5KI + KIO_3 \longrightarrow 6CH_3COOK + 3H_2O + 3I_2$$
$$3I_2 + 6Na_2S_2O_3 \longrightarrow 3Na_2S_4O_6 + 6NaI$$
$$\therefore \quad 6CH_3COOH \equiv KIO_3 \equiv 3I_2 \equiv 6Na_2S_2O_3$$

or, $Na_2S_2O_3 \equiv CH_3COOH$

1 ml of 0·1 M, $Na_2S_2O_3 \equiv$ 1 ml, 0·1 M CH_3COOH
                    $\equiv 6·0$ mg CH_3COOH

1 ml of 0·01 M, $Na_2S_2O_3 \equiv 0·60$ mg CH_3COOH

[Mol. wt of CH_3COOH is 60,

1000 ml, 1 M CH_3COOH soln contains 60 g of acid

1000 ml, 0·1 M CH_3COOH soln contains 6·0 g of acid

1 ml, 0·1 M CH_3COOH soln contains 6·0 mg of acid]

(Iodometric titration will be studied in greater detail in Chapter 10.)

Experiment 8·5

Quantitative analysis of a mixture of NaOH and Na_2CO_3 by titration with HCl.

Discussion

In the titration of NaOH (say of concentration 0·1 M) with 0·1 M HCl, the change in pH near the equivalence point is 4·5 to 9·5 and phenolphthalein can be used as an indicator (see 8·11·1).

Sodium carbonate reacts with HCl in two stages as shown by :

$$Na_2CO_3 + HCl \longrightarrow NaCl + NaHCO_3 \qquad \qquad ...(A)$$
$$NaHCO_3 + HCl \longrightarrow NaCl + H_2O + CO_2 \qquad \qquad ...(B)$$

It has been seen in 8·18·1, that the pH at the first end point (corresponding to reaction A) is 8·35 and that at the completion of the reaction B is 3·93. The first end point can, therefore, be detected by means of phenolphthalein and the second end point by using methyl orange as indicator.

Procedure

    Take a known volume of the given soln, containing a mixture of NaOH and Na_2CO_3, by means of a pipette into a conical flask.

2. Add 2 drops of phenolphthalein soln (because the soln is alkaline, hence the colour of the soln will be pink).

3. Gradually add 0·1 M HCl (or some other soln of known strength) from a burette and keep on swirling the flask. Stop adding HCl when the soln just becomes colourless and record the volume of HCl by noting burette reading ; suppose it is T ml. (These T ml of HCl will be required for the complete neutralisation of NaOH and for completing reaction A).

4. Add 2 drops of methyl orange soln (the pH at the first end point is 8·35, hence methyl orange will have its alkaline colour, *i.e.*, yellow colour).

5. Continue the addition of HCl until the soln becomes just red. Note the burette reading ; suppose it is $(T+t)$ ml.

6. Calculations :

$(T+t)$ ml HCl used for complete neutralisation of NaOH and Na_2CO_3.

T ml HCl used for complete neutralisation of NaOH and half nentralisation of Na_2CO_3 (carbonate to bicarbonate—reaction A).

∴ $(T+t)-T=t$ ml HCl will be used for the half neutralisation of Na_2CO_3.

∴ $2t$ ml HCl used for the complete neutralisation of Na_2CO_3.

∴ $(T-2t)$ ml HCl used for the neutralisation of NaOH.

Note. Phenolphthalein soln is prepared by weighing 1 g of the indicator, dissolving in 50 ml of alcohol and diluting with water to 100 ml. Methyl orange is prepared by dissolving 0·05 g of the indicator in 100 ml water.

Example 8(v)

25·0 ml of a mixture containing NaOH and Na_2CO_3 was titrated with 0·1 N HCl. The first end point with phenolphthalein was obtained when 20·0 ml HCl was added. On continuing the titration, the second end point with methyl orange was observed when a total of 25·0 ml HCl was added. Calculate meq of NaOH and Na_2CO_3 present in the mixture.

1. Total volume of HCl used up is 25·0 ml. This **corresponds** to the complete neutralisation of NaOH and Na_2CO_3.

2. The volume of HCl at the first end point is 20·0 ml. This corresponds to the complete neutralisation of NaOH and half neutralisation of Na_2CO_3.

3. The volume of HCl **required** for half neutralisation of Na_2CO_3 will, therefore, be equal to (25·0 −20·0)=5·0 ml.

4. The volume of HCl required for the complete neutralisation of Na_2CO_3 will be, therefore, equal to $5.0 \times 2 = 10.0$ ml.

5. The total volume of HCl consumed is 25.0 ml. Out of this, 10.0 ml are consumed by Na_2CO_3 and the rest, *i.e.*, $(25.0 - 10.0) = 15.0$ by NaOH. Thus :

15.0 ml, 0.1 N HCl consumed by NaOH

and   10.0 ml, 0.1 N HCl consumed by Na_2CO_3

Now, 1000 ml, 1 N HCl = 1 g eq

1000 ml, 0.1 N HCl = 0.1 g eq

1 ml, 0.1 N HCl = 0.1 meq (milligram eq).

$\therefore$ 15.0 ml, 0.1 N HCl = $0.1 \times 15 = 1.5$ meq

and   10.0 ml, 0.1 N HCl = $0.1 \times 10 = 1.0$ meq.

Hence, the mixture will contain 1.5 meq of NaOH and 1.0 meq of Na_2CO_3. (For Na_2CO_3, mol wt = 2 eq wt, or 2 g eq are equal to a mole, or 2 milligram equivalents are equal to 1 millimole. Hence, in the mixture the amount of Na_2CO_3 will be, $\frac{1}{2}$ *i.e.*, 0.5 millimole).

A mixture containing Na_2CO_3 and $NaHCO_3$ can also be quantitatively analysed by making use of phenolphthalein and methyl orange indicators.

9

Acid-Base Titrimetry in Non-Aqueous Solvents

It is well known that water can act as a solvent for a large number of substances of different nature. Although water itself is poorly dissociated and so has poor conducting ability but it dissolves so many electrolytes. The aqueous solution of electrolytes contain ions, hence these can take part in ionic reactions. Now, ionic reactions are generally quite rapid, hence they are very useful in developing quantitative methods of analysis. Besides, the use of water is economical and aqueous solutions are easy to handle. For these reasons, water is preferred as a solvent and most of the analytical work involves reactions in aqueous medium. However, there are certain cases where the use of non-aqueous solvents is advantageous.

9.1. PROBLEMS IN THE ALKALIMETRIC DETERMINATION OF WEAK ACID IN AQUEOUS MEDIUM

In sections 8.11 and 8.12, the change of pH during the neutralisation of strong and weak acids with alkali was studied. It was seen that when 0.1 N HCl is titrated with 0.1 N NaOH, the jump in pH (inflection) at the equivalence point is from 4.3 to 9.7, i.e., by 5.4 pH units. But if a weak acid, such as CH_3COOH, is taken in place of HCl, the inflection is 7.7 to 10.0, i.e., by only 2.3 pH units. As the dissociation constant (which is a measure of strength of an acid) of the acid becomes smaller the pH jump also decreases. Furthermore, when acid and alkali solutions used in the titration are dilute the inflection on the pH-neutralisation curve becomes still smaller (see Fig. 8.2). Now it has been shown that when this inflection is smaller than 2 pH units, the change in colour of the indicator at the end point cannot be judged. This is the reason that when a dilute soln (concentration less than 0.01 N) of a weak acid is titrated with alkali, there is difficulty in judging the end point so, there is considerable titration error.

It has been seen in 8·12 that phenolphthalein is a suitable indicator in the titration of a weak acid with strong base. When a small amount of a weak acid is given we have to use a dilute soln of NaOH for the titration. It has been observed that if 0·01 N or more dilute soln of NaOH is used, the pink colour of the indicator fades away rapidly at the end point. This presents difficulty in the recognition of the end point. (A faint pink colour first appears. Now, it is necessary to shake the soln so that there is a thorough mixing of the added titrant. When this is done the pink colour practically disappears. This creates a doubt that the end point has not been reached. In order to confirm the end point, a drop or two of the titrant are then added when soln again appears to be faint pink but on shaking it fades away rapidly. This is known as fleeting end point. Due to this problem, more titrant has to be added to locate the end point than required stoichiometrically).

Another problem in the titration of a dilute soln of a weak acid is the interference due to atmospheric CO_2. Hence the titration is done at a higher temperature to drive out the dissolved CO_2. But if the acid under question is volatile, a part of the acid will be lost.

The difficulties encountered in the titration of a dilute soln of a weak acid with alkali soln can be summarised as :

(i) the inflection on the pH-neutralisation curve is small,

(ii) the phenolphthalein colour fades away at the end point,

and

(iii) interference due to atmospheric CO_2.

The above difficulties can be overcome if by some means the dissociation constant of the weak acid can be increased so that it behaves like a strong acid. This can be done by using a suitable non-aqueous solvent in place of water. In order to understand the increase in the dissociation of a weak acid in a suitable solvent we must study the concept of acids and bases suggested by Bronsted.

9·2. ACID-BASE CONCEPT OF BRONSTED AND LOWRY

It was seen in 8·1 that according to Arrhenius an acid is a compound which dissociates in water to give H^+ ions and a base is one which gives OH^- ions. The theory of Arrhenius is quite successful in explaining acid-base reactions in aqueous medium but it has certain shortcomings, moreover, it is restricted to acid base reactions only in aqueous medium.

It has been known, for a long time, that the bare proton (H^+) does not exist in soln but like other ions is solvated (or hydrated if water is the solvent). Thus in aqueous soln we do not have H^+ but it is associated with water molecules ; the ion can be represented as $H(H_2O)_n^+$, where n may be large. However, the hydrated proton is generally represented as H_3O^+ called *hydronium ion* (also hydro-xonium or oxonium ion). We know that hydrogen chloride gas (HCl gas) contains covalent molecules and because H^+ ions are not present so HCl gas does not show acidic property. But when this gas is dissolved in water, a proton is taken out from the HCl mole-cule by a water molecule :

$$HCl + H_2O \rightarrow H_3O^+ + Cl^- \qquad \qquad ...(9\text{·}1)$$

Hence, the soln of HCl gas in water (called hydrochloric acid) behaves like an acid. If dry HCl gas is dissolved in dry benzene, the resultant soln will not act like an acid because benzene molecules are not capable of accepting protons from HCl molecules.

In 1923, Bronsted and Lowry, independently, defined acids and bases in terms of proton transfer ; an acid being a substance which donates proton whereas a base acts as an acceptor of proton. Thus, the concept of Arrhenius has been considerably modified and extended to include many substances that were not considered as acids or bases in the original theory. For example, in the reaction

$$NH_4^+ + H_2O \rightarrow NH_3 + H_3O^+ \qquad \qquad ...(9\text{·}2)$$

ammonium ion is giving a proton to a water molecule, hence according to Bronsted-Lowry theory, NH_4^+ is an acid and H_2O is a base. The protonic definition of a base is also quite different from that proposed by Arrhenius. In Arrhenius theory a base must be a hydroxyl compound which should give hydroxyl ions in aqueous soln. But the Bronsted model does not require any parti-cular type of compound or a particular solvent. Any substance in any medium will be called a base if it can accept a proton. Thus ammonia and pyridine will also be called base because they can accept proton although they do not contain hydroxyl group.

$$NH_3 + H_2O \rightarrow NH_4^+ + OH^- \qquad \qquad ...(9\text{·}3)$$
$$NH_3 + HCl \rightarrow NH_4^+ + Cl^- \qquad \qquad ...(9\text{·}4)$$

9·2·1. Conjugate Acid and Conjugate Base

Suppose we have a compound HB which gives **off** a proton (hence HB is an acid), the remaining part B will have some affinity for proton, *i.e.*, it can accept a proton, hence it will be a base :

$$\underset{\text{Acid}}{HB} \rightleftharpoons H^+ + \underset{\text{Base}}{B^-} \qquad \qquad ...(9\text{·}5)$$

B is said to be conjugate base of the acid HB. Thus an acid differs from its conjugate base only by a proton. The acid HB can be electrically neutral (HCl) or a cation (NH_4^+) or an anion (HSO_4^-), as shown by :

$$HCl + H_2O \rightleftharpoons H_3O^+ + Cl^- \qquad ...(9\cdot6)$$
$$NH_4^+ + H_2O \rightleftharpoons H_3O^+ + NH_3 \qquad ...(9\cdot7)$$
$$HSO_4^- + H_2O \rightleftharpoons H_3O^+ + SO_4^{2-} \qquad ...(9\cdot8)$$

In above equations HCl, NH_4^+ and HSO_4^- are acids and Cl^-, NH_3 and SO_4^{2-} respectively are their conjugate bases. An acid can donate proton only when there is a base present to accept it. For the simple dissociation of an acid, the solvent will act as a base :

$$\underset{\text{Acid I}}{HCl} + \underset{\text{Base I}}{H_2O} \rightleftharpoons \underset{\text{Acid II}}{H_3O^+} + \underset{\text{Base II}}{Cl^-} \qquad ...(9\cdot9)$$

The pair Acid I-Base II or Base I-Acid II are said to be conjugates.

9·3. SOME PROPERTIES OF SOLVENTS

The acidic or basic behaviour of a solute dissolved in a given solvent depends upon :

(i) acid-base properties of the solvent relative to the solute,

(ii) autoprotolysis constant of the solvent, and

(iii) dielectric constant of the solvent.

First of all let us consider the different types of solvents and their influence on acid-base behaviour of a solute.

Amphiprotic Solvents

These solvents can accept as well as donate protons hence are able to act as Bronsted-Lowry acid or base. Water is a well known example of an *amphiprotic solvent* as shown by :

$$\underset{\text{Acid I}}{H_2O} + \underset{\text{Base I}}{H_2O} \rightleftharpoons \underset{\text{Acid II}}{H_3O^+} + \underset{\text{Base II}}{OH^-} \qquad ...(9\cdot10)$$

Here one water molecule donates a proton thus acts as an acid and after giving a proton forms its conjugate base OH^-. The other water molecule accepts the proton hence is a base : its conjugate acid is H_3O^+. In this way water is behaving as an acid and also as a base. Methanol and ethanol are also amphiprotic solvents which under go auto-protolysis :

$$CH_3OH + CH_3OH \rightleftharpoons CH_3OH_2^+ + CH_3O^-$$
$$C_2H_5OH + C_2H_5OH \rightleftharpoons C_2H_5OH_2^+ + C_2H_5O^-$$

The term *autoprotolysis* means that no other substance is needed in the proton transfer process.

Inert or Aprotic Solvents

Certain solvents do not donate or accept protons hence do not show acidic or basic properties. These are known as *aprotic* or *inert* solvents. Benzene and carbon tetrachloride are examples of this class of solvents.

Protophilic Solvents

If a substance dissolved in a solvent has to show acidic properties it must donate protons and this is possible when the solvent acts as a proton acceptor, *i.e.*, it must have basic character. Such a solvent is known as *protophilic* solvent ; examples of this type of solvent are water, alcohol, liquid ammonia and amines.

Protogenic Solvents

A solvent which has a tendency to give protons and so exhibit acidic character is known as a *protogenic* solvent. Examples of this class of solvents include water, alcohol pure formic, acetic and **sulphuric acid.**

9·4. THE ROLE OF SOLVENT

One of the important contributions of Bronsted theory is its emphasis on the role of the solvent in the dissociation of acids and bases. According to Bronsted an acid is any species having a tendency to lose a proton and this will happen only when another substance is present to accept protons ; this substance then acts as a base. Consider an acid HB which is dissolved in a solvent S capable of accepting proton then we can write :

$$\underset{\text{Acid 1}}{HB} + \underset{\text{Base II}}{S} \rightleftharpoons \underset{\text{Acid II}}{HS^+} + \underset{\text{Base I}}{B^-} \qquad ...(9\cdot11)$$

Here, $HB-B^-$ and HS^+-S are two conjugate acid-base pairs. If HB has a greater tendency to give protons as compared to HS^+, the equilibrium (9·11) will lie on the right side. Thus the relative tendency of furnishing protons is a measure of the relative strength of two acids. If HB is very much stronger than HS^+ the equilibrium will lie far to the right and HB will be almost 100 per cent dissociated so that [HB] will be practically zero. For example, if $HClO_4$ (perchloric acid) is dissolved in water the following equilibrium can be written :

$$HClO_4 + H_2O \rightleftharpoons H_3O^+ + ClO_4^- \qquad ...(9\cdot12)$$

The tendency of $HClO_4$ to lose proton is very much greater than that of H_3O^+, hence $HClO_4$ will be almost completely dissociated and will behave like a strong acid in aqueous medium. Now if the solvent is changed from water to glacial acetic acid, the equilibrium will be given by :

$$HClO_4 + CH_3COOH \rightleftharpoons CH_3COOH_2^+ + ClO_4^- \qquad .. (9\cdot13)$$

According to Arrhenius theory $HClO_4$ and CH_3COOH both are acids. But $HClO_4$ has a stronger tendency for losing protons as compared to that of CH_3COOH so under pressure CH_3COOH will have to accept protons supplied by $HClO_4$; thus CH_3COOH which according to Arrehenius theory should always act as an acid will play the role of a base if Bronsted concept is applied. Further, $CH_3COOH_2{}^+$ (protonated acetic acid) is a stronger acid as compared to H_3O^+. Hence, $CH_3COOH_2{}^+$ will put up a greater resistance to the proton donating capability of $HClO_4$ as compared to the opposition provided by H_3O^+. This is the reason why the dissociation of $HClO_4$ will not be 100 per cent in glacial acetic acid. It follows that the dissociation of $HClO_4$ will be greater in water than in glacial acetic acid, i.e., $HClO_4$ is a stronger acid in water than in glacial acetic acid medium.

In aqueous medium $HClO_4$ and HCl both dissociate practically completely provided the soln is not very concentrated. Hence, both of them will appear to be equally strong. This is known as *leveling effect*. But in a less basic solvent, such as glacial acetic acid, the dissociation of these acids will not be complete ; it will be greater for $HClO_4$ than for HCl so that we can say that $HClO_4$ is a stronger acid than HCl. Because CH_3COOH can differentiate between the strengths of the two acids, it is known as *differentiating solvent*.

Let us consider the acid-base behaviour of CH_3COOH in three solvents namely anhydrous H_2SO_4, water and dimethylformamide (DMF). In H_2SO_4 medium, the proton giving ability of H_2SO_4 is greater than that of CH_3COOH so it will have to accept protons furnished by H_2SO_4, i.e., CH_3COOH will act as a base. In water soln the proton donating capacity of CH_3OOH will be greater than that of water, hence CH_3COOH will donate protons to water and will behave as an acid.

$$CH_3COOH + H_2O \rightleftharpoons H_3O^+ + CH_3COO^-$$

In the above case CH_3COOH is a stronger acid than H_3O^+, hence the equilibrium will lie slightly to the right so that in aqueous soln CH_3COOH will behave like a weak acid. If DMF is used as a solvent it has a strong tendency to accept protons so it will promote the dissociation of CH_3COOH. Thus in a basic solvents (protophilic solvent) like DMF or ethylenediamine (EDA) even carboxylic acids behave like mineral acids in water. Thus acetic acid in DMF or EDA will act like a strong acid.

9·5. THE AUTOPROTOLYSIS CONSTANT

Suppose SH is an amphiprotic solvent, then its autoprotolysis can be written as :

$$SH + SH \rightleftharpoons HSH^+ + S^- \qquad \qquad ...(9·14)$$

The equilibrium constant for (9·14) is given by

$$Ks = \frac{a_{HSH^+} \times a_{S^-}}{a^2_{SH}}$$

Now, by convention the activity of the pure solvent is taken to be unity and making the approximation that activity is equal to concentration we can write :

$$Ks = [HSH^+] \times [S^-] \qquad \text{(autoprotolysis constant)}$$

For water the autoprotolysis constant at 25°C is given by :

$$Ks = Kw = [H_3O^+] \times [OH^-] = [H^+] \times [OH^-]$$
$$= 1·00 \times 10^{-14}$$

or $pKw = 14·00$

For ethanol pKs is 19·1, for methanol it is 16·7. It can be shown that smaller the value of autoprotolysis constant greater is the inflection on the pH-neutralisation curve. Hence, in titrating a weak acid with alkali we should use a solvent whose autoprotopsis constant is smaller.

9·6. THE DIELECTRIC CONSTANT

The dielectric constant of a solvent is a measure of the ease of separation of two oppositely charged ions or the ease of dissociation of an ion-pair in that solvent. The effect of dielectric constant on the strength of the dissolved acid can be understood by studying the acidic behaviour of CH_3COOH in water and in ethanol. The dielectric constant of water at 25°C is 78·5 while it is only 24·3 for ethanol. Hence, the dissociation of CH_3COOH will be greater in water than in ethanol, *i.e.*, CH_3COOH will act as a weaker acid in ethanol as compared to that in water. In general, while selecting a non-aqueous solvent for acid-base titrimetry its behaviour (protogenic, protophilic, amphiprotic or aprotic), the value of its autoprotolysis constant and that of its dielectric constant must be taken into consideration.

9·7. TITRATIONS IN BASIC SOLVENTS

It was pointed out in 9·1 that the titration of a dilute soln of a weak acid with standard alkali does not give accurate results. In 9·4 it has been shown that in a basic solvent the dissociation constant of a weak acid is increased and so even a weak carboxylic acid in such a solvent behaves like a strong acid. Among the common basic solvents are butylamine, ethylenediamine, dimethylformamide and liquid ammonia. These solvents have a strong tendency to accept protons. This is the reason that if HCl and CH_3COOH are dissolved in a basic solvent like butylamine, the solvent extracts protons from both the acids so that they are virtually completely ionised :

$$HCl + C_4H_9NH_2 \rightleftharpoons C_4H_9NH_3^+Cl^-$$

$$CH_3COOH + C_4H_9NH_2 \rightleftharpoons C_4H_9NH_3^+OOCH_3^-$$

Because butylamine has a low dielectric constant the two acids exist as undissociated ion-pairs. Acetic acid whlch is weak acid in water is leveled to the strength of a strong acid in butylamine. Thus both HCl and CH_3COOH will behave like strong acids in a basic solvent.

When simple alcohols like ethanol or methanol are used as solvents for the titrimetric determination of carboxylic acids, the titrant generally used are sodium methoxide or sodium ethoxide (C_2H_5ONa, prepared by the reaction of pure sodium metal and anhydrous ethyl alcohol). Tetraalkylemmonium hydroxides are also used as titrants in a number of solvents such as alcohols and benzene-alcohol mixture.

The advantage of these basic solvents and titrants is that there is a good inflection on the pH-neutralisation curve. But there is a problem with handling and storage of strongly basic titrants and solvents because these quickly absorb atmospheric carbon dioxide and other acidic impurities. Furthermore, these should be protected from the absorption of moisture.

The problem of end point detection in non-aqueous titrimetry is not very simple. It should be noted that the pH ranges during which an indicator changes colour in non-aqueous solvents is different from those in water. The whole concept of a pH scale has to be modified for solvents other than water. (Note that for water autoprotolysis constant is 10^{-14} and the pH scale extends from 0 to 14, but this is not the case when we use some other solvent such as ethanol whose autoprotolysis constant is 7.9×10^{-20}). However, several well known acid-base indicators such as methyl red, phenolphthalein and thymolphthalein have been found to function satisfactorily in certain non-aqueous titrations.

The number of compounds which have been titrated in non-aqueous media is quite large. Very weak acids, such as phenols, have been titrated in a strong basic solvent like ethylenediamine. Weak bases, like amines and amino acids can be titrated with perchloric acid in an acidic solvent like glacial acetic acid. In glacial acetic medium even a weak base will behave like a strong base.

10

Redox Titrimetry

An oxidation-reduction titration (or redox titration) is one in which the substance to be determined is either oxidised or reduced by means of the soln with which the titration is made. The detailed study of redox reactions started at a much later date as compared to other types of chemical reactions. In spite of this, titrimetric determinations based on oxidation-reduction reactions are most widely used methods in the quantitative analysis of inorganic as well as organic compounds. In order to understand the theory of redox titrimetry, we must know such terms as oxidation, reduction, oxidising agent or oxidant and reducing agent or reductant. In a titrimetric procedure, a reagent soln of known normality is needed. For preparing such a soln the eq wt of the reagent must be known. Hence, we must know how the eq wt of the reagent is related to its mol wt. These problems will be discussed in this chapter and then some redox titration will be described.

10·1. OXIDATION AND REDUCTION

Originally oxidation meant addition of oxygen, such as :

$$C + O_2 \longrightarrow CO_2$$

or,
$$2Mg + O_2 \longrightarrow 2MgO$$

Reduction which was just the opposite of oxidation, meant removal of oxygen usually through the use of hydrogen such, as :

$$CuO(hot) + H_2 \longrightarrow Cu + H_2O$$

Such a definition has a very limited scope, hence a wider definition was then proposed. According to this definition, oxidation involved an increase in valency. For example, when $FeSO_4$ is converted into $Fe_2(SO_4)_3$, it is a case of oxidation because during this conversion the valency of iron increases from 2 to 3. Change of

$Fe_2(SO_4)_3$ to $FeSO_4$ will be called reduction because now the valency decreases from 3 to 2.

A more general definition of oxidation and reduction can be obtained by considering the electron transfer during these processes. Consider the reaction between ferric chloride and stannous chloride :

$$2FeCl_3+SnCl_2 \longrightarrow 2FeCl_2+SnCl_4 \qquad \text{...(10.1)}$$

or in terms of ions :

$$2Fe^{3+}+6Cl^-+Sn^{2+}+2Cl^- \longrightarrow 2Fe^{2+}+4Cl^-+Sn^{4+}+4Cl^-$$

or,
$$2Fe^{3+}+Sn^{2+} \longrightarrow 2Fe^{2+}+Sn^{4+} \qquad \text{...(10.2)}$$

Equation (10.2) can be divided into two parts :

$$2Fe^{3+} \longrightarrow 2Fe^{2+} \qquad \text{...(10.3)}$$

and,
$$Sn^{2+} \longrightarrow Sn^{4+} \qquad \text{...(10.4)}$$

Equation (10.3) is not balanced with respect to charge. There are $2\times3=6$ positive charges on the left hand side and only $2\times2=4$ on the right hand side. This equation can be balanced if we add 2 electrons to the left hand side :

$$2Fe^{3+}+2e \longrightarrow 2Fe^{2+} \text{ (partial equation for reduction) ...(10.5)}$$
$$+6 \quad +(-2) \qquad +4$$

or,
$$Fe^{3+}+e \longrightarrow Fe^{2+}$$

The conversion Fe^{3+} to Fe^{2+} ion involves a decrease of valency from +3 to +2, hence it is a case of reduction. At the same time there is a gain of electron so we can relate reduction with gain of electrons. Thus, *reduction* is defined as a process accompanied by a gain of one or more electrons by atoms or ions. Equation (10.5) is a part of the overall equation (10.2) and because it represents reduction so it can be called the *partial equation for reduction.*

The other change is Sn^{2+} to Sn^{4+} which involves an increase in valency from +2 to +4, hence, it is a case of oxidation. It will also be seen that to balance equation (10.4) it is necessary to write :

$$Sn^{2+} \longrightarrow Sn^{4+}+2e$$
$$+2 \qquad +4 + (-2)$$

or, $Sn^{2+}-2e \longrightarrow Sn^{4+}$ (partial equation for oxidation) ...(10.6)

In this way the change Sn^{2+} to Sn^{4+} is oxidation and it involves a loss of electrons. Therefore, *oxidation* is defined as the process involving a loss of electrons.

In the following processes, there is a loss of one or more electrons, hence the ion concerned is said to be oxidised :

$$(i) \quad Fe^{2+} - e \longrightarrow Fe^{3+}$$

$$(ii) \quad Sn^{2+} - 2e \longrightarrow Sn^{4+}$$

$$(iii) \quad I^- - e \longrightarrow \tfrac{1}{2}I_2$$

$$(iv) \quad Cl^- - e \longrightarrow \tfrac{1}{2}Cl_2$$

$$\cdots(10.7)$$

In above examples, Fe^{2+} is oxidised to Fe^{3+}, Sn^{2+} to Sn^{4+}, I^- to I_2 and Cl^- ion is oxidised to chlorine.

In the following examples, there is a gain of electrons consequently, the ions or atoms are said to be reduced :

$$(i) \quad Sn^{4+} + 2e \longrightarrow Sn^{2+}$$

$$(ii) \quad \tfrac{1}{2}Cl_2 + e \longrightarrow Cl^-$$

$$(iii) \quad MnO_4^- + 8H^+ + 5e \longrightarrow Mn^{2+} + 4H_2O$$

$$(iv) \quad Cu^{2+} + e \longrightarrow Cu^+$$

$$\cdots(10.8)$$

In above processes, Sn^{4+}, Cl_2, MnO_4^- and Cu^{2+} ions are reduced.

During electrolysis, the negative electrode (cathode) supplies electrons which are gained by ions which are discharged at the cathode. The process taking place at the cathode is, therefore, reduction. For example, when a soln of $CuSO_4$ is electrolysed, the process at the cathode is given by :

$$Cu^{2+} + 2e \longrightarrow Cu$$

Thus, Cu^{2+} ions are reduced to copper at the cathode.

At the positive electrode (anode), oxidation takes place. For example, in the electrolysis of HCl soln, the process at the anode is given by :

$$Cl^- - e \longrightarrow \tfrac{1}{2}Cl_2$$

Thus, Cl^- ions are oxidised to chlorine at the anode.

10.2. OXIDANT AND REDUCTANT

Oxidant (or oxidising agent) is a substance which gains electrons and itself gets reduced. In equations (10.8), Sn^{4+}, Cl_2, MnO_4^- and Cu^{2+} ions are gaining electrons and getting reduced, hence these are *oxidants*.

On the other hand, reductant (or reducing agent) is a substance which loses electrons and itself gets oxidised. In equation (10.7),

Fe^{2+}, Sn^{2+}, I^- and Cl^- ions are losing electrons and are themselves oxidised (to Fe^{3+}, Sn^{4+}, I_2 and Cl_2 respectively), hence these are called *reductants*.

It is thus seen that a reductant supplies electrons which are received by an oxidant. We also know that in oxidation electrons are lost but electrons cannot be lost unless there is some substance present to accept them ; this acceptance of electrons is reduction. It is, therefore, concluded that oxidation and reduction are complementary processes, one cannot take place without the other. A redox reaction is thus a chemical change in which electrons are transferred from atoms or ions (called reductant) to other atoms or ions (called oxidant).

10·3. OXIDATION NUMBER

The concept of oxidation number can be used to find out valency of an element in a compound (the valency so determined may be hypothetical) and also in finding out eq wt of oxidants and reductants. For example, $KMnO_4$ in presence of dilute H_2SO_4, is reduced to manganous sulphate :

$$+1 \quad +7 \quad -8 \quad \text{equal to zero}$$

$$K \quad Mn \quad O_4$$

$$+2 \quad +6 \quad -8 \quad \text{equal to zero}$$

$$Mn \quad S \quad O_4$$

Element (In $KMnO_4$)	Valency	No. of atoms	Oxidation number	
K	+1	1	+1 ⎫	+1−8=−7
O_2	−2	4	−8 ⎬	
Mn	+7	1	+7	−7+7=0
In MnSO₄				
S	+6	1	+6 ⎫	+6−8=−2
O_2	−2	4	−8 ⎬	
Mn	+2	1	+2	−2+2=0

Thus, oxidation state of manganese is $+7$ in $KMnO_4$ and $+2$ in $MnSO_4$. During the reduction of $KMnO_4$ to $MnSO_4$, oxidation number of manganese is decreased by 5 units per molecule of $KMnO_4$. This information can be used for finding out a relation between eq wt and mol wt of $KMnO_4$ as given by :

$$\text{eq wt of } KMnO_4 = \frac{\text{mol wt}}{5}$$

In general, eq wt of an oxidant

$$= \frac{\text{mol wt of the oxidant}}{\text{change in oxidation no. per molecule of the oxidant}} \quad \text{...(10-A)}$$

Ferrous sulphate in presence of dilute H_2SO_4 is oxidised to ferric sulphate :

$$\overset{+4\ -4}{2Fe\ SO_4} \longrightarrow \overset{+6\ -6}{Fe_2\ (SO_4)_3}$$

(Valency of ferrous ion is $+2$ and that of sulphate ion is -2. On the left hand side, for two ferrous ions we write, $+2 \times 2 = +4$, at the top of Fe. For two sulphate ions, we put $-2 \times 2 = -4$ at the top of SO_4. Note that the total $+4 + (-4) = 0$. On the right hand side, for three sulphate ions we write $-2 \times 3 = -6$. Hence, the oxidation number of two ferric ions must be $+6$ or valency of ferric ion must be $+3$). It is seen that the oxidation number of iron increases from $+4$ to $+6$, i.e., by 2 units for two molecule of $FeSO_4$. Hence, for one molecule, the change in oxdation number will be only by one unit. So,

$$\text{eq wt of } FeSO_4 = \frac{\text{mol wt}}{1} \text{ (eq wt=mot wt)}$$

In general, eq wt of a reductant

$$= \frac{\text{mol wt of reductant}}{\text{change in oxidation no. per molecule of reductant}} \quad \text{...(10-B)}$$

Example 10(i)

In presence of dilute H_2SO_4, $K_2Cr_2O_7$ is reduced to $Cr_2(SO_4)_3$. Find out the valency of Cr in $K_2Cr_2O_7$ and also eq wt of $K_2Cr_2O_7$.

In potassium dichromate ($K_2Cr_2O_7$) :

Valency of K is $+1$ and oxidation no. is $+1 \times 2 = 2$; valency of O_2 is -2 and oxidation no. is $-2 \times 7 = -14$. The total of these oxidation, no. is $(+2 - 14) = -12$ hence the oxidation no. of chromium will be $+12$, so that we can write :

$$\overset{+2\ +12\ -14}{K_2\ \ Cr_2\ \ O_7} \longrightarrow \text{Total is zero}$$

Since in $K_2Cr_2O_7$ there are two chromium, atoms hence valency of chromium will be $12/2 = 6$.

In chromic sulphate $[Cr_2(SO_4)_3]$:

Valency of SO_4^{2-} ion is -2 and oxidation no. is $-2 \times 3 = -6$.

∴ Oxidation no. of chromium will be $+6$, so that we can write :

$$\overset{+6}{Cr_2} \overset{-6}{(SO_4)_3}$$

It is thus seen that when $K_2Cr_2O_7$ changes to $Cr_2(SO_4)_3$, the oxidation number of two chromium atoms decreases from $+12$ to $+6$, *i.e.*, by 6 units. Hence,

$$\text{eq wt of } K_2Cr_2O_7 = \frac{\text{mol wt}}{6}$$

Example 10(*ii*)

In acidic medium oxalic acid $(H_2C_2O_4)$ is oxidised to CO_2. Find out the valency of carbon in $H_2C_2O_4$ and eq wt of the acid.

We know that valency of hydrogen is 1 and that for oxygen is -2, hence, we can write :

$$\overset{+2}{H_2} \overset{+6}{C_2} \overset{-8}{O_4} \longrightarrow 2 (\overset{+4}{C} \overset{-4}{O_2})$$

The oxidation number of carbon in $H_2C_2O_4$ is $+6$, because the acid molecule contains two carban atoms so ; valency of carbon in $H_2C_2O_4$ will be $6/2 = 3$.

When $H_2C_2O_4$ changes to CO_2, the oxidation number of carbon increase from $+6$ to $+8$, *i.e.*, by 2 units per molecule of $H_2C_2O_4$ (there are two molecules of CO_2, hence oxidation number of two carbon atoms will be $+4 \times 2 = +8$). So,

eq wt of $H_2C_2O_4$

$$= \frac{\text{mol wt}}{\text{increase in oxidation no. per molecule of } H_2C_2O_4}$$

$$= \frac{\text{mol wt}}{2}$$

The mol wt of $H_2C_2O_4.2H_2O$ is $126\cdot07$ so its eq wt will be $126\cdot07/2 = 63\cdot04$.

Note. The oxidation number method can give incorrect result for the valency of an element. For example, in the above example, valency of carbon in $H_2C_2O_4$ is found to be $+3$ by oxidation number method whereas the correct value is $+4$. However, the eq wt can be correctly calculated.

10·4. ION-ELECTRON METHOD

A more satisfactory method of studying redox reaction is the ion-electron method. Application of this method to a redox reaction involves the following five steps :

(i) finding out the products of the reaction ;

(ii) setting up a partial equation for oxidation ;

(iii) setting up a partial equation for reduction ;

(iv) multiplying each partial equations by such factors so that electrons cancel out when the two equations are added ;

(v) cancelling out substances which appear on both sides of the equation.

Example 10(iii)

The reduction of ferric chloride with stannous chloride.

(i) The products of the reaction are ferrous chloride and stannic chloride as shown by the equation :

$$2FeCl_3 + SnCl_2 \rightarrow 2FeCl_2 + SnCl_4$$

or

$$2Fe^{3+} + Sn^{2+} \rightarrow 2Fe^{2+} + Sn^{4+}$$

The valency of iron decreases from $+3$ to $+2$ so it is reduced whereas the valency of tin increases from $+2$ to $+4$, hence, it is oxidised.

(ii) The process representing reduction is :

$$Fe^{3+} \rightarrow Fe^{2+}$$

The above equation is balanced atomically but not with respect to electric charge as there are $+3$ charges on left and only $+2$ on the right. If an electron is added to the left side, the equation is completely balanced :

$$Fe^{3+} + e \rightarrow Fe^{2+} \qquad \qquad ...(10·9)$$

Charge on the left is now $+3-1=2$ and that on the right is also '2. Equation (10·9) shows a gain of electron, hence it is called *partial equation for reduction.*

(iii) The process representing oxidation is :

$$Sn^{2+} \rightarrow Sn^{4+}$$

In order to balance this equation with respect to electric charge we must add 2 electrons to right hand side :

$$Sn^{2+} \rightarrow Sn^{4+} + 2e$$

or

$$Sn^{2+} - 2e \rightarrow Sn^{4+} \qquad \qquad ...(10·10)$$

The charge on the left is $+2-(-2)=2+2=4$. The charge on the right is 4. Equation (10·10) shows a loss of electrons so it is known as *partial equation for oxidation.*

\

(*iv*) Equations (10·9) and (10·10) are multiplied by such factors so that the electrons cancel out when the equations are added :

Equation (10·9) $\times 2 = 2Fe^{3+} + 2e \rightarrow 2Fe^{2+}$

Equation (10·10) $\times 1 = Sn^{2+} - 2e \rightarrow Sn^{4+}$

$$2Fe^{3+} + Sn^{2+} \rightarrow 2Fe^{2+} + Sn^{4+} \qquad ...(10·11)$$

In this way by applying the ion-electron method to the reaction between $FeCl_3$ and $SnCl_2$ we can build up a balanced equation (10·11) for the reaction and can find out that :

(*a*) Fe^{3+} ion is reduced, hence it is the oxidant, and

(*b*) Sn^{2+} ion is oxidised, hence it is the reductant.

This method also gives a relation between the eq wt and mol wt of an oxidant and reductant.

$$eq\ wt\ of\ an\ oxidant = \frac{mol\ wt\ of\ the\ oxidant}{no.\ of\ electrons\ gained\ by\ a\ molecule\ of\ the\ oxidant} \quad ...(10\text{-}C)$$

Thus,

$$eq\ wt\ of\ FeCl_3 = \frac{mol\ wt\ of\ FeCl_3}{1}$$

(one molecule of $FeCl_3$ gives a ferric ion which gains one electron)

$$eq\ wt\ of\ a\ reductant = \frac{mol\ wt\ of\ the\ reductant}{no.\ of\ electrons\ lost\ per\ molecule} \quad ...(10\text{-}D)$$

Thus,

$$eq\ wt\ of\ SnCl_2 = \frac{mol\ wt\ of\ SnCl_2}{2}$$

(one molecule of $SnCl_2$ gives a Sn^{2+} ion which loses two electrons)

Example 10(*iv*)

Reaction between potassium permanganate and oxalic acid in presence of dilute sulphuric acid.

The products of the reaction are K_2SO_4, $MnSO_4$, H_2O and CO_2.

For the change $KMnO_4$ to $MnSO_4$, the following equation can be written.

$$\underset{\substack{permanganate \\ ion}}{MnO_4^-} \rightarrow \underset{\substack{manganous\ ion}}{Mn^{2+}} \qquad (unbalanced)$$

$$MnO_4^- + 8H^+ \rightarrow Mn^{2+} + 4H_2O \qquad (unbalanced)$$

The above equation is balanced with respect to number and kind of atoms (H^+ ions are supplied by dilute H_2SO_4 present in the reaction mixture). To balance this equation with respect to electric charge, we must add 5 electrons to the left side.

$$MnO_4^- + 8H^+ + 5e \rightarrow Mn^{2+} + 4H_2O \quad \text{(balanced)}$$
$$...(10\cdot12)$$

$$-1 \ +8-5 \rightarrow +2$$
$$+2 \rightarrow +2$$

Equation $(10\cdot12)$ shows a gain of electrons and so it is a partial equation for reduction. Also, eq wt of $KMnO_4$ will be mol wt/5, because a molecule of $KMnO_4$ gives a permanganate ion which gains 5 electrons.

$$KMnO_4 \equiv MnO_4^- \text{ which gains 5 electrons.}$$

$$\text{eq wt of } KMnO_4 = \frac{\text{mol wt}}{5}$$

It should be noted that because MnO_4^- ion is gaining electrons, hence it is an oxidant.

For the change oxalate ion to carbon dioxide, the equation can be written as :

$$C_2O_4^{2-} \rightarrow 2CO_2 \quad \text{(unbalanced)}$$

$$C_2O_4^{2-} - 2e \rightarrow 2CO_2 \qquad ...(10\cdot13)$$

Equation $(10\cdot13)$ is the partial equation for oxidation. Now,

$$H_2C_2O_4 \equiv C_2O_4^{2-} \text{ which loses 2 electrons.}$$
$$\text{(hence it is a reductant)}$$

$$\text{eq wt of } H_2C_2O_4 = \frac{\text{mol wt}}{2}$$

If equation $(10\cdot12)$ is multiplied by 2 and $(10\cdot13)$ by 5 and the resultant equations are added we get :

Eq. $(10\cdot12) \times 2 = 2MnO_4^- + 16H^+ + 10e \rightarrow 2Mn^{2+} + 8H_2O$

Eq. $(10\cdot13) \times 5 = 5C_2O_4^{2-} \qquad -10e \rightarrow 10CO_2$

$$2MnO_4^- + 16H^+ + 5C_2O_4^{2-} \rightarrow 2Mn^{2+} + 8H_2O + 10CO_2$$
$$...(10\cdot14)$$

In this example MnO_4^- is gaining electrons, hence it is the oxidant and oxalic acid is the reductant.

Example 10 (v)

Reaction between potassium dichoromate and potassium iodide in presence of dilute sulphuric acid.

The products of the reaction are K_2SO_4, $Cr_2(SO_4)_3$, H_2O and I_2. For the change $Cr_2O_7^{2-}$ to Cr^{3+}, the equation can be written as :

$$Cr_2O_7^{2-} \rightarrow 2Cr^{3+} \text{ (unbalanced)} \quad ...(10\cdot15)$$

$$Cr_2O_7^{2-}+14H^+ \rightarrow 2Cr^{3+}+7H_2O$$
$$\text{(balanced atomically)}$$

$$Cr_2O_7^{2-}+14H^++6e \rightarrow 2Cr^{3+}+7H_2O$$
$$\text{(completely balanced)}$$

$$-2 \quad +14 \quad -6 \rightarrow +6 \quad\quad ...(10\cdot16)$$

Equation $(10\cdot16)$ is the partial eqution for reduction.

$$K_2Cr_2O_7 \equiv Cr_2O_7^{2-} \text{ which gains 6 electrons, hence it is an}$$
$$\text{oxidant,}$$

and eq wt of $K_2Cr_2O_7 = \dfrac{\text{mol wt}}{6}$

For the change iodide ion to iodine, the equation is :

$$I^- \rightarrow I_2 \text{ (unbalanced)}$$
$$2I^- \rightarrow I_2 \text{ (balanced atomically)}$$
$$2I^--2e \rightarrow I_2 \text{ (completely balanced)} \quad ...(10\cdot17)$$

Equation $(10\cdot17)$ is the partial equation for oxidation. Now, $KI \equiv I^-$ which loses one electron so, it is a reductant and :

$$\text{eq wt of } KI = \frac{\text{mol wt}}{1}$$

Eq $(10\cdot16) \times 1 = Cr_2O_7^{2-}+14H^++6e \rightarrow 2Cr^{3+}+7H_2O$
Eq $(10\cdot17) \times 3 = 6I^- \quad\quad\quad -6e \rightarrow 3I_2$
_____

$$Cr_2O_7^{2-}+14H^++6I^- \rightarrow 2Cr^{3+}+7H_2O+3I_2 \quad ...(10\cdot18)$$

In terms of molecules the reaction can be written as :

$$K_2Cr_2O_7+7H_2SO_4+6KI \rightarrow 4K_2SO_4+Cr_2(SO_4)_3+7H_2O+3I_2$$
$$...(10\cdot19)$$

Example 10(vi)

Reaction between copper sulphate and potassium iodide.

The products of the reaction are Cu_2I_2 (cuprous iodide), K_2SO_4 and I_2. The partial equation for reduction is :

$$Cu^{2+}+e \rightarrow Cu^+ \quad\quad ...(10\cdot20)$$

and, partial equation for oxidation is :

$$I^--e \rightarrow 1/2\ I_2 \quad\quad ...(10\cdot21)$$

The total reaction can, therefore, be written as :

$$Cu^{2+}+I^- \rightarrow Cu^++1/2\ I_2 \quad\quad ...(10\cdot22)$$

(or $\quad\quad 2Cu^{2+}+4I^- \rightarrow Cu_2I_2+I_2)$ $\quad\quad ...(10\cdot23)$

Also,

$$\text{eq wt of } CuSO_4 = \frac{\text{mol wt}}{1}$$

(Oxidant)

$$\text{eq wt of } KI = \frac{\text{mol wt}}{1}$$

Note. In the reaction between $CuSO_4$ and KI, the Cu^{2+} ions (from $CuSO_4$) are reduced to cuprous state (in Cu_2I_2) so that valency of Cu reduces from $+2$ to $+1$. In the reduction process

$$Cu^{2+} + e \rightarrow Cu^+ \qquad \qquad ...(10\cdot24)$$
$$\underset{\substack{\text{Cupric} \\ \text{ion}}}{} \qquad \underset{\text{cuprous ion}}{}$$

H^+ ions are not involved. Hence, when KI soln is added to $CuSO_4$ soln, there is liberation of I_2 as seen in equation ($10\cdot23$); the presence of acid is not necessary. But when KI is added to a soln of $K_2Cr_2O_7$ or KIO_3, there is no liberation of iodine unless acid is added. This is because for the reduction processes :

$$Cr_2O_7{}^{2-} + 14H^+ + 6e \rightarrow 2Cr^{3+} + 7H_2O$$
and $\qquad \qquad IO_3{}^- + 6H^+ + 5e \rightarrow 3H_2O + 1/2\,I_2$

the presence of H^+ ions is necessary.

Example 10(*vii*)

Reaction between sodium thiosulphate ($Na_2S_2O_3$) and iodine.

The products of the reaction are $Na_2S_4O_6$ (sodium tetrathionate) and NaI. The partial equation for reduction is :

$$I_2 \rightarrow I^-$$
$$1/2\,I_2 \rightarrow I^-$$
$$1/2\,I_2 + e \rightarrow I^- \text{ (balanced)} \qquad ...(10\cdot25)$$
(or $\qquad \qquad I_2 + 2e \rightarrow 2I^-$) $\qquad \qquad ...(10\cdot26)$

Because iodine is gaining electrons, it will be the oxidant and its eq wt will be given by :

$$\text{eq wt of } I_2 = \frac{\text{mol wt}}{2}$$

(**Note** : that a molecule of iodine gains 2 electrons.)

The partial equation for oxidation is :

$$S_2O_3{}^{2-} \rightarrow S_4O_6{}^{2-} \text{ (unbalanced)}$$
$$\underset{\substack{\text{thiosulphate} \\ \text{ion}}}{} \quad \underset{\substack{\text{tetrathionate} \\ \text{ion}}}{}$$
$$2S_2O_3{}^{2-} \rightarrow S_4O_6{}^{2-} \text{ (unbalanced)}$$

$$2S_2O_3^{2-} - 2e \rightarrow S_4O_6^{2-} \text{ (balanced)} \qquad ...(10\cdot27)$$

(or $\qquad S_2O_3^{2-} - e \rightarrow 1/2\ S_4O_6^{2-}$)

Thiosulphate ion is losing electron, hence it is a reductant and because one electron is lost per molecule of $Na_2S_2O_3$:

$$\text{eq wt of } Na_2S_2O_3 = \frac{\text{mol wt}}{1}$$

The chemical equation for the reaction between $Na_2S_2O_3$ and I_2 can be obtained by summing up the partial equations :

$$I_2 + 2e \rightarrow 2I^-$$
$$2S_2O_3^{2-} - 2e \rightarrow S_4O_6^{2-}$$

_____

$$I_2 + 2S_2O_3^{2-} \rightarrow S_4O_6^{2-} + 2I^- \qquad ...(10\cdot28)$$

or $\qquad I_2 + 2Na_2S_2O_3 \rightarrow Na_2S_4O_6 + 2NaI$

10·5. DEPENDENCE OF EQUIVALENT WEIGHT ON THE REACTION

It has already been mentioned that the eq wt of a substance is not a constant quantity but depends upon the reaction in which it is taking part.

Example 10(*viii*)

When $FeSO_4$ is oxidised to $Fe_2(SO_4)_3$ (say by $KMnO_4$ in presence of H_2SO_4) the partial equation for oxidation is :

$$Fe^{2+} - e \rightarrow Fe^{3+}$$

Now, $FeSO_4 \equiv Fe^{2+}$ which loses one electron,

$$\therefore \quad \text{eq wt of } FeSO_4 = \frac{\text{mol wt}}{1}$$

But, in a precipitation reaction, such as,

$$FeSO_4 + BaCl_2 \rightarrow BaSO_4 + FeCl_2$$

$$\text{eq wt of the reactant} = \frac{\text{mol wt}}{\text{valency of precipitating ion}}$$

In this reaction, $FeSO_4$ is the precipitating reagent which contains the precipitating sulphate ion whose valency is 2, hence

$$\text{eq wt of } FeSO_4 = \frac{\text{mol wt}}{2}$$

(see Chapter 11 for precipitation titrations)

It is thus seen that in the first case (oxidation reaction) the eq wt of $FeSO_4$ is equal to its mol wt but in the second case (precipitation reaction) the eq wt of $FeSO_4$ is half its mol wt. Hence, $FeSO_4$ soln which is $0\cdot1$ N in a redox titration will be $0\cdot2$ N in a precipitation titration.

Even in similar type of reactions a compound can have different eq wts.

Example 10(ix)

The permanganate ion gets reduced to different products depending upon the reaction conditions. In alkaline medium manganate ions are formed, in neutral medium the product is manganese dioxide, whereas in acidic soln, manganous ions are produced as shown by the following equations :

$$MnO_4^- + e \rightarrow MnO_4^{2-} \text{ (alkaline medium)}$$
$$MnO_4^- + 4H^+ + 3e \rightarrow MnO_2 + 2H_2O \text{ (neutral medium)}$$
$$MnO_4^- + 8H^+ + 5e \rightarrow Mn^{2+} + 4H_2O \text{ (acidic medium)}$$

All the three equations represent reduction of permanganate ion, but $KMnO_4$ will have different values of eq wt in three cases :

In the first case, eq wt of $KMnO_4 = \dfrac{\text{mol wt}}{1}$

In the second case, eq wt of $KMnO_4 = \dfrac{\text{mol wt}}{3}$

In the third case, eq wt of $KMnO_4 = \dfrac{\text{mol wt}}{5}$

10·6. IODIMETRY AND IODOMETRY

Oxidation and reduction reactions involving iodine are very useful in titrimetric analysis because iodine can be very conveniently and accurately titrated with standard thiosulphate soln. Titrimetric methods involving iodine are of two types :

(i) *Iodimetry* which describes titrations in which a standard iodine soln is used.

(ii) *Iodometry* deals with titrations in which the iodine liberated during chemical reactions is titrated.

10·6·1. Iodimetric Determinations

Iodine is a weak oxidant which can be reduced by reductants, such as stannous chloride, sodium thiosulphate, sulphurous acid and arsenious oxide. The reductants react rapidly and completely with iodine. In the following cases, the reduction of iodine is fast and stoichiometric :

(i) $Sn^{2+} + I_2 \rightarrow Sn^{4+} + 2I^-$
(ii) $2S_2O_3^{2-} + I_2 \rightarrow S_4O_6^{2-} + 2I^-$
(iii) $SO_3^{2-} + I_2 + H_2O \rightarrow SO_4^{2-} + 2H^+ + 2I^-$
(iv) $H_3AsO_3 + I_2 + H_2O \rightarrow H_3AsO_4 + 2H^+ + 2I^-$

In an iodimetric method, a known volume of a soln of the reductant is taken in a glass-stoppered conical flask (iodine flask). About 1 ml of starch soln in added as an indicator and a standard soln of iodine is gradually added through a burette, swirling the flask frequently during the titration. When the titration soln just becomes blue, the addition of iodine is stopped and burette reading is noted. In this titration, at the end point, the indicator colour changes from colourless to blue. It has been found that the change, blue to colourless is easier to observe rather than colourless to blue. Hence, in iodimetric titrations, generally, a known volume of standard iodine soln is taken in an iodine flask and it is titrated with a soln of the reductant whose concentration is to be determined. Starch is used as an indicator which shows a change blue to colourless at the end point. Volume and normality of iodine soln are known, volume of the analyte soln is found out by the titration and so its normality can be calculated. It should be noted that in all iodimetric procedures iodine is reduced to iodide ion as given by :

$$I_2 + 2e \rightarrow 2I^- \qquad \qquad ...(10\cdot29)$$

In these processes a molecule of iodine gains two electrons, hence it is an oxidant and its eq wt is given by :

$$\text{eq wt of } I_2 = \frac{\text{mol wt}}{2}$$

10·6·2. Iodometric Determinations

Suppose we have a soln (say 25 ml) of a strong oxidant, such as $CuSO_4$, KIO_3, $K_2Cr_2O_7$ or $KMnO_4$. If to this soln, we add a large excess of KI soln (usually in the presence of acid), the iodide ions are oxidised to iodine as shown by the equation :

$$2I^- - 2e \rightarrow I_2 \qquad \qquad ...(10\cdot30)$$

Electrons are given out by I^- ions (reductant). The oxidant accepts these electrons and thereby gets reduced. For example, if oxidant is $CuSO_4$ then :

$$2Cu^{2+} + 2e \rightarrow 2Cu^+ \qquad \qquad ...(10\cdot31)$$

Cu^{2+} ions (oxidant) accept electrons supplied by iodide ions (reductant) and themselves get reduced to cuprous state [Cu(II) is reduced to Cu(I)]. On adding partial equations (10·30) and (10·31) we get :

$$2Cu^{2+} + 2I^- \rightarrow 2Cu^+ + I_2$$

or $\qquad \qquad 2Cu^{2+} + 4I^- \rightarrow Cu_2I_2 + I_2 \qquad \qquad ...(10\cdot32)$

Because I^- ions are present in large excess, the quantity of iodine liberated will be equivalent to concentration of Cu^{2+} (or amount of $CuSO_4$). Thus,

$$2CuSO_4 \equiv 2Cu^{2+} \equiv I_2$$

Two molecules of $CuSO_4$ will produce a molecule of iodine. Hence, if we find out the quantity of the liberated iodine, the amount of Cu^{2+} ions or that of $CuSO_4$ can be calculated. The quantity of liberated iodine is found out by titration with standard thiosulphate soln.

$$I_2 + 2Na_2S_2O_3 \rightarrow Na_2S_4O_6 + 2NaI$$

Thus,

$$2CuSO_4 \equiv I_2 \equiv 2Na_2S_2O_3$$

Iodometric method can be applied for determining several substances as shown by the following reactions :

$$2MnO_4^- + 16H^+ + 10I^- \rightarrow 2Mn^{2+} + 5I_2 + 8H_2O$$

$$IO_3^- + 6H^+ + 5I^- \rightarrow 3H_2O + 3I_2$$

$$BrO_3^- + 6H^+ + 6I^- \rightarrow Br^- + 3I_2 + 3H_2O$$

$$2Cu^{2+} + 4I^- \rightarrow Cu_2I_2 + I_2 \qquad \qquad ...(10\cdot33)$$

$$Cr_2O_7^{2-} + 14H^+ + 6I^- \rightarrow 2Cr^{3+} + 3I_2 + 7H_2O$$

$$2Ce^{4+} + 2I^- \rightarrow 2Ce^{3+} + I_2$$

$$IO_4^- + 8H^+ + 7I^- \rightarrow 4I_2 + 4H_2O$$

Potassium permanganate, potassium iodate, potassium bromate, copper sulphate. potassium dichromate, ceric sulphate, potassium periodate can be determined by iodometric titrations. The procedure is that a known volume of a soln of the substance to be determined is taken in an iodine flask and an excess of KI soln and dil H_2SO_4 are added. [It is seen in above equations that in most cases H^+ ions are involved in the reaction]. After the reaction is complete, the liberated iodine is titrated with a standard thiosulphate soln using starch as indicator. The amount of thiosulphate (A) is thus found out so that the quantily (B) of the liberated iodine is determined. Then with the help of a stoichiometric equation (such as those given above), the amount of the substance that liberated amount (B) of iodine can be calculated. [In the case of $CuSO_4$, addition of H_2SO_4 is not required].

10·7. APPLICATION OF REDOX REACTIONS IN TITRIMETRIC ANALYSIS

It has been seen that the reactions in which electrons are transferred from one atom or molecule or ion to another are called oxidation-reduction or redox reactions. (It should be remembered that oxidation and reduction cannot take place independently but occur simultaneously by transfer of electron from the reductant to the oxidant.)

There are many elements which exist in different oxidation states. For example, oxidation state (oxidation number or valency) of manganese is :

$+7$ in permanganate ion (MnO_4^-),

$+6$ in manganate ion (MnO_4^{2-}),

$+5$ in hypomanganate ion (MnO_4^{3-}),

$+4$ in manganese dioxide (MnO_2);

$+3$ in manganic ion (Mn^{3+}), and

$+2$ in manganous ion (Mn^{2+}).

(There is evidence even for monovalent manganese in certain complexes.

The change in the oxidation state of an element can be brought about by electron transfer. For example, when Sn^{4+} ion receives two electrons, its oxidation state changes from that of $+4$ to $+2$:

$$Sn^{4+} + 2e \rightarrow Sn^{2+}$$

Similarly, if Fe^{2+} loses an electron the change in oxidation state will be $+2$ to $+3$ [iron (II) to iron (III)] :

$$Fe^{2+} - e \rightarrow Fe^{3+}$$

The purpose of the above discussion was to make it clear that several elements, which exist in different valency states, take part in redox reactions. Fortunately most of these reactions are fast and quantitative, hence are very suitable for developing titrimetric methods for determining many compounds of these elements. (It should be noted that redox reactions involving organic compounds are not always fast and quantitative, and steps are to be taken to speed them up and make them quantitative). This is the reason why a very large number of redox titrations are available for determining a large number of compounds.

In redox titrimetry fewer titrants are needed because a strong oxidant, such as, $KMnO_4$ or $K_2Cr_2O_7$ can be used to titrate a large number of reducing agents. Likwise, a strong reducing agent can be used in the titration of a number of oxidants.

10.7.1. Oxidimetric Methods

When a standard soln of an oxidant is used in a titration, the procedure is called an oxidimetric method. For example, a standard soln of $K_2Cr_2O_7$ (Oxidant) can be used for titrating $FeSO_4$ (reductant). The methods using a standard soln of reducing agent (reductimetric method) are fewer in number because it is difficult to protect a soln of a reducing agent from atmospheric oxidation.

10·7·2.   Some Common Oxidants and Reductants

Some common oxidising and reducing agents used in redox titrations are given below.

Oxidising agents. Potassium permanganate, potassium dichromate, potassium iodate, potassium bromate, ceric sulphate, iodine, lead dioxide and potassium periodate.

Reducing agents. Ferrous sulphate, sodium thiosulphate, stannons chloride, oxalic acid, titanous sulphate and sodium arsenite.

Potassium iodate (KIO_3), potassium bromate ($KBrO_3$), potassium dichromate ($K_2Cr_2O_7$), potassium bi-iodate [$KH(IO_3)_2$] iodine (I_2), arsenious oxide (As_2O_3) and sodium oxalate [$Na_2C_2O_4$] can be used as primary standards, hence their standard solutions can be prepared by direct method, *i.e.*, by dissolving a known amount of the dried substance in water and then making up to a known volume in a measuring flask.   The concentration of such a soln, in general, is given in terms of molarity, such as, 0·1 M or 0·01 M. (Eq wt is not a fixed quantity, hence a soln which is 0·1 N in a particular reaction may not have the same normality in some other reaction).

10·8.   LABORATORY EXERCISES

Experiment 10·1

Preparation of a 0·1 M $KMnO_4$ soln.

Although $KMnO_4$ of high purity is available, it cannot be used as a primary standard.   Potassium permanganate in neutral soln slowly decomposes :

$$4MnO_4^- + 2H_2O \rightarrow 4MnO_2 + 4OH^- + 3O_2$$

Manganese dioxide produced, catalyses the decomposition, *i.e.*, the decomposition reaction is autocatalytic.   Even if MnO_2 is not present in $KMnO_4$ as impurity, the reducing impurities of water used to prepare the soln react with $KMnO_4$ to produce MnO_2. Thus an aqueous soln of $KMnO_4$ is unstable and its concentration decreases with time.   In acidic or alkaline medium or in the presence of light the decomposition is further increased.   An approximate soln is, therefore, prepared which is then standardised.   The mol wt of $KMnO_4$ is 157·94, it means 1 litre of 0·1 M soln must contain 15·794 g $KMnO_4$.   To prepare such a soln, the following steps are taken :

1.   Preparation of an approximate soln of $KMnO_4$

Dissolve approximately 16 to 17 g $KMnO_4$ in a litre of distilled water and keep on a steam bath for about an hour (to oxidise all the impurities present in water). Cool, filter through glass wool and store the soln in a grease free, glass stoppered, dark glass bottle (to protect soln from light).

The approximate soln prepared in step 1 can be standardised with a number of reagents, such as, sodium oxalate, arsenious oxide, potassium hexacyanoferrate (II) etc. Here, we will describe standardisation with sodium oxalate.

2. Standardisation of $KMnO_4$ soln with $Na_2C_2O_4$

Weigh out accurately 6·701 g $Na_2C_2O_4$, transfer it to a 250 ml volumetric flask, dissolve in water and make up to the mark. Shake the soln well. Pipette out 25·0 ml of the soln into a conical flask and add 150 ml of 2N H_2SO_4. Gradually add $KMnO_4$ soln from the burette with constant shaking until the soln becomes pink. Allow to stand the soln until it again becomes colourless. Warm the soln to 50—60°C and continue titration until the soln becomes just pink.

3. Calculations

Suppose, 25 ml $Na_2C_2O_4$ soln requires 19·5 ml of $KMnO_4$ soln.

(a) **Calculation of normality of $Na_2C_2O_4$ soln**

250 ml soln contains 6·701 g $Na_2C_2O_4$

$$\therefore \quad 1000 \text{ ml} \quad ... \quad \frac{1000}{250} \times 6\cdot701$$

$$= 26\cdot804 \text{ g } Na_2C_2O_4/\text{litre}$$

Now, mol wt of $Na_2C_2O_4$ = 134·02.

In the present reaction, oxalate ion is oxidised according to the equation :

$$C_2O_4^{2-} - 2e \rightarrow 2CO_2$$

It means that a molecule of $Na_2C_2O_4$

($\equiv C_2O_4^{2-}$) loses 2 electrons so that :

$$\text{eq wt of } Na_2C_2O_4 = \frac{\text{mol wt}}{2} = \frac{134\cdot02}{2} = 67\cdot01$$

$$\text{Now, normality} = \frac{\text{wt present per litre}}{\text{-eq wt}}$$

$$\text{normality of } Na_2C_2O_4 \text{ soln} = \frac{26\cdot804}{67\cdot01} = 0\cdot4$$

(b) **Calculation of normality of $KMnO_4$ soln**

normality of $KMnO_4$ $= N_{KMnO_4}$

volume of $KMnO_4$ $= 19\cdot5$

normalitty of $Na_2C_2O_4$ $= 0\cdot4$

$$\text{volume of } Na_2C_2O_4 \qquad = 25 \cdot 0 \text{ ml}$$

$$N_{KMnO_4} \times 19 \cdot 5 \qquad = 0 \cdot 4 \times 25 \cdot 0$$

or

$$N_{KMnO_4} = \frac{0 \cdot 4 \times 25 \cdot 0}{19 \cdot 5} = 0 \cdot 5128.$$

In the reaction, MnO_4^- ion is reduced as shown by the equation :

$$MnO_4^- + 8H^+ + 5e \rightarrow Mn^{2+} + 4H_2O$$

It means that a molecule of $KMnO_4 (\equiv MnO_4^-)$ gains five electrons. hence,

$$\text{eq wt of } KMnO_4 = \frac{\text{mol wt}}{5}$$

Now,

$$\text{molarity} \times \text{no. of electrons transferred per molecule} = \text{normality.}$$

$$\cdots(10\text{-}E)$$

The normality of $KMnO_4$ has been found to be $0 \cdot 5128$, and number of electrons gained by a molecule of $KMnO_4$ is 5. Substituting these values in (10-E) we get

$$\text{molarity} \times 5 = 0 \cdot 5128$$

$$\text{Molarity} = \frac{0 \cdot 5128}{5} = 0 \cdot 1025$$

4. Preparation of exact 0·1 M KMnO₄

The molarity of $KMnO_4$ soln prepared in step 1 is $0 \cdot 1025$ or its normality in this particular reaction is $0 \cdot 1025 \times 5 = 0 \cdot 5128$. We want to prepare exact $0 \cdot 1$ M (or $0 \cdot 5$ N) soln. This can be done by finding out that what volume of $0 \cdot 1025$ M soln will be equivalent to 1000 ml of $0 \cdot 1$ M soln :

$$V \times 0 \cdot 1025 = 1000 \times 0 \cdot 1$$

or

$$V = \frac{1000 \times 0 \cdot 1}{0 \cdot 1025} = 975 \text{ ml.}$$

It means that 975 ml of $KMnO_4$ soln prepared, should be diluted to 1000 ml to obtain exact $0 \cdot 1$ M soln.

The same result can be obtained by taking into consideration the normality. We have a soln of normality $0 \cdot 5128$ and we want to prepare a soln whose normality is exactly $0 \cdot 5N (= 0 \cdot 1$ M).

$$V \times 0 \cdot 5128 = 0 \cdot 5 \times 1000$$

or

$$V = \frac{0 \cdot 5 \times 1000}{0 \cdot 5128} = 975 \text{ ml}$$

That is, to 975 ml of $KMnO_4$ soln ($0 \cdot 5128$ N) 25 ml of water should be added and the soln should be thoroughly shaken to obtain exactly $0 \cdot 5$ N or $0 \cdot 1$ M $KMnO_4$ soln.

Note : 0.1 M soln of $KMnO_4$ will not always be equal to its 0.5 N soln. Consider the following different ways in which $KMnO_4^-$ ion can be reduced :

$$MnO_4^- + e \quad \rightarrow MnO_4^{2-} \quad ; \ 0.1 \text{ M soln} = 0.1 \text{ N soln.}$$
$$MnO_4^- + 4H^+ + 3e \rightarrow MnO_2 + 2H_2O \ ; \ 0.1 \text{ M soln} = 0.3 \text{ N soln.}$$
$$MnO_4^- + 8H^+ + 5e \rightarrow Mn^{2+} + 4H_2O \ ; \ 0.1 \text{ M soln} = 0.5 \text{ N soln.}$$

Experiment 10·2

Titrimetric determination of calcium as calcium oxalate by permanganimetric method.

Discussion

Calcium (and also some other metals, such as Cu, Zn, Pb) gives insoluble oxalates. To a soln containing Ca^{2+} ions, ammonium oxalate is added when CaC_2O_4 is precipitated (see expt. 6·5). The ppt is filtered, washed and dissolved in dilute H_2SO_4.

$$CaC_2O_4 + H_2SO_4 \rightarrow CaSO_4 + H_2C_2O_4$$

Oxalic acid produced during the reaction is titrated with a standard $KMnO_4$ soln.

$$2KMnO_4 + 3H_2SO_4 + 5H_2C_2O_4 \rightarrow K_2SO_4 + 2MnSO_4 + 8H_2O + 10CO_2$$

Thus,

$$CaC_2O_4 \equiv H_2C_2O_4$$

and
$$5H_2C_2O_4 \equiv 2KMnO_4$$

Hence, we can write :

$$2KMnO_4 \equiv 5H_2C_2O_4 \equiv 5CaC_2O_4 \equiv 5Ca \text{(at wt } 40.1)$$

2 litre, 1 M $KMnO_4 = 5 \times 40.1 = 200.5$ g Ca

1 litre, 1 M $KMnO_4 \qquad = \dfrac{200.5}{2} = 100.25$ g Ca

1 litre, 0.1 M $KMnO_4 \qquad = \dfrac{100.25}{10} = 10.025$ g Ca

1 ml, 0.1 M $KMnO_4 \qquad = 10.025$ mg Ca

1 ml, 0.1 N $KMnO_4 \qquad = \dfrac{10.025}{5} = 2.005$ mg Ca.

(Note that for $KMnO_4$, eq wt = mol wt/5 in this reaction).

Experiment 10·3

Preparation and standardisation of a thiosulphate soln with potassium iodate.

Discussion

It has been seen in 10·6 that many substances can be titrimetrically determined by iodimetric and iodometric methods. The advantage of these methods is that a very small concentration of I_2 can be detected either by its own colour or by the blue colour produced by starch indicator. A soln of I_2 in KI has an intense brown colour which becomes yellow if soln is diluted. With more dilute iodine soln, starch indicator can be used which gives an intense blue colour even with very low I_2 concentrations. (When I_2 is dissolved in KI soln it forms KI_3). Several compounds, like arsenious acid, stannous chloride and sulphurous acid can be directly titrated with iodine ; these are oxidised by iodine. On the other hand, a large number of compounds oxidise KI (usually in acidic medium) to I_2 which can be very conveniently and accurately titrated with a standard thiosulphate soln. Such iodometric determinations form a very useful class of redox titrations. In almost all of these titrations, $Na_2S_2O_3$ soln is used to titrate iodine and starch is employed as an indicator.

Starch is cheap and is very sensitive to I_2, *i.e.*, gives blue colour even with very small I_2 concentrations. Its disadvantages are :

(*i*) It is insoluble in water (so its suspension in boiling water is prepared),

(*ii*) Its suspension in water is unstable (so a fresh starch soln is used),

(*iii*) In dilute soln of iodine, the blue colour with starch becomes faint or disappears on keeping (so the first appearance of the blue colour is taken as the end point),

(*iv*) Starch with iodine forms a water-insoluble complex. If the I_2 concentration is high, some iodine remains adsorbed on it (so the starch indicator is added just before the end point when I_2 concentration is very small, hence loss of iodine due to adsorption is negligible).

If sodium starch glycollate is used as the indicator, most of the disadvantages observed with starch are absent. Hence, sodium starch glycollate can be used, as a better alternative for starch, as an indicator in iodine titrations.

Procedure

(*i*) *Preparation of starch indicator soln.* Make a paste of 1 g of soluble starch with little water. Pour this paste, with constant stirring, into a beaker containing 100 ml of boiling water and boil for 1 minute. Cool the soln.

By the above method we get a suspension in water which is not very stable, hence a freshly prepared starch soln is used.

(*ii*) *Preparation of approximately 0·1 M thiosulphate soln.* Sodium thiosulphate, $Na_2S_2O_3.5H_2O$, (mol wt 248·20) is available in pure form but there is always some uncertainty about its water content, therefore, it is not used as a primary standard. An approximate soln is first prepared which is then standardised with KIO_3 or $K_2Cr_2O_7$.

The thiosulphate ion loses electrons as shown by :
$$2S_2O_3^{2-} - 2e \rightarrow S_4O_6^{2-}$$
$$\text{(reductant)}$$

$$2Na_2S_2O_3 \equiv 2S_2O_3^{2-} \quad \text{(loses 2 electrons)}$$
or $\quad Na_2S_2O_3 \equiv S_2O_3^{2-} \quad \text{(loses 1 electron)}$

$$\text{eq wt of } Na_2S_2O_3 = \frac{\text{mol wt}}{1} = \frac{248 \cdot 20}{1} = 248 \cdot 20$$

For $Na_2S_2O_3.5 H_2O$, mol wt and eq wt are equal, hence its $0 \cdot 1$ M soln is the same as its $0 \cdot 1$ N soln. For the preparation of approximately $0 \cdot 1$ M thiosulphate soln :

Dissolve about 25 to 26 g of sodium thiosulphate in water and make up the volume in a 1 litre measuring flask. Shake well.

(iii) *Preparation of $0 \cdot 1$ N $(0 \cdot 1/6 = 0 \cdot 0167$ M) KIO_3 soln.* A.R. KIO_3 is 99·9 per cent pure, is non-hygroscopic, can be dried at 120°C and its aqueous soln is quite stable, hence it is an excellent primary standard for standardising $Na_2S_2O_3$ soln.

The iodate ion oxidises I^- ions in presence of H^+ ions to iodine :
$$IO_3^- + 6H^+ + 5I^- \rightarrow 3H_2O + 3I_2 \qquad \qquad ...(10 \cdot 34)$$
$$KIO_3 \equiv IO_3^- \equiv 3I_2 (\equiv 6H)$$
$$\text{eq wt of } KIO_3 = \frac{\text{mol wt}}{6} = \frac{214 \cdot 02}{6} = 35 \cdot 67$$

It means that for $0 \cdot 1$ N soln, $3 \cdot 567$ g KIO_3 should be present in a litre of soln. The molarity of this soln will be :

$$\frac{\text{wt in 1 litre}}{\text{mol wt}} = \frac{3 \cdot 567}{214 \cdot 02} = 0 \cdot 0167,$$

In order to prepare $0 \cdot 1$ N KIO_3 soln :

Dissolve exactly $3 \cdot 567$ g of KIO_3 (dried at 120°C for 1 hour and then cooled in a desiccator) in water and dilute it to 1 litre in volumetric flask, shake the soln. (This soln is highly stable).

(iv) *Standardisation of $Na_2S_2O_3$ soln.* Pipette out $25 \cdot 0$ ml of standard KIO_3 soln [prepared in step (iii)] into a 250 ml glass-stoppered flask (also known as iodine flask). Add 2 g of pure KI and 5 ml of 2N H_2SO_4. (The soln will become dark brown due to the liberation of I_2). Gradually add through a burette $Na_2S_2O_3$ soln that is to be standardised [the soln prepared in step (ii)]. Swirl the conical flask. (As $Na_2S_2O_3$ is gradually added, it neutralises iodine ;' so, the colour becomes light brown, yellow and then light yellow or straw-yellow). When the soln becomes straw-yellow, add about 100 ml water and 1 ml of starch soln. (The soln will appear deep blue). Continue dropwise addition of $Na_2S_2O_3$ until soln just becomes colourless. (On keeping a blue colour may appear again but this is to be ignored ; the first disappearance of blue colour should be noted). Record the burette reading.

(v) *Calculations.* Suppose,

$$25 \text{ ml, } 0\cdot1 \text{ N } KIO_3 \equiv 24\cdot5 \text{ ml, } Na_2S_2O_3$$

then,

$$N_{Na_2S_2O_3} = \frac{N_{KIO_3} \times V_{KIO_3}}{V_{Na_2S_2O_3}}$$

$$= \frac{0\cdot1 \times 25}{24\cdot5} = 0\cdot1020$$

(vi) *Preparation of exact $0\cdot1$ N $Na_2S_2O_3$ soln.* Now, we have a standard soln of $Na_2S_2O_3$ which can be used for titrating iodine. The normality of the soln is $0\cdot1020$. If we want 1 litre of $Na_2S_2O_3$ soln of exact $0\cdot1000$ normality (this simplifies titrimetric calculations considerably), it can be done with the help of the relationship :

$$V \times 0\cdot1020 = 1000 \times 0\cdot1$$

$$V = \frac{1000 \times 0\cdot1}{0\cdot1020} = 980\cdot4 \text{ ml}$$

($980\cdot4$ ml of $0\cdot1020$ N $Na_2S_3O_3$ on dilution to $1000\cdot0$ ml will give $0\cdot1$ N $Na_2S_2O_3$).

Experiment 10·4

Standardisation of a thiosulphate soln with potassium dichromate.

Discussion

Potassium dichromate $K_2Cr_2O_7$ (mol wt $294\cdot21$) is used as a primary standard for standardising $Na_2S_2O_3$ soln. Dichromate ion accepts electrons and gets reduced :

$$Cr_2O_7^{2-} + 14H^+ + 6e \rightarrow 2Cr^{3+} + 7H_2O$$

$$\therefore \quad \text{eq wt of } K_2Cr_2O_7 = \frac{\text{mol wt}}{6}$$

$$= \frac{294\cdot21}{6} = 49\cdot035$$

When a known amount of $K_2Cr_2O_7$ is **treated** with an excess of KI and H_2SO_4, $K_2Cr_2O_7$ oxidises iodide to indine :

$$Cr_2O_7^{2-}+14H^++6I^- \rightarrow 2Cr^{3+}+7H_2O+3I_2 \qquad ...(10\cdot35)$$

Because KI and H_2SO_4 are in excess, the amount of liberated iodine will depend only on the quantity of $K_2Cr_2O_7$ present. (If $K_2Cr_2O_7$ and H_2SO_4 are in excess, the amount of liberated iodine will depend upon the quantity of KI.) The liberated iodine is **then titrated** with $Na_2S_2O_3$ soln which is to be standardised.

$$6Na_2S_2O_3+3I_2 \rightarrow 6NaI+3Na_2S_4O_6 \qquad ..(10\cdot36)$$

By combining equations (10·35) and (10·36) we can write :

$$K_2Cr_2O_7 \equiv Cr_2O_7^{2-} \equiv 3I_2 \equiv 6Na_2S_2O_3$$

[The amount (A g) of $K_2Cr_2O_7$ taken for the titration is known. The amount of iodine (B g) liberated by A g of $K_2Cr_2O_7$ can be found out with the help of equation (10·35). From equation (10·36), we can calculate the quantity (C g) of $Na_2S_2O_3$ which must have reacted with B g of iodine. Suppose V ml of $Na_2S_2O_3$ soln are required for titrating B g iodine, then V ml of thiosulphate soln will contain C g of $Na_2S_2O_3$. Thus the exact concentration of $Na_2S_2O_3$ soln will become known, *i.e*, the soln will be standardised.]

Procedure

(*i*) *Preparation of approximately 0·1 M $Na_2S_2O_3$.* Dissolve about 25 g of sodium thiosulphate in water and make up the volume in a 1 litre-measuring flask.

(*ii*) *Preparation of 0·1 N (0·1/6=0·0167 M) $K_2Cr_2O_7$ soln.* Dissolve exactly weighed 4·9035 g of $K_2Cr_2O_7$ in water and dilute it to 1000 ml in a volumetric flask. Shake well.

(*iii*) *Standardisation of $Na_2S_2O_3$ soln.* Pipette out 25·0 ml of $K_2Cr_2O_7$ soln in an iodine flask. Add about 50 ml water, 3 g KI and 4 ml concentrated HCl. Stopper the flask and allow to stand in dark for about 5 minutes so that the reaction is complete. Titrate the liberated I_2 with $Na_2S_2O_3$ soln taken in a burette and constantly rotate the flask so that the solutions are thoroughly mixed. When most of the I_2 has reacted (Colour will change from brown to pale yellow), add 1 ml of starch soln ; the colour of the soln will become blue. Continue dropwise addition of $Na_2S_2O_3$ and swirling the flask constantly, until one drop of the titrant changes the colour from greenish blue to light green (due to Cr^{3+} ions). The end point is sharp. Repeat the titration with 25 ml water in place of $K_2Cr_2O_7$ soln (known as blank determination)—if some $Na_2S_2O_3$ is consumed, it should be subtracted from the titre value. For example, suppose the experimental titre is 24·4 ml and blank titre is 0·2 ml, then the corrected titre will be (24·4 −0·2)

$=24\cdot2$ ml of $Na_2S_2O_3$ soln. The normality of $Na_2S_2O_3$ soln can be calculated as follows :

$$N_{Na_2S_2O_3} \times 24\cdot2 = 0\cdot1 \times 25\cdot0$$

$$N_{Na_2S_2O_3} = \frac{0\cdot1 \times 25\cdot0}{24\cdot2} = 0\cdot1033$$

Notes :

(1) The reaction between $K_2Cr_2O_7$ and KI (in presence of HCl) is not instantaneous, hence sometime is allowed for the reaction to go to completion.

(2) The reaction between KI and acid produces HI which de-composes into iodine in presence of light that is why the reaction mixture is allowed to stand in the dark. The photo-oxidation of

$$2HI + O \rightarrow H_2O + I_2 \qquad \qquad ...(10\cdot37)$$

HI can be prevented if the titration is carried out in an atmosphere of carbon dioxide gas.

Experiment 10·5

Iodometric determination of KIO_3.

Pipette out $25\cdot0$ ml of the given KIO_3 soln into an iodine flask. Add 20 ml water, 3 g KI and 5 ml 2N H_2SO_4. Swirl the flask. Titrate the liberated iodine with a standardised soln of $Na_2S_2O_3$ using starch as an indicator. The reactions involved are :

$$KIO_3 + 3H_2SO_4 + 5KI \rightarrow 3K_2SO_4 + 3H_2O + 3I_2$$

$$3I_2 + 6Na_2S_2O_3 \rightarrow 3Na_2S_4O_6 + 6NaI$$

$\therefore \quad 6Na_2S_2O_3 \equiv 3I_2 \equiv KIO_3 \quad$ (mol wt $214\cdot02$)

so that,

$$6000 \text{ ml, } 1 \text{ M } Na_2S_2O_3 = 1000 \text{ ml, } 1 \text{ M } KIO_3$$
$$= 214\cdot02 \text{ g } KIO_3$$
$$6000 \text{ ml, } 0\cdot1 \text{ M } Na_2S_2O_3 = 21\cdot402 \text{ g } KIO_3$$
$$1000 \text{ ml, } 0\cdot1 \text{ M } Na_2S_2O_3 = \frac{21\cdot402}{6} = 3\cdot567 \text{ g } KIO_3$$
$$1 \text{ ml, } 0\cdot1 \text{ M } Na_2S_2O_3 = 3\cdot567 \text{ mg } KIO_3$$

(**Note** that for $Na_2S_2O_3$, eq wt = mol wt, hence its $0\cdot1$ M soln is the same as its $0\cdot1$ N soln.) If $18\cdot7$ ml, $0\cdot1$ N, $Na_2S_2O_3$ soln is required in the titration, the amount of KIO_3 in 25 ml of the given soln will be :

$$3\cdot567 \times 18\cdot7 = 66\cdot703 \text{ mg } KIO_3.$$

Experiment 10·6

Iodometric determination of $K_2Cr_2O_7$.

Pipette out 25·0 ml of the given $K_2Cr_2O_7$ soln into an iodine flask. Add 20 ml water, 3 g KI and 5 ml 2N H_2SO_4. Swirl the flask and keep it in dark for 5 min. Titrate the liberated iodine with a standard $Na_2S_2O_3$ soln. The reactions involved are :

$$Cr_2O_7{}^{2-}+14H^++6e \rightarrow 2Cr^{3+}+7H_2O$$

$$6I^--6e \rightarrow 3I_2$$

$$Cr_2O_7{}^{2-}+14H^++6I^- \rightarrow 2Cr^{3+}+7H_2O+3I_2$$
$$3I_2+6Na_2S_2O_3 \rightarrow 3Na_2S_4O_6+6NaI$$

So that,

$$6Na_2S_2O_3 \equiv 3I_2 \equiv K_2Cr_2O_7 \text{ (mol wt 294·2)}$$

or $\quad Na_2S_2O_3 \equiv 1/2\ I_2 \equiv 1/6\ K_2Cr_2O_7$ (divide throughout by 6)

$$1000\text{ ml, 1 M } Na_2S_2O_3 = \frac{294\cdot21}{6} = 49\cdot035\text{ g } K_2Cr_2O_7$$

1000 ml, 0·1 M $Na_2S_2O_3$=4·9035 g $K_2Cr_2O_7$

1 ml of 0·1 M (or 0·1 N)$Na_2S_2O_3$=4·9035 mg $K_2Cr_2O_7$.

Experiment 10·7

Iodometric determination of $CuSO_4$.

Discussion

Cupric ions react with iodide ions as shown by :

$$2Cu^{2+}+4I^- \rightarrow Cu_2I_2+I_2$$

A cupric ion receives an electron and gets reduced to cuprous state so cupric ion acts as an oxidant which oxidises iodide to iodine ; iodide acts as a reducing agent (see 10·6·2). To the given soln of $CuSO_4$ an excess of KI is added and the liberated iodine titrated with $Na_2S_2O_3$ soln.

$$2Cu^{2+} \equiv I_2 \equiv 2Na_2S_2O_3$$

or, $\quad Na_2S_2O_3 \equiv Cu^{2+} \equiv Cu$ (at wt 63·54)

1 ml 0·1 N, $Na_2S_2O_3$ soln=6·354 mg Cu.

Procedure

Pipette out 25 ml of the given $CuSO_4$ soln into a 250-ml iodine flask. Add 10 ml of a 10 per cent KI soln. Titrate the liberated I_2 with standard $Na_2S_2O_3$ soln. Repeat the titration until two readings agree within 0·1 ml.

Notes :

(1) In the iodometric determination of Cu^{2+} there is no need to add acid to $CuSO_4$ soln along with KI as was necessary in the case of KIO_3 and $K_2Cr_2O_7$. The reason is that the reduction does not

$$Cu^{2+}+e \longrightarrow Cu^+ \qquad ...(10\cdot38)$$

involve any H^+ ions [compare this equation with $(10\cdot34)$ and $(10\cdot35)$]. On the other hand, if an acid is present in the given $CuSO_4$ soln, it should be neutralised. Because the acid would react with KI to give HI which in presence of light decomposes to give I_2 [see equation $(10\cdot37)$]. This would give an error because our method is based upon the measurement of I_2.

(2) It has been found that the normality, of thiosulphate soln determined by titration with KIO_3 or $K_2Cr_2O_7$, is slightly different from that obtained by titration with a standard soln containing Cu^{2+} ions. This difference is due to the fact that some of the liberated iodine gets adsorbed on the cuprous iodide and is thus not available for titration with thiosulphate. It is for this reason that $Na_2S_2O_3$ soln used in the iodometric titration of $CuSO_4$ is standardised not with KIO_3 but with a standard soln of Cu^{2+} ions as described below.

Weigh out accurately about $0\cdot25$ g of A.R. copper turnings into a 250 ml iodine flask. Add 10 ml of HNO_3 (1 : 3, i.e., 30 ml concentrated HNO_3 diluted to about 90 ml) to dissolve the copper turnings. Dilute to 25 ml and heat to boiling, add 1 g urea, again boil for 1-2 minutes. The urea reacts with nitrous acid and oxide of nitrogen produced during the reaction between Cu and HNO_3. (The nitrite ion present in the soln reacts with iodide to produce I_2 which causes error). Cool the soln and add NH_4OH (1 : 1) until a slight turbidity due to $Cu(OH)_2$ is seen. (This would neutralise the excess HNO_3 present in the soln.) Add CH_3COOH until the turbity is clear and then add 20 ml of a 10 per cent KI soln. Keep the iodine flask for 1 minute. The soln becomes dark brown due to the liberated iodine. Add $Na_2S_2O_3$ soln to be standardised through a burette while swirling the flask. When the soln becomes pale yellow, add 1 ml of starch soln and continue the titration with shaking until a drop of $Na_2S_2O_3$ changes the colour from blue to white (or slightly yellowish—this colour is due to adsorption of some iodine on the white ppt of cuprous iodide).

A.R. copper sulphate (mol wt=eq wt=$249\cdot69$) can also be used for the standardisation of thiosulphate if it is to be used for the iodometric titration of Cu^{2+} ions. The reaction is :

$$2CuSO_4+4KI \longrightarrow Cu_2I_2+2K_2SO_4+I_2$$
$$I_2+2Na_2S_2O_3 \longrightarrow 2NaI+Na_2S_4O_6$$

Experiment 10'8

Iodometric determination of $KMnO_4$.

Pipette out 20 ml of the given $KMnO_4$ soln into an iodine flask, add 25 ml, N H_2SO_4 and 5 g of KI. Swirl the flask and keep in dark for 10 minutes. Titrate the liberated iodine with a standard $Na_2S_2O_3$ soln. The reactions involved are :

$$2KMnO_4+8H_2SO_4+10KI \longrightarrow 6K_2SO_4+2MnSO_4+8H_2O+5I_2$$
$$5I_2+10Na_2S_2O_3 \longrightarrow 10NaI+5Na_2S_4O_6$$
$$10Na_2S_2O_3 \equiv 5I_2 \equiv 2KMnO_4 \quad \text{(mol wt 157'94)}$$

10 litre, M $Na_2S_2O_3 = 157'94 \times 2 = 315'88$ g $KMnO_4$

1 litre M $Na_2S_2O_3 \equiv 31'588$ g $KMnO_4$

1 litre 0'1 M (or 0'1 N) $Na_2S_2O_3 \equiv 3'16$ g $KMnO_4$

1 ml 0'1 N $Na_2S_2O_3 \equiv 3'16$ mg $KMnO_4$.

Experiment 10'9

Preparation of a standard soln of iodine (potassium tri-iodide)..

Iodine has a poor solubility in water but it readily dissolves in a concentrated soln of KI to form a complex ion :

$$I_2+I^- \longrightarrow [I_3]^- \quad \text{(tri-iodine ion)}$$
or
$$I_2+KI \longrightarrow KI_3 \quad \text{(potassium tri-iodide)}$$

Iodine soln for titration purposes is therefore prepared by adding KI.

In most redox reactions, a molecule of iodine gains two electrons [see equation (10'28)] so that eq wt of I_2 is half of its mol wt and normality of I_2 soln is double the molarity.

Thus, the normality of 0'05 M soln of iodine will be $0'05 \times 2$ $=0'1$. Commercially available iodine contains certain impurities. It can be purified by sublimation. Iodine is mixed up with solid KI and heated. The iodine vapours are allowed to deposit on a cold surface. Iodine so obtained is quite pure. Resublimed iodine can be used as a primary standard but the difficulty is that I_2 is volatile even at room temperature, hence there can be loss in weight during weighing.

The following three methods are generally used for preparing a standard soln of iodine.

(A) BY WEIGHING. Weigh approximately 20 g of KI in a weighing bottle and dissolve it in about 5 ml of water. Wait for some time so that the soln acquires room temperature, close the bottle and weigh it accurately on an analytical balance. Transfer some resublimed iodine (in the range of 13 to 14 g) into the weighing bottle, quickly close it and again weigh accurately. The difference between two weight readings is the weight of I_2. Carefully stir the mixture until all the iodine has dissolved. Transfer the soln through a funnel into a measuring flask, carefully wash the weighing bottle so that the transfer is complete. Make up to the mark with water and shake thoroughly. Suppose :

wt of weighing bottle+KI soln=38·3256 g

wt of weighing bottle+KI soln+I_2=52·3588 g

wt of iodine=(52·3588−38·3256)=14·0332 g

If this much iodine is dissolved and diluted to 1 litre ; the normality of the soln will be :

$$\frac{14·0332}{127·0}=0·1105$$

This soln can be suitably diluted if we want to prepare exactly 0·1 N soln of iodine (see expt. 10·1).

Remember

$$normality= \frac{wt\ per\ litre}{eq\ wt}$$

mol wt of iodine=253·84

$$eqwt= \frac{mol\ wt}{2} = \frac{253·84}{2}$$

$$=126·92\ (or\ 127·0)$$

In method [B] and [C], an approximate soln of iodine is prepared. About 25 g KI is taken in a conical flask and dissolved in a small volume of water (about 10 ml) so that a concentrated soln of KI is obtained. To this soln about 14 to 15 g resublimed iodine is added and soln agitated so that I_2 is completely dissolved. (Do not use a large volume of water otherwise KI soln will be dilute and dissolution of iodine will be difficult). The soln is then completely transferred to a 1 litre measuring flask, volume made up to the mark, soln is thoroughly shaken and standardised by one of the following methods.

[B] **STANDARDISATION BY TITRATION WITH A STANDARD THIOSULPHATE SOLN.**

[C] **STANDARDISATION WITH ARSENIOUS OXIDE**

Discussion. Arsenious oxide of A.R. (Analytical grade) variety is 99·9 per cent pure and can be used as a primary standard for standardising iodine soln. Arsenic(III) oxide (As_2O_3 ; mol wt 197·82) is not soluble in water but dissolves in NaOH soln :

$$As_2O_3+2NaOH \longrightarrow 2NaAsO_2+H_2O \qquad ...(10·39)$$

(or, $$As_2O_3+2OH^- \longrightarrow 2AsO_2^-+H_2O)$$

On neutralising the excess NaOH by HCl and then adding iodine to the resultant soln, the reaction is :

$$HAsO_2 + I_2 + 2H_2O \longrightarrow H_3AsO_4 + 2H^+ + 2I^- \qquad ...(10\text{·}40)$$
$$(or, \quad AsO_2^- + I_2 + 2H_2O \longrightarrow AsO_4^{3-} + 4H^+ + 2I^-) \qquad ...(10\text{·}41)$$
$$(or \ HAsO_2 + I_3^- + 2H_2O \longrightarrow H_3AsO_4 + 2H^+ + 3I^-) \qquad ...(10\text{·}42)$$

[Note that iodine has been dissolved in KI soln, I_2 and KI combine to give the tri-iodide ion (I_3^-). Hence, reaction (10·40) can also be written in the form shown by (10·42).]

The value for equilibrium constant for the reaction (10·42) is given by :

$$K = \frac{[H_3AsO_4] \times [H^+]^2 \times [I^-]^3}{[HAsO_2] \times [I_3^-]} = 0\text{·}17 \qquad ...(10\text{·}43)$$

The value of K is very small so we can conclude that reaction will be incomplete and hence cannot be used in quantitative analysis (see 4·1·1).

If in a reaction [product] = 10,000 [reactant], then it would be 99·99 per cent complete. If we put $[H_3AsO_4] = 10,000$ and $[HAsO_2] = 1$ in equation (10·43) and calculate $[H^+]$, we find that is comes out to $5\text{·}5 \times 10^{-5}$ g ion per litre (corresponding to pH 4·26). It means if the pH of the reaction mixture is kept at 4·3, the oxidation reaction (10·42) will go to completion. But at this pH, the rate of the reaction is slow. However, at pH between 7 to 9, the reaction is fast and complete. If we neutralise arsenic oxide soln and add $NaHCO_3$, the pH then becomes 7 to 8 and this soln can be successfully titrated with iodine soln. This case provides an example, how theoretical considerations guide us to search suitable experimental conditions for developing a quantitative analytical method.

By combining reactions (10·39) and (10·40) it is possible to write :

$$As_2O_3 \equiv 2AsO_2^- \equiv 2I_2 (\equiv 4H).$$

or,
$$eq \ wt \ of \ As_2O_3 = \frac{mol \ wt}{4}$$
$$= \frac{197\text{·}82}{4} = 49\text{·}46$$

Procedure

(i) *Preparation of a standard soln of As_2O_3.* Dry about 5 to 6 g of As_2O_3 at 110°C for about 1 hour and then cool in a desiccator.

(ii) *Weigh out exactly 2·473 g of As_2O_3.* (It is not necessary to take exactly 2·473 g of the substance. The only condition is that the weight taken should be near about this weight but the weight of the substance used for preparing soln should be exactly known). Transfer accurately weighed As_2O_3 into a 400 ml beaker and dissolve it in a soln of NaOH prepared by dissolving 2 g alkali in 20 ml water. Dilute the soln to 200 ml and neutralise with 1 N HCl soln using a litmus paper (blue litmus paper should turn red ; the soln will be slightly acidic). Transfer the soln completely to a 500 ml volumetric flask, add 2 g of $NaHCO_3$. Shake and make up the volume to the mark, shake the soln thoroughly. Suppose 2·4958 g As_2O_3 is taken to prepare 500 ml soln. Then weight of As_2O_3 per litre will be $2·4958 \times 2 = 4·9916$ g.

$$\text{normality of soln} = \frac{\text{wt in 1 litre}}{\text{eq wt}}$$

$$= \frac{4·9916}{49·46} = 0·1009$$

(iii) *Standardisation of iodine soln.* Measure out 25·0 ml of arsenite soln from a burette into a 250 ml conical flask. (Do not use pipette as the soln is poisonous). Add about 20 ml water, 5 g $NaHCO_3$ and 2 ml of starch soln. Swirl, the flask, to dissolve $NaHCO_3$ and titrate slowly with iodine soln which is to be standardised. Swirl the flask during the titration. The first appearance of blue colour shows the end point. (It is also possible to titrate 25·0 ml of iodine soln taken in a conical flask with arsenite soln).

(iv) *Calculation of normality of iodine soln.* Normality of arsenite soln is known, hence that of iodine soln can be calculated.

Notes :

1. If an exact 0·1 N soln of arsenite is required, exactly 2·473 g As_2O_3 should be weighed.

2. Standard iodine soln can be used in the iodimetric determination of thiosulphate, tin(II), H_2S, As(III) compounds (arsenites) and Sb(III) compounds (antimonites).

10·9. REDOX SYSTEM AND REDOX POTENTIAL

A system containing an oxidant and its reduced form is called a *redox system.* For example, if we have a soln containing Fe^{3+} ions (oxidant) and also Fe^{2+} ions (reduced form of Fe^{3+} ion), it will form a redox system. If an inert electrode such as a platinum electrode, is dipped into such a soln, it acquires certain potential known as *redox potential.*

10·9·1. Expression for Redox Potential

We have seen that an oxidant (Ox) receives electrons and gets converted into its reduced form (Red). A reversible oxidation-reduction reaction can be written as :

$$Ox + ne \rightleftharpoons Red$$

The potential acquired by a platinum electrode dipping in a soln containing oxidant and its reduced form, is given by :

$$E_{Redox} = E°_{Redox} + \frac{RT}{nF} \log_e \frac{a_{Ox}}{a_{Red}} \qquad ...(10.44)$$

where,

E_{Redox} = Redox potential of the system

$E°_{Redox}$ = Standard redox potential of the system

R = Gas constant ; T = Absolute temperature

n = Number of electrons gained by a molecule of the oxidant in getting converted into the reductant

F = Faraday (96,500 coulombs)

a_{Ox} = Activity of the oxidant

a_{Red} = Activity of the reductant.

If we have a dilute soln the activity terms can be replaced by concentration of the oxidant and reductant :

$$E_{Redox} = E°_{Redox} + \frac{RT}{nF} \log_e \frac{[Ox]}{[Red]}$$

Remember

In dil soln

$f = 1$ (see 4.1)

$\therefore a = c$

Substituting the known values of R and F, changing from natural logarithms to common logarithms ($\log_e$ to $\log_{10}$) and taking the temperature of the soln as 25°C we can write :

$$E_{Redox} = E°_{Redox} + \frac{0.059}{n} \log_{10} \frac{[Ox]}{[Red]} \qquad ...(10.45)$$

If in a redox system [Ox] = [Red],

$$E_{Redox} = E°_{Redox} + \frac{0.059}{n} \log 1$$

Remember

$\log_e a = 2.303 \times \log_{10} a$

or, $E_{Redox} = E°_{Redox}$ ...(10.46)

and, log 1 = 0

The standard redox potential of a system is thus equal to its redox potential when in the system, the concentration of the oxidant is equal to that of its reduced form.

Suppose we have a soln in which $[Fe^{3+}] = [Fe^{2+}]$. Now, we dip a platinum electrode into this system and measure its potential with reference to a standard hydrogen electrode (whose potential is taken to be zero). Then the measured potential of the platinum electrode will be known as the standard redox potential of the ferric-ferrous redox system (the value has been found to be $+0.75$ volt). Thus, for the redox system involving Fe^{3+} and Fe^{2+} ions we can write :

$$Fe^{3+}+e \to Fe^{2+} \; ; \; E°=0.75 \text{ V}$$

Standard redox potentials of certain redox systems have been given in Table 10.1

Table 10.1. Standard Redox Potentials of Some Redox Systems

Electrode	*Electrode reaction*	*E° (volts)*
MnO_4^-, Mn^{2+}/Pt	$MnO_4^-+8H^++5e \to Mn^{2+}+4H_2O$	$+1.52$
Ce^{4+}, Ce^{3+}/Pt	$Ce^{4+}+e \to Ce^{3+}$	$+1.45$
$Cr_2O_7^{2-}$, Cr^{3+}/Pt	$Cr_2O_7^{2-}+14H^++6e \to 2Cr^{3+}+7H_2O$	$+1.36$
Cl_2, Cl^-/Pt	$Cl_2+2e \to 2Cl^-$	$+1.36$
Br_2, Br^-/Pt	$Br_2+2e \to 2Br^-$	$+1.07$
I_2, I^-/Pt	$I_2+2e \to 2I^-$	$+0.53$
Sn^{4+}, Sn^{2+}/Pt	$Sn^{4+}+2e \to Sn^{2+}$	$+0.15$
H^+, H_2/Pt	$2H^++2e \to H_2$	0.0000
Cd^{2+}, Cd/Pt	$Cd^{2+}+2e \to Cd$	-0.40
Zn^{2+}, Zn/Pt	$Zn^{2+}+2e \to Zn$	-0.76

The standard potentials given in Table 10.1 are measured at 25°C and in a soln 1 M in H^+. The magnitude of $E°$ is a measure of the oxidising power of an oxidant. For example, the standard oxidation potential of Cl_2, Cl^- system is $+1.36$ and that of Br_2, Br^- is $+1.07$ V, hence chlorine is more powerful oxidant than bromine. Similarly, it can be seen that bromine is a more powerful oxidant than iodine. This is the reason that the following reactions are possible.

$$Cl_2+2Br^- \to 2Cl^-+Br_2 \quad (Cl_2 \text{ oxidises } Br^- \text{ to } Br_2)$$
$$Cl_2+2I^- \to 2Cl^-+I_2 \quad (Cl_2 \text{ oxidises } I^- \text{ to } I_2)$$
$$Br_2+2I^- \to 2Br^-+I_2 \quad (Br_2 \text{ oxidises } I^- \text{ to } I_2)$$

But the reverse reactions are not possible. For example, I_2 cannot oxidise Cl^- to Cl_2 or Br^- to Br_2. [Note that in the detection of I$^-$ ion, some CCl_4 and Cl_2 water are added when the CCl_4 layer becomes violet. The I$^-$ ions are oxidised by Cl_2 to I_2 which dissolves in CCl_4 to produce a violet soln. In the case of Br$^-$, Br_2 is produced which forms a brown soln with CCl_4.]

10·10. CALCULATION OF EQUILIBRIUM CONSTANT OF A REDOX REACTION

It should be remembered that only those reactions can be used in titrimetric analysis which go to completion at the equivalence point. In order to know whether or not a reaction will go to completion, we must find out the value of equilibrium constant, K, of the reaction under the given conditions. If the value of K is quite high the reaction would go to virtual completion (see 3·1·5).

Suppose we want to titrate ferrous iron with Ce^{4+} ions, then there are two requirements which must be fulfilled.

1. The reaction between Fe^{2+} and Ce^{4+} should be fast and complete.

2. A suitable indicator should be available to show when the reaction is just complete.

The reaction between Fe^{2+} and Ce^{4+} is given by :

$$Fe^{2+} + Ce^{4+} \rightarrow Fe^{3+} + Ce^{3+} \qquad ...(10·47)$$

The equilibrium constant is given by :

$$K = \frac{[Ce^{3+}] \times [Fe^{3+}]}{[Ce^{4+}] \times [Fe^{2+}]}$$

Reaction (10·47) may be regarded as taking place in a voltaic cell which has two electrodes ; I, the Fe^{3+}, Fe^{+2} electrode and II, the Ce^{4+}, Ce^{3+} electrode. Thus we can write two electrode reactions :

A. $Fe^{2+} - e \rightarrow Fe^{3+}$ (oxidation) for the electrode I. The standard redox potential of this electrode is denoted by $E°_I$ (its value has been found to be 0·75 volt).

B. $Ce^{4+} + e \rightarrow Ce^{3+}$ (reduction) for electrode II. The standard potential of this electrode is represented by $E°_{II}$ (its value has been found to be 1·45 volt).

The two electrode potentials at 25°C can be given by :

$$E_I = E°_I + \frac{0·059}{1} \log \frac{[Fe^{3+}]}{[Fe^{2+}]}$$

$$E_{II} = E°_{II} + \frac{0·059}{1} \log \frac{[Ce^{4+}]}{[Ce^{3+}]}$$

For both the electrode reactions

$n = 1$
see equation (10·45)

If reaction (10.47) which is regarded as taking place in a cell is allowed to proceed to equilibrium, the e.m.f. of the cell will be zero, i.e., the potentials of the two electrodes will be equal $(E_I = E_{II})$:

$$0.75 + 0.059 \log \frac{[Fe^{3+}]}{[Fe^{2+}]} = 1.45 + 0.059 \log \frac{[Ce^{4+}]}{[Ce^{3+}]}$$

or, $0.059 \log \frac{[Fe^{3+}]}{[Fe^{2+}]} - 0.059 \log \frac{[Ce^{4+}]}{[Ce^{3+}]} = 1.45 - 0.75$

or, $0.059 \left(\log \dfrac{[Fe^{3+}]}{[Fe^{2+}]} + \log \dfrac{[Ce^{3+}]}{[Ce^{4+}]} \right)$
$\qquad\qquad\qquad = 1.45 - 0.75$

$0.059 \times \log \dfrac{[Fe^{3+}] \times [Ce^{3+}]}{[Fe^{2+}] \times [Ce^{4+}]}$
$\qquad\qquad\qquad = 1.45 - 0.75$

or $\quad \log K = \dfrac{1.45 - 0.75}{0.059} = 11.84$

or $\qquad K = 7 \times 10^{11}$

> *Remember*
>
> $-\log \dfrac{a}{b} = +\log \dfrac{b}{a}$
>
> $\log \dfrac{a_1}{b_1} + \log \dfrac{a_2}{b_2}$
>
> $= \log \dfrac{a_1 \times a_2}{b_1 \times b_2}$

The value of K is quite high, hence the oxidation of Fe^{2+} with Ce^{4+} ions will go to virtual completion, hence this reaction can] be used in redox titrimetry.

In general, suppose we have a redox reaction involving the redox systems I and II having standard potentials $E°_I$ and $E°_{II}$ and n is the number of electrons involved in the reaction. Then the equilibrium constant for the reaction is given by :

$$\frac{[E°_I - E°_{II}] \times n}{0.059} = \log K$$

Example 10(x)

Calculate the equilibrium constant for the reaction :

$$MnO_4^- + 5Fe^{2+} + 8H^+ \rightarrow Mn^{2+} + 5Fe^{3+} + 4H_2O$$

(the [H^+] is 1 molar : the standard potential for ferric-ferrous electrode is 0.77 volt and that for permanganate-manganous system is 1.52 volt).

The equilibrium constant for the reaction can be written as :

$$K = \frac{[Mn^{2+}] \times [Fe^{3+}]^5}{[MnO_4^-] \times [H^+]^8 \times [Fe^{2+}]^5}$$

The complete reaction can be divided into two parts :

$$MnO_4^- + 8H^+ + 5e \rightarrow Mn^{2+} + 4H_2O \ ; \ (I), \ E_I° = 1.52v$$
$$Fe^{2+} - e \rightarrow Fe^{3+} \ ; \ (II), \ E_{II}° = 0.77v$$

These equations are called partial equations or half-cell reactions or electrode reactions. The half-cell reaction (II) should be multiplied by 5 so that the same number of electrons are involved as in (I) :

$$5Fe^{2+} - 5e \rightarrow 5Fe^{3+}$$

$$E_{II} = E^\circ_{II} + \frac{0·059}{5} \log \frac{[Fe^{+3}]^5}{[Fe^{2+}]^5}$$

Thus, the potential for system (II) will be :

$$E_{II} = 0·77 + \frac{0·059}{5} \log \frac{[Fe^{3+}]^5}{[Fe^{2+}]^5}$$

Similarly, the potential for the half-cell reaction (I) is given by :

$$E_I = 1·52 + \frac{0·059}{5} \log \frac{[MnO_4^-] \times [H^+]^8}{[Mn^{2+}]}$$

Combining the two electrodes and allowing the reaction to proceed to equilibrium, when the two potentials will be equal $(E_I = E_{II})$:

$$1·52 + \frac{0·059}{5} \log \frac{[MnO_4^-] \times [H^+]^8}{[Mn^{2+}]}$$

$$= 0·77 + \frac{0·059}{5} \log \frac{[Fe^{3+}]^5}{[Fe^{2+}]^5}$$

$$\frac{(1·52 - 0·77) \times 5}{0·059} = \log \frac{[Fe^{3+}]^5}{[Fe^{2+}]^5} - \log \frac{[MnO_4^-] \times [H^+]^8}{[Mn^{2+}]}$$

$$= \frac{0·75 \times 5}{0·059}$$

$$= \log \frac{[Fe^{3+}]^5}{[Fe^{2+}]^5} + \log \frac{[Mn^{2+}]}{[MnO_4^-] \times [H^+]^8}$$

$$\frac{3·75}{0·059} = \log \frac{[Mn^{2+}] \times [Fe^{3+}]^5}{[MnO_4^-] \times [H^+]^8 \times [Fe^{2+}]^5}$$

$$63·5 = \log K \text{ or } K = 4·7 \times 10^{63}$$

The large value of K tells us that the oxidation of Fe_2^+ ions by acidic $KMnO_4$ goes to completion.

10·11. CHANGE OF POTENTIAL DURING REDOX TITRATION

In section 10·10, a procedure has been described for calculating the value of equilibrium constant (K) of a redox reaction. If its value is large the reaction is suitable to act as a basis of a titrimetric method. For example, the value of K for the reaction between Fe^{2+} and Sn^{4+} is 7×10^{11} so that the reaction will be practically complete at the equivalence point. The next problem is to choose a suitable indicator which will show when the reaction of Fe^{2+} with Sn^{4+} is just complete. In order to understand how indicators are selected for redox titrations, it is necessary to study the change in electrode potential during a redox titration.

Let us consider the titration of 100 ml, 0·1 N ferrous soln (titrand) with 0·1 N ceric soln (titrant). The half reaction for the titrand is written as :

$$Fe^{2+} - e \rightarrow Fe^{3+}$$

The half reaction for the titrant is :

$$Ce^{4+} + e \rightarrow Ce^{3+}$$

Thus we have two redox systems :

I, ferric-ferrous system   ($E_I° = 0·75$ V) and

II, ceric-cerous system   ($E_{II}° = 1·45$ V).

The complete reaction between Fe^{2+} and Ce^{4+} is given by

$$Fe^{2+} + Ce^{4+} \rightarrow Fe^{3+} + Ce^{3+}$$

In this titration, the potential (of the platinum electrode dipping in the titration mixture) upto the equivalence point is calculated from $E_I°$. Because when the titration is not complete all the Ce^{4+} ions added are reduced to Ce^{3+}, so, the soln contains Fe^{2+}, Fe^{3+} and Ce^{3+} ions. As there are no Ce^{4+} ions, only ferric-ferrous system exists. After the equivalence point, all the Fe^{2+} ions have been converted into Fe^{3+} and now Ce^{4+} ions are present in excess. Hence, the soln contains Fe^{3+}, Ce^{3+} and Ce^{4+} ions, so, now only ceric-cerous system exists. The potential after the equivalence point is therefore calculated from $E_{II}°$. Let us now calculate potential at the different stages of the titration.

(i) 50 ml, Ce^{4+} soln added (reaction 50% complete).

$[Fe^{3+}]$ = 50 ml, 0·1 N ; $[Ce^{3+}]$ = 50 ml, 0·1 N

$[Fe^{2+}]$ = 50 ml, 0·1 N ; $[Ce^{4+}]$ = zero

Note that only ferric-ferrous system is present and the amount of cerous formed is equal to the amount of ferric ion. The potential at this stage is given as :

$$E_I = E_I° + 0·06 \ \log \ \frac{[Fe^{3+}]}{[Fe^{2+}]} = 0·75 + 0·06 \times \log 1$$

$$= 0·75 \text{ V} \qquad \begin{bmatrix} (\log 1 = 0) \\ (0·059) \approx 0·06) \end{bmatrix}$$

(ii) 90 ml Ce^{4+} soln added (reaction 90% complete) :

$[Fe^{3+}]$ = 90 ml, 0·1 N ; $[Ce^{3+}]$ = 90 ml, 0·1 N

$[Fe^{2+}]$ = 10 ml, 0·1 N ; $[Ce^{4+}]$ = zero

$$E_I = 0.75 + 0.06 \log \frac{90}{10} \approx 0.75 + 0.06 \log \frac{100}{10}$$

$$= 0.75 + 0.06 \log 10 = 0.75 + 0.06 \times 1$$

$$= 0.75 + 0.06 = 0.81 \text{ V} \mid [\log 10 = 1].$$

(iii) *99 ml Ce⁴⁺ soln added (reaction 99% complete)* :

$[Fe^{3+}] = 99$ ml, 0.1 N ; $[Ce^{3+}] = 99$ ml, 0.1 N

$[Fe^{2+}] = 1$ ml, 0.1 N ; $[Ce^{4+}] = $ zero

$$E_I = 0.75 + 0.06 \log \frac{99}{1} \approx 0.75 + 0.06 \log 100 \mid [\log 100 = 2]$$

$$= 0.75 + 0.06 \times 2 = 0.75 + 0.12 = 0.87 \text{ V}$$

(iv) *99.9 ml Ce⁴⁺ soln added (reaction 99.9% complete)* :

$[Fe^{3+}] = 99.9$ ml, 0.1 N ; $[Ce^{3+}] = 99.9$ ml, 0.1 N

$[Fe^{2+}] = 0.1$ ml, 0.1 N ; $[Ce^{4+}] = $ zero

$$E_I = 0.75 + 0.06 \log \frac{99.9}{0.1} \approx 0.75 + 0.06 \log \frac{100}{0.1}$$

$$= 0.75 + 0.06 \log \frac{1000}{1} = 0.75 + 0.06 \times 3 \mid (\log 1000 = 3)$$

$$= 0.75 + 0.18 = 0.93 \text{ V}$$

(v) *100.0 ml Ce⁴⁺ soln added (reaction 100% complete)* :

$[Fe^{3+}] = 100$ ml, 0.1 N ; $[Ce^{3+}] = 100$ ml, 0.1 N

$[Fe^{2+}] = $ zero   ; $[Ce^{4+}] = $ zero

It can be shown that the potential at the equivalence point is the arithmatic mean of the two standard redox potentials.

$$E_{e.p} = \frac{E_I° + E_{II}°}{2} = \frac{0.75 + 1.45}{2} = \frac{2.20}{2} = 1.10 \text{ V}$$

(vi) *100.1 ml Ce⁴⁺ soln added* :

$[Fe^{3+}] = 100$ ml, 0.1 N ; $[Ce^{3+}] = 100$ ml, 0.1 N

$[Fe^{2+}] = $ zero   ; $[Ce^{4+}] = 0.1$ ml, 0.1 N

Note that 100 ml, 0.1 N Ce⁴⁺ soln is used up in converting 100 ml. 0.1 N, Fe²⁺ soln to Fe³⁺ ions. There are no Fe²⁺ ions left, 0.1 ml 0.1 N Ce⁴⁺ ions are present as excess and Ce³⁺ ions are already there in the soln. Hence, ceric-cerous system exists and the potential will be calculated from $E_{II}°$.

$$E_{II} = 1.45 + 0.06 \log \frac{[Ce^{4+}]}{[Ce^{3+}]} = 1.45 + 0.06 \log \frac{0.1}{100}$$

$$= 1.45 + 0.06 \log \frac{1}{1000} = 1.45 + 0.06 \log 10^{-3}$$

$$=1\cdot45+(0\cdot06\times -3)\mid (\log 10^{-3}=-3)$$
$$=1\cdot45+(-0\cdot18)=1\cdot27 \text{ V}.$$

(vii) 101 ml Ce^{4+} soln added :

$[Fe^{3+}]=100$ ml, $0\cdot1$ N ; $[Ce^{3+}]=100$ ml, $0\cdot1$ N

$[Fe^{2+}]=$ zero   ; $[Ce^{4+}]=1$ ml, $0\cdot1$ N

$$E_2=1\cdot45+0\cdot06 \log \frac{1}{100}=1\cdot45+0\cdot06 \log 10^{-2}$$

$$=1\cdot45+(0\cdot06\times -2)=1\cdot45-0\cdot12=1\cdot33 \text{ V}$$

By similar calculations it can be shown that when 110 ml, Ce^{4+} soln is added the potential is $1\cdot39$ volt and when 200 ml, Ce^{4+} soln is added, the potential will be $1\cdot45$ volt. These calculations have been summarised in Table 10·2.

Table 10·2.   Change of Potential During Titration of 100 ml, 0·1 N Fe^{2+} with 0·1 N Ceric Solution

Ce^{4+} added ml	Potential volt	Change of Potential per ml
50·0	0·75	
90·0	0·81	0·06/40=0·0015
99·0	0·87	0·06/9 =0·0067
99·9	0·93	0·06/0·9=0·0667
100·0	1·10	0·17/0.1=1·7000
100·1	1·27	0·17/0·1=1·7000
101·0	1·33	0·06/0·9=0·0667
110·0	1·39	0·06/9=0·0067
200·0	1·45	0·06/90=0·0006

From the results of Table 10·2, it is evident that potential rises slowly in the initial stages of the titration but near the equivalence point there is a sudden change of potential. These results have been graphically shown in Fig. 10·1. (Compare this curve with pH-neutralisation curves obtained in acid-base titrations).

From Fig. 10·1, it is clear that an ideal indicator for the titration of Fe^{2+} with Ce^{4+} ions should show a colour change at $1\cdot10$ volt. However, even if the colour change takes place at $0\cdot93$ volt, the error will be only $0\cdot1$ per cent. Similarly, if the colour of an indicator changes at 1·27 volt, the titration error will be again 0·1 per cent. Thus, for this titration we should select such an indicator which will show a colour change between 0·93 to 1·27 volt.

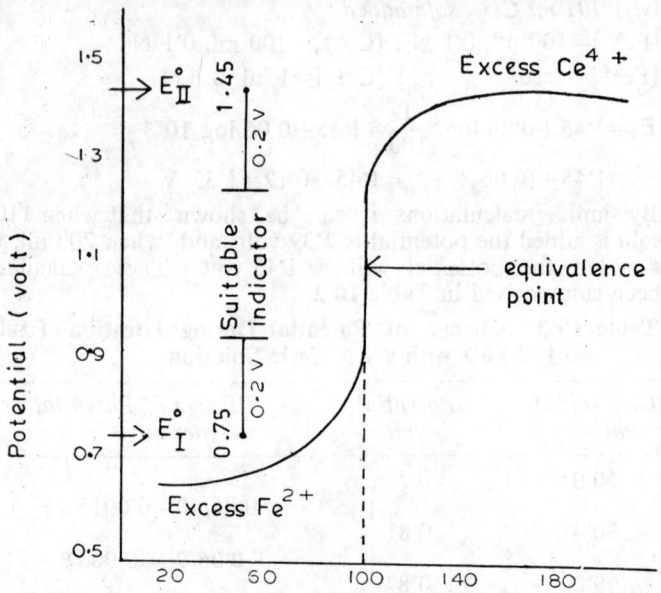

Fig. 10·1. Change of potential in the titration of 100 ml 0·1N Fe²⁺ with 0 1N Ce⁴⁺ soln.

10·12. REDOX INDICATORS

Three types of visual indicators are used in redox titrimetry :

    (*i*) reagent serving as its own indicator (self indication),
    (*ii*) external indicator,
    (*iii*) internal indicator.

Apart from these visual indicators, end point can also be detected by potential measurement (potentiometric titrations — see Chapter 14).

10·12·1. Self Indicator

The well known example is that of $KMnO_4$. For example, in the titration of Fe^{2+} with standard $KMnO_4$ soln, the completion of the reaction is shown by pink colour due to the unreacted $KMnO_4$. Another example is that if we are using 0·1 N iodine soln as titrant, a light yellow colour will be observed at the end point. The drawback in such cases is that a slight excess of the oxidant is always present at the equivalence point. Hence, for accurate work, indicator blank should be determined.

Example 10(xi)

In titrating 25 ml of Fe^{2+} soln, 29·3 ml of a standard $KMnO_4$ soln was required. The titration was then repeated in an identical manner by taking 25 ml water in place of iron (II) soln. This time 0·2 ml $KMnO_4$ soln was required to produce the same intensity of colour which was observed in the first titration. Then 0·2 ml will be the indicator blank and the corrected titre will be (29·3−0·2) =29·1 ml.

10·12·2. External Indicator

In a redox titration using an external indicator, the indicator is not added to the titrand soln but the titration liquid is taken out from time to time and added to the indicator soln kept out side.

Example 10(xii)

Titration of Fe^{2+} soln with standard $K_2Cr_2O_7$ soln.

Take 25 ml of Fe^{2+} soln whose normality is to be determined. Add 10 ml 4N, H_2SO_4 and titrate with a standard $K_2Cr_2O_7$ soln taken in a burette. Add a small volume of $K_2Cr_2O_7$ soln, shake and take out a drop of the titration liquid from the conical flask and add it to a few drops of potassium ferricyanide soln placed on a spot plate. If blue colour appears, it means Fe^{2+} ions are still present and the titration is not complete. Add little more of $K_2Cr_2O_7$ and repeat the test. Continue the titration until the titration liquid does not give any blue colour with potassium ferricyanide. Repeat the titration 3 or 4 times to correctly locate the end point.

10·12·3. Internal Redox Indicator

It has already been seen that acid-base indicators have different colours in acidic and alkaline soln. Similarly a redox indicator has one colour in an oxidising medium and a different colour when it is added to a soln of a reductant. A redox indicator is a compound which has different colours in the oxidised and reduced forms. The oxidation and reduction of the indicator is reversible. For example, ortho-phenanthroline ferrous ion has a red colour in the reduced form. If a few drops of this indicator are added to $K_2Cr_2O_7$ soln, its reduced form will be oxidised by $K_2Cr_2O_7$ and the soln will become blue (colour of the oxidised form) :

$$[Fe (C_{12}H_8N_2)_3]^{2+}-e \rightarrow [Fe(C_{12}H_8N_2)_3]^{3+}$$
reduced form (red)   oxidised form (blue)

If to this soln an excess of $FeSO_4$ soln is added, the oxidised form of the indicator will be reduced, hence the soln will again become red. Thus, we can say that this indicator undergoes reversible oxidation.

In general,

$$In_{ox}+ne \rightleftharpoons In_{red}$$

where In_{ox} and In_{red} are oxidised and reduced forms of the indicator. The potential of the indicator system is given by (see 10'9'1) :

$$E_{In} = E^{\circ}_{In} + \frac{0.059}{n} \log \frac{[In_{ox}]}{[In_{red}]}$$

Suppose $n=1$ and $[In_{ox}] = 10 [In_{Red}]$, then :

$$E_{In} = E^{\circ}_{In} + 0.06 \log \frac{10}{1} = E^{\circ}_{In} + 0.06 \log 10$$

$$= E^{\circ}_{In} + 0.06 \times 1 = E^{\circ}_{In} + 0.06$$

If the potential is $(E^{\circ}_{In} + 0.06)$, then most of the indicator will be in the oxidised form, hence colour of the oxidised form will be exhibited. It can be shown that when potential is $(E^{\circ} - 0.06)$, $[In_{Red}] = 10 (In_{xo}]$ and the colour of the soln will be clearly that of the reduced form. In the potential range $(E^{\circ} + 0.06)$ to $(E^{\circ} - 0.06)$ volt, the colour will be in between that of the oxidised and the reduced form. For example, E°_{In} for ferroin is 1'14 volt. If this indicator is added to a redox system whose potential is less than $(1'14 - 0'06) = 1'08$ volt, the soln will be clearly red. If the potential is greater than $(1'14 + 0'06) = 1'20$ volt, the soln will be distinctly blue. In the potential range 1'08 to 1'20 volt, the colour will be a mixture of red and blue. The range $(E^{\circ} - 0'06)$ to $(E^{\circ} + 0'06)$ is, therefore, called the indicator range.

10'13. CHOICE OF REDOX INDICATOR

In section 10'11, we have seen that in the titration of Fe^{2+} soln with Ce^{4+} ions, the potential at the end point is 1'10 volt (mean of E°_I and E°_{II}, i.e., $\frac{0.75 + 1.45}{2} = 1.10$ V). Hence, it appears that only that indicator will be suitable which will show a colour change at 1'10 volt. But a careful examination of results of Table 10'2 reveals that any indicator which shows a colour change between 0'93 volt (reaction 99'9%, error 0'1%) and 1'27 volt (reaction 100'1% ; error 0'1%) is suitable for this titration. It should be noted that in this titration two redox systems are involved. Their standard potentials are 0'75 volt (E°_I for ferric-ferrous-system) and 1'45 volt (E°_{II} for ceric-cerous system). The colour change is required between 0'93 and 1'27 volt, i e., E°_{In} should differ from E°_I and E°_{II} by about 0'2 volt provided that $n=1$. The value of E°_{In} for ferroin is 1'10 volt, this differs from 0'75 by more than 0'2 volt $[(1'10 - 0'75) > 0'2]$, similarly it differs from 1'45 by more than 0'2 volt $[(1'45 - 1'10) > 0'2]$. Hence, ferroin is a suitable indicator for the titration of ferrous iron with ceric soln.

11

Precipitation and Complexation Titrations

Titrations involving precipitation reactions are much smaller in number as compared to those based on acid-base or redox reactions. The limited application of precipitation reactions to titrimetric analysis is due to the following reasons :

(i) Lack of suitable indicators.

(ii) In some cases, particularly in the titration of dilute solutions, the rate of reaction is too slow for a convenient titration.

(iii) Composition of the precipitate sometimes is not fixed due to coprecipitation so that the stoichiometry of the reaction is not definite causing error.

11.1. REQUIREMENTS FOR PRECIPITATION TITRATIONS

In a precipitation titration we find out that what quantity of the added precipitant would be chemically equivalent to the substance being precipitated. For example, if we are given a soln of $AgNO_3$, we will gradually add a standard soln of KCNS (potassium thiocyanate which acts as a precipitant) through a burette until the precipitation of AgCNS is just complete. Since we have used a standard KCNS soln, the amount of KCNS (X g) required in the titration can be calculated. Now, the reaction of $AgNO_3$ with KCNS can be represented by :

$$AgNO_3 + KCNS \rightarrow AgCNS + KNO_3 \qquad ...(11.1)$$
$$\begin{matrix} 169.89 & 97.18 & 165.96 & 101.11 \\ \text{(analyte)} & \text{(reagent)} & \text{(ppt)} & \end{matrix}$$

With the help of equation (11.1) we can calculate what amount of $AgNO_3$ must have reacted with X g of KCNS. Thus the amount of

$AgNO_3$ in the given soln can be determined without collecting, washing, drying and weighing the ppt.

A precipitation reaction can act as a basis of a titrimetric method only when it satisfies the following conditions.

(*i*) The rate of reaction between the precipitant and the substance to be precipitated must be fast. In a gravimetric determination, the rate of precipitation can be increased by using an excess of the precipitant. But this is not possible in precipitation titration. Near the equivalence point the concentrations of the analyte and the reagent become quite small so that the reaction rate also slows down.

(*ii*) The reaction between the analyte and the reagent should proceed according to a definite stoichiometric relationship. Such as in equation (11·1) 169·89 g of $AgNO_3$ react with 97·18 g of KCNS to produce 165·96 g AgCNS and 101·11 g KNO_3. This fact is used in titrimetric calculations.

(*iii*) There should be no coprecipitation. It should be noted that in a gravimetric procedure, coprecipitation can be avoided by reprecipitation, digestion and washing. But this cannot be done during a precipitation titration.

(*iv*) A suitable indicator should be available to locate the end point of the titration. Apart from visual indicators, the end point can also be identified by measuring some physical property such as electrical conductance or light scattering etc.

11·2. THEORY OF PRECIPITATION TITRATIONS

The most important precipitation reactions in titrimetric analysis are those which involve the use of silver nitrate ; these are called *argentimetric determinations*.

Let us construct the titration curve for the titration of 50·0 ml. of 0·100 M NaCl with 0·100 M $AgNO_3$.

(*i*) *At the start of the titration* (0·0 ml $AgNO_3$ added)

$$[Cl^-] = 0·100 \text{ g ion}/l = 10^{-1} \text{ g ion}/l$$

$\therefore$ $-\log [Cl^-] = p \, Cl = -\log 10^{-1} = -(-1) = 1·00$

(*ii*) *After adding 10·0 ml AgNO$_3$* (reaction 20% complete)

Chloride ions left in the soln = 40·0 ml, 0·100 M and total volume 50 + 10 = 60 ml.

$\therefore$ $[Cl^-]$ will be given by :

$$40 \times 0·1 = 60 \times [Cl^-]$$

or $$[Cl^-] = \frac{40 \times 0·1}{60} = 0·067 \text{ g ion}/l$$

or $\qquad$ $pCl = -\log[Cl^-] = -\log[0.067] = 1.17$

(iii) *After adding 49.9 ml AgNO$_3$* (reaction 99.8% complete)

Chloride ion left $= 0.1$ ml, 0.100 M

Total volume $\quad = 50 + 49.9 = 99.9 \approx 100$ ml

$$0.1 \times 0.1 = 100 \times [Cl^-]$$

$\therefore \qquad [Cl^-] = \dfrac{0.1 \times 0.1}{100} = 10^{-4} \text{ g ion}/l$

$$pCl = -\log 10^{-4} = -(-4) = 4.00$$

(iv) *After adding 50.0 ml AgNO$_3$* (Equivalence point). Neither Cl^- nor Ag^+ ions are in excess, and concentration of these ions is given by the square root of SAgCl (solubility product of AgCl)

$$[Ag^+] \times [Cl^-] = SAgCl = 1.0 \times 10^{-10}$$

and since $\qquad [Ag^+] = [Cl^-]$

$$[Cl^-]^2 = 1.0 \times 10^{-10} \qquad \Big| \qquad AgCl \rightleftharpoons Ag^+ + Cl^-$$

or $\qquad [Cl^-] = 1.0 \times 10^{-5} \qquad \Big| \quad \therefore \quad [Ag^+] = [Cl^-]$

$$pCl = -\log 10^{-5}$$
$$= 5.00$$

(v) *After adding 60.0 ml AgNO$_3$*

Excess silver ions in the soln $= 10.0$ ml, 0.100 M

Total volume $\qquad\qquad = 50 + 60 = 110$ ml.

$$10 \times 0.1 = 110 \times [Ag^+]$$
$$[Ag^+] = \frac{10 \times 0.1}{110} = 9.1 \times 10^{-3} \text{ g ion}/l$$

Now, $\qquad [Ag^+] \times [Cl^-] = 1.0 \times 10^{-10} \text{ (SAgCl)}$

Substituting for $[Ag^+]$, we get,

$$[Cl^-] = \frac{1.0 \times 10^{-10}}{9.1 \times 10^{-3}} = 1.1 \times 10^{-8}$$
$$pCl = -\log(1.1 \times 10^{-8}) = 7.96$$

In this way it is possible to calculate chloride ion concentration at different stages. The values so obtained have been shown in Table 11.1.

Table 11·1. Titration of 50 ml, 0·1 M NaCl with 0·1 M AgNO₃

AgNO₃ added ml	Reaction %	pCl
0·0	0·0	1·00
10·0	20·0	1·17
20·0	40·0	1·37
30·0	60·0	1·60
40·0	80·0	1·96
49·0	98·0	3·00
49·9	99·8	4·00
50·0	100·0	5·00
51·0	100·0	7·00
60·0	100·0	7·96

The data of Table 11·1 can be plotted to obtain a titration curve as shown in Fig. 11·1. It will be seen that the shape of the titration curves for precipitation reactions is similar to those obtain-

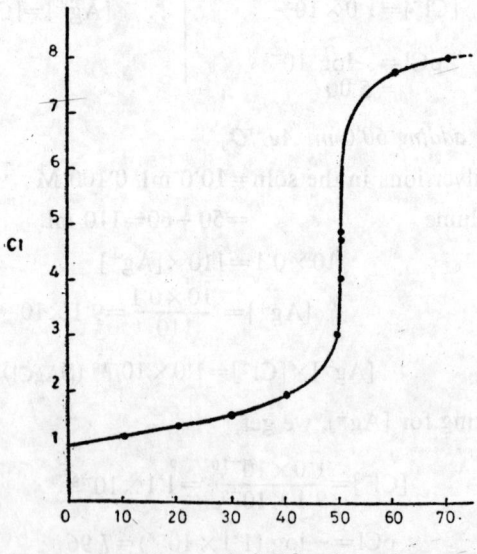

Fig. 11·1. Titration curve for the titration of 50·0 ml of a 0·100 M NaCl with a 0·100 M AgNO₃ solution.

-ed for acid-base or redox raactions. More the steepness of the titration curve, more accurately the equivalence point can be located. The steepness or sharpness of the curve depends upon the concentrations of the solutions used in the titration and on the solubility product value of the ppt formed. Greater the concentrations of the solutions involved and lesser the solubility of the ppt, greater is the accuracy in the location of the end point. (Note that the smaller the value of solubility product, greater is the value of equilibrium constant for the precipitation reaction). It is, therefore, concluded that for an accurate titration, the titrand and the titrant soln should not be very dilute further, the solubility product value of the ppt formed should be very small.

11`3. EQUIVALENT WEIGHT CALCULATION IN PRECIPITATION TITRATION

The eq wt of a precipitant in a precipitation titration is given by the relationship :

$$\text{eq wt of precipitant} = \frac{\text{mol wt}}{\text{valency of precipitating ion}} \quad \text{...(11-A)}$$

For example, KCl is used as precipitant for precipitating AgCl from $AgNO_3$ soln. Here the precipitating ion is Cl^- ion whose valency is one, so,

$$\text{eq wt of KCl} = \frac{\text{mol wt}}{1}$$

The eq wt of the substance containing the ion which is precipitated is given by :

$$\text{eq wt} = \frac{\text{mol wt}}{\text{valency of ion that is precipitated}} \quad \text{...(11-B)}$$

For example, when KCl is added to $AgNO_3$, Ag^+ ion is precipitated as AgCl, hence,

$$\text{eq wt of } AgNO_3 = \frac{\text{mol wt}}{\text{valency of } Ag^+ \text{ ion}} = \frac{\text{mol wt}}{1}.$$

11`4. LABORATORY EXERCISES

Experiment 11`1

Determination of normality of the given chloride solution by Mohr titration.

Discussion

In the Mohr titration, the given chloride soln is titrated with a standard $AgNO_3$ soln when Cl^- ions are precipitated as AgCl. A small amount of K_2CrO_4 (potassium chromate) is added to the chloride soln which acts as an indicator. When $AgNO_3$ is gradually added, the end-point is signaled by the first permanent appearance of a brick red coloured ppt of Ag_2CrO_4.

It is necessary that the precipitation of the indicator should take place at or near the equivalence point. When $AgNO_3$ soln is added to the titrand soln containing Cl^- and CrO_4^{2-} ions, chloride ions react first and when practically all the chloride ions have been precipitated then only the formation of Ag_2CrO_4 begins. The equilibria involved in this method are as follows :

$$Ag^+ + Cl^- \rightleftharpoons AgCl \qquad ...(11\cdot2)$$
$$2Ag^+ + CrO_4^{2-} \rightleftharpoons Ag_2CrO_4 \qquad ...(11\cdot3)$$

The solubility product values at ordinary temperature for $AgCl$ and Ag_2CrO_4 are $1\cdot0 \times 10^{-10}$ and $1\cdot7 \times 10^{-12}$ respectively. Note that $S_{Ag_2CrO_4}$ is smaller but it dissolves to give three ions so its solubility is greater. Hence, for a small concentration of CrO_4^{2-} ions in presence of relatively large amount of Cl^- ions, $AgCl$ is precipitated first because the free Ag^+ ion concentration never becomes high enough to cause the solubility product of Ag_2CrO_4 to be exceeded. After Cl^- ions are completely precipitated, on adding a drop of $AgNO_3$ soln, there is an excess of Ag^+ ions which form red coloured Ag_2CrO_4 and thus indicate the end point of the titration.

Procedure

(1) Dry some A.R. $AgNO_3$ at 150°C for 2 hours and allow to cool it in a desiccator. Weigh out accurately $4\cdot248$ g, dissolve it in water and make up to 250 ml in a volumetric flask. This gives $0\cdot100$ N or $0\cdot100$ M soln (note that for $AgNO_3$ in the precipitation reaction involved, eq wt=mol wt.)

(2) Dissolve 5 g of A.R. K_2CrO_4 in 100 ml of water.

(3) Pipette out $25\cdot0$ ml of the given chloride in a clean conical flask placed over a white tile or paper. Add 1 ml of K_2CrO_4 soln. Add $AgNO_3$ soln gradually through a burette with constant swirling of the flask. A stage will come when on adding a drop of $AgNO_3$ soln a red colour will appear which will slowly disappear on shaking ; this indicates that we are near the end point. Continue dropwise addition of $AgNO_3$ with thorough shaking until a permanent red colour persists. Determine the indicator blank by repeating the titration by taking 25 ml of water in place of the chloride soln. The indicator blank should be deducted from the volume of $AgNO_3$ required in the titration. Now, in this titration :

$$AgNO_3 \equiv KCl \ (mol \ wt = 74\cdot47)$$
$$1000 \ ml, \ 1 \ N \ AgNO_3 = 74\cdot47 \ g \ KCl$$
$$1 \ ml, \ 1 \ N \ AgNO_3 = 74\cdot47 \ mg \ KCl$$
$$1 \ ml, \ 0\cdot1 \ N \ AgNO_3 = 7\cdot447 \ mg \ KCl$$

In this titration, an adsorption indicator, such as sodium fluoresceinate can also be used as described in 11·6).

Experiment 11·2

Determination of silver by Volhard method.

Discussion

The Volhard method for the determination of silver involves the titration of Ag^+ ions in acidic soln (containing a small amount of ferric ions as indicator) with a standard potassium thiocyanate soln. Silver ions react with thiocyanate ion to form AgCNS (silver thiocyanate). After all the silver ions have been precipitated, the addition of extra drop or two of thiocyanate combine with Fe^{3+} to form a blood-red-coloured complex which marks the end point. The reaction involved in the titration is :

$$Ag^+ + CNS^- \rightarrow \underset{\text{(white ppt)}}{AgCNS} \qquad ...(11·4)$$

The solubility product of AgCNS is $1·0 \times 10^{-12}$. The indicator soln is added before starting the titration and its amount is such that it reacts with CNS^- ion only after Ag^+ ions have been completely precipitated.

Procedure

(1) Prepare 0·1000 N $AgNO_3$ soln as described in experiment 11·1.

(2) Weigh out about 11 g of KCNS and dissolve it in 1 litre of water in a measuring flask, shake well.

(3) Prepare a cold saturated soln of A.R. ferric ammonium sulphate (this is about 40%) in water and add little nitric acid to it. This is the indicator soln.

(4) Pipette 25 ml of 0·1 N $AgNO_3$ soln into a 250 ml conical flask, add 5 ml of 6 N HNO_3 and 1 ml of the indicator soln. Add KCNS soln from a burette. A white ppt of AgCNS is formed and the soln appears milky. With the addition of each drop of KCNS a reddish brown spot is formed which disappears on shaking. Near the end point the white ppt settles down and the final drop produces a faint brown colour which does not disappears on shaking. This is the end point. The indicator blank is also determined (as described in Experiment 11·1) and it is subtracted from the volume of KCNS used in the titration. Repeat the titration with two other 25 ml portions of $AgNO_3$ soln. The difference between titre values obtained should not be more than 0·1 ml. Suppose 24·8 ml KCNS soln is required in the titration then its normality is calculated as :

$$25 \times 0·1 = 24·8 \times N_{KCNS}$$

$$N_{KCNS} = \frac{25 \times 0·1}{24·8} = 0·1008.$$

Thus KCNS soln is standardised. (By suitably diluting this soln exactly 0·1000 N KCNS soln can be obtained—see Experiment 8·1, step 5).

(5) Pipette out 25·0 ml of the given AgNO₃ soln in a 250 ml conical flask and add 5 ml, 6N HNO₃ and 1 ml indicator soln and titrate with standardised KCNS soln in a manner described in step 4.

$$KCNS \equiv AgNO_3$$
$$1000 \text{ ml, 1 N KCNS} \equiv 169·89 \text{ g AgNO}_3$$
$$1 \text{ ml, 0·1 N KCNS} \equiv 16·989 \text{ mg AgNO}_3 \text{ or}$$
$$10·788 \text{ mg Ag.}$$

11·5. APPLICATIONS OF VOLHARD'S METHOD

1. **Determination of chlorides.** A known volume of given chloride soln in presenee of dilute HNO₃ is treated with a known excess of a standard AgNO₃ soln. The ppt of AgCl obtained is filtered and washed. To the combined filtrate and washing, 1 ml of a saturated ferric alum soln is added and the unused Ag⁺ ions are titrated with a standardised KCNS soln. Knowing the amount of AgNO₃ consumed, the quantity of chloride in the given soln is calculated by using the relationship :

$$1 \text{ ml of 0·1 N AgNO}_3 \equiv 3·546 \text{ mg Cl.}$$

Example 11(i)

To a given chloride soln, 30 ml of 0·1 N AgNO₃ soln was added. After filtering off AgCl, the residual AgNO₃ in the filtrate required 5·0 ml of 0·05 N KCNS soln. Calculate the amount of chloride in the given soln.

30·0 ml, 0·1 N AgNO₃ added ≡ 30·0 ml, 0·1 N KCNS
$$= 60·0 \text{ ml, 0·05 N KCNS.}$$

(Note that AgNO₃ ≡ KCNS)

After the reaction AgNO₃ left unreacted = 5·0 ml, 0·05 N

AgNO₃ consumed = (60·0 − 5·0) = 55·0 ml, 0·05 N

$$= \frac{55·0}{2} = 27·5 \text{ ml 0·1 N}$$

Now, 1 ml, 0·1 N AgNO₃ ≡ 3·546 mg Cl

∴   27·5 ml ≡ 27·5 × 3·546 mg Cl
$$\equiv 97·515 \text{ mg Cl.}$$

(The Volhard titration method can also be used for determining bromides and iodides. In these determinations it is not necessary to filter the precipitates of AgBr and AgI. Because AgBr and AgI are less soluble than AgCl.)

2. Determination of thiocyanate with Hg (II). In this deter-mination, the thiocyanate containing ferric alum indicator is titrated with Hg(II) soln, the reaction involved is :

$$2CNS^- + Hg^{2+} \rightarrow Hg(CNS)_2 \text{ (weakly ionised)}$$

The soln is red in the colour in the beginning of the titration. As mercuric nitrate soln is added, Hg_2^+ ions react with CNS^- and at the end point the red colour disappears.

This reaction can also be used in the titration of Hg^{2+} ions with thiocyanate soln using ferric alum as indicator. In this case, appearance of red colour marks the end point. This method is quite similar to one used for titrating silver by Volhard's method.

11'6. ADSORPTION INDICATORS

There are certain organic dyes which are strongly adsorbed by colloidal precipitates. In a percipitation titration this adsorption may be greater prior to equivalence point or the indicator may be more strongly adsorbed after the equivalence point. In some cases the dye undergoes a sudden change of colour in the process of being adsorbed. This may act as a means of locating the end point in a precipitation titration. For example, sodium salt of fluorescein, sodium fluoresceinate, can be used as an indicator in the titration of chloride with $AgNO_3$ soln in a neutral or slightly basic medium. The chloride soln becomes yellowish green due to the addition of the indicator. Now, sodium fluoresceinate ionises to give Na^+ and fluoresceinate ion (Ind^-). If a small volume of $AgNO_3$ is added, some AgCl is formed. Before equivalence point, Cl^- ions are in excess and these form a primary adsorbed layer on AgCl particle (see Fig. 6'1) and the secondary layer will consist of positive ions such as Na^+ and H^+ ions. After the equivalence point, Ag^+ ions will be in excess hence now they form the primary adsorbed layer and the secondary layer is mostly made of Ind^- ions. When Ind^- ions are adsorbed the ppt particles become pink. Thus a colour change from yellowish green to pink marks the end point of the titration.

11'7. COMPLEXOMETRIC OR COMPLEXATION TITRATIONS

Reactions involving complex formation have also been utilized for developing titrimetric methods. The required condition is that the dissociation of the complex formed should be negligibly small, *i.e.* the complex should be stable. For example, Ag^+ ion reacts with CN^- ions to form $Ag(CN)_2^-$ (dicyanoargentate I ion) as shown by :

$$Ag^+ + 2CN^- \rightleftharpoons Ag(CN)_2$$

In this example, $Ag(CN)_2^-$ is a stable complex of silver. Such complexes involve a reaction of a metal ion with a cation or anion or a neutral molecule. The metal ion in the complex is called the central atom and the group attached to it is known as *ligand*. The number of bonds formed by the central atom is called the *coordination number* of the metal. In the above case silver is the central atom, its coordination number is 2 (because 2 cyanide ions are attached) and cyanide is ligand. A complexometric titration involves the titration of a metal ion with a standard soln of a suitable complexing agent or ligand which forms a *stable* complex with the metal ion.

11·8. REQUIREMENTS FOR COMPLEXOMETRIC TITRATIONS

In order that a reaction may act as a basis of a complexation titration, it must fulfil the same conditions as described in the case of acid-base, redox or precipitation titrations. The complex formation reaction under consideration should be rapid, should proceed according to well defined stoichiometry and an indicator should be available for identifying the end point. The value of equilibrium constant for the complex forming reaction should be quite high so that the reaction goes to completion.

11·9. LABORATORY EXERCISES

Experiment 11·3

Determination of the concentration of a cyanide soln by titration with $AgNO_3$ soln.

Discussion

The titration of cyanide with silver ions, known as Liebig titration, is based on the complex forming reaction.

$$Ag^+ + 2CN^- \rightleftharpoons Ag(CN)_2^- \qquad \qquad ...(11·5)$$

A soln containing cyanide ion is titrated with Ag^+ ions, the end point is shown by a permanent turbidity due to the formation of slightly soluble silver dicyanoargentate (I) :

$$Ag(CN)_2^- + Ag^+ \rightarrow Ag[Ag(CN)_2] \qquad ...(11·6)$$
$$\text{(white ppt)}$$

(The ppt is sometimes considered as silver cyanide, note that $Ag[Ag(CN)_2]$ may be regarded as equivalent to 2AgCN). The value of equilibrium constant for reaction (11·5) is quite high ($1·26 \times 10^{21}$), hence, the reaction goes practically to completion and the reverse reaction is negligible. The value of solubility product of AgCN is $1·6 \times 10^{-14}$. As $AgNO_3$ is added to a cyanide soln reaction (11·5) takes place and because the solubility product of AgCN is not exceeded. hence, its precipitation does not take place. The addition of a drop of $AgNO_3$ soln just after the equivalence point provides Ag^+ ions and since there are no CN^- ions to react with it, the precipitation of AgCN takes place [see reaction (11·6)] so that the soln becomes turbid ; this can be taken as the end point. But it is not very sharp so it is not easy to locate the end point accurately. Hence, to the cyanide soln, NH_4OH, and KI soln are added before the titration. Silver cyanide is soluble in ammonia soln but the yellow ppt of AgI does not dissolve. After the equivalence point, the first excess of Ag^+ ions combine with I^- ions to form a yellow ppt of AgI. Thus the appearance of yellow ppt marks the end point.

For this titration the eq wt of $AgNO_3$ is calculated as :

$$\text{eq wt} = \frac{\text{mol wt}}{\text{valency of metal ion forming complex}} \qquad ...(11\text{-}C)$$

$$\text{eq wt of } AgNO_3 = \frac{\text{mol wt}}{\text{valency of } Ag^+}$$

$$= \frac{\text{mol wt of } AgNO_3}{1}$$

According to equation (11·5), 2 cyanide ions react with a Ag^+ ion which is monovalent, so :

$$Ag^+ \equiv AgNO_3 \equiv 2KCN \equiv 2CN^-$$

A molecule of $AgNO_3$ is thus chemically equivalent to 2 molecules of KCN, so :

1 g eq of $AgNO_3 \equiv 2$ g mole of $KCN \equiv 1$ g eq of KCN

eq wt of $KCN \equiv 2 \times$ mol wt of KCN

Procedure

1. Transfer 25 ml of given cyanide soln from a burette into a 250 ml conical flask (KCN is a deadly poison, hence its soln should not be taken out by means of a pipette). Add about 50 ml water, 5 ml 6 N ammonia soln and 2 ml of 10 per cent KI soln.

2. Place the conical flask on a black paper. Run in a standard $AgNO_3$ soln from a burette with constant swirling of the conical flask. Near the equivalence point a drop of $AgNO_3$ soln added produces a yellow spot which slowly disappears on shaking. At this stage, add $AgNO_3$ soln dropwise and when a drop produces a permanent turbidity, the end point has been reached. [The turbidity is seen in the black background]

1 ml of 0·1 N $AgNO_3 \equiv 5·204$ mg CN^- [∵ $AgNO_3 \equiv 2KCN$]

$\equiv 13·04$ mg KCN.

Experiment 11·4

Determination of silver by Liebig titration.

Procedure

1. Pipette out 25 ml of given $AgNO_3$ soln in a 250 ml conical flask and add a known excess of a standard KCN soln (by means of a burette).

2. Back titrate the unreacted KCN with a standard AgNO₃ soln. The amount of KCN consumed is thus found out and from this, the quantity of AgNO₃ in the sample soln can be calculated.

$$2KCN \equiv AgNO_3 \equiv Ag \text{ (at wt} = 107\cdot88)$$
$$2000 \text{ ml, } 1 \text{ M KCN} = 107\cdot88 \text{ g Ag}$$
$$1000 \text{ ml, } 1 \text{ M KCN} = 53\cdot94 \text{ g Ag}$$
$$1 \text{ ml, } 1 \text{ M KCN} = 53\cdot94 \text{ mg Ag}$$
$$1 \text{ ml, } 0\cdot1 \text{ M KCN} = 5\cdot394 \text{ mg Ag}$$

Example 11(*ii*)

To a given AgNO₃ soln, 40 ml of 0·1 N KCN soln was added. The excess KCN required 10 ml of 0·1 N AgNO₃ soln. Calculate the amount of Ag in the given sample soln.

$$KCN \text{ added} = 40 \text{ ml, } 0\cdot1 \text{ N}$$
$$KCN \text{ left} = 10 \text{ ml, } 0\cdot1 \text{ N}$$
$$KCN \text{ consumed} = (40 - 10) = 30 \text{ ml, } 0\cdot1 \text{ N}$$
$$= 60 \text{ ml, } 0\cdot1 \text{ M}$$

(Note that 0·1 N KCN means 0·2 M KCN because eq wt of KCN = 2 × mol wt of KCN in this reaction).

Now, 1 ml, 0·1 M KCN = 5·394 mg Ag

∴ 60 ml, 0·1 M KCN = 60 × 5·394 mg Ag
$$= 323\cdot64 \text{ mg or } 0\cdot3236 \text{ g Ag}$$

Experiment 11·5

Determination of mercuric nitrate with standard KCl soln.

Discussion

Many of the soluble mercuric salts (mercury II salts) are weakly ionised. However, mercuric nitrate [Hg(NO₃)₂], and mercuric perchlorate [Hg(ClO₄)₂] are strongly dissociated. When Hg(NO₃)₂ soln is added to a chloride soln (containing little sodium nitroprusside as indicator) Hg²⁺ ions from Hg(NO₃)₂ combine with Cl⁻ ions to form weakly ionised HgCl₂ as shown by :

$$Hg^{2+} + 2Cl^- \rightarrow HgCl_2 \text{ (weakly ionised)} \quad \ldots (11\cdot7)$$

Since HgCl₂ is weakly ionised it will not furnish enough Hg²⁺ ions to produce turbidity by reacting with the indicator. After the equivalence point, the first excess of Hg(NO₃)₂ soln will combine with sodium nitroprusside as shown by :

$$Hg^{2+} + Fe(CN)_5NO^{2-} \rightarrow HgFe(CN)_5NO \quad \ldots (11\cdot8)$$
$$\text{(white ppt)}$$

The appearance of white turbidity of mercuric nitroprusside marks the end point of the titration.

Procedure

1. Dry some finely powdered NaCl at 250 to 300°C for 1 to 2 hours in an electric oven and allow to cool in a desiccator. Weigh out exactly 2·923 g of pure and dry salt, dissolve it in water and make up the volume to 500 ml in a measuring flask. This gives exactly 0·1000 M NaCl soln.

2. Pipette out 25 ml of 0·1 M NaCl soln into a 250 ml conical flask and add to it sodium nitroprusside soln (1 ml, 1 per cent) as indicator. Titrate with the given soln of $Hg(NO_3)_2$ until a permanent turbidity is observed. Determine the blank correction also (experiment 11·1).

Example 11(*iii*)

For the titration of 25 ml of 0·1 M NaCl, 20 ml of given mercuric nitrate soln was required. Calculate the weight of mercuric nitrate present per litre.

The reaction between mercuric nitrate and sodium chloride can be written as :

$$Hg(NO_3)_2 + 2NaCl \rightarrow HgCl_2 + 2NaNO_3$$

Thus : $2NaCl \equiv Hg(NO_3)_2$ (mol wt = 324·63)

2000 ml, 1 M NaCl = 324·63 g $Hg(NO_3)_2$

1000 ml, 1 M NaCl = 162·315 g $Hg(NO_3)_2$

1 ml, 1 M NaCl = 162·315 mg $Hg(NO_3)_2$

1 ml, 0·1 M NaCl = 16·2315 mg $Hg(NO_3)_2$

∴   25 ml, 0·1 M NaCl ≡ 16·2315 × 25 = 405·78 mg

= 0·4058 g $Hg(NO_3)_2$

Now, 20 ml soln contains 0·4058 g $Hg(NO_3)_2$

1000 ml soln contains $\dfrac{1000 \times 0·4058}{20}$

= 20·29 g $Hg(NO_3)_2$ per litre.

(A bromide soln can also be titrated in a similar manner with mercury (II) soln).

Experiment 11·6

Determination of iodide by titration with mercury (II) soln.

Discussion

On adding Hg (II) soln to an iodide soln, a soluble colourless compound is obtained :

$$4I^- + Hg^{2+} \rightarrow HgI_4^{2-} \qquad \qquad ... (11·9)$$

Prior to the equivalence point, I^- ions are in excess so reaction (11·9) takes place. For this reaction the value of equilibrium constant is quite high so the reaction is quantitative. Addition of a drop of mercury (II) soln (say $Hg(NO_3)_2$ or $HgCl_2$ soln) just after the equivalence point produces a red turbidity due to mercuric iodide :

$$HgI_4^{2-} + Hg^{2+} \rightarrow 2HgI_2 \text{ (red ppt)} \qquad ...(11·10)$$

So long as I^- ions are in excess (before the equivalence point), reaction (11·9) takes place. When all the iodide ions have been converted into the stable complex HgI_4^{2-}, the addition of extra Hg (II) soln causes the precipitation of a red ppt of HgI_2. The theory of this titration is similar to that for Liebig titration.

11·10. COMPLEX-FORMING REACTIONS OF EDTA

Of the several complexing agents in titrimetric analysis, ethylenediaminetetraacetic acid, abbreviated as EDTA has the widest application because of its powerful complexing action and commercial availability. With several metal ions it forms stable five membered rings (the process of ring formation is called *chelation* and the reagent is called *chelon*). EDTA (also known as versene) is an aminopolycarboxylic acid containing four carboxyl and two amino groups. EDTA behaves like a tetrabasic (tetraprotic) acid dissociating in four stages. It is written as H_4Y to show its tetraprotic character. The acid is sparingly soluble in water so its disodium salt (written as Na_2H_2Y) which is relatively more soluble and commercially available is used in titrimetric work ; the reacting species in an aqueous soln of Na_2H_2Y is H_2Y^{2-} ion. This ion reacts with several metals in a 1 : 1 ratio, such as :

$$M^{2+} + H_2Y^{2-} \rightarrow MY^{2-} + 2H^+ \qquad \text{(with bivalent metal ion)}$$
$$M^{3+} + H_2Y^{2-} \rightarrow MY^- + 2H^+ \qquad \text{(with trivalent metal ion)}$$
$$M^{4+} + H_2Y^{2-} \rightarrow MY + 2H^+ \qquad \text{(for tetravalent metal ion)}$$

In general,

$$M^{n+} + H_2Y^{2-} \rightarrow MY^{(n-4)+} + 2H^+$$

It is seen that one mole of complex forming ion H_2Y^{2-} reacts with one mole of the metal ion in each case and two moles of H^+ ions are formed. Hence, the dissociation of the resultant complex depends on H^+ ion concentration or pH. The formation of H^+ ions as a reaction product will decrease the pH of the soln and the reverse reaction may start taking place. This can be prevented by adding a buffer to regulate the pH of the soln at a desired value. The only condition is that buffer itself should not take part in the chemical reaction. This is the reason why most metal-EDTA titrations are carried out in neutral or alkaline soln. (Note, according to Le Chatelier-Braun principle, if product is removed, the reaction moves in the forward direction—see section 4·2).

11·11. TITRATION OF CALCIUM WITH EDTA

We know that only that reaction can act as a basis of a titrimetric method which is rapid and goes to completion. It means that the reaction :

$$Ca^{2+} + H_2Y^{2-} \rightarrow CaY^{2-} + 2H^+ \qquad \qquad ...(11·11)$$

should be quantitative. In order to push equation (11·11) to completion, H^+ ions must be removed. Hence, a buffer containing ammonia-ammonium ion is added and thus the pH of the soln is maintained at 10. As a soln containing Ca^{2+} ions is added to a soln of Na_2H_2Y, the H_2Y^{2-} reacts with Ca^{2+} ions. But just after the equivalence point, the added Ca^{2+} ions do not have any H_2Y^{2-} ions to react with, hence they react with oxalate ions which are added as indicator, to give a white turbidity ; this can be taken as the end point.

$$Ca^{2+} + C_2O_4^{2-} \rightarrow CaC_2O_4 \quad \text{(white ppt)}$$

11·11·1. The Titration Curve

Let us consider the titration of 0·1000 M Ca^{2+} ion with a 0·1000 M soln of Na_2H_2Y. If we calculate the concentration of Ca^{2+} ions at different stages of the titration and plot various values of pCa ($-\log [Ca^{2+}]$) against volume of Na_2H_2Y added, a curve similar in shape to that shown in Fig. 11·1 is obtained. The graph shows that the value of pCa changes slowly in the beginning of the titration but there is a sudden change in its value near the equivalence point, i.e., the value jumps suddenly in the vicinity of the equivalence point. The greater the jump, greater is the sharpness of the titration curve and more accurately and conveniently end point of titration can be judged.

11·12. TITRATION WITH EDTA REAGENT

Several metal ions can be determined by using a standard soln of EDTA. Some of the determinations are described here to illustrate the general procedure followed, various buffers and indicators used in the titrimetric determination with EDTA reagent.

Preparation of standard EDTA soln

EDTA is sparingly soluble in water so its sodium salt disodium dihydrogenethylenediaminetetraacetate (Na_2H_2Y), which is more soluble and available commercially, is used in titrimetric work. The salt is dried at 80°C to remove any moisture that might be present. But this cannot be regarded as a primary standard, i.e., its standard soln cannot be prepared by direct weighing but has to be standardised. For preparing 0·1 M soln of Na_2H_2Y, 37·224 g of the dried salt is dissolved in water and soln made up to 1000 ml in a volumetric flask ; this soln is standardised by titration with a standard soln of Zn^{2+} or Mg^{2+} ion.

Buffer solutions

In many titrations with EDTA it is very necessary to control the pH of the soln in order to obtain satisfactory results. A pH meter is generally used to measure pH of the soln. Many EDTA titrations are performed in presence of a buffer such as a tartrate or citrate or a buffer containing ammonia and ammonium ion. The pH is thus kept in general between 8 to 10.

Indicator solution

Several indicators are used in complexometric titrations. Since these indicators form stable, brightly coloured complexes with most metal ions, these are called *metallochromic indicators*. One of the most widely used indicators is Eriochrome Black T which acts as a triprotic acid and can therefore be represented as H_3In. This indicator dissociates in three stages giving H_2In^-, HIn^{2-} and In^{3-} species which are red, blue and orange respectively.

Let us try to understand the behaviour of the indicator by considering the titration of Zn^{2+} with Na_2H_2Y in an ammonia-ammonium ion buffer containing a small amount of Eriochrome Black T as indicator. Prior to the equivalence point soln has a red colour because of Zinc-Eriochrome Black T complex ($ZnIn^-$). The added Na_2H_2Y reacts with the indicator complex to form zinc-EDTA complex as shown by :

$$\underset{\text{(red)}}{Zn\,In^-} + H_2Y^{2-} \rightleftharpoons ZnY^{2-} + \underset{\text{(blue)}}{HIn^{2-}} + H^+ \qquad ...(11\cdot12)$$

According to the above reaction HIn^{2-} ions are formed which show a blue colour. Thus, a change of colour from wine-red to blue gives the end point when Zn^{2+} soln is titrated with that of Na_2H_2Y. The indicator soln is prepared by dissolving $0\cdot2$ g of solid reagent grade Eriochrome Black T in 20 ml of ethanol ; a fresh soln should be used. The blue colour appears on the completion of the reaction ($11\cdot12$).

11·13. LABORATORY EXERCISES

Experiment 11·7

Determination of a given soln of Zn^{2+} with EDTA using Eriochrome Black T indicator.

Procedure

1. Take a known weight of A.R. zinc pellets ($6\cdot538$ g are required for preparing $0\cdot1$ M soln), dissolve it in pure dilute H_2SO_4,

neutralise excess acid and make up the volume to 1 litre. (De-ioni-sed water is used for preparing all solutions required in EDTA titration and this de-ionised water is prepared using distilled water).

2. Prepare a buffer soln by dissolving 7 g NH_4Cl in 60 ml concentrated reagent grade (15 M) ammonia and then diluting to 100 ml.

3. Pipette out 25 ml of zinc soln into a 250 ml Erlenmeyer flask. Add 10 ml of buffer and 5 drops of Eriochrome Black T solution and titrate with 0·1 M Na_2H_2Y soln (37·224 g salt per litre of soln). The end point is shown by a change of colour from wine red to blue. From this titration the exact normality of Na_2H_2Y soln is calculated, i.e., its soln is standardised.

4. Pipette out 25 ml of given zinc soln and titrate it with standardised Na_2H_2Y soln in an exactly similar manner described in step 3.

$$1 \text{ ml, } 0·1 \text{ M } Na_2H_2Y \text{ soln} \equiv 6·538 \text{ mg Zn.}$$

Experiment 11·8

Titrimetric determination of calcium with EDTA involving back-titration with magnesium.

Discussion

Calcium ions react with EDTA to form a relatively stable complex. The value of equilibrium constant (called formation constant in complex formation reactions) is high, hence the reaction is suitable to act as a basis of a titrimetric method for the determination of Ca^{2+} ion. The next problem is selection of a suitable indicator.

Like zinc, calcium also forms a wine-red-coloured complex with Eriochrome Black T (shown as $CaIn^-$ complex). So if we directly titrate a soln containing Ca^{2+} ions with Na_2H_2Y reagent the soln should be red before the equivalence point and should become blue just after the equivalence point due to the reaction :

$$\underset{\text{(red)}}{CaIn^-} + H_2Y^{2-} \rightleftharpoons CaY^{2-} + \underset{\text{(blue)}}{HIn^{2-}} + H^+ \qquad ...(11\cdot13)$$

The formation of Ca-Eriochrome Black T complex ($CaIn^-$) may be written as :

$$Ca^{2+} + In^{3-} \rightleftharpoons CaIn^- \qquad ...(11\cdot14)$$

The value of formation constant for $CaIn^-$ (which is equal to the value of equilibrium constant for the reaction (11·14)) is $2·51 \times 10^5$ whereas that for $ZnIn^-$ is $7·95 \times 10^{12}$. It means that the reaction :

$$Zn^{2+} + In^- \rightleftharpoons ZnIn^- \qquad ...(11.15)$$

proceeds more towards completion as compared to reaction (11·14) In other words Ca In⁻ complex is much less stable than ZnIn⁻. For this reason, in the direct titration of Ca^{2+} ion with EDTA the colour change red to blue at the equivalence point is not sharp and so a titration error is observed. This difficulty can be solved in the following manner.

1. The titration error can be minimised by using a standard soln of Ca^{2+} to standardise Na_2H_2Y titrant soln under identical conditions to those used in the analysis of unknown calcium soln. [The sources of systematic errors (indicator error in this case) can thus be neutralised].

2. Eriochrome Black T indicator can be replaced by another metallochromic indicator namely Eriochrome Blue Black B which gives a more accurate end point.

3. Another approach is to add a measured excess of EDTA reagent to sample soln of calcium and then back-titrate the reagent with a standard Mg^{2+} soln using Eriochrome Black T as indicator. This procedure is based on the following theoretical considerations.

(a) When an excess of EDTA is added to calcium soln the reaction is :

$$Ca^{2+}+H_2Y^{2-} \rightleftharpoons CaY^{2-}+2H^+ \qquad ...(11·16)$$

The Ca-EDTA complex is less stable, i.e., the reection does not proceed to completion. But if this reaction is carried out in the presence of ammonia-ammonium ion buffer (at pH 10), H^+ ions are removed so that the reaction proceeds to completion. Thus, the first condition is that reaction (11·16) should be carried out at pH 10. The reagent is in excess so the colour of the soln will be blue because the free indicator has a blue colour between pH 7 to 11.

(b) To the excess reagent a standard Mg^{2+} soln is gradually added when the following reaction takes place :

$$Mg^{2+}+H_2Y^{2-} \rightleftharpoons MgY^{2-}+2H^+ \qquad ...(11·17)$$

Note that MgY^{2-} is less stable than CaY^{2-}. [In other words, the value of equilibrium constant is greater for (11·16) than for the reaction (11·17).] Hence, the added Mg^{2+} ions will not disturb equilibrium (11·16) but will simply react with the excess-reagent. [The reaction

$$CaY^{2-}+Mg^{2+} \rightleftharpoons MgY^{2-}+Ca^{2+} \qquad ...(11·18)$$
(more stable)   (less stable)

is not possible, hence the main reaction (11·16) is not disturbed.]

(c) When all the excess reagent has been used up in the formation of MgY^{2-}, the first excess of Mg^{2+} will react with the indicator as shown by :

$$HIn^{2-}+Mg^{2+} \rightleftharpoons Mg\ In^-+H^+ \qquad ...(11.19)$$
$$\underset{\text{(blue)}}{} \qquad\qquad \underset{\text{(red)}}{}$$

Thus, a change of colour from blue to red will be observed at the equivalence point. [Note that Ca-EDTA complex is more stable than Mg-EDTA complex but Ca-Indicator complex is less stable than Mg-Indicator complex. Hence, in the titration of the reagent with Ca^{2+} ion, a sharp end point is not observed but if the reagent is titrated with Mg^{2+} soln, a sharp end point is obtained.]

Procedure

1. Dissolve a known weight of pure magnesium in HCl (2·4305 g for 0·1 M soln) neutralise the excess acid and make up the volume to 1000 ml in a measuring flask.

2. Weigh out 37·224 g dried A.R. Na_2H_2Y reagent in water and dilute to 1 litre.

3. Prepare a buffer soln containing ammonia and ammonium ion as described in experiment 11·3.

4. Pipette out 25 ml Na_2H_2Y reagent soln in a 250 ml conical flask. Adjust the pH of the soln to 10 with the help of ammonia-ammonium ion buffer and add 5 drops of Eriochrome Black T indicator. Add standard magnesium soln gradually from a burette with constant swirling of the flask until the colour changes from blue to red. Thus the reagent soln is standardised.

5. Pipette a known volume of sample calcium soln in a 250 ml conical flask adjust its pH to 10 and add 5 drops of indicator soln. Add reagent soln from a burette until the colour changes from red to blue. (This is the approximate end point for calcium titration). Add about 20 per cent reagent in excess. Finally back-titrate the excess reagent with standard magnesium soln. The end point is marked by a change of colour from blue to red.

11·14. APPLICATIONS OF EDTA REAGENT IN TITRIMETRIC ANALYSIS

EDTA forms chelates with several metals ; these are called metal chelonates and the complexing agent EDTA is called *chelon*. The titrations involving the use of chelons are termed *chelometric titrations*. EDTA has been used for the titrimetric determination of several metals, for example, Ca^{2+}, Mg^{2+}, Zn^{2+}, Ba^{2+}, Cu^{+2}, Fe^{3+}, etc. These methods involve either direct titration with standard EDTA soln or the addition of a known excess of EDTA reagent and back-titration of the unused reagent. Procedures have also been developed for quantitatively analysing mixtures of cations.

Determination of anions

Anions do not form complexes directly with EDTA but methods can be worked out for determining several anions, such as halides, thiocyanates, phosphates, sulphates etc. These determinations consist of adding a measured excess of a cation which reacts with the anion to be determined. The unreacted cation is then determined by titration with standard EDTA soln. Knowing the amount of cation consumed, the quantity of anion in the test soln can be calculated.

12

Quantitative Analysis of Some Minerals, Ores and Alloys

In nature, metals occur either in free state or in a state of combination (in the form of their compounds). For example, metals such as platinum, gold, etc., occur in free state. But generally metals are found in the form of their compounds which are formed when a metal combines with other elements. Such compounds along with sand and other impurities are found below the earth's surface ; these are called *minerals*. There are some minerals from which extraction of a metal is economically profitable ; these are called *ores*. A homogeneous mixture of metals is called an *alloy*. A profitable extraction of a metal depends upon a suitable metallurgical process and also upon the percentage of a metal in its ore. The properties of an alloy depends upon its composition. Thus analytical chemistry plays an important role in the preparation of metals and alloys.

12'1. ANALYSIS OF REAL MATERIAL

So far we have studied the analysis of samples containing a chemical compound or a mixture of compounds ; such samples are prepared in the laboratory by mixing various chemicals. In this type of analytical work, accepted theories, standard reactions and well known techniques are used. The purpose of these exercises is to provide training to a beginner of various operations involved in analytical chemistry. For example, in the gravimetric determination of Ba as $BaSO_4$, we have used a standard reaction :

$$Ba^{2+}+SO_4^{2-} \rightarrow BaSO_4$$

The other operations such as precipitation, filtration, washing and drying of the ppt are all well known. The sample soln for the exercise is prepared by taking a known weight of barium chloride. This is not real analytical chemistry or it cannot be regarded as analysis of real material. A trained analytical chemist has to deal with unknown samples which may be connected with different fields such as industry, agriculture, medicine etc. A sample of urine, blood, alloy, ore, rock etc., may be required to be analysed ; this is the analysis of real material.

Usually a sample has a history that provides some idea about what it contains. Another point is whether a complete analysis is needed or only one or two components are to be determined. The next consideration is how much accuracy is required ? Taking these points into account an analytical chemist searches for a suitable method for the analysis of the sample. Suppose a sample contains constituents A, B and C. First of all a method for determining one of the constituents, say B, will be selected. The method should be such that it will not be interferred by A and C. After that the next constituent, say C, will be determined by a method which will be applicable to the determination of C in presence of A. Sometimes such methods may not be available. In such cases the different constituents of the sample are separated and then individually estimated. The analysis of certain real materials is described below.

12.2. DETERMINATION OF MANGANESE CONTENT IN PYROLUSITE

Discussion

Manganese dioxide occurs in nature as the mineral pyrolusite. For many purposes it is necessary to find out the percentage of MnO_2 in pyrolusite. Since MnO_2 has oxidising properties its determination can be done by a suitable redox reaction. Manganese dioxide quantitatively oxidises ferrous sulphate, oxalic acid and arsenious oxide as shown by :

$$MnO_2 + 2FeSO_4 + 2H_2SO_4 \rightarrow Fe_2(SO_4)_3 + MnSO_4 + 2H_2O \quad \cdots(12.1)$$

$$MnO_2 + H_2C_2O_4 + H_2SO_4 \rightarrow MnSO_4 + 2CO_2 + 2H_2O \quad \cdots(12.2)$$

$$2MnO_2 + As_2O_3 + 2H_2SO_4 \rightarrow 2MnSO_4 + As_2O_5 + 2H_2O \quad \cdots(12.3)$$

The determination of MnO_2 involves reaction with a known excess of a reducing agent such as $FeSO_4$, $H_2C_2O_4$ (or $Na_2C_2O_4$) or As_2O_3, after the completion of the reaction, the remaining quantity of the reducing agent is determined by a suitable titrimetric method. Knowing the amount of the reducing agent consumed, the quantity of MnO_2 in the given weight of the sample material is calculated by means of stoichiometric equations such as (12.1) and (12.2). If $FeSO_4$ is used the difficulty is that the procedure should be carried out in an atmosphere of CO_2 because O_2 present in air oxidises iron (II) to iron (III) sulphate. Both As_2O_3 and $Na_2C_2O_4$ are primary standards and their solutions are stable in air so are more convenient.

Procedure

(i) Weigh out accurately 6·701 g of $Na_2C_2O_4$, transfer it to a 1000-ml volumetric flask and make up to the mark. Shake well ; this gives 0·1 N sodium oxalate soln. Also prepare 0·1 N $KMnO_4$ soln as described in Experiment 10· 1.

(ii) Dry some finely powdered pyrolusite at 120°C for about 30 minutes, cool in a desiccator and weigh. Again heat, cool and weigh. Repeat the process until the weight of the sample becomes constant. Then weigh out accurately about 0·2 g of the dried sample into a conical flask, add 50 ml, 0·1 N $Na_2C_2O_4$ and 50 ml 4 N H_2SO_4. Boil the mixture carefully until no black particles are visible. Cool the soln and titrate the unreacted $Na_2C_2O_4$ with 0·1 N $KMnO_4$ soln and calculate the amount of $Na_2C_2O_4$ consumed in the reaction and from this the quantity of MnO_2 in the pyrolusite.

$$1 \text{ ml}, 0·1 \text{ N } KMnO_4 \equiv 1 \text{ ml}, 0·1 \text{ N } Na_2C_2O_4$$
$$\equiv 4·346 \text{ mg of } MnO_2$$

Example 12(i)

A pyrolusite sample weighing 0·1152 g was allowed to react with 40 ml, 0·1 N $Na_2C_2O_4$ in presence of dilute H_2SO_4. The residual $Na_2C_2O_4$ required 17·5 ml, 0·1 N $KMnO_4$. Calculate the percentage of MnO_2 in the pyrolusite sample.

40 ml, 0·1 N $Na_2C_2O_4 \equiv 40$ ml, 0·1 N $KMnO_4$

$Na_2C_2O_4$ consumed $= (40-17·5) = 22·5$ ml, 0·1 N $Na_2C_2O_4$

The amount of MnO_2 in the sample will be

$22·5 \times 4·346 = 97·785$ mg or 0·0978 g MnO_2.

0·1152 g pyrolusite contains 0·0978 g MnO_2

$\therefore$ 100 g pyrolusite contains $\dfrac{100 \times 0·0978}{0·1152} = 84·89\%$

12·3. ANALYSIS OF DOLOMITE

Discussion

Limestone mainly contains $CaCO_3$ along with some $MgCO_3$. Strictly speaking, in dolomite $CaCO_3$ and $MgCO_3$ are present in equimolar ratio. But all carbonate rocks containing sufficient magnesium are called dolomite. Apart from Ca and Mg which are major constituents, the usual minor constituents of dolomite are Fe, Al, Ti, Mn, Si, Na, K, S and organic matter. The mineral dolomite has many industrial uses and for judging the suitability of a particular sample it is not generally necessary to carry out a complete analysis. A shorter analysis involving the determination of the following constituents may be suitable to derive the necessary informations.

(*i*) Loss on ignition, *i.e.*, determination of volatile matter.

(*ii*) Determination of insoluble matter.

(*iii*) Determination of combined oxides such as Fe_2O_3, Al_2O_3 along with phosphate.

(*iv*) Determination of Ca.

(*v*) Determination of Mg.

Procedure

(*i*) *Determination of loss on ignition.* Dry some finely powdered dolomite sample in air and weigh out accurately about 1 g of this sample into a weighed platinum or porcelain crucible. Heat the crucible to 110°C for 1 hour, cool in a desiccator and weigh. The loss in weight gives the amount of adsorbed moisture in the sample. The percentage of moisture can thus be calculated. Then heat the crucible and its contents first gently and then at 1000-1100°C for 1 hour. Cool and weigh. Repeat the process until constant weight. Note that cooling should be done in a desiccator containing concentrated H_2SO_4. Calculate the percentage loss on ignition.

(*ii*) *Determination of insoluble matter.* Transfer the ignited residue from step (*i*) into a covered porcelain dish. Add 5 ml, 1 : 1 HCl to the crucible to dissolve the sticking material and rinse the soln to the porcelain dish. Add 5 ml concentrated HCl and 1 ml of concentrated HNO_3. Stir to dissolve the solid in the porcelain dish and keep it on a steam bath to evaporate the soln to dryness. Add 20 ml water and again warm on a steam bath with stirring for 5 minutes. Filter through a Whatman no. 41 filter paper. Wash the ppt with 1 per cent HCl and finally twice with water. Evaporate the filtrate and washings to dryness, heat the residue to 110°C. Cool and dissolve the solid in 1-2 ml concentrated HCl and then add 10 ml of water. Filter through another filter paper and wash the ppt as before. Keep the combined filtrate and washings for step (*iii*). Place the two filter papers containing ppt in a weighed porcelain crucible. Dry, ignite, cool and weigh, calculate the percentage of the insoluble matter. The purpose of repeated warming of the sample is to ensure that all the acid soluble material goes into soln.

(*iii*) *Determination of combined oxide.*

(*a*) Dilute the filtrate from step (*ii*) to 200 ml (dilution prevents adsorption of foreign ions which may be adsorbed or occluded on the desired ppt).

(*b*) Add 5 g NH_4Cl to prevent precipitation of $Mg(OH)_2$ on adding ammonia soln (see common ion effect in sections 4·5 and 5·6),

(*c*) Heat to boiling (to obtain bigger particles of the ppt).

(d) Add 2 drops of methyl red indicator and then gradually 1 : 1 ammonia soln until the soln is just yellow. Boil for about 2 minutes and filter through a quantitative filter paper. Transfer the ppt completely to the filter paper and wash with hot 2 per cent NH_4NO_3 soln. (If the ppt obtained is large, dissolve it in a small volume of hot 1 : 1 HCl soln, add few drops of indicator and reprecipitate with ammonia soln.) Keep the filtrate and washings for step (iv). Place the filter paper containing the washed ppt in a weighed porcelain crucible, dry, ignite, cool and weigh to constant weight. Calculate the percentage of combined oxides.

(iv) *Determination of calcium.* Add HCl to the filtrate and washings from step (iii) so that it becomes slightly acidic (as shown by red colour of the indicator) and evaporate the soln so that the volume becomes about 250 ml. Add 1 ml of concentrated HCl, heat the soln to about 80°C and add 4 per cent hot $(NH_4)_2C_2O_4$ soln slowly with constant stirring. Add 1 : 10 ammonia soln dropwise until the soln is just alkaline as shown by yellow colour of the indicator. Test for complete precipitation by adding **little** oxalate soln to the supernatant liquid. After the **precipitation**, filter and wash the ppt and either weigh as $CaC_2O_4.H_2O$ or **convert** it to $CaCO_3$ or CaO and weigh as described in experiment 6·5. Report the weight of calcium in terms of CaO. Calculate the percentage of CaO.

(v) *Determination of magnesium.* The filtrate and washings from step (iv) contains excess of oxalate ion and ammonium salt ; this gives higher results for Mg when it is gravimetrically determined as $MgNH_4PO_4.6H_2O$ (magnesium ammonium phosphate). To avoid this error the filtrate is heated with HNO_3 when oxalate is oxidised to CO_2 and ammonium salts to oxides of nitrogen and water.

To the filtrate from step (iv) add 50 ml of concentrated HNO_3 and evaporate to dryness on a steam bath. Dissolve the residue in 2-3 ml of concentrated HCl and 20 ml of water and dilute to 150 ml. Add few drops of methyl red indicator and 10 ml of 20 per cent freshly prepared A.R. $(NH_4)_2HPO_4$ (diammonium hydrogen phosphate) soln. Now add concentrated ammonia soln slowly while stirring the soln until it turns yellow. Continue stirring the soln for 5 minutes, add ammonia soln to keep the soln yellow and finally add 5 ml of ammonia soln as excess. Allow the soln to stand for at least 4 hours or preferably overnight. The ppt may be weighed either as $MgNH_4PO_4.6H_2O$ or as $Mg_2P_2O_7$ (magnesium pyrophosphate).

(a) **Weighing as $MgNH_4PO_4.6H_2O$.** Filter through a weighed sintered-glass crucible and wash the ppt with small portions of 1 : 9 ammonia soln until free from Cl⁻ ions as tested by adding HNO_3 and $AgNO_3$ soln. Now, wash three times with rectified spirit using each time 5 ml of the wash liquid. Drain well after each washing to remove most of the water from the ppt. Finally wash five times (each time use 5 ml of wash liquid) with anhydrous ether. Drain well after each washing and then draw air through the crucible for 10 minutes. Wipe outside of the crucible with clean linen cloth. Dry for 20 minutes in a desiccator and weigh. From the difference in weight find out the weight of $MgNH_4PO_4.6H_2O$.

(b) **Weighing as $Mg_2P_2O_7$.** Filter through a gravimetric filter paper and wash the ppt several times with cold 1·5 M ammonium hydroxide soln. When the washing does not give any turbidity on treatment with HNO_3 and $AgNO_3$ soln, transfer the ppt on the filter paper. Dry the ppt at 100°C and place it in a previously weighed platinum or porcelain crucible. Char the paper and burn the carbon at a low temperature. Keep the lid slightly open so that air can come in. Then heat in an electric furnace at about 1100°C until constant weight. Find out the weight of $Mg_2P_2O_7$ and then calculate the percentage of MgO in the sample (For more satisfactory result a porcelain filter crucible should be used).

(vi) *Determination of carbon dioxide.* Weight out accurately about 0·5—0·6 g of dry sample into a flat bottom flask fitted with a thistle funnel and a delivery tube. Connect the delivery tube to a bubbler containing A.R. syrpy phosphoric acid and then to two previously weighed U tubes containing soda lime. Add phosphoric acid to the sample through the thistle funnel and regulate the temperature of the flask so that about 2 bubbles of gas pass through the bubbler per second. After about 40 minutes draw in air (CO_2 free) slowly through the flask so that all the CO_2 is driven out. Weigh the U tubes containing soda lime. The increase in their weight gives the amount of CO_2.

12·4.   ANALYSIS OF CEMENT

Discussion

The chief constituents of cement are silica, lime, alumina, ferric oxide, magnesia, small amounts of oxides of alkali metals, sulphuric anhydride and carbonic anhydride. The industrial analysis of cement involves determination of insoluble matter, silica, alumina and ferric oxide, lime, magnesia, sulphuric anhydride and loss upon ignition.

Procedure

(i) *Determination of loss upon ignition.* Weigh out accurately about 1 g of cement into a weighed platinum crucible, cover with the lid, heat gradually and then strongly at about 1000°C for about 30 minutes. Cool in a desiccator and weigh. Calculate percentage loss upon ignition.

(ii) *Determination of insoluble matter.* Weigh out accurately about 1 g of cement into a porcelain dish, add 10 ml water and 5 ml of concentrated HCl and quickly cover with a clock-glass. **Warm, add 40 ml water and digest upon a steam bath until the decomposition is complete. Filter and wash the residue with hot water.** Transfer the filter paper along with its contents to a pyrex beaker, add 30 ml of 5 per cent Na_2CO_3 soln and heat to about 80—90°C for 15 minutes. Filter, wash with cold water, then with 1 : 10 HCl and finally with hot water. Place the filter paper and its contents in a weighed porcelain crucible, burn off the paper and then ignite to red heat for about 30 minutes, cool in a desiccator and weigh. Calculate the percentage of insoluble mater.

(*iii*) *Determination of silica.* Weigh out accurately about 0·5 g of the sample into a porcelain dish, add 30 ml water, stir and then add 10 ml of concentrated HCl, stir well. Cover the dish and heat on a water bath until the sample is decomposed. Evaporate to dryness on the water bath. Heat the residue at 11C—120°C for 1 hour. Add dilute HCl to the residue and warm. Filter and wash the ppt with hot water. Evaporate the filtrate and washings to dryness. Heat the residue at 110—120°C, then add dilute HCl, warm and filter. Wash the ppt with warm water until free from Cl^- ions and keep the combined filtrate and washings for step (*iv*). Combine the two washed precipitates and place them in a weighed platinum crucible. Heat the crucible to 1050—1100°C for 1 hour cool and weigh. Calculate the percentage of SiO_2 present.

(*iv*) *Determination of alumina and ferric oxide.* Dilute the filtrate from step (*iii*) to 200 ml, add 5 g NH_4Cl (to prevent precipitation of $Mg(OH)_2$) then 3 ml of bromine water (to oxidise iron to ferric state). Add 2 drops of methyl red indicator, boil the soln and add 1 : 1 ammonia soln until the soln turns yellow. Filter and collect the filtrate in a 500 ml beaker. Wash the ppt with 2 per cent NH_4Cl soln. Dissolve the ppt in 1 : 1 HCl, dilute to 150 ml and reprecipitate with ammonia soln. Transfer the ppt to a quantitative filter paper and wash with 2 per cent NH_4NO_3 soln. Combine the two filtrates and washings and keep them for step (*v*). Transfer the filter paper containing the ppt to a weighed platinum crucible and ignite, cool and weigh the crucible until constant weight is observed. Calculate the percentage of $Fe_2O_3 + Al_2O_3$.

(*v*) *Determination of lime.* Acidify the combined filtrate and washings from step (*iv*) with HCl and evaporate so that the volume of the soln reduces to about 150 ml. Boil and precipitate by adding $(NH_4)_2C_2O_4$ followed by an excess of ammonia soln. Filter and then dissolve the ppt in dilute HCl and reprecipitate by adding $(NH_4)_2C_2O_4$ soln and ammonia soln. Filter and wash the ppt with dilute $(NH_4)_2C_2O_4$ soln. Weigh calcium as CaC_2O_4 or CaO as described in step (*iv*) of section 12·3. Keep the two filtrates and washings for step (*vi*).

(*vi*) *Determination of magnesia.* Acidify the combined filtrates and washings from step (*v*) with HCl, evaporate the soln to 150 ml and oxidise excess of oxalate and ammonium salt with HNO_3. Determine magnesium by double precipitation with diammonium hydrogen phosphate. Weigh magnesium as $MgNH_4PO_4.6H_2O$ or $Mg_2P_2O_7$ as described in step (v) of section 12.3. Calculate the percentage of MgO. (Organic precipitants can also be used for the gravimetric estimation of Mg).

(vii) *Determination of sulphuric anhydride.* Weigh out accurately about 0.5 g of the cement sample into a 250 ml porcelain dish, add 30 ml water and 10 ml concentrated HCl and heat until the cement is decomposed. Evaporate to dryness and heat the residue to 110—120°C for 1 hour. Add dilute HCl to the residue and warm. Filter and wash the ppt with water. Determine the sulphate in the filtrate by adding $BaCl_2$ soln as described in experiment 6.4. Express the result as percentage of SO_3.

12.5. ANALYSIS OF BRASS

Discussion

The percentage of the important constituents of brass have generally the following values.

Cu	Zn	Sn	Pb	Fe
50—90%	20—40%	0—6%	0—2%	0—1%

The quantitative analysis of brass involves treatment of the sample with HNO_3 when a ppt of hydrated tin oxide $SnO_2.nH_2O$ (stannic acid) is obtained and Cu, Zn, Pb and Fe go into soln. The ppt of stannic acid is filtered, washed, ignited and weighed as SnO_2. The filtrate after separating Sn is evaporated with excess of H_2SO_4 to expel HNO_3 and then diluted when $PbSO_4$ is precipitated which is filtered and weighed as $PbSO_4$. The copper present in the filtrate is estimated electrolytically or gravimetrically as $Cu_2(CNS)_2$. After precipitating Cu, the filtrate is treated with Br_2 water to oxidise iron to ferric state and is then separated from Zn by double precipitation with ammonia ; ferric hydroxide obtained is ignited and weighed as Fe_2O_3. Finally Zn is precipitated as $ZnNH_4PO_4$ and is weighed as $ZnNH_4PO_4$ or after ignition as $Zn_2P_2O_7$.

Procedure

The sample should be in the form of drillings or turnings. If the sample is not clean, wash it with ether and dry in air.

(i) *Determination of tin.* Weigh out accurately about 1 g of brass turnings into a 150 ml beaker, add 10 ml water and 15 ml of concentrated HNO_3. Keep the beaker covered with a clock-glass until the vigorous reaction is over. Evaporate slowly (in about 1 hour) on a water-bath until the volume becomes 5—10 ml. Dilute to 50 ml and again warm on water bath for 10-20 minutes to dissolve all the soluble salts. Filter hot through a Whatman filter paper no. 42 and collect the filtrate in a beaker. (Refilter if the filtrate is turbid). Wash the ppt ten times with hot 1 per cent HNO_3. Keep the filtrate and washings for step (ii). Place the filter paper containing the ppt in a weighed platinum crucible and char the filter paper at a low temperature. Finally ignite at about 1000°C for 30 minutes, cool in a desiccator and weigh as SnO_2. Repeat the ignition until constant weight is obtained. Calculate the percentage of tin.

(ii) *Determination of lead.* Add 3-4 ml of concentrated H_2SO_4 to the filtrate from step (i) and evaporate slowly until white fumes come out. Cool, dilute to 25 ml and again evaporate until white fumes are evolved. The purpose of this process is to expel all the nitric acid. Cool, add 25 ml water, heat to about 90—95°C and stir so that all the soluble salts pass into soln. Add 50 ml water, stir and allow to stand for 1 hour. Filter through a weighed porcelain filter crucible. Keep the filtrate for step (iii). Wash the ppt of $PbSO_4$ with cold 1 : 50 H_2SO_4. Ignite the lead sulphate to constant weight at 500—600°C, cool in a desiccator and weigh as $PbSO_4$. Calculate the percentage of lead. (Lead can also be gravimetrically estimated with organic precipitant salicylaldoxime).

(iii) *Determination of copper.* Evaporate the filtrate from step (ii) to about 50 ml and neutralise the free acid with ammonia soln. Add 2-3 ml of a saturated soln of H_2SO_3 (sulphorous acid). Dilute to 150 ml, heat to boiling and add gradually with constant stirring a slight excess of NH_4CNS (ammonium thiocyanate) soln. Allow to stand for 3-4 hours or overnight. Filter through a weighed sintered crucible. Wash 10—15 times with 0˙1 per cent NH_4CNS soln containing few drops of H_2SO_3 soln. Then wash several times with 20 per cent alcohol. Reserve the filtrate and washings for step (iv). Dry the ppt to constant weight at 110—120°C and weigh as $Cu_2(CNS)_2$ (cuprous thiocyanate). Calculate the percentage of copper in the sample.

(iv) *Determination of iron.* To the filtrate from step (iii) add 30 ml of concentrated HNO_3 and 15 ml of concentrated HCl and evaporate the soln to near dryness. (This process is necessary to remove the excess of thiocyanate, sulphite and ammonium salts). Cool ond add 3 ml of concentrated HCl, warm and dilute to 75 ml. Heat to boiling and add a concentrated ammonia soln until a ppt is obtained and then about 10 ml in excess. Determine iron as Fe_2O_3 as described in experiment 6˙6. Calculate the percentage of Fe.

(v) *Determination of zinc.* Neutralise the filtrate obtained after the precipitation of $Fe(OH)_3$, with HCl, add 5 g NH_4Cl and 10 ml 2N CH_3COONa and dilute to about 150 ml. (If the expected amount of Zn in this soln is more than 0˙1 g then soln is made up to 250 ml in a volumetric flask and 100 ml of this soln is taken for the determination of Zn). Heat nearly to boiling and add slowly with constant stirring 25 ml of 10 per cent A.R. $(NH_4)_2HPO_4$ (diammonium hydrogen phosphate) ; for $0\cdot1$ g of Zn expected to be present in the sample. Heat to boiling for 30—60 minutes when the ppt settles down. Cool to room temperature and filter through a porcelain filter crucible. Wash first with 1 per cent $(NH_4)_2HPO_4$ soln and then several times with cold water. Dry to constant weight at 100—150°C and weigh as $ZnNH_4PO_4$. (To weigh as $Zn_2P_2O_7$, heat the filter crucible first slowly and then to 900°C to constant weight.

12·6.   ANALYSIS OF A SILVER COIN

A silver coin contains Ag, Cu, Ni along with little zinc.

Procedure

(i) *Determination of silver.*   Rub a piece of the coin with sand paper, wash with acetone and then weigh out accurately about $0\cdot4$ g of the alloy into a 500 ml beaker. Add about 5 ml water and 5—10 ml concentrated HNO_3. Warm the beaker slowly on a water-bath to dissolve the alloy (the minimum quantity of HNO_3 required for dissolution should be used). Dilute to 250 ml, heat to 70°C and quantitatively precipitate Ag as AgCl by gradually adding $0\cdot2$ N HCl. Complete the determination of Ag as described in experiment 6·2. Keep the filtrate and washings for step (ii).

(ii) *Determination of copper.*   To the combined filtrate and washings from step (i), add 3-4 ml concentrated H_2SO_4 and evaporate until white fumes of SO_3 come out. Cool, wash down the sides of the beaker with water and dilute to 100 ml. Neutralise the soln with 1 : 1 ammonia soln, add 5 ml of freshly prepared saturated soln of H_2SO_3 and then add 10 per cent NH_4CNS soln to completely precipitate Cu as $Cu_2(CNS)_2$. Complete the determination as described in step (iii) of section 12·5.

(iii) *Determination of nickel.*   Evaporate the filtrate after the separation of Cu as $Cu_2(CNS)_2$, to 50 ml. Add 35 ml of concentrated HNO_3 and 15 ml of concentrated HCl and evaporate the soln to a small volume to destroy the excess of thiocyanate. Heat the soln on a water-bath to dryness to expel HNO_3. Add 1 ml of concentrated HCl, 150 ml water (to dissolve the residue), 5 g NH_4Cl (to prevent the precipitation of Zn) and then 1 : 1 ammonia soln until the soln is slightly alkaline. Determine Ni as nickel dimethylglyoxime as descriced in section 6·9·1.

(iv) *Determination of zinc.*   Determine Zn in the filtrate from step (iii) by the method described in step (v) of section 12·5.

12·7.   ANALYSIS OF BRONZE

Bronze mainly consists of Cu (60—97%) and Sn (1—35%) but small amounts of Pb, Fe and Zn may also be present. Different types of bronze can be obtained by varying the amounts of different constituents.

(a) *Gun metal* contains about 90% Cu and 10% Sn along with small amounts of Zn, Pb, Fe and traces of phosphorus.

(b) *Phosphor bronze* has a similar composition as gun metal but contains 0·2—1·5% phosphorus and traces of antimony.

(c) *Aluminium bronze* consists of about 90% Cu and 10% Al and may contain small amounts of iron and other metals.

(d) *Manganese bronze* contains 55—60% Cu, 30—40% Zn, 0—2% Sn, 0—1·5% Pb, 1—2% Fe, 0—3% Al and about 1% of Mn.

For the analysis of different varieties of bronze, the experimental details are similar to those described for the analysis of brass in section 12·5.

PART IV
SEPARATIVE TECHNIQUES

13

Separative Techniques

When a sample contains several components, its analysis becomes complicated. For analysing such a sample, a method should be available to determine a particular component in presence of others. Thus for each species an analytical method should be available which will be specifically applicable for the determination of that particular species and it should not be interfered by the other constituents present in the mixture. Such a condition is not always fulfilled. There are two ways to deal with such problems. The interference of a particular substance can be eliminated by adding a complexing agent which reacts selectively with the interfering substance (but not with the species to be determined) so that now it does not disturb the main reaction on which the analytical procedure under consideration is based ; this technique is known as *masking*. Another approach is to isolate the interfering species from the sample mixture by some separative technique such as solvent extraction, ion-exchange or chromatography. It should be remembered that a total separation of the interfering substance from the species to be determined is not possible but the concentration level of the interfering substance can be lowered to such an extent that then, it does not cause any interference.

13'A. SOLVENT EXTRACTION

In solvent extraction, usually an aqueous soln is shaken with another solvent which is generally organic and is immiscible with water, in order to bring about a transfer of a solute from aqueous to organic medium. For example, if an   soln of I_2 in water is shaken with CCl_4, most of the I_2 will be transferred from water to CCl_4. This separation technique is advantageous because it is quick and many separations can be achieved by using only a separatory (or separating) funnel (see Fig. 13'1). A constituent can also be separated by adding a suitable reagent which will precipitate out the interfering substance but this separation is not as clean as achieved by solvent extraction. In separations by precipitation there are many problems such as contamination of the separated ppt by post-precipitation, surface adsorbption, occlusion etc., which do not permit a clean separation.

13·A·1. DISTRIBUTION LAW

When a solute 'A' is shaken with two immiscible solvents 1 and 2, the solute dis-. tributes or partitions itself between these two liquids and a dynamic equilibrium as shown below is established :

$$A_1 \rightleftharpoons A_2$$

where A_1 and A_2 are concentrations of the solute A in solvents 1 and 2 respectively. If the solute exists in the same molecular or ionic form in both the solvents, Nernst distribution law states that :

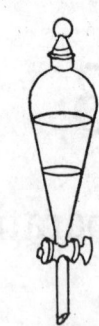

Fig. 13·1. Separating funnel.

$$\frac{A_1}{A_2} = K_D \qquad \qquad ...(13·1)$$

where K_D is a constant at a particular temperature known as *partition* or *distribution constant*. (Strictly speaking activities should be taken but in dilute solutions activity is regarded as approximately equal to concentration).

The distribution law can be successfully applied only if the solutions formed are very dilute. With increasing amounts of the solute the value of the partition constant shows fluctuations. Further, if there is a change in the molecular state of the solute in one of the solvents, the distribution law as expressed by (13·1) will not be applicable. For example, C_6H_5COOH (benzoic acid) in water shows its normal mol wt but in benzene its two molecules associate so that its mol wt in benzene is twice the value in water.

$$2\ C_6H_5COOH \rightleftharpoons (C_6H_5COOH)_2$$
$$\text{in water} \qquad \qquad \text{in benzene}$$

In this case the following form of the distribution law will be applicable :

$$\frac{A_1}{\sqrt{A_2}} = K.$$

Similarly if the solute undergoes dissociation in either phase, the distribution law has to be modified.

In the practical applications of solvent extraction we are not interested whether the solute, in any of the solvent, is in the associated or dissociated form, but our primary interest is to know the fraction of the total solute in one or the other solvent. Hence, a term *distribution ratio* (D) or *extraction coefficient* (E) is used which is given by :

$$D = \frac{(C_A)_1}{(C_A)_2} \qquad \qquad ...(13\cdot2)$$

where $(C_A)_1$ is the concentration of the solute A in solvent 1 ; this includes all forms of A in which it is present in solvent 1 and which is determined analytically. Likewise, $(C_A)_2$ is the concentration of A in solvent 2 as determined analytically.

Example 13(*i*)

20 g of an organic substance A is present in 100 g of its aqueous soln. If it is shaken with 100 g of ether, how much of A will be transferred to ether. Given that the solubility of A in ether is double the solubility of A in water, *i.e.*, the partition coefficient of A between water and ether is 2 in favour of ether.

Now, $\dfrac{(C_A)\text{water}}{(C_A)\text{ether}} = \dfrac{1}{2}$

Suppose on shaking 100 g of aqueous soln of A with 100 g of ether, w g of A is transferred to ether layer. Then, concentration of A in water $= \dfrac{20-w}{100} = (C_A)\text{water}$. and concentration of A in ether

$= \dfrac{w}{100} = (C_A)\text{ether}.$

$\dfrac{(20-w)/100}{w/100} = \dfrac{1}{2}$ or, $\dfrac{20-w}{w} = \dfrac{1}{2}$

or, $40 - 2w = w$ or, $3w = 40$

or, $w = 40/3 = 13\cdot33$ g.

Thus 13·33 g of A will be in the ether layer and remainder 6·67 g will be in the aqueous layer.

Let us see the result if we extract A from its aqueous soln twice, each time using 50 g of ether. Suppose in the first extraction of A with 50 g ether, w_1 g of A is transferred to ether.

Then, $(C_A)\text{water} = (20-w_1)/100$

$(C_A)\text{ether} = (w_1/50)$

Now, $\dfrac{(20-w_1)/100}{w_1/50} = \dfrac{1}{2}$

or, $$\frac{(20-w_1)}{w_1} \times \frac{50}{100} = \frac{20-w_1}{2w_1} = \frac{1}{2}$$

or, $$40-2w_1 = 2w_1$$

or, $$4w_1 = 40 \quad \text{or,} \quad w_1 = 10 \text{ g}$$

Thus in the first extraction 10 g of A will be transferred to ether and 10 g will remain in aqueous phase.

If in the second extraction with 50 g of ether, w_2 g of A is transferred to ether then,

$$(C_A)_{water} = (10-w_2)/100$$

$$(C_A)_{ether} = (w_2/50)$$

Now, $$\frac{(10-w_2)/100}{w_2/50} = \frac{10-w_2}{w_2} \times \frac{50}{100} = \frac{1}{2}$$

or, $$\frac{10-w_2}{2w_2} = \frac{1}{2}$$

or, $$20-2w_2 = 2w_2 \quad \text{or,} \quad 4w_2 = 20$$

or, $$w_2 = 5 \text{ g}$$

In the first extraction 10 g of A was transferred to ether and in the second extraction 5 g more passes to the ether phase. Thus, 15 g of A will be extracted by 100 g ether during two extractions with two 50 g portions. If only one extraction with 100 g ether is done the amount of A extracted is only 13·33 g. These calculations show that it is more advantageous to use a given quantity of the solvent in as many instalments as practicable. It should also be clear that a total transfer of a solute from one solvent to another is not possible however large the number of extractions may be. The partition involves an equilibrium process, hence, every time some quantity, however small, will be left behind in the solvent from which extraction is being done.

13·A·2. APPLICATIONS OF DISTRIBUTION LAW

The uneven distribution of a substance between two immiscible liquids has been made use of in several analytical operations. For example, iodine is much more soluble in CS_2, CCl_4 or $CHCl_3$ as compared to that in water. Suppose we have a very dilute soln of iodine in water, then its yellow colour will be so faint that we will not be able to see it. But if we add a drop of CS_2 or CCl_4 and shake, most of the iodine will be transferred to the organic layer which will therefore become violet. Thus, a very small quantity of iodine present in aqueous medium can be detected.

In testing iodide radical in a given aqueous soln, we add a few drops of CCl_4 and then Cl_2 water. Chlorine oxidises iodide to iodine. On shaking, most of the iodine passes into CCl_4 layer making it distinctly violet. If we do not add CCl_4, the small amount. of iodine formed will remain in aqueous medium giving it a very faint yellow colour which is not easily visible. Hence, we will not be sure that iodide radical is present in the given soln.

In Andrew's titration, a soln of a reductant in presence of HCl and CCl_4 is titrated with a standard soln of KIO_3. During the titration IO_3^- is reduced first to I_2 which is then converted to ICl (iodine monochloride). The end point is reached when all the liberated I_2 is converted to ICl. Now both I_2 and ICl are brownish-yellow in aqueous soln, hence, the change I_2 to ICl cannot be seen. Fortunately I_2 is purple in CCl_4 but ICl remains yellow. Hence, about 2-3 ml of CCl_4 is added to the titration mixture and flask is shaken when CCl_4 layer becomes purple due to I_2. Dropwise addition of KIO_3 is continued with thorough shaking. When the titration is complete, the CCl_4 layer loses the last trace of purple colour and becomes pale yellow showing that all the iodine has been converted into ICl.

Suppose a soln contains constituents A and B, and B interferes with the method for determining A. The solvent extraction technique can be used for removing B from the sample soln. In order to achieve this such a solvent is selected in which the solubility of B is very high but that of A is negligibly small. If the distribution coefficient of B (K_{DB}) is 100 and that of A (K_{DA}) is 0·1 and the volume of the soln and that of the solvent used for extraction is the same then, 99 per cent of B and 9 per cent of A will be extracted by the solvent. If the value of K_{DB} is 200 and that of K_{DA} is 0·01, using the same volume of the solvent as that of the soln, 99·5 per cent of B and 1 per cent of A will be transferred to the solvent. By repeating the extraction with fresh solvent the amonut of B in the sample soln can be further decreased.

Iron (III) can be separated from several monovalent and bivalent cations by preparing its soln in 6N HCl and then extracting with diethyl ether. In a single extraction about 99 per cent of iron (III) is extracted into ether.

The most important type of analytical application of solvent extraction involves metal chelates which are readily soluble in organic solvents but only sparingly soluble in water. For example, by adding dimethylglyoxime to an aqueous soln of Ni(II) at pH between 5-12, nickel dimethylglyoximate is quantitatively precipitated which can be extracted with chloroform. The red soln in chloroform so obtained is examined spectrophotometrically and the amount of nickel present in the sample soln can be determined.

13·B. ION-EXCHANGE

It has been known for a long time that certain minerals can exchange one ion for another. Aluminosilicates were found to possess this property. The earlier ion exchange studies involved mainly Na^+, K^+, NH_4^+ and Ca^{2+} ions. Naturally occurring and artificially prepared zeolites (sodium aluminium silicates) were used for softening hard water. When hard water is precolated through zeolite, Ca^{2+} and Mg^{2+} ions present in hard water are exchanged with Na^+ ions of zeolite. Thus Ca^{2+} and Mg^{2+} ions of hard water which are responsible for the hardness of water are replaced by Na^+, hence hard water becomes soft. After a prolonged use the water-softening capacity of zeolite is decreased and it has to be regenerated ; regeneration is done by treatment with NaCl soln. A simple ion exchange column has been shown in Fig. 13·2.

The phenomenon of ion exchange provides a means of separating ionic species. In most cases a solid, ion exchanger is used which contains ions of its own and has such structure that permits a free flow of ions and solvent molecules through it. For most analytical work synthetic organic ion exchangers are generally used. The ion exchange resins are complex organic polymers. By varying the structure and functional groups of these polymers the properties of resins can be controlled in regard to the rate of exchange, exchange capacity and selectivity.

13·B·1. CATION EXCHANGE RESINS

In cation exchange resins, anionic groups are firmly held in the resin structure while the cation is diffusable hence takes part in ion exchange. Most of the cation exchange resins contain sulphonic or carboxylic acids which exchange their H^+ ions with other cations as shown by :

$$(Res.A^-)B^+ + C^+(soln) \rightleftharpoons (Res.A^-)C^+ + B^+(soln)$$

The extent of exchange of ions between an ion exchange resin and a soln depends upon a number of factors. At low concentra-

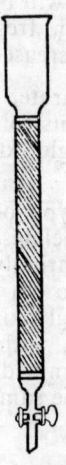

Fig. 13 2. (Ion-exchange colum).

tions and at ordinary temperature, the extent of exchange increases with increasing valency of the exchanging ion, *i.e.*,

$$Na^+ < Ca^{2+} < Al^{3+}$$

For the same valency and under similar conditions the extent of exchange increases with increasing atomic number, *i.e.*,

$$Li^+ < Na^+ < K^+$$

The extent of exchange also depends upon the nature of the resin and the solvent, temperature and concentration of the soln.

13·B·2. ANION EXCHANGE RESINS

Anion exchange resins generally contain substituted amines as functional groups. A primary amine in aqueous soln reacts to form a hydroxyl compound :

$$Res.NH_2 + H_2O \rightleftharpoons (Res.NH_3^+)OH^-$$

The hydroxyl ion can then be exchanged with other anions :

$$(Res.NH_3^+)OH^- + Cl^-(soln) \rightleftharpoons (Res.NH_3^+)Cl^- + OH^-$$

Also, anions other than OH^- can exchange with one another :

$$2(Res.NH_3)^+.Cl^- + SO_4^{2-} \rightleftharpoons (Res.NH_3^+)_2.SO_4^{2-} + 2Cl^-$$

13·B·3. APPLICATIONS OF ION-EXCHANGE

Ion exchange process is applied in several cases for separation of ions ; a few examples are given here. We have already seen that zeolite can be used as an ion exchanger for softening hard water. Ion exchange finds several applications in analytical chemistry. The ionic species of opposite charge can be separated by a cation or anion exchanger. Suppose we have a soln which contains A^+ and B^- ions and we want to remove A^+, then we will use a suitable cation exchange resin that will take up A^+ ions and so these will be separated from B^- ions. A soln containing ions of the same charge can also be separated by choosing a resin having exchange affinity for the ion to be separated. Thus ions that interfere in many analytical procedures may be removed. Phosphate ions interfere in qualitative analysis after Group II ; this ion can be removed by using a suitable anion exchange resin.

13·C. CHROMATOGRAPHY

Chromatography is a separative process which is very useful for separating molecular mixtures. In this technique advantage is taken of the differential adsorption of different components of a mixture by an adsorbent. For example, suppose a petroleum ether extract of green leaves is allowed to flow down (under the influence of gravity) through a glass tube filled with $CaCO_3$ powder (called adsorption column). The ether extract is a mixture of different components derived from green leaves such as green pigments (chlorophylls), yellow pigments (xanthophylls) and another yellow substance (carotene). The green pigments are more strongly adsorbed and so are more firmly held by the powder consequently they are not able to move much down the column and remain near the top of the column. Yellow pigments are less strongly adsorbed so they move farther down the column. The adsorption material has the least adsorption tendency for carotenes, hence, they pass through the column without being adsorbed. The various molecular components present in green leaves can thus be separated by means of a very simple method. The adsorption column along with its coloured bands containing separated material is called a chromatogram and this technique of separation is known as chromatography (see Fig. 13·3).

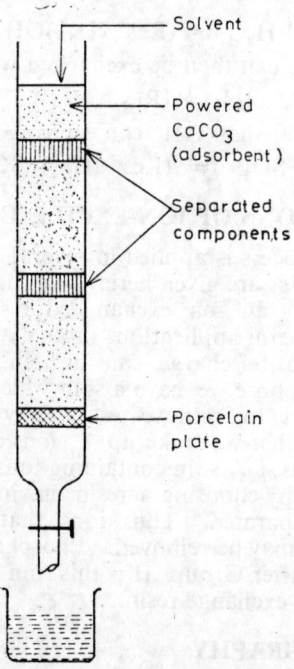

Fig. 13·3. Adsorption column.

13·C·1. CLASSIFICATION OF CHROMATOGRAPHIC PRO-CESSES

One of the ways of classifying chromatographic processes is on the basis of the physical states of the two phases involved. In the example given in 13·C, the adsorbing material (powdered

$CaCO_3$) is a solid that does not move, this forms a *stationary phase*. The petroleum ether, containing the various components to be separated, is capable of moving through the adsorbing material, hence, this constitutes the *mobile phase*. The stationary phase may be either liquid or solid and the mobile phase either gas or liquid. In naming different types of chromatographic processes, the name of the physical state of the mobile phase is placed first. Liquid-solid chromatography means the mobile phase is liquid and the stationary phase is solid.

Mobile phase	Stationary phase	Type
1. gas	liquid	gas-liquid chromatography
2. gas	solid	gas-solid chromatography
3. liquid	liquid	liquid-liquid chromatography
4. liquid	solid	liquid-solid chromatography

The first two types (1 and 2) are generally referred to as gas-phase chromatography or simply gas chromatography and the last two as liquid-phase chromatography.

Chromatographic processes can also be classified on the basis of mechanism by which separation is achieved (not taking into consideration the physical states of the mobile and stationary phases). According to this classification there are three classes of chromatographic separation techniques ; these are adsorption, partition and ion exchange chromatography.

13·C·2. ADSORPTION CHROMATOGRAPHY

In this type of separation process an adsorption column is used. For liquid-solid chromatography, an ordinary glass tube packed with solid particles is used; these particles act as the stationary phase. The soln of mixture moves down the column. Various adsorbents, such as $CaCO_3$, $CaSO_4$, $MgCO_3$, MgO, CaO, charcoal, starch, cellulose can be used. These substances differ considerably from one another in their adsoption characteristics and in their chemical reactivity. The choice of adsorbent depends upon the nature of the substance to be separated. The common solvents used are organic acids, water alcohols, chloroform, benzene, ether, carbon disulphide, carbon tetrachloride and petroleum ether.

The soln containing the mixture to be separated is placed on the top of the column, a solvent is poured from the top and it is allowed to flow down under gravity. The solvent selected to act as a mobile phase is called *eluent* and the process of continuous movement of the sample material through the column due to continuous flow of the mobile phase (solvent) is known as *elution*. The liquid coming out of the column is the *eluate* which contains the solvent and separated components of the mixture. As the solution moves down the column along with the solvent, the different components present in the sample material are adsorbed by the adsorbent to different extents. The component which is least adsorbed will move relatively rapidly through the column along with the solvent and can be collected. The different components are held by the adsorbent to different extent, hence, they require different time to travel the length of the adsorption column ; this is known as the *retention time*. Since the different components have different retention times, they come out of the column one after another and thus get separated. The retention time depends upon the nature of the adsorbent, substance that is adsorbed, the solvent, the diameter and length of the adsorption column, mode of packing of the column, solvent flow rate and temperature. The adsorbent, the solvent and other experimental conditions are so selected that the different components have different retention time.

The earliest applications of this separation technique involved coloured substances hence the name chromatography (Greek, meaning colour and to write) was given to this technique. However, it can be applied to coloured as well as colourless substances. If the separated components are coloured we can see when a particular component has completely passed through the column so that we can change the receiver, placed at the bottom of the column. In case the separated components are colourless a suitable reagent can be used which would produce different colours with different components. For example, we have a soln containing As^{3+}, Sb^{3+} and Bi^{3+}, the soln along with a suitable solvent is made to flow through an adsorption column when the three ions get separated. Now, if H_2S water is poured through the column three differently coloured bands will appear ; a yellow band due to the formation of As_2S_3, an orange band due to Sb_2S_3 and a brownish-black band as a result of formation of Bi_2S_3. Each band will move with different rate through the column and can be separately collected by elution.

13·C·2·1. Theoretical Basis of Separation by Adsorption

If a solid adsorbent is brought in contact with a soln containing a solute, A, then the solute is distributed between the adsorbent and the soln and there is the following dynamic equilibrium :

$$A_{soln} \rightleftharpoons A_{adsorb}$$

where A_{soln} and A_{adsorb} are the amounts of A in soln and adsorbent respectively. The relation between A_{soln} and A_{adsorb} is given by the adsorption isotherm :

$$\left[\; K = \frac{m}{C^{1/n}} \;\right]$$

where K and n are constants, m is mass of the substance adsorbed per unit mass of adsorbent and C is the concentration of the substance in the soln phase. For a successful separation of two components A and B of a mixture by adsorption, the solid phase should adsorb practically all of A and a negligible amount of B. In column chromatography there is a continuous flow of solvent, hence, B continuously moves down leaving behind A in the column. Thus, if we have components with different retention times, they can be separated by column chromatography.

Several practical applications of adsorption chromatography have been developed especially in the separation of complex natural and commercial products including foods, drugs etc. This technique is also useful in qualitative analysis for identifying constituents of a mixture and also for checking the purity of a substance.

13·C·3. FLUID PARTITION CHROMATOGRAPHY

Basically partition chromatography is similar to adsorption chromatography. The only difference is that in partition chromatography the solid adsorbent is coated with a liquid (L_1) which acts as a stationary phase (the adsorbent simply serves as a support for the non-mobile phase). Another liquid (L_2) which is immiscible with L_1 acts as a mobile phase which passes through the non-mobile liquid phase. A gas can also act as a mobile phase. In each case distribution of solute takes place between absorbed stationary liquid phase and a mobile fluid that is in intimate contact with stationary liquid.

13·C·3·1. Paper Chromatography

Let us consider the separation of a mixture of amino acids by means of a strip of a filter paper. A drop of a soln containing the mixture of amino acids is placed at one end of the strip, is allowed to dry and its position on the paper is marked with a pencil. Equal volumes of phenol and water are shaken in a separatory funnel. The upper layer (I) consists of water (containing some phenol) which is used as stationary phase while the lower layer (II) consists of phenol (containing some water) and this is used as the mobile phase. (The strip of the filter paper provides support for the stationary phase). The strip is hung in a gas jar, as shown in Fig. 13·4, with its upper end (at which a drop of soln is placed) dipping in a trough. The mixture in layer I (containing mostly water with little phenol) is placed at the bottom of the jar so that the air inside becomes saturated with it and the paper strip also gets conditioned to mixture I. The liquid in layer II (containing mostly phenol with

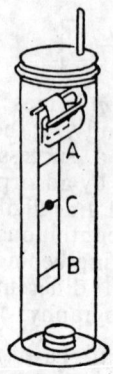

Fig. 13·4. Paper chromatography.

little water) which acts as the mobile phase (it is called developer), is now placed in the trough and the gas jar is closed. The developer moves into the paper by capillary action and then under gravity passes down over the test mixture placed at A. As the developer flows down, the different amino acids, present in the mixture, also move down with different characteristic rates. When the developer reaches almost to the lower end of the strip the gas jar is opened, the paper strip removed, the position of the developer B marked and the strip is dried. Since amino acids are colourless the strip is sprayed with 0·1 per cent soln of nyn-hydrin and warmed when different spots of purple colour are observed. The distance (AB) between A and B is measured. Suppose the distance between A and the centre of a spot at C is AC, then the R_F value for the substance reaching up to point C is given by :

$$R_F = \frac{AC}{AB}$$

Since R_F values are characteristic of different components, they can be used to identify the component. For a good separation the R_F values ef different components should be quite different from one another. A better resolution can be obtained by two-dimensional paper chromatography. In this case the mixture to be separated is placed on the corner of a sheet of filter paper and developed in one direction as described above. Later, the paper is turned through 90° and again developed. Thus the movement of the components is now along two directions perpendicular to each other. By this method mixtures of several similar amino acids have been resolved.

In circular paper chromatography (Fig. 13·5), a circular sheet ·of filter paper (D) is placed on a glass vessel (A). A drop (E) of

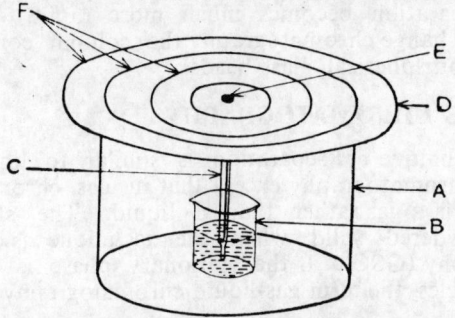

Fig. 13·5.   Circular paper chromatography.

:a soln containing the mixture is placed at the centre of the sheet D. A beaker (B) containing the developer is placed in the vessel A. By capillary action, the developer rises through a wick (C) and reaches the spot·E. As the developer moves through the paper, it carries along the components of the test soln. The different components move with their own characteristic rates and so get separated. The resulting chromatogram shows a series of concentric rings (F). From the measurement of the radius of a particular ring, the component producing that ring can be identified. If the components are colourless, the paper is treated with a suitable reagent which will form coloured compounds with the components. The intensity of the colour of a ring is a measure of the concentration of the component producing that ring.

13·C·4. THIN LAYER CHROMATOGRAPHY

In this technique an adsorbent, coated on a glass plate, acts as the stationary phase. The mobile phase (developer) percolates through the adsorbent and carries along with it various components of a mixture which move with different speeds and thus get separated. Silica gel or cellulose powder is very often used as adsorbents. The adsorbent should be such that different components should have different values of R_F in it. The plate is dipped in a solvent (mobile phase) placed at the bottom of a glass chamber which is then covered. The chromatogram is developed by ascending technique, i.e., the solvent moves in upward direction.

13·C·5. HIGH PERFORMANCE LIQUID CHROMATOGRAPHY (HPLC)

In ordinary column liquid chromatography, the mobile liquid phase moves down the column slowly through the stationary phase under the influence of gravity ; this requires much time for the separation of various components. In HPLC, the eluent (mobile liquid phase) is pumped through the column packed with adsorbent, hence, the separation becomes much more rapid. In high performance ion exchange chromatography the column contains exchange resin coated on spherical glass beads.

13·C·6. GAS CHROMATOGRAPHY

This technique of separation is similar to liquid-liquid and liquid-solid chromatography except that in gas chromatography the mobile phase is a gas rather than a liquid. The stationary phase can be a powdered solid when the technique is called gas-solid chromatography (GSC). If the stationary phase is a liquid coated on solid particles, the term gas-liquid chromatography (GLC) is used.

In GLC, a column is used which is packed with solid particles acting as a support for the stationary liquid phase. For separating particular components, the nature of the solid support and of the liquid phase, method of packing the column, length, diameter and temperature of the column are the factors which must be taken into account. The entire column is heated to a suitable constant temperature. The mobile phase is a gas called the carrier gas. The carrier gas used is either helium, nitrogen, hydrogen or argon. The sample soln is introduced from the top of the column. The carrier gas at constant pressure, regulated by a flow meter, is also sent through the column. The component that is held less strongly by the stationary phase moves more rapidly along with the carrier gas and thus different components get separated. The gas coming out of the column is sent to thermal conductivity detector which records the chromatogram showing the various components present is test sample.

13·C·7. ION EXCHANGE CHROMATOGRAPHY

In ion exchange chromatography, a column filled with ion exchange resin (see 13·B) is used for the separation process. Suppose we have to separate two components A and B present in a sample soln. If we have such a resin which has a distinct preference for one of the components, say A, then A will be taken up by the resin during ion exchange process and B will be left in the soln and so the two will get separated.

13·D. · SEPARATION BY ELECTROLYSIS

When a metal is dipped in a soln containing its own ions, a potential difference is developed between the metal electrode and the electrolyte soln containing its ions. This potential is called the electrode potential of the metal, its value depends upon the nature of the metal, temperature and the concentration (more correctly activity) of the metal ions in the soln. When the concentration of ions is unity the potential acquired by the metal electrode is known as its standard potential. The standard electrode potentials, at ordinary temperature, of Cu and Zn are $+0.34$ and -0.77 volt respectively. Suppose we have a soln in which Cu^{2+} and Zn^{2+} ions are at unit concentration. If this soln is electrolysed the deposition of Cu, at the cathode, will begin when the cathode potential exceeds $+0.34$ volt in the negative direction, *i.e.*, it is less than 0.34 volt. Thus in a molar $CuSO_4$ soln, the deposition or discharge potential of Cu is $+0.34$ volt. The deposition of Zn at the cathode will start only when its potential becomes more negative than -0.77 volt. It is obvious that if we properly control the cathode potential, we can separate Cu and Zn from a soln containing Cu^{2+} and Zn^{2+} ions. For a successful separation the values of deposition potentials of metals to be separated must not be close.

13 E. SEPARATION BY VOLATALISATION

If a sample mixture contains a volatile component. it can be separated by heating the mixture to a suitable temperature when the volatile component leaves the mixture in vapour form which can be then cooled separately, collected and weighed. Determination of moisture content of a sample is based on this principle.

13 F. SEPARATION BY PRECIPITATION

If one of the components forms an insoluble compound with a reagent (while the other components remain in soln), it can be precipitated and separated from the soln containing other components by filtration. For example, suppose we have a soln containing Cu^{2+} and Ba^{2+}. On adding H_2SO_4, $BaSO_4$ will be precipitated and can be filetred out, the Cu^{2+} ions will pass into the filtrate.

Experiment 13 1

Determination of partition coefficient of iodine between water and carbon tetrachloride.

Chemicals required. Carbon tetrachloride, iodine, potassium iodate, potassium iodide, sodium thiosulphate, sulphuric acid and starch.

Apparatus required. Six clean and dry glass bottles with tight glass stoppers, burette, 2 and 10 ml pipettes, weighing bottle, conical flasks and measuring flasks.

Discussion

It has been seen in 13 A 1 that when a solute A is shaken with two immiscible solvents (those solvents which do not mix with each other) the solute (which has solubility in both the solvents 1 and 2) distributes itself between these two solvents. When a mixture containing solute A, solvent 1 and solvent 2 is thoroughly shaken for a sufficient period of time, an equilibrium is attained. Now, if the concentration (C_1) of the solute in solvent 1 and that (C_2) in the solvent 2 is determined, the ratio $C_1/C_2 = K_D$ known as distribution or partition coefficient has been found to be constant provided the temperature is maintained constant. It is important to note that the value of K_D is independent of the amounts of the solute, solvent 1 and solvent 2 taken so long as the temperature remains constant. The present experiment is so designed that in different bottles, the quantities of iodine, water and carbon tetrachloride are different yet when we determine the concentration of iodine in water and that in carbon tetrachloride layer, the ratio of the concentrations in all the cases remains the same at constant temperature. In this experiment two solvents used are immiscible and iodine has solubility in both these solvents.

Preparation of Solutions

1. **Saturated soln of iodine in carbon tetrachloride.** Take about 200 ml of carbon tetrachloride in a clean and dry bottle and go on adding iodine with constant shaking until no more iodine dissolves. Filter and collect the filtrate which is a saturated soln of iodine in carbon tetrachloride.

2. **Thiosulphate soln.** Prepare 0·1 N thiosulphate soln by titration with a standard soln of potassium iodate as described in Experiment 10·3. Prepare 0·005 N thiosulphate soln also by diluting (20 times) 0·1 N soln. (10 ml of 0·1 N thiosulphate soln should be diluted to 200 ml in a volumetric flask).

Procedure

(i) Clean and dry six glass bottles with tight glass stoppers, number them and introduce into these bottles water and saturated soln of iodine in carbon tetrachloride according to the following scheme :

Bottle no.	1	2	3	4	5	6
ml of water	65	60	55	50	45	40
ml of saturated soln of I_2 in CCl_4	10	15	20	25	30	35

It should be noted that in these bottles, the quantities of iodine, water and carbon tetrachloride are different from one another.

(ii) Put the glass stopper on each bottle tightly so that no liquid can leak out of the bottle. Shake these six bottles for about 30 minutes by means of an electrical shaker. (If a thermostat is available place these bottles for about one hour with occassional shaking). After shaking keep the bottles for about 10 minutes when the two layers are clearly separated. The upper layer consists of aqueous soln of iodine while the lower layer contains soln of iodine in carbon tetrachloride. (Note that CCl_4 is heavier than water).

(*iii*) Take bottle no. 1, close the upper tip of a 2 ml pipette with your thumb and dip the lower tip of the pipette right down to the bottom of the bottle. (By doing so the water soln cannot enter the pipette). Then remove the thumb and take out exactly 2 ml of the CCl_4 layer by means of the pipette and introduce it into a conical flask. Add 10 ml of 10% KI, shake well and titrate with 0.1 N thiosulphate soln using starch as indicator. (On adding KI the iodine is transferred from CCl_4 layer to aqueous layer and titration with thiosulphate can be conveniently done). Note the titre value. Since the normality and volume of thiosulphate soln and the volume of CCl_4 soln is known, the normality of iodine in CCl_4 layer (N_{CCl_4}) can be calculated.

(*iv*) Pipette out 10 ml of aqueous layer into a conical flask, add little KI soln and titrate with 0.005 N thiosulphate soln using starch indicator. Calculate the normality of iodine in aqueous soln (N_{H_2O}).

(*v*) In this way calculate the normality of iodine in water and that in CCl_4 in all the six cases. The ratio N_{CCl_4}/N_{H_2O} will give the value of the partition coefficient of iodine between water and carbon telrachloride. The six values so obtained should be constant.

Example

In bottle 1 :

2.0 ml of CCl_4 layer required 5.0 ml, 0.1 N thiosulphate soln ; then

$$2 \times N_{CCl_4} = 5 \times 0.1$$

or

$$N_{CCl_4} = \frac{5 \times 0.1}{2} = 0.25$$

10.0 ml of water layer required 6.0 ml of 0.005 N thiosulphate soln ; then

$$10 \times N_{H_2O} = 6 \times 0.005$$

or

$$N_{H_2O} = \frac{6 \times 0.005}{10} = 0.003$$

∴ Partition coefficient

$$K_D = \frac{N_{CCl_4}}{N_{H_2O}} = \frac{0.25}{0.003}$$

$$= 83.33$$

Similarly the value of the partition coefficient of iodine between water and carbon tetrachloride can be calculated in all the six cases. From the above value of partition coefficient it is evident that iodine is much more soluble in CCl_4 than in water. This is the reason that we use a more concentrated thiosulphate soln for titrating iodine in the CCl_4 layer.

Alternative Calculation

$$2 \cdot 0 \text{ ml of } CCl_4 \text{ layer} \equiv 5 \cdot 0 \text{ ml } \frac{N}{10} \text{ thio soln}$$

$$\therefore \quad 10 \cdot 0 \quad ,, \quad ,, \quad \equiv (5 \times 5) = 25 \cdot 0 \text{ ml } \frac{N}{10} \text{ thio}$$

$$\therefore \quad 10 \cdot 0 \quad ,, \quad ,, \quad \equiv (25 \times 20) = 500 \text{ ml } \frac{N}{200} \text{ thio}$$

$$\text{and} \quad 10 \cdot 0 \text{ ml of water layer} \equiv 6 \cdot 0 \text{ ml } \frac{N}{200} \text{ thio}$$

$$\therefore \quad \text{Partition coefficient} \quad = \frac{500 \cdot 0}{6 \cdot 0} = 83 \cdot 33$$

Note :

1. In the alternative calculation, it is seen, that the normality of iodine in CCl_4 or water layer has not been used. We have simply applied similar conditions, *i.e.*, 10 ml soln has been considered in both the cases and the normality of thiosulphate soln has also been made equal in the calculations. It is therefore not necessary to prepare a standard solution of thiosulphate. What we need to know is :

(*a*) volume of CCl_4 layer taken for the titration,

(*c*) volume of water layer taken for the titration, and

(*c*) how many times thiosulphate soln is diluted while titrating the aqueous layer.

2. While titrating iodine in CCl_4 and water layer, the volume of the soln taken for the titration and concentration of the thiosulphate soln should be so chosen that the titre value ranges between about 5 to 25 ml.

Experiment 13·2

Verification of Freundlich adsorption isotherm.

Chemicals required. Oxalic acid, sodium hydroxide, activated charcoal and phenolphthalein indicator soln.

Apparatus required. : clean and dry glass bottles with tight glass stoppers, pipette, burette, weighing bottle, conical flasks and measuring flasks.

Discussion

The molecules present at the surface of a solid or a liquid have unsatisfied valencies, hence, they are in a state of tension giving rise to surface forces. These molecules, therefore, have a tendency to attract and hold other molecules which come in their contact. This results in the accumulation of a foreign substance (called adsorbate) on the surface of a solid or a liquid (called adsorbent). The process of accumulation of gases, liquids, solutes etc., at the *surface* of a solid or a liquid is known as adsorption. For example, if a solid is an adsorbent and a gas adsorbate, the molecules of the gas will be concentrated on the surface of the solid. The molecules of the gas will said to be *adsorbed* on the solid surface. This phenomenon will be distinguished from the penetration of the gas throughout the body of the solid which is called *absorption*.

The adsorption at the surface of an adsorbent depends upon the nature of the surface forces involved. If these forces are weak and physical in nature, the adsorption is termed physical adsorption. If the forces are strong and chemical in nature, the adsorption is called *chemisorption*.

It has been observed that the extent of adsorption decreases with increasing temperature. If the temperature and amount of adsorbent is kept constant, the extent of adsorption increases with the increase in the concentration of adsorbate. Freundlich has given a relation between the extent of adsorption and equilibrium concentration of the adsorbate—it is known as Freundlich adsorption isotherm :

$$\frac{x}{m} = K.C^{1/n}$$

where x is the amount adsorbed by m g of adsorbent, C is the equilibrium concentration of the adsorbate.' K and n are empirical constants. The present experiment is so planned that the amount of adsorbent and temperature is kept fixed but the amount of adsorbate is gradually increased. The graph between $\log x/m$ and $\log C$ is plotted which gives a straight line showing a direct proportionality between adsorption and concentration of adsorbate.

Preparation of Solutions

1. Prepare 0·5 N oxalic acid soln by dissolving exactly 7·875 g of pure oxalic acid in small amount of water and then making up the volume to 250 ml in a measuring flask.

2. Prepare 0·1 N sodium hydroxide soln as described in experiment 8·1.

Procedure

(i) Clean and dry five bottles with tight glass stoppers, number them from 1 to 5 and introduce into each bottle accurately weighed

2·0 g of finely powdered activated charcoal. (The given charcoal should be dried in an oven at about 100°C for 1 hour and then cooled in a desiccator—this is known as activated charcoal). Add oxalic acid soln and water to each bottle (by means of a burette) according to the following scheme :

Bottle no.	1	2	3	4	5	6
Ml of 0·5 N oxalic acid	50	40	30	20	10	0
Water (ml)	0	10	20	30	40	50

(ii) Stopper the bottles and shake them for about 30 minutes by means of an electric shaker so that an equilibrium is attained. (If a theimostat is available suspend these bottles into it for about 1 hour with intermittent shaking).

(iii) Take bottle no. 1 and filter the supernatant liquid using a dry filter paper (reject first 5 ml of the filtrate). Collect the filtrate in a clean and dry conical flask. Pipette out 10 ml of this soln to another conical flask and titrate it with 0·1 N sodium hydroxide soln using phenolphthalein indicator. Repeat this titration.

(iv) Repeat step (iii) with all the six bottles.

Calculations

Let us try to understand the calculations by taking for example bottle no. 3. In this bottle, 30 ml of 0·5 N oxalic acid has been diluted to 50 ml (30 ml acid+20 ml water). Hence, the normality N of oxalic acid in this bottle, before adsorption has taken place, is given by :

$$50 \times N = 30 \times 0·5$$

$$\therefore \quad N = \frac{30 \times 0·5}{50} = 0·3 \text{ g eq/litre}$$

(initial concentration)

Now equivalent weight of oxalic acid is 63·0, hence weight of oxalic acid per litre will be :

$$0·3 \times 63·0 = 18·9 \text{ g /litre}$$

Suppose after shaking with charcoal and filtration, 10 ml of acid requires 25 ml of 0·1 N NaOH, the normality of the acid be :

$$10 \times N' = 25 \times 0·1$$

$$N' = \frac{25 \times 0·1}{10} = 0·25$$

(normality after adsorption)

∴ 0·25 g eq/litre   =equilibrium concentration.

The weight of oxalic acid present per litre is

$$0·25 \times 63·0 = 15·75 \text{ g/litre}$$
(equilibrium concentration)

The difference in the initial and equilibrium concentration is :

(18·90 − 15·75) g/litre = 3·15 g

For 1000 ml, the amount of acid adsorbed is 3·15 g

∴ 50 ml   ...   ... $\dfrac{50}{1000} \times 3·15$

$$= 0·1575 \text{ g } (=x)$$

This in bottle no. 3, the value of x, *i.e.*, the quantity of oxalic acid adsorbed is 0·1575 g ; the value of m is 2g, hence,

$$\frac{x}{m} = \frac{0·1575}{2·000}$$

Similarly the value of x/m for all the six cases can be calculated.

The different values of log x/m are plotted against corresponding values of log of equilibrium concentrations when a straight line is obtained. Thus Freundlich adsorption isotherm is verified.

Note. The concentration of sodium hydroxide soln used for titrating oxalic acid soln in different cases should be so chosen that the titre value ranges from 5 to 20 ml.

PART V

PHYSICO-CHEMICAL
OR
INSTRUMENTAL METHODS OF
QUANTITATIVE ANALYSIS

PART V

Physico-Chemical or Instrumental Methods of Quantitative Analysis

It has already been stated (see sections 1·3·7 and 1·3·8) that the methods of quantitative analysis can be divided into two major categories ; classical methods and instrumental or physicochemical methods. Gravimetric and volumetric procedures constitute the classical methods of analysis. Those methods in which quantitative analysis is achieved by measuring physical properties such as current strength, electrical conductance, electrical potential, polarisation, optical rotation, scattering of light, intensity of light, absorbance of radiations etc., are termed physicochemical methods. These are also sometimes called instrumental methods since they involve the use of instruments in addition to balances, pipettes, measuring flasks etc. It should be noted that the volumetric and gravimetric procedures require only simple instruments like burettes, pipettes, measuring flasks, balances, beakers, conical flasks, crucibles, funnels, filtration assemblies etc. Furthermore, these methods are based on the measurement of either the weight or volume. Such methods are simple, give accurate results and because no special equipment is needed hence are not very expensive and are therefore quite useful to ordinary laboratories. Instrumental methods, on the other hand, require costly equipment but they are normally quite rapid, very sensitive and, therefore, are extremely useful while dealing with micro samples. Thus both categories of methods have their own advantages and disadvantages and it is wrong to think that one is superior to another. As a matter of fact they are supplementary to each other. An instrumental method requires calibration which is done with the help of solutions of known concentrations. Such standard solutions are generally prepared by standardisation using titrimetric procedures. Once the instrument has been calibrated, it can then be used with great advantage for the microanalysis where a visual titrimetric method may not give accurate results due to inefficiency of the indicator in very dilute solution.

Part-V describes some of the important physicochemical or instrumental methods used in quantitative analysis. These can be broadly classified into the following types :

(A) Methods based on the measurement of electrical properties.

(B) Methods based on the measurement of radiant energy.

(C) Methods based on the measurement of radioactivity.

(D) Methods based on the measurement of other physical properties such as viscosity, surface tension etc.

14

Quantitative Analytical Methods Based on the Measurement of Electrical Properties

The methods of quantitative analysis based on the measurement of electrical properties are briefly called electrical methods of analysis. The main techniques employed in these electrical methods are :

A. Potentiometric titration

B. Conductometric titration

C. Polarographic, polarometric, or amperometric titration

D. Coulometry (coulometric titrations)

Electrometric titrations

E. Electrogravimetric analysis

14·A. POTENTIOMETRIC TITRATION METHOD

14·A·1. THEORY

When a metal electrode is dipped in a solution containing its own ions, there are two opposite processes which take place at the metal-soln junction. The metal atoms have a tendency to pass into soln in the form of metal ions. For a monovalent metal, M, this process (ion-formation process) can be represented as :

$$M - e \rightarrow M^+ \text{ (or, } M \rightarrow M^+ + e) \qquad \ldots(14·1)$$

At the same time, the metal ions, M^+, present in the soln have a tendency to get discharged on the surface of the metal electrode. This process known as ion-discharge process can be represented as :

$$M^+ + e \rightarrow M \qquad \qquad ...(14\cdot2)$$

If the process $(14\cdot1)$ is predominant, more electrons will be produced than are consumed in the process $(14\cdot2)$. Hence, the electrons will be in excess and these will be deposited on the metal surface consequently the metal electrode will acquire a negative charge. On the other hand, if the process $(14\cdot2)$ is predominant, more electrons will be required than supplied by the process $(14\cdot1)$. These extra electrons are supplied by the metal electrode. Now, the metal is made of atoms which are electrically neutral. If electrons are taken out from these neutral atoms, the metal will be left with a positive charge. Thus, when a metal is dipped in a soln containing its own ions, it acquires certain potential which is known as the *electrode*

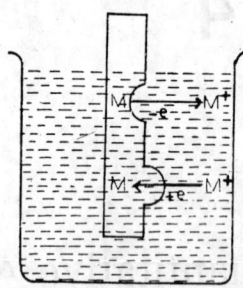

Fig. 14·1. Formation and discharge of ions.

potential. The sign of the potential depends upon the nature of the metal of which the electrode is made. In certain metals like Zinc, the ion-formation process is predominant hence it will have a negative potential. (Zinc can easily give out electrons hence it will have reducing properties). In copper, for example, the ion-discharge process is predominant so it will have a positive potential and since Cu^{2+} has a tendency to accept electrons this ion will have oxidising properties.

When a metal is placed in a soln of its ions, ion-formation and ion-discharge processes take place at different rates. But after some time the rate of formation of ions becomes equal to the rate of their discharge. The electrode is then said to be in equilibrium and the potential it acquires under such condition is referred to as its *reversible potential* which is shown by E and is given by :

$$E = E^\circ + \frac{RT}{nF} \ln {}^a M^{n+} \qquad \qquad ...(14\cdot3)$$

E° = standard electrode potential of the metal

R = gas constant

T = temperature

n = valency of the metal ion

F = Faraday

$^a M^{n+}$ = activity of the metal ion in the soln.

If $^aM^{n+}$ is unity, then

$$E = E° + \frac{RT}{nF} \ln 1$$

$$\ln 1 (= \log_e 1) = 0$$

$$E = E°$$

The standard electrode potential of a metal is thus equal to its electrode potential when the metal electrode is placed in a soln containing its own ions at unit activity. In dilute solutions activity can be taken to be equal to concentration (see section 4'1). If values of R and F are substituted, temperature is taken to be 25°C, $\log_e$ is converted into $\log_{10}$, and activity is replaced by concentration, expression (14'3) reduces to :

$$E = E° + \frac{0'059}{n} \log [M^{n+}] \qquad \qquad ...(14'4)$$

$[M^{n+}]$ = concentration of metal ion in the soln. Thus, the value of E depends upon the metal ion concentration in the soln.

Example 14'A(i)

If a piece of pure Ag metal is dipped in 0'1 M $AgNO_3$ soln, the potential (E) assumed by the silver piece will be called electrode potential of Ag in 0'1 M $AgNO_3$. Similarly if 0'01 M $AgNO_3$ soln is taken, the potential (E) of the silver metal will be called the electrode potential of Ag in 0'01 M $AgNO_3$. Note that the two values of the electrode potential will be different because the metal is immersed in two $AgNO_3$ solutions of different concentrations. If the concentration of $AgNO_3$ soln is 1 M, then the potential (E°) acquired by a Ag electrode, dipped in it will have a definite value at a constant temperature and it will be called the standard electrode potential of Ag at the given temperature.

14'A'1'1. Measurement of Electrode Potential

Potential of a single electrode cannot be measured. It is, therefore, coupled with another electrode whose potential is known ; this is called *reference electrode*. The two electrodes, *i.e.*, experimental electrode whose potential is to be found out and the reference electrode constitute a cell (X) whose e.m.f. can be measured by a potentiometer.

Fig. 14'2 shows various components of a potentiometer. At first the standard cell is connected through key K_2, the moving contact M is moved along the wire AB and that position of M is found out which gives no deflection in the galvanometer. The length AM on the scale is noted. Then the standard cell is removed from the circuit and the unknown cell is connected. Again the position M' of the moving contact is found out for no deflection in G. The

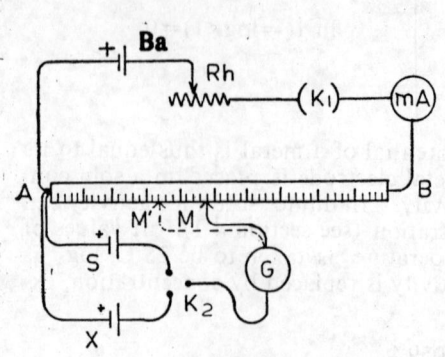

AB = metal wire
Ba = battery
Rh = rheostat
K_1 = key
mA = milliammeter
S = standard cell (having known e.m.f.)

X = unknown cell formed by combining experimental and reference electrode

K_2 = two way key
G = galvanometer
M = moving contact

Fig. 14·2. Potentiometer.

length AM′ is also recorded. Now, if E_s is the e.m.f. of the standard cell and E_x is that of the unknown cell, then :

$$\frac{E_x}{E_s} = \frac{AM'}{AM}$$

or,

$$E_x = E_s \times \frac{AM'}{AM}$$

The value of E_s is known, AM′ and AM are also known, hence the value of E_x can be calculated. The e.m.f. of the unknown cell, E_x, is the algebraic sum of the potentials of the experimental and reference electrode. The value of E_x and the potential of the reference electrode are known so the value of the potential of the experimental electrode can be calculated.

14·A·1·2. Indicator and Reference Electrode

It has been seen in section 14·A·1 that when a metal electrode is immersed in a soln containing its own ions, the metal attains equilibrium with its ions. The electrode is then said to be reversible with respect to its ions, and the potential assumed by the electrode is known as its reversible potential in that particular soln. From equation (14·4) it is evident that this potential depends upon the metal ion concentration in the soln. Thus the magnitude of the electrode potential is indicative of the metal ion concentration of the soln in which the electrode is placed, hence, this electrode is known as *indicator electrode*. If we measure the electrode potential, we can calculate the metal ion concentration in the soln in which the metal electrode is placed with the help of equation (14·4).

Consider pure H_2 gas at 1 atmosphere in contact with H^+ ions in presence of a platinum foil ; this forms a hydrogen electrode (Fig. 14·3). The electrode reaction at the platinum surface is :

$$\tfrac{1}{2}H_2 - e \rightleftharpoons H^+ \qquad \qquad ...(14·5)$$

The potential of the hydrogen electrode will be given by

$$E_{H_2} = E_{H_2}^\circ + \frac{0.059}{1} \log [H^+]$$

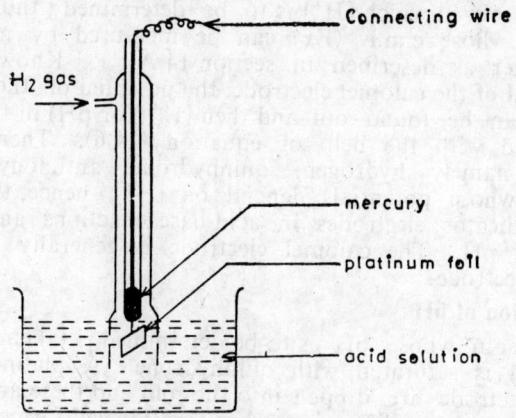

Fig. 14·3. Hydrogen electrode.

The standard electrode potential of hydrogen electrode ($E_{H_2}^\circ$) is taken to be zero by convention so that we can write :

$$E_{H_2} = 0.059 \log [H^+] \qquad\qquad ...(14·6)$$

Thus if we know the value of E_{H_2} we can calculate the H^+ ion concentration of the soln in which the hydrogen electrode is placed. Now, it has already been mentioned in 14·A·1·1 that potential of a single electrode cannot be measured. Hence, if we want to measure the potential of the hydrogen electrode then it must be coupled with another electrode whose potential is known (and constant) and does not depend on [H⁺] of the soln in which it is placed ; such an electrode is called a *reference electrode*. In the present case calomel electrode shown in Fig. 14·4 can be used as a

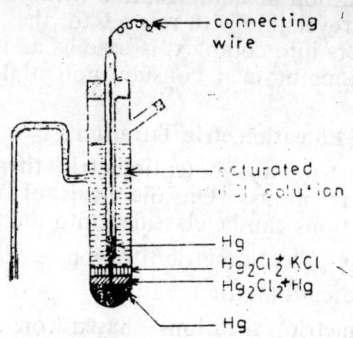

Fig. 14·4. Calomel electrode.

reference electrode. The potential of hydrogen electrode depends upon [H⁺], hence, it is an indicator electrode in this particular case while calomel electrode (whose potential does not depend upon [H⁺]) can act as a reference electrode. These two electrodes are dipped in a soln in which [H⁺] is to be determined ; thus a cell is constituted whose e.m.f. (Ex) can be measured by means of a potentiometer as described in section 14 A 1 1. Knowing Ex and the potential of the calomel electrode, the potential of the hydrogen electrode can be found out and then [H⁺] (or pH) in the soln can be calculated with the help of equation (14·6). There are four electrodes namely hydrogen, quinhydrone, antimony and glass electrodes whose potentials depend on [H⁺], hence, these can be used as indicator electrodes in acid-base reactions and also for finding out pH. The calomel electrode is generally used as the reference electrode.

Determination of pH

The soln whose pH is to be determined is taken in a 100 ml beaker and is saturated with quinhydrone. A platinum and a calomel electrode are dipped into the soln and these are connected to a potentiometer. If E$_{obs}$ is the e.m.f. of the cell formed by these electrodes, the pH of the soln is given by :

$$pH = \frac{0·4533 - E_{obs}}{0·0591}$$

It has been seen in section 10·9, that when a platinum electrode is dipped in a soln containing an oxidant and its reduced form (redox system), its potential depends upon [O$_X$]/[Red], $i.e.$, the ratio of the concentrations of the oxidant and reductant present in the system. When a reductant is titrated with an oxidant, the ratio [O$_X$]/[Red] changes during the course of the titration hence the potential of the platinum electrode will also change. Thus a platinum electrode is used as an indicator electrode for redox titrations and calomel electrode is employed as reference electrode.

In a precipitation or complexation titration, generally a metal electrode, which is reversible with respect to the metal ion that is precipitated or enters into complex, is used as an indicator electrode. An electrode which maintains a constant potential can be used as a reference electrode.

14 A 1 3.   Types of Potentiometric Titration

Like visual titrimetry, potentiometric titrations also use four types of chemical reactions. On the basis of this consideration, potentiometric titrations can be classified into the following types :

(i) Acid-base potentiometric titration.

(ii) Redox potentiometric titration.

(iii) Potentiometric titrations based on precipitation and complexation reactions.

14·A·1·4.   Change of Electrode Potential During a Titration

It was seen in 10·11 (Fig. 10·1) that during a redox titration the potential of the indicator platinum electrode changes slowly in the beginning but there is a sudden jump of potential at the equivalence point. It is true not only for redox titrations but for other types of titrations also and this fact is the basis of potentiometric titration methods.

14·A·2.   POTENTIOMETRIC TITRATION

In a potentiometric titration, the soln (10-25 ml) to be titrated is taken in a 100 ml beaker and a suitable indicator and a reference electrode are immersed in the soln (if the electrodes do not dip properly some distilled water is added to the soln). The electrodes are connected to a potentiometer. The titrant soln is gradually added from a burette. After each addition, the soln is stirred, prefer-

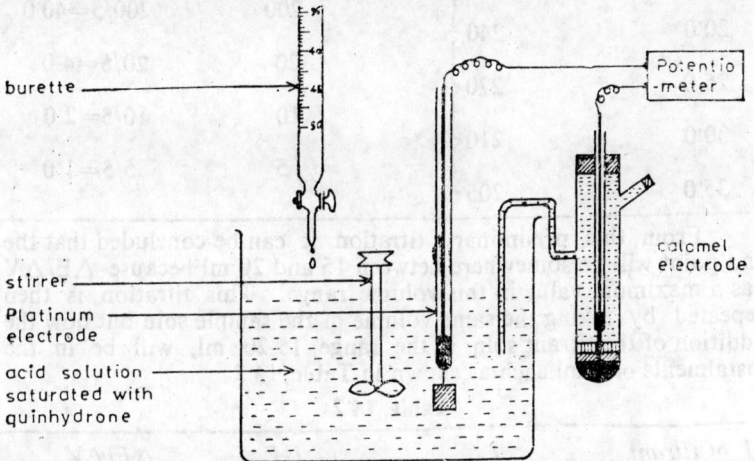

burette

stirrer

Platinum electrode

acid solution saturated with quinhydrone

Potentio-meter

calomel electrode

Fig. 14·5.   Potentiometric titration assembly.

ably by means of an electrical stirrer and potentiometer reading is recorded. Since the potential of the reference electrode remains constant throughout the titration, the change in e.m.f. shown by the potentiometer is actually the change in the potential of the indicator electrode during the titration. Suppose ΔE represents the change in potential when a volume ΔV of the titrant is added. If a graph between different values of $\Delta E/\Delta V$ against corresponding values of volume of the titrant added is plotted, a sharp peak (see Fig. 14·6) is obtained which gives the end point of the titration.

14·A·2·1.   Location of End Point, in a Potentiometric Titration

If we take 20 ml of a sample soln and titrate it with a suitable titrant, we have no idea as to what volume of the titrant would be needed for the titration. We shall, therefore, add the titrant soln in instalments of 5 ml and record the potentiometer reading after each addition. The pattern of readings will be something like that shown in the following table.

Table 14·1. Pattern of Readings in a Potentiometric Titration

Vol. of titrant added (ml)	Potential (E) (mV)	Change in Potential (ΔE)	$\Delta E/\Delta V$
0·0	450		
5·0	448	2	2/5=0·4
10·0	445	3	3/5=0·6
15·0	440	5	5/5=1·0
20·0	240	200	200/5=40·0
25·0	220	20	20/5=4·0
30·0	210	10	10/5=2·0
35·0	205	5	5/5=1·0

From this preliminary titration it can be concluded that the end point will be somewhere between 15 and 20 ml because $\Delta E/\Delta V$ has a maximum value in this volume range. This titration is then repeated by taking the same volume of the sample soln but now the addition of the titrant soln, in the range 15-20 ml, will be in the instalments of 1 ml each as shown in Table 14·2.

Table 14·2

Vol. of titrant (ml)	E (mV)	ΔE	$\Delta E/\Delta V$
0·0	450		
10·0	445	5	5/10=0·5
15·0	440	5	5/5=1·0
16·0	430	10	10/1=10·0
17·0	385	45	45/1=45·0
18·0	375	10	10/1=10·0
19·0	370	5	5/1=5·0
20·0	367	3	3/1=3·0
21·0	365	2	2/1=2·0
22·0	364	1	1/1=1·0

The second titration shows that the end point is between 16 and 17 ml. A third and the final titration is then performed in which the addition of titrant, in the volume range 16 to 17 ml, is done in instalments of 0·1 ml. A graph is then plotted between $\Delta E/\Delta V$ and corresponding volume of the added titrant when a sharp peak is obtained which gives the end point of the titration.

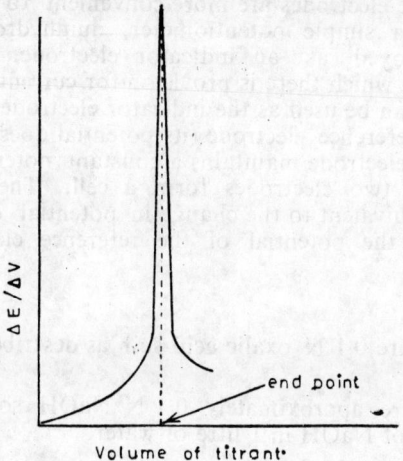

Fig. 14·6. Location of end point in a potentiometric titration.

14·A·2·2. Advantages of Potentiometric Titration

Potentiometric titrations can be used to titrate coloured soln where visual indicators cannot work. Furthermore, in the visual titration of very dilute solutions the colour change of an indicator cannot be located but by using potentiometric technique the equivalence point of the titration can be accurately determined.

14·A·3. LABORATORY EXERCISES

Experiment 14·1

Potentiometric titration of given HCl soln with an alkali soln using quinhydrone-calomel electrode system.

Discussion

When an acid is titrated with an alkali soln, the H^+ ions of the acid react with OH^- ions supplied by the alkali, hence as the titration progresses $[H^+]$ goes on decreasing. Suppose an electrode which is reversible with respect to H^+ ions (an electrode whose potential depends upon $[H^+]$, i.e., an indicator electrode in this case) is dipped in the titration liquid. Now, as we go on adding the alkali soln from the burette, $[H^+]$ will change and so the potential of the indicator electrode. If the rate of change of potential ($\triangle E / \triangle V$) is plotted against the volume of the alkali added, a graph as shown in Fig. 14·6 is obtained from which the end point of the titration is located.

In acid-base titrations hydrogen, quinhydrone, antimony and glass electrodes can act as indicator electrodes. Out of these, glass and quinhydrone electrodes are more convenient to use. If we are working with a simple potentiometer, quinhydrone electrode is generally employed as an indicator electrode. (If we have a potentiometer in which there is provision for current amplification— glass electrode can be used as the indicator electrode). It is coupled with calomel reference electrode (its potential does not deped upon [H⁺] hence this electrode maintains a constant potential during the titration). The two electrodes form a cell. The change in e.m.f. of this cell is equivalent to the change in potential of the indicator electrode since the potential of the reference electrode remains unchanged.

Procedure

(*i*) Prepare 0·1 N oxalic acid soln as described in Experiment 8·1.

(*ii*) Prepare approximately 0·1 N NaOH soln by dissolving roughly 4·5-5 g of NaOH in 1 litre of water.

(*iii*) Pipette out 25 ml of 0·1 N oxalic acid soln into a 100 ml beaker. Add little quinhydrone to this soln and stir by means of a glass rod. In this way go on adding small amounts of quinhydrone gradually with stirring until a saturated soln is obtained. Dip a clean platinum electrode (cleaned with chromic acid and then washed several times with distilled water) into the soln ; now it will be called a quinhydrone electrode. Dip a calomel reference electrode also. Connect the two electrodes to a potentiometer. Perform the titration with NaOH soln [prepared in step (*ii*)] as described in section 14·A·2. Suppose 20·2 ml of alkali soln is required for this titration, the normality of NaOH soln will be :

$$N_{NaOH} \times 20·2 = 0·1 \times 25$$

$$N_{NaOH} = \frac{0·1 \times 25}{20·2} = 0·1238$$

The soln of NaOH is thus standardised potentiometrically by titration with a standard soln of oxalic acid.

(*iv*) Pipette out 25 ml of the given HCl soln and titrate it potentiometrically with standardised NaOH soln in an identical manner as described in the case of oxalic acid in step (*iii*). Suppose 22·5 ml of NaOH soln is required for this titration.

$$25 \times N_{HCl} = 22·5 \times 0·1238$$

$$N_{HCl} = \frac{22 \cdot 5 \times 0 \cdot 1238}{25} = 0 \cdot 1114$$

The normality of given HCl soln will be $0 \cdot 1114$.

Note :

The titre readings should be somewhere between 20 to 30 ml. If the titre volume is too small (say 1 or 2 ml) or too large (say 70 or 100 ml), the strength of the oxalic acid and NaOH soln prepared should be so selected that the titre reading is more than 20 ml and less than about 30 ml.

Experiment 14·2

Potentiometric titration of a given ferrous sulphate soln with potassium dichromate soln.

Discussion

The potential of a platinum electrode dipping in a soln containing an oxidant and also its reduced form (say Fe^{3+} and Fe^{2+} ions) is given by (see sections 10·9, 10·11, equations 10·44 and 10·45) :

$$E_{Redox} = E^{\circ}_{Redox} + \frac{RT}{nF} \ ln \ \frac{[O_X]}{[Red]}$$

The redox potential depends upon the ratio $[O_X]/[Red]$. Now, during a redox titration the ratio $[O_X]/[Red]$ changes, hence, the potential of the platinum electrode dipping in the titration liquid will also change in the course of the titration. In the present titration as $K_2Cr_2O_7$ soln is added to $FeSO_4$ soln more and more Fe^{2+} ions will be converted into Fe^{3+} ions, therefore, the ratio $[Fe^{3+}]/[Fe^{2+}]$ and hence the potential of a platinum electrode dipping in the titration liquid will change. Thus the platinum electrode can act as an indicator electrode. A calomel electrode can be used as a reference electrode because its potential remains constant.

Procedure

(*i*) Dissolve exactly weighed $4 \cdot 9035$ g $K_2Cr_2O_7$ in water, dilute it to 1000 ml in a 1 litre measuring flask. Shake well. This will give $0 \cdot 0167$ M (or $0 \cdot 1$ N) $K_2Cr_2O_7$ soln.

(*ii*) Pipette out 25 ml of the given iron (II) soln into a 100 ml beaker and add about 10 ml of 4N H_2SO_4. Dip a platinum and a calomel electrode into the soln and connect them to a potentiometer. Gradually add $K_2Cr_2O_7$ soln from a burette. Stir the soln after each addition and take the potentiometer reading. The reaction taking place is :

$$6Fe^{2+} + Cr_2O_7^{2-} + 14H^+ \longrightarrow 6Fe^{3+} + 2Cr^{3+} + 7H_2O$$
$$6Fe^{2+} \equiv Cr_2O_7^{2-} \equiv K_2Cr_2O_7$$

(Note that H_2SO_4 is added because H^+ ions take part in the reaction). The end point of the titration is graphically located by plotting $\Delta E/\Delta V$ against volume of $K_2Cr_2O_7$ soln added. If 20·0 ml of $K_2Cr_2O_7$ are used in the titration then :

$$N_{FeSO_4} \times 25 = 0·1 \times 20$$

$$N_{FeSO_4} = \frac{0·1 \times 20}{25} = 0·08$$

The normality of the given ferrous sulphate soln will be 0·08.

Note :

The concentration of the $K_2Cr_2O_7$ soln prepared should be such that the titre value lies between 20 to 30 ml.

14·B. CONDUCTOMETRIC TITRATION METHOD
14·B·1. THEORY

From the view point of electrical conduction substances can be divided into two categories. Those substances which permit the passage of current through them (conduct electric current), are called *conductors*, while substances which do not conduct electricity are known as *insulators*. For the conduction of electricity the presence of charged particles is necessary. Depending upon the nature of the charged particles present in conductors, they can be divided into the following three types :

(*i*) *Metallic or electronic conductors*, such as a piece of Cu or Ag ; in these conductors electrons carry electric current.

(*ii*) *Electrolytic or ionic conductors*, such as an aqueous soln of NaCl or $CuSO_4$; here ions act as carriers of current.

(*iii*) *Mixed conductors*, in which current is partly carried by ions and partly by electrons as is the case with a soln of an alkali metal in liquid ammonia.

According to Ohm's law, the current (C) flowing through a conductor is proportional to the applied voltage (E).

$$C \propto E \quad \text{or,} \quad CR = E \quad \text{or,} \quad C = E/R$$

where R is a constant for a given conductor and is called its *resistance*. The reciprocal of resistance is termed *conductance*, thus :

$$\text{Conductance} = \frac{1}{\text{Resistance}}$$

It means that greater the resistance of a conductor, smaller is its conducting power. The resistance of a conductor is directly proportional to its length (*l*) and inversely proportional to its area of cross-section(s) :

$$R \propto l \quad \text{and} \quad R \propto 1/s \quad \text{so that} \quad R \propto l/s$$

or, $R = \rho \dfrac{l}{s}$ (ρ is a Greek letter pronounced as row)

where ρ is a constant called *specific resistance* of the conductor. If l is 1 cm and s is 1 sq. cm, then

$$R = \rho$$

Thus, specific resistance of a conductor is equal to the resistance of its cube whose each side is equal to 1 cm, *i.e.*, unit cube of that conductor. The reciprocal of specific resistance is called *specific conductance* (κ) of the conductor (κ is a Greek letter pronounced as kapa).

$$\kappa = 1/\rho$$

If we have a solid conductor its unit cube (whose volume is one cubic centimeter) can be prepared and its resistance can be measured ; this will be its specific resistance and its reciporocal will give the specific conductance of the conductor. But if we have a conductor in the form of an electrolyte soln, a special cell, known as *conductivity cell*, has to be used for measuring the specific resistance of the soln conductor. A conductivity cell used for

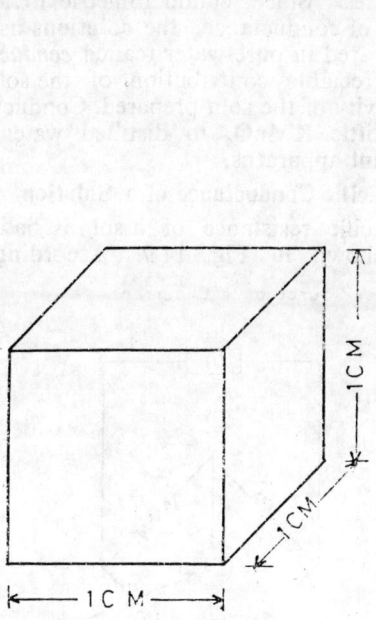

Fig. 14·7. Unit cube.

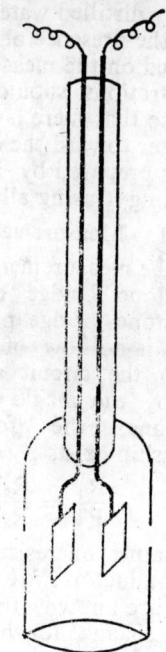

Fig. 14·8. Dip type conductivity cell.

performing a conductometric titration consists of two vertical platinum electrodes each of one square centimeter area and separated by a distance equal to 1 centimeter (Fig. 14·8). This cell is dipped into the soln whose specific conductance is to be determined. The two electrodes between them cover exactly 1 cubic centimeter of soln. The resistance between the two electrodes is measured which gives the value of specific resistance of the soln. The reciprocal of the specific resistance will give the specific conductance or specific conductivity of the electrolyte soln under consideration.

[Note. In a conductivity cell, the area of each electrode may not be exactly 1 sq cm or the distance between them may not be exactly 1 cm. Such a cell cannot measure the specific resistance of a soln accurately. A correction factor, called *cell constant*, has to be determined for the conductivity cell in question. By multiplying the observed specific conductance with the cell constant, the correct value of specific conductance can be calculated. However, it is not necessary to know the cell constant of a conductivity cell used in a conductometric titration because we need not know the exact value of specific conductance. What we want to measure is the change in specific conductance as the titration progresses.]

Pure water has a very poor conductance power, but if we take ordinary distilled water it will have relatively more conducting power due to the presence of impurities. Since conductometric titrations are based on the measurement of conductance, the solutions used in these titrations should be prepared in pure water (called *conductivity water*) so that there is no appreciable contribution of the solvent, *i.e.*, water toward the conductivity of the soln prepared. Conductivity water is prepared by adding little $KMnO_4$ to distilled water and redistilling it using all glass joint apparatus.

14·B·1·1. Measurement of Specific Conductance of a Solution

The measurement of specific resistance of a soln is based on Wheatstone bridge circuit shown in Fig. 14·9. According to Wheatstone bridge principle, if there is no flow of current through the circuit as indicated by the magic eye or headphone, the following relationship exists :

$$\frac{R_1}{R_2} = \frac{R_3}{R_4}$$

If the values of resistance of three conductors, *i.e.*, R_1, R_2 and R_3 are known, the value of the resistance for the fourth (R_4) can be calculated. The apparatus shown in Fig. 14·10, is used for the measurement of specific resistance of a soln.

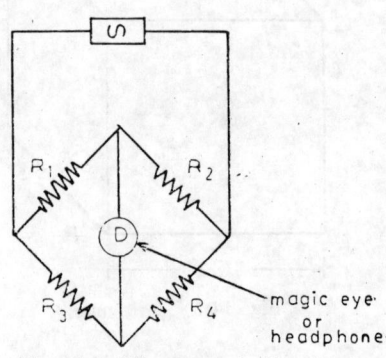

Source of A C current

Fig. 14·9. Wheatstone bridge circuit.

A suitable resistance is introduced by means of the resistance box and moving contact M is moved along the wire AB to a point when there is no flow of current as indicated by the headphone (at this point the sound intensity in the headphone is minimum). The length AM and BM are recorded. Now, according to Wheatstone's bridge principle :

$$\frac{\text{Resistance in conductivity cell C}}{\text{Resistance in resistance box R.B.}} = \frac{BM}{AM}$$

Knowing the resistance of resistance box and lengths AM and BM, the specific resistance of the soln placed in the conductivity cell can be calculated. The reciprocal of the specific resistance will give the observed specific conductance (if this is multiplied by the cell constant, the correct specific conductance can be calculated).

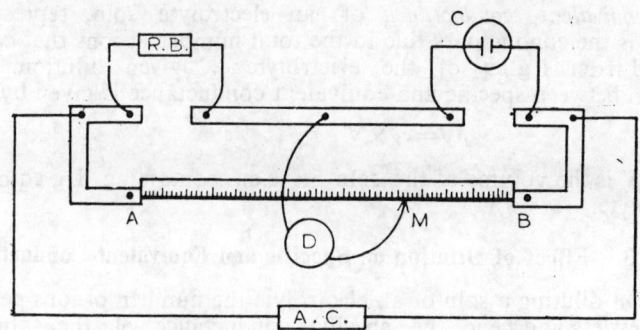

AB = manganin wire of uniform thickness.

RB = resistance box.

C = conductivity cell containing electrolyte solution.

AC = source of A.C. current.

D = detector magic eye or headphone.

M = moving contact.

Fig. 14·10. Measurement of conductance of an electrolyte solution.

14·B·1·2. Specific, Molecular and Equivalent Conductance

It has been seen in 14·B·1 that specific conductance of a soln of an electrolyte means the conductivity of ions present in 1 c.c. of that soln ; this is represented by κ. Now, if 1 g mole of electrolyte is present in 75 c.c. of its soln then conductivity due to all the ions present in 75 c.c. of the soln will be equal to $75 \times \kappa$; this is known as the *molecular conductance* of the electrolyte at given concentration and temperature and is represented by μ. Thus the following relationship exists :

$$\mu_V = \kappa_V \times V$$

where K_V and μ_V are specific and molecular conductance of the electrolyte soln at given dilution and V is the volume in c.c. of the soln containing 1 g mole of the electrolyte.

Example 14·B(i)

In 1000 c.c. of a soln, 0·1 g mole of an electrolyte is present, *i.e.*, the concentration of soln is M/10 or 0·1 M. If the specific conductance of this soln is $\kappa_{M/10}$, calculate its molecular conductance, *i.e.*, $\mu_{M/10}$.

0·1 g mole electrolyte is present in 1000 c.c.

∴   1 g mole electrolyte is present in 10,000 c.c.

$$\mu_{M/10} = \kappa_{M/10} \times 10,000$$

The *equivalent conductance* of an electrolyte soln, represented as Λ_V, is the conductivity due to the total number of ions that can be derived from 1 g eq of the electrolyte at given dilution. The relation between specific and equivalent conductance is given by :

$$\Lambda_V = \kappa_V \times V$$

where V is the volume of the soln in c.c., containing 1 g eq of the electrolyte.

14·B·1·3.   Effect of Dilution on Specific and Equivalent Conductance

On diluting a soln of an electrolyte the number of ions per c.c. becomes less and hence the specific conductauce of the soln also decreases. But as the soln is diluted, the equivalent conductance goes on increasing and eventually reaches a maximum value called equivalent conductance at infinite dilution represented as Λ_∞ or Λ_0. There are two reasons for this increase. Firstly, on diluting an electrolyte soln, the degree of dissociation of the electrolyte increases hence more and more ions become available for conductance. Since equivalent conductance includes conductivity of all the ions, it will increase with dilution of the soln. Furthermore, in a dilute soln the attraction between positive and negative ions is small hence they move at a faster rate in a dilute soln placed between two electrodes ; this is also the reason for the increase in the conductance of an electrolyte soln on dilution.

Kohlrausch showed that the equivalent conductance at infinite dilution of an electrolyte is made of two parts, the contribution to conduction by positive ions and the contribution by negative ions :

$$\Lambda_\infty = \lambda_+^\circ + \lambda_-^\circ$$

where λ_+° and λ_-° are known as the *ionic conductances* of cation and anion respectively.

Table 14'3. Ionic Conductance at Infinite Dilution of Some Ions in Ohm^{-1} cm^2

Cation		Anion	
H$^+$	349·82	OH$^-$	198·0
K$^+$	73·52	Br$^-$	78·4
NH$_4^+$	73·4	Cl$^-$	76·34
Na$^+$	50·11	NO$_3^-$	71·44
1/2 Ba^{2+}	63·64	1/2 SO$_4^{2-}$	79·8

The data given in Table 14·3 show that different ions have different conducting power.

14·B·1·4. Change of Conductance During a Titration

Suppose we take a known volume of HCl soln in a beaker, dip a conductivity cell into it and measure the conductance of the soln by means of a conductivity meter. If a small volume of NaOH soln is added to HCl soln, the reaction will be :

$$(H^+ + Cl^-) + (Na^+ + OH^-) \rightarrow (Na^+ + Cl^-) + H_2O$$

Prior to equivalence point, NaOH will not be in excess and some of the HCl will be converted into NaCl. During this change H$_2$O will also be formed but it has very small conductance which can be neglected. Now Cl$^-$ ion is common to HCl and NaCl, so from conductivity point of view the only change is that H$^+$ ions are replaced by Na$^+$ ions. From Table 14·3, it is seen that the ionic conductance of H$^+$ is much greater than that of Na$^+$ ion, hence as H$^+$ ions are being replaced by Na$^+$ ions, the conductance of the soln will go on decreasing as shown by the conductivity meter. Thus, as we go on adding NaOH soln to HCl soln the conductance will also go on decreasing. After the equivalence point there is no HCl left for NaOH to react with and NaCl formed also does not react with NaOH. Hence, the addition of NaOH after the equivalence point will increase the number of Na$^+$ and OH$^-$ ions so the conductivity would start increasing.

14·B·1·5. Change in Volume During Conductometric Titration

If we take 25 ml of 0·1 M HCl and titrate it with 0·1 M NaOH, the total volume at the equivalence point is 50 ml, *i.e.*, there would be 100 per cent increase in volume. We know that specific conductance of a soln depends upon number of ions present per c.c. of that soln. If the volume of the soln changes during the titration then its specific conductance will also change. Now, we want to record the change in conductance due only to the chemical reaction that takes place during the titration. But if volume is allowed to change it would also contribute toward the change in conductance. It is, therefore, necessary that the volume of the titration liquid must not increase appreciably so that the recorded change in the specific conductance is only due to ionic reaction between the titrand and the titrant. This can be achieved by using a titrant soln which is 100 times stronger than the soln to be titrated, i.e., the titrand soln. For example, if we titrate 50 ml of 0·01 M HCl with 1 M NaOH, the total volume at the end point will be 50+0·5=50·5 ml, i.e., only 1 per cent increase in volume will take place.

14·B·2. CONDUCTOMETRIC TITRATION

Apart from acid-base reactions, those ionic reactions in which there is a sudden change in conductance after the completion of the reaction, can act as a basis of conductometric titration method. Such reactions can be precipitation or complexation reactions. The following assembly is generally used for performing a conducto-metric titration (Fig. 14·11).

A known volume (25 to 50 ml) of the soln to be titrated is taken in a 100 ml beaker. A stirrer and a conductivity cell is dipped into it. The two ends of the cell are connected to a conductivity meter. The titrant soln, which should be about 10 times more concentrated than the titrand soln, is taken in a microburette. The titrant soln in small portions is added through a microburette. The soln is stirred after each addition and its conductance is measured. A graph is then plotted between the observed conductance values and the corresponding volumes of the titrant soln added. The graph gives two straight lines. The point of intersection of these lines indicate the end point of the titration.

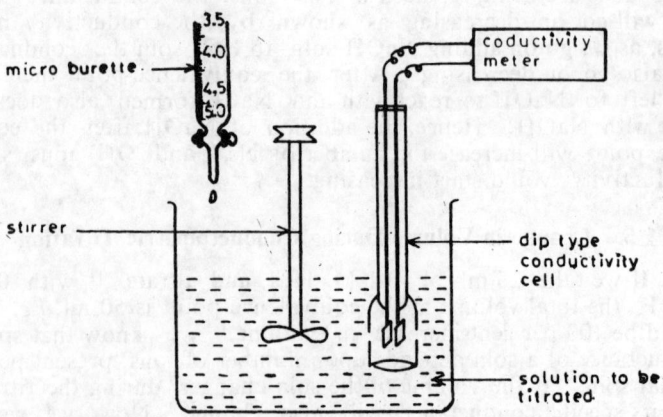

Fig. 14·11. Apparatus for conductometric titration.

14·B·2·1. Applications of Conductometric Titrations

Some typical conductometric titration curves have been shown in Fig. 14·12 *a* to *d*.

(*a*) **Titration of a strong acid with a strong base (HCl-NaOH).** On adding NaOH to HCl, the more conducting H^+ ions of HCl are replaced by less conducting Na^+ ions, hence, the conductivity falls up to the equivalence point. But, thereafter the addition of NaOH causes increase in the conductivity of the soln. The graph obtained for such a titration has been shown in Fig.14·12 *a*.

(*b*) **Titration of a strong acid with a weak base (HCl-NH₄OH).** When NH₄OH soln is gradually added to a soln of HCl, there is replacement of highly conducting H^+ ions by less conducting NH_4^+ ions so the conductivity of the titration liquid goes on decreasing. At the equivalence point all the HCl is converted into NH₄Cl and

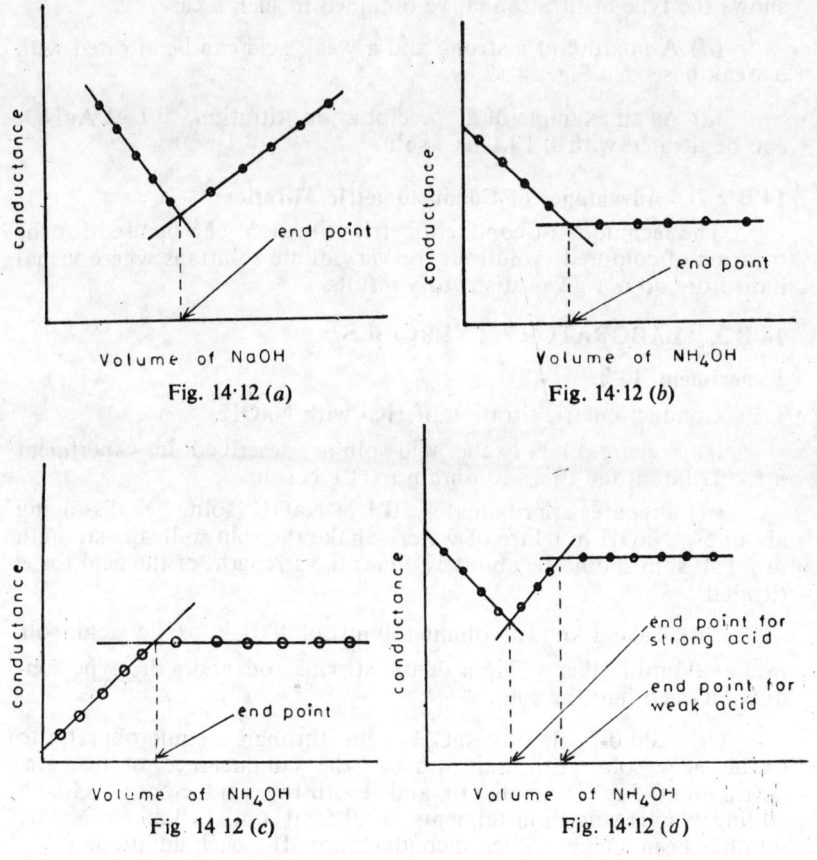

Fig. 14·12 (*a*)

Fig. 14·12 (*b*)

Fig. 14·12 (*c*)

Fig. 14·12 (*d*)

further addition of NH_4OH does not cause any chemical reactions. Since NH_4OH is a weak electrolyte its addition after the equivalence point will not cause any appreciable increase in conductance (note the difference from case (a) where NaOH has been used as the titrant). The graph obtained in this case has been given in Fig. 14·12b.

(c) **Titration of a weak acid with a weak base** ($CH_3COOH—NH_4OH$). Since CH_3COOH is a weak acid, the conductivity of CH_3COOH soln taken for the titration will be quite small. On adding NH_4OH there is formation of the salt CH_3COONH_4 which is a strong electrolyte so conductance will go on increasing until the equivalence point is reached. After the equivalence point, the addition of NH_4OH would not cause any appeciable change in the conductance of the titration liquid because it does not undergo any chemical reaction and is itself a weak electrolyte. Figure 4·12 c shows the type of titration curve obtained in such a case.

(d) A mixture of a strong and a weak acid can be titrated with a weak base (see Fig. 14·12 d).

(e) As an example of a precipitation titration, 0·1 M $AgNO_3$ can be titrated with 0·1 M KCl soln.

14·B·2·2   Advantages of Conductometric Titrations

The technique of conductometric titration can be used for the titration of coloured solutions or very dilute solutions where visual indicators do not give satisfactory results.

14·B·3.   LABORATORY EXERCISES

Experiment 14·3

Conductometric titration of HCl with NaOH.

(i) Prepare 0·1 N oxalic acid soln as described in experiment 8·1. Dilute it ten times to obtain a 0·01 N soln.

(ii) Prepare approximately 0·1 N NaOH soln by dissolving about 5 g NaOH in 1 litre of water. Shake the soln well (the strength of alkali soln should be about 10 times the strength of the acid to be titrated).

(iii) Take a known volume (50 ml) of 0·01 N oxalic acid soln into a 100 ml beaker. Dip a glass stirring rod and a dip type conductivity cell into the soln.

(iv) Add 0·5 ml of NaOH soln through a microburette to oxalic acid soln. Stir and measure the conductance of the soln. Again add 0·5 ml of alkali, stir and record the conductance. Go on adding NaOH soln in instalments of 0·5 ml until 10 ml of NaOH soln has been added. Record conductance after each addition.

(v) Plot different values of conductance against the corresponding volumes of added alkali. Draw two straight lines, the point of intersection will give the volume of the alkali required for the titration.

(vi) Calculate the normality of NaOH soln from the above titration.

(vii) Take 50 ml of given HCl soln (whose normality is near about 0·01 N) and titrate it conductometrically with the standardised NaOH as described for oxalic acid in step (iv). The normality of NaOH is known, hence, that of the given HCl can be calculated.

Experiment 14·4

Conductometric titration of HCl with NH_4OH.

(i) Prepare 0·1 N oxalic acid soln. Dilute it to obtain 0·01 N soln.

(ii) Prepare approximately 0·1 N NH_4OH soln and find out its correct normality by conductometric titration as described in the case of NaOH in experiment 14·3.

(iii) Titrate the given HCl soln conductometrically with standardised NH_4OH soln and calculate the normality of HCl soln.

Experiment 14·5

Conductometric titration of CH_3COOH with NH_4OH.

Standardise NH_4OH soln (0·1 N) with oxalic acid as described in experiment 14·4. Find out the normality of CH_3COOH soln by titrating it conductometrically with NH_4OH soln.

14·C. POLAROGRAPHY AND AMPEROMETRIC TITRATIONS
14·C·1. THEORY

It has been mentioned in 14·A·1 that when at a metal electrode, the rate of formation of ions is equal to the rate of their discharge, the electrode is said to be in equilibrium. The potential acquired by the electrode under such a condition is called its reversible (or equilibrium) potential and is represented by E. When the electrode is in equilibrium there is no flow of current through the electrode. Now, if such conditions are created that there is an actual passage of current through the electrode then, it will be disturbed from its equilibrium condition; this disturbance of equilibrium associated with the flow of current is called *electrolytic polarisation*.

Example 14. C(i)

Consider a copper electrode dipping in a soln of $CuSO_4$. When the copper electrode attains equilibrium, the rate of formation of Cu^{2+} ions is equal to the rate of their discharge so, there is no flow of current through the electrode. The potential assumed by copper electrode under these conditions, E_{Cu}, will be called the reversible potential of copper in the given soln of $CuSO_4$ at experimental temperature. Imagine that a platinum electrode is also dipped into $CuSO_4$ soln and it is connected to the positive terminal while the copper electrode is connected to the negative terminal of a battery. The platinum and copper electrodes dipping in $CuSO_4$ soln constitute an electrolytic cell. When battery is switched on, the current passes through the cell. At the cooper cathode, now, there is an actual passage of current and the rate of discharge of ions is greater than the rate of formation of ions, hence, the electrode will not be in equilibrium and its potential will also be now different from E_{Cu}. The electrode, therefore, will said to be polarised. The greater the difference between the electrode potential and its reversible value, the greater will be the extent of polarisation. Suppose the reversible potential of a copper electrode in a given $CuSO_4$ soln is 0.32 volt. This electrode is then made cathode of an electrolytic cell and current is made to pass through   the copper electrode when its potential changes to 0.30 volt. Since the actual potential (0.30 volt) differs from the reversible value (0.32 volt), the electrode is said to be polarised. The difference between the two values, $(0.32—0.30)=0.02$ volt, is small so the extent of polarisation will also be small. If the applied e.m.f. is increased so that the potential of the copper electrode (cathode potential) becomes 0.15 volt, the difference from the reversible value, $(0.32—0.15)=0.17$ volt, is relatively large and, hence, the extent of polarisation will be greater in the second case.

14·C·1·1.   Decomposition Voltage

Consider two smooth platinum electrodes dipping in a soln of 1 M H_2SO_4. By moving the moving contact M along the wire AB (from A to B) the applied voltage can be gradually increased. If a small voltage say 0.5 volt is applied to the electrodes, the milliammeter

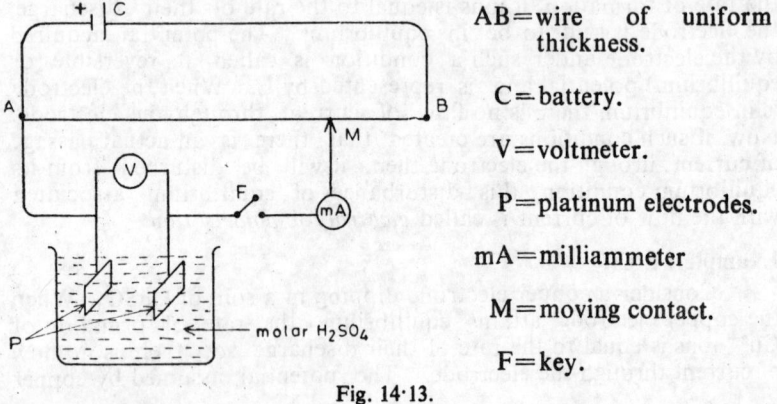

AB = wire   of   uniform thickness.

C = battery.

V = voltmeter.

P = platinum electrodes.

mA = milliammeter

M = moving contact.

F = key.

Fig. 14·13.

(mA) shows a deflection which after a short time becomes zero. On gradually increasing the applied voltage there is only a slight increase in current as shown by the milliammeter. But after a certain value of the applied voltage, the current suddenly increases rapidly, bubbles of gas start coming out freely from the electrodes and continuous electrolysis begins. Upon plotting the current against applied voltage, a curve of the type shown in Fig. 14·14 is obtained. The minimum external voltage that must be applied in order to bring about continuous electrolysis is called the *decomposition voltage*. In the example under consideration, when the applied voltage reaches 1·7 volt, there is a sudden rise in current and bubbles of gases start coming out from the electrode surface, hence the value of decomposition potential will be 1·7 volt. The value of the decomposition voltage depends upon the nature of the metal of which the electrodes are made. For example, the decomposition voltage for molar H_2SO_4 with smooth platinum electrodes is 1·7 volt but with lead electrodes this value is 2·2 volt.

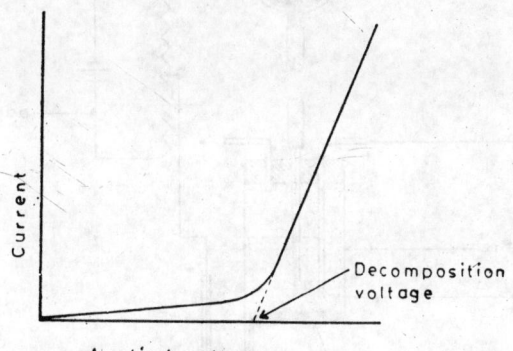

Fig. 14·14.

[**Over voltage**—It has been mentioned in the above paragraph that when a small voltage is applied, milliammeter shows a flow of current for a short period. This means that the electrolysis takes place at this stage and there is liberation of H_2 at the cathode and O_2 at the anode. The liberated H_2 gets deposited at the platinum cathode, H^+ ions are present in the soln—thus a hydrogen electrode is set up. Similarly an oxygen electrode is set up at the platinum anode. The hydrogen and oxygen electrodes constitute a hydrogen-oxygen cell whose e.m.f. (which has a value of 1·23 volt) opposes the applied e.m.f. This is the reason why the current does not increase in the beginning on increasing the applied voltage. The e.m.f. of hydrogen-oxygen cell is, therefore, called *back* or *counter* e.m.f. Since the value of back e.m.f. is 1·23 volt it is reasonable to expect that if 1·23 volt are applied from a battery then the resistance of hydrogen-oxygen cell can be overcome. It means that the value of the decomposition voltage should also be 1·23 volt. But the observed value is 1'7 volt. The difference between the observed value of the decomposition voltage and the back e.m.f. is called over voltage or over potential. In the present example, the value of over voltage will be (1'7−1'23)=0'47 volt. If any of the steps in the ion-discharge or ion-formation process is slow an extra energy is needed to speed it up—this is the reason for the existence of the over voltage. The total over voltage is the sum of the over voltages at the cathode and at the anode].

14'C.1'2. Polarography

A glass vessel C shown in Fig. 14'15 is known as a polarographic cell. It contains a large quantity of mercury at its bottom

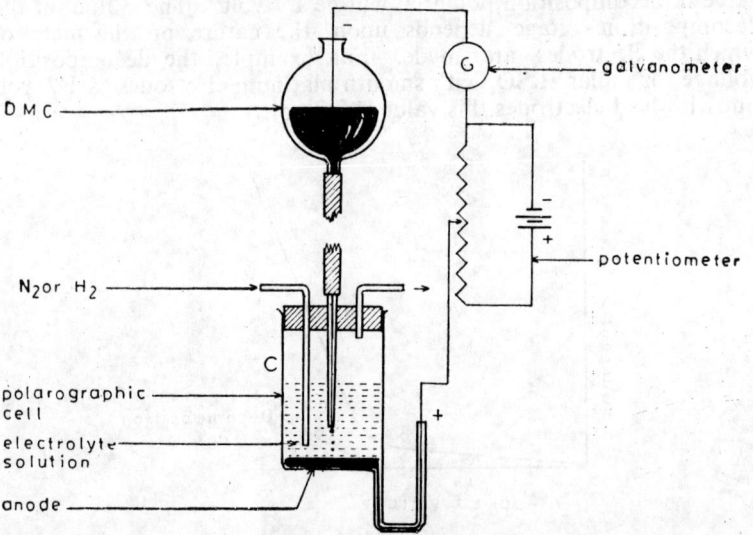

Fig. 14·15. Polarograph.

which acts as an anode. Because of its large area the mercury anode does not get polarised. A dropping mercury cathode (DMC) which consists of a succession of small mercury drops falling slowly from a fine capillary tube is used as an indicator electrode. This is the electrode which is made of very fine drops whose area is small; hence, this electrode gets polarised. The electrolyte is a dilute soln of the electroactive material to be analysed (say $CdCl_2$ soln), to which a large quantity of an indifferent electrolyte such as KCl has been added (note that KCl does not react with $CdCl_2$, hence, can act as an indifferent electrolyte in this case). The function of the *indifferent* or *supporting* or *base* electrolyte is to increase the conductance of the soln. Pure N_2 or H_2 gas is bubbled through the soln to drive out the dissolved oxygen. Cadmium ions are discharged at the cathode :

$$Cd^{2+}+2e \rightarrow Cd$$

We can also say that Cd^{2+} ions are reduced ; thus cadmium ions will be called *electro-reducible material*.

The voltage applied to the polarographic cell is gradually increased and for each value of applied voltage the corresponding value of current is recorded by means of galvanometer G. A graph is then plotted between applied voltage and current ; this gives what is known as current-voltage curve (in brief C-V curve shown in Fig. 14·16). The curves so obtained are a graphical representation of the polarisation of the dropping mercury cathode, hence, these C-V curves are called *polarograms* and the apparatus used to obtain these curves is known as a *polarograph*. From the examination of the C-V curve, it is possible to identify electroactive material

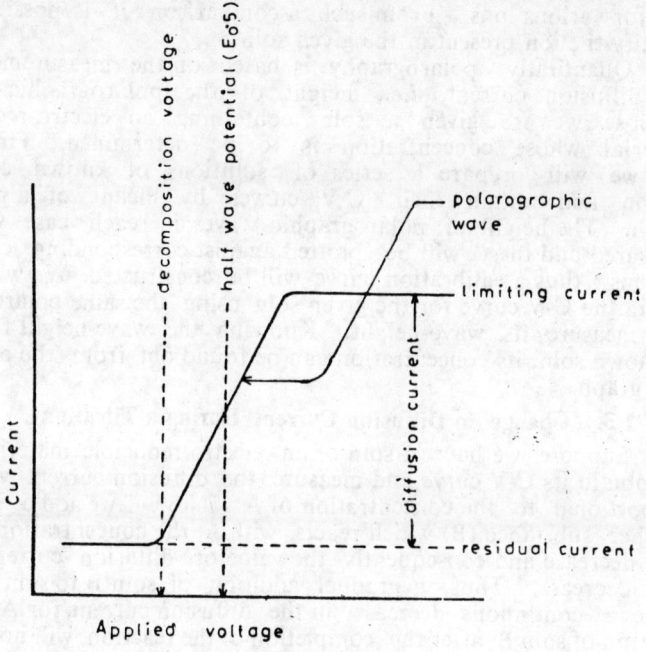

Fig. 14·16.   C-V curve.

present in the soln and its amount can also be determined. The half-wave potential is characteristic of the reacting material ; this is the basis of *qualitative polarography*. The diffusion current (which is equal to the height of the polarographic wave) is proportional to the amount of the reacting material ; this is the basis of *quantitative polarography*.

It will be seen in Fig. 14·16 that when the voltage applied to a polarographic cell (containing soln of an electroactive material such as $CdCl_2$, $ZnCl_2$ or $MnCl_2$) is increased, the current in the circuit remains practically constant ; this is called *residual current*. When the voltage reaches the value E_D (decomposition voltage for the electroreducible matter taken in the cell), the current suddenly starts flowing. On further increasing the voltage, current rises very rapidly and eventually becomes constant ; this is known as the *limiting current*. The difference between the limiting and residual current is termed *diffusion current* ; this is equal to the height of the polarographic wave. The midpoint of this wave gives the half-wave potential ($E_{0.5}$). Each electro-reducible ion has a definite value for its half-wave potential. Suppose we are given a soln containing a metal ion which is to be identified. First, we will obtain C-V curve with the help of a polarograph and find out the value of $E_{0.5}$ for the given ion. This value will then be compared with known values of $E_{0.5}$ for various ions. From such a comparison it is possible to identify the ion present in the given soln.

Quantitative polarography is based on the measurement of the diffusion current, *i.e.*, height of the polarographic wave. Suppose we are given a soln containing an electro-reducible material whose concentration is to be determined. First of all, we will prepare a series of solutions of known concentration and obtain their C-V curves by means of a polarograph. The height of polarographic wave in each case will be measured and these will be plotted against corresponding concentrations ; thus a calibration curve will be constructed. We will then obtain the C-V curve for the given soln using the same polarograph and measure its wave-height. Knowing the wave-height for the unknown soln, its concentration can be found out from the calibration graph.

14C.1.3. Change in Diffusion Current During a Titration

Suppose we have a soln of an electro-reducible material (A). We obtain its C-V curve and measure the diffusion current which is proportional to the concentration of A. Now, if we add a soln of another substance (B) which reacts with A, the concentration of A will decrease and consequently the value of diffusion current will also decrease. Thus, a gradual addition of soln B to soln A will cause a continuous decrease in the diffusion current for A. The addition of soln B, after the completion of the reaction, will not cause any change, hence, the value of diffusion current will remain constant. If the different values of diffusion current are plotted against corresponding values of the volume of soln B added, a sudden change in diffusion current is observed at the completion of the reaction. This is the basis of what are known as *amperometric*, or *polarographic* titrations. Different types of titration curves are obtained depending upon the nature of the titrand and titrant soln ; these will be discussed in section 14C.2.1.

14C.2. AMPEROMETRIC TITRATION METHOD

An amperometric titration can be performed in a polarographic cell of the type shown in Fig. 14.17. A known volume of the soln

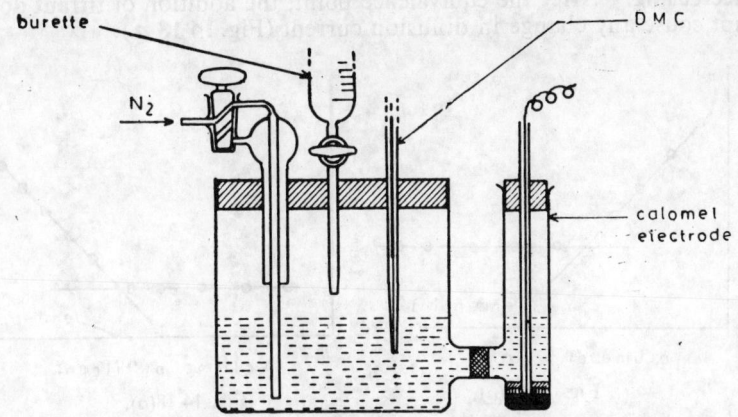

Fig. 14·17. Amperometric titration.

to be titrated is taken in this cell, a large amount of an indifferent electrolyte and little agar-agar are added. Pure N_2 gas is bubbled through the soln to expel the dissolved O_2. The titrant soln, whose concentration should be 10 times than that of the soln to be titrated (titrand), is taken in a microburette. A dropping mercury cathode (DMC) is used as an indicator electrode and a calomel electrode as a reference electrode. A suitable voltage is applied to the polarographic cell so that the maximum value of diffusion current is obtained, which is measured by a galvanometer placed in the circuit. A small volume of the titrant soln is added through a microburette, N_2 gas is bubbled through the soln and galvanometer reading is recorded. This procedure is repeated to obtain several current readings which are plotted against the corresponding volumes of the titrant added. The point of intersection of two straight lines in the graph gives the end point of the titration.

14·C·2·1. Location of End Point in Amperometric Titration

Some of the typical curves in amperometric titrations have been shown in Fig. 14·18 a-c. If the C-V curves of titrant and titrand are not known then these must be obtained by separate experiments. This helps in finding out the suitable voltage-range in which the titration should be performed. The voltage applied in the beginning of the titration must be such that the total diffusion current of the titrand, or of the titrant or of both is obtained. The titration curves obtained in different cases are discussed below.

(a) *The titrand gives the diffusion current but the titrant does not* :—A suitable voltage is applied so that the total diffusion current of the titrand is obtained. On adding the titrant, the concentration of the titrand and, hence, the diffusion current goes on decreasing. After the equivalence point, the addition of titrant does not cause any change in diffusion current (Fig. **14·18 a**).

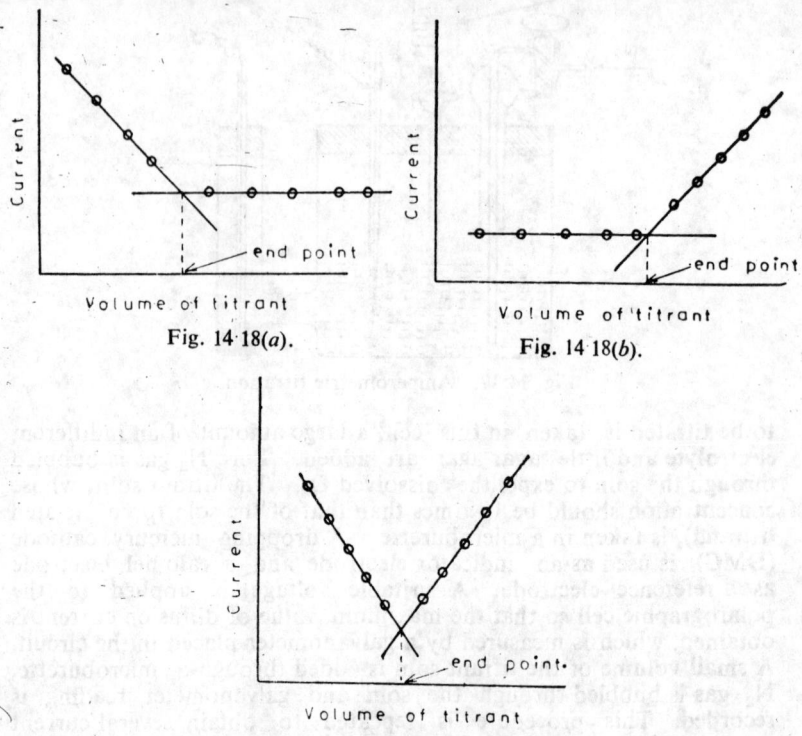

Fig. 14·18(*a*).

Fig. 14·18(*b*).

Fig. 14·18(*c*).

(*b*) *The titrant gives the diffusion current but the titrand does not* :—In this case (Fig. **14·18 b**) there is no diffusion current up to the equivalence point. After the reaction is complete, the titrant is in excess and gives diffusion current. As the volume of titrant, added, is increased the diffusion current also increases.

(*c*) *The titrand and titrant, both give diffusion current* :—As the titrant is added the concentration of the titrand **decreases** and so the diffusion current. At the equivalence point the diffusion current is minimum. After the equivalence point, the addition of the titrant causes increase in the diffusion current (Fig. 14·18 *c*).

14·C·3. COMPARISON OF POTENTIOMETRIC, CONDUCTO-METRIC AND AMPEROMETRIC TITRATIONS

It has been seen in sections 14·A, 14·B and 14·C that potentio-metric titrations are based on the measurement of potential, **conduc-**

tometric titrations on that of conductance and measurement of current is the basis of amperometric titrations. Since these three types of titrations are based on the measurement of electrical properties, these are called *eletrometric titrations*. Coulometric titrations described in 14·D·4 are also a type of electrometric titrations. Some of the similarities and dissimilarities between them are mentioned below.

In potentiometric titrations the readings near the equivalence point are important. But it is not so in conductometric and amperometric titrations because here the end point is located graphically as the point of intersection between two straight lines giving the change of conductance or current strength before and after the equivalence point.

In conductometric and amperometric titrations the concentration of the titrant soln should be atleast $^-10$ times than that of the soln to be titrated. This is not necessary in a potentiometric titration.

If in a precipitation titration, the ppt formed has some solubility, then accurate results cannot be obtained by means of a potentiometric titration. But amperometric or conductometric titration will still give satisfactory results because readings near the equivalence point are not very important.

A number of amperometric titrations can be carried out at high dilutions (with 10^{-3} to 10^{-4} N solutions) at which visual or potentiometric titrations no longer give satisfactory results.

14·C·4. LABORATORY EXERCISE

Experiment 14·6

Amperometric titration of lead nitrate with potassium dichromate.

Discussion

At an applied voltage of 1 volt both Pb^{2+} and $Cr_2O_7^{2-}$ ions give diffusion current. As $K_2Cr_2O_7$ soln is added to $Pb(NO_3)_2$ soln, the diffusion current due to Pb^{2+} ions goes on **decreasing** and after the equivalence point it again increases due to increasing concentration of $Cr_2O_7^{2-}$ ions. Thus a V shape curve (see Fig 14·18·c) is obtained.

Procedure

(i) Prepare a 0·01 M $Pb(NO_3)_2$ soln by weighing. Dilute it 10 times to obtain 0·001 M soln.

(ii) Prepare a 0·05 M $K_2Cr_2O_7$ soln by weighing. Dilute it 10 times to obtain a 0·005 M soln.

(iii) Prepare a 0·01 M KNO_3 soln by weighing.

(*iv*) Assemble a polarograph as shown in Fig. 14·17.

(*v*) Set up a dropping mercury cathode and allow the mercury drops to fall into distilled water for about 5 minutes. Pipette out 25 ml of 0·001 M $Pb(NO_3)_2$ soln into the polarographic cell. Add little gelatin and 25 ml of 0·01 M KNO_3 soln and bubble pure N_2 gas through the soln. Introduce DMC into the cell. Apply 1 volt to the polarographic cell by means of the potentiometer. Note the galvanometer reading. Add 0·5 ml of 0·005 M $K_2Cr_2O_7$ soln, bubble N_2 gas through the soln and again note the galvanometer reading. Repeat this process to take sufficient current readings so that two straight lines are obtained in the graph between current against volume of $K_2Cr_2O_7$ soln added. Since the volume of the titration liquid changes after each addition of $K_2Cr_2O_7$ soln, a volume correction is applied. Multiply the observed current reading with $(V+x)/V$, where V is the initial volume of the soln and x is the volume of the titrant added. Plot the values of the corrected current readings on Y axis and corresponding volume of the titrant on X axis. Draw two straight lines and note the point of intersection of these lines which gives the end point of the titration (see Fig. 14·18 *c*). The concentration of $K_2Cr_2O_7$ is known, hence, that of the given $Pb(NO_3)_2$ can be calculated.

14·D. COULOMETRY

14·D·1.   THEORY

According to Faraday's first law of electrolysis, the extent of chemical reaction at an electrode is directly proportional to the quantity of electricity passing through the electrode. Consider two Cu electrodes dipping in $CuSO_4$ soln, and connected to a battery. On passing electric current, Cu is deposited on Cu cathode. If *w* g Cu is deposited in *t* seconds then by passing the current of the same strength for 2 *t* seconds, 2 *w* g of Cu will be deposited.

A coulomb is the quantity of electricity given by the flow of one ampère of current for one second. It has been found that for liberating 1 g eq of a substance at an electrode, 96,487 coulombs are required ; this quantity of electricity is called a *Faraday* and is represented by F.

Example 14·D(*i*)

Atomic weight of Ag is 107·87, its valency is one, hence, its equivalent weight will also be 107·87. On passing 96,487 coulombs of electricity through a $AgNO_3$ soln containing Ag electrodes, 107·87 g of Ag (1 g eq of Ag) will be deposited. Atomic weight of Cu is 63·54 and its valency is two, hence, its equivalent weight will be 63·54/2=31·77. One Faraday of electricity (96,487 coulombs) will, therefore, liberate 31·77 g of Cu at a cathode when $CuSO_4$ soln is electrolysed.

14·D·1·1. Coulometers

We know that the amount of a substance liberated at an electrode is related to the quantity of electricity passed through the electrode. If we determine the amount of the substance formed at the electrode, it is possible to calculate the quantity of electricity which passed through the electrode. The extent of chemical reaction can thus be used for measuring the quantity of electricity. This is the principle of a *coulometer*. A number of coulometers employing different chemical reactions have been developed ; these include the silver coulometer, the iodine coulometer etc.

A silver coulometer consists of a clean, dry and weighed platinum basin. A 10 per cent $AgNO_3$ soln is placed in the basin and a pure Ag rod is dipped into this soln. The platinum basin acts as a cathode and the silver rod as an anode. Increase in the weight of the platinum basin gives the weight of the silver deposited on it. Knowing the weight of the silver deposited, the quantity of electricity passed through the electrode can be calculated. The iodine coulometer contains a pair of platinum electrodes immersed in a KI soln. When electricity is passed, there is liberation of iodine at the anode :

$$I^- - e \rightarrow \tfrac{1}{2} I_2$$

The liberated iodine is determined by titration with a standard $Na_2S_2O_3$ soln. Knowing the amount of iodine the quantity of electricity passed can be calculated.

Example 14·D(ii)

On passing electricity through a silver coulometer, the amount of silver deposited was found to be 0·0108 g, calculate the quantity of electricity passed.

108 g Ag are deposited by 96,487 coulombs

$$\therefore \quad 0·0108 \text{ g are deposited by } \frac{0·0108}{108} \times 96,487$$

$$= 9·6487 \text{ coulombs.}$$

14·D·2. COULOMETRIC ANALYSIS

Suppose a substance A is formed at an electrode during electrolysis then we can develop a coulometric method for determining the substance A. A soln of the substance A to be determined is placed in an electrolytic cell which is connected in series to a coulometer. Electricity by means of a battery is passed through the cell as well as through the coulometer. After the completion of the reaction in the electrolytic cell, the quantity of electricity used in the dertermination is found out by means of the coulometer. Knowing the quantity of electricity used, the amount of the substance A present in the given soln can be calculated.

14·D·2·1.   Completion of Reaction in Coulometric Analysis

In coulometric analysis it is important to find out when the reaction is complete so that the supply of electricity can then be stopped and quantity of electricity measured by the coulometer. It has been found that in a coulometric analysis at controlled potential, the current generally decreases exponentially with time according to the equation :

$$I_t = I_o.10^{-kt}$$

where I_o is the initial current, I_t the current at time t and k is a constant. Strictly speaking a reaction is never complete, however, when the ratio I_t/I_o falls to 0.001, the reaction may be assumed to be complete and the passage of electricity should be stopped at this stage.

Example 14·D(iii)

A $CuSO_4$ soln is given in which the amount of Cu is to be determined by coulometry ; this can be done in the following manner :

(i) Dip two clean platinum electrodes into the given $CuSO_4$ soln ; this will form an electrolytic cell.

(ii) Connect the cell to a battery through a coulometer and an ammeter.

(iii) Switch on the battery and note the current (I_o) in the ammeter. When the current value becomes $I_o/1000$ (reduces to one thousandth of its original value), switch off the battery.

(iv) Find out the quantity of electricity used from the coulometer

Suppose 0.0108 g of Ag is deposited in the silver coulometer. Then the quantity of electricity used can be calculated as follows :

108 g Ag are deposited by 96,487 coulombs

$$\therefore \quad 0.0108 \text{ g are deposited by } \frac{0.0108}{108} \times 96,487$$

$$= 9.6487 \text{ coulombs.}$$

Now, 96,487 coulombs deposit 31.77 g Cu

$$\therefore \quad 9.6487 \text{ coulombs deposit } \frac{9.6187}{96,487} \times 31.77$$

$$= 0.003177 \text{ g of Cu.}$$

Thus the amount of Cu present in the $CuSO_4$ soln will be 0.003177 g.

14·D·3. SECONDARY COULOMETRIC ANALYSIS

In primary coulometric analysis the substance being determined directly undergoes reaction at one of the electrodes. In example 14·D(iii), the substance being determined is Cu which directly undergoes reaction at the cathode $(Cu^{2+}+2e \rightarrow Cu)$: This is an example of *primary coulometric analysis.* In secondary coulometric analysis the substance being determined reacts with another substance which is generated by an electrode reaction.

Example 14·D(iv)

A $Na_2S_2O_3$ soln is given whose concentration is to be determined by secondary coulometric analysis ; this can be done in the following manner.

(i) Take the given $Na_2S_2O_3$ soln in a beaker and add KI and starch soln to it. Dip two platinum electrodes into the soln ; this forms an electrolytic cell.

(ii) Connect the cell in series to a coulometer and then to a battery.

(iii) Switch on the battery, iodine will be generated, due to the electrolysis of KI, at the anode which will react with $Na_2S_2O_3$ present in the soln. After all the $Na_2S_2O_3$ has reacted, the first excess of I_2 will turn the soln blue due to the presence of starch.

(iv) Switch off the battery as soon as the soln becomes blue. Find out the quantity of electricity used from the coulometer. Knowing the quantity of electricity, the amount of liberated iodine can be calculated and then the quantity of $Na_2S_2O_3$ present in the given soln from the following equation :

$$2Na_2S_2O_3+I_2 \rightarrow 2NaI+Na_2S_4O_6$$

14·D·4 COULOMETRIC TITRATIONS

In a coulometric titration, the reagent soln is not added from a burette as is done in titrimetric analysis but is generated electrically at an electrode. For instance, in example 14·D(iv), the reagent I_2 is electrically generated which then reacts with $Na_2S_2O_3$ present in the soln. Starch shows the end point of the titration.

There are two important conditions which must be fulfilled :

(a) The primary reaction (taking place at the electrode) must take place with 100 per cent efficiency. It means that 1 Faraday of electricity must generate exactly 1 g eq of the reagent.

[Note that 96,487 coulombs liberate exactly 1 g eq (127 g) of I_2, hence, the efficiency of this reaction is 100 per cent].

(b) The reaction between the substance being determined and the electrically generated reagent must be rapid and stoichometric

ANALYTICAL CHEMISTRY

(such as the reaction between $Na_2S_2O_3$ and I_2). Coulometry has the following advantages.

(i) Standard solutions are not needed and in their place coulomb acts as the primary standard.

(ii) Even unstable reagents can be used because they are produced at the electrode and are immediately consumed.

(iii) There is no need to store reagent soln.

(iv) The sample soln does not get diluted because reagent soln is not added from outside. (Note that at greater dilution the detection of end point by indicators becomes difficult).

14·E ELECTROGRAVIMETRIC ANALYSIS

This technique of analysis has already been discussed in section 6·10. The difference between ordinary gravimetric analysis and electrogravimetry is that in the latter electricity is used as a precipitating reagent.

15

Analytical Methods Based on the Measurement of Radiant Energy

It was mentioned in section 1·3·8 that analytical methods may be broadly classified into the following two types :

(i) *Those based on matter-matter interaction.* These involve reactions between a substance being determined and another substance which acts as a reagent. For example, in the titrimetric determination of HCl with NaOH, the analysis is based on the reaction of one substance (HCl) with another substance (NaOH).

(ii) *Those based on matter-energy interaction.* These methods involve interaction between matter and energy. For example, when light is passed through a soln of a substance A, the amount of light absorbed is proportional to the quantity of A present ; this can form a basis of a method for the determination of A. Such a method would involve the measurement of light which is a form of radiant energy.

Several analytical techniques have been developed which involve the measurement of radiant energy. Some of these will be briefly discussed in this chapter ; these are :

(a) Emission spectrography
(b) Colorimetry
(c) Fluorimetry
(d) Turbidimetry and Nephelometry
(e) Spectrophotometry
(f) Flame photometry
(g) Atomic absorption spectroscopy
(h) Polarimetry.

15`A.   EMISSION SPECTROGRAPHY

When sodium chloride is introduced in the flame of a Bunsen burner, a yellow colour is seen. Similarly, a barium salt imparts yellowish green colour and a calcium salt a red colour to the flame. This observation made by Bunsen and Kirchhoff, is the basis of flame test for identifying certain metals. If the light from a flame containing a metal salt is examined by a spectroscope several lines, known as *spectral lines*, are seen. The wavelengths of these lines are characteristic of the metal producing them. For example, a sodium flame examined by a spectroscope will always show two very prominant lines of wavelengths 5890 and 5896 Å. Thus, it is possible to identify a metal by measuring the wavelengths of its spectral lines ; this is the basis of *qualitative emission spectroscopy*. By measuring the intensity of the spectral lines, it is possible to estimate the amount of metal producing these lines ; this is the basis of *quantitative emission spectroscopy*.

15`A`1   Spectroscope

A spectroscope has three essential components. A light source, a dispersing device such as a prism or a grating and a means of observing or recording the spectral lines which form the spectrum. A simple spectroscope has been shown in Fig. 15`1. White light

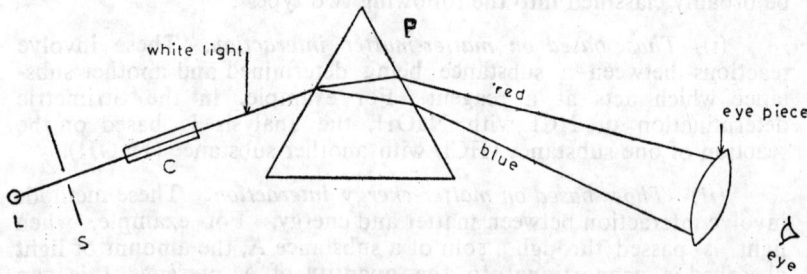

Fig. 15`1. Spectroscope.

from a source L is passed through a slit S to obtain a narrow beam of light. The function of collimator C is to provide a parallel beam of white light which then falls on prism P. If a white screen or a telescope is placed on the other side of the prism a band of seven colours is seen. This separation of light into different colours, of which it is made, is called *dispersion* and the pattern observed is known as *spectrum*. In the narrow beam of white light there are several rays of different wavelengths, these during their passage through the prism bend to different extent that is why they get separated. If in place of a screen, a photographic plate is placed, we can get a permanent record of the spectrum ; the instrument is then called a *spectrograph*.

15˙A˙2 Electromagnetic Spectrum

Light consists of electromagnetic radiations of wavelengths between 4000 to 7600 Å (Å is called Angstrom which is equal to 10^{-8} cm) ; only these wavelengths can affect our eyes hence this wavelength range constitutes *visible region* of spectrum. When the wavelength of a radiation is greater than 7600Å, it is called *infrared* radiation. For still greater wavelengths the term *radiowaves* is used. On the lower side, as the wavelength becomes smaller and smaller we have *ultraviolet, x-rays* and *γ-rays*. Thus we have what is known as the *electromagnetic spectrum*. The visible spectrum forms a very small part (covering 4000 to 7600 Å) of the electromagnetic spectrum.

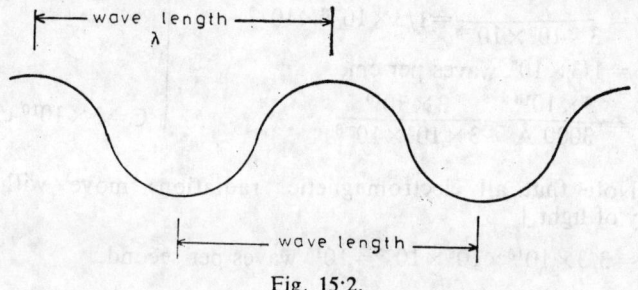

Fig. 15˙2.

Fig. 15˙2 shows the wavelength of an electromagnetic radiation. The reciprocal of wavelength is called wave number and is represented by $\bar{\nu}$, it means number of waves in 1 cm.

$$\frac{1}{\lambda} = \bar{\nu} \qquad \qquad \dots(15˙1)$$

$$\lambda \times \bar{\nu} = C \quad \text{or,} \quad \nu = \frac{C}{\lambda} \qquad \qquad \dots(15˙2)$$

where, λ is the wavelength, $\bar{\nu}$ is the wave number, ν is the frequency of the radiation, C is the velocity of light which is equal to 2.99793×10^8 meters per second. The frequency of radiation means number of waves passing from a point in one second. The units of wavelength in common use are :

Angstrom unit (Å) $= 10^{-10}$ meter or 10^{-8} cm.

Nanometer　(nm) $= 10^{-9}$ meter or 10^{-7} cm.

$$= 10 \text{ Å}$$

Example 15A (i)

The wavelength of a radiation is 3000 Å, calculate its wavelength in meter, centimeter and nanometer. Also calculate its wave number and frequency.

$3000\text{Å}=3000\times10^{-8}$ cm $=3\times1000\times10^{-8}$ cm
$\qquad =3\times10^3\times10^{-8}$ cm $=3\times10^{-5}$ cm

$\dfrac{3\times10^{-5}\text{ cm}}{(3000\text{Å})}=\dfrac{3\times10^{-5}}{100}$ m $=3\times10^{-5}\times10^{-2}$ m

$\qquad\qquad =3\times10^{-7}$ **meter**

3000 Å $=\dfrac{3000}{10}$nm $=$ **300 nm**

$\bar{\nu}=\dfrac{1}{\lambda}=\dfrac{1}{3000\text{ Å}}=\dfrac{1}{3000\times10^{-8}}$

$\qquad =\dfrac{1}{3\times10^3\times10^{-8}}=1/3\times10^{-3}\times10^{+8}$

$\qquad =1/3\times10^5$ waves per cm.

$\nu=\dfrac{C}{\lambda}=\dfrac{3\times10^{10}}{3000\text{ Å}}=\dfrac{3\times10^{10}}{3\times10^3\times10^{-8}}$

> *Remember*
>
> $1\text{Å}=10^{-8}$ cm
>
> 100 cm $=1$m
>
> 1 cm $=\left(\dfrac{1}{100}\text{m}\right)$
>
> $10\text{Å}=1$ nm
>
> $1\text{Å}=\left(\dfrac{1}{10}\text{nm}\right)$
>
> $C=3\times10^{10}$ cm/sec

[Note that all electromagnetic radiations move with the velocity of light.]

$\nu=3/3\times10^{10}\times10^8\times10^{-3}=10^{15}$ waves per second.

15'A'3. Different Types of Spectra

(A) Emission Spectra

When a solid is heated to a high temperature or electricity is passed through a gas (this process is known as excitation), there is emission of light. If this emitted light is examined by means of a spectroscope, the pattern observed will be called an emission spectrum. Emission spectra can be divided into three types.

(i) *Continuous spectrum.* Suppose a solid is strongly heated and the light emitted by it is examined by means of a prism. The spectrum produced will be similar to that given by sunlight. It will show all the colours from red to violet and the spectrum will be continuous, i.e., it will not be possible to find out exactly where one colour ends and the other begins ; such a spectrum would be called a continuous spectrum.

(ii) *Line or atomic spectrum.* If electricity is made to pass through a gas (say for example H_2 gas) taken in a discharge tube, the tube will give out light. On examining this emitted light by means of a spectroscope a pattern will be seen in which bright lines will be separated by dark space. Such spectra are produced by atoms hence are called line or atomic spectra. A flame containing a sodium salt (sodium flame) when viewed through a spectroscope will show two very bright yellow lines (at wavelength positions 5890 and 5896 Å) separated by a dark space.

(iii) *Band or molecular spectrum.* These are produced by molecules and consist of a group of closely packed lines forming a band that is why they are known as band or molecular spectra.

(B) Absorption Spectra

Consider a spectroscope in which a sodium flame is acting as a source of light. The light emitted by the sodium flame on passing through a prism would produce a line spectrum of sodium containing two bright yellow lines of wavelenghs 5890 and 5896 Å ; this would be called the emission line spectrum of sodium. Now, if an electric arc is placed before the sodium flame, a continuous spectrum (like that produced by white light) will be seen which will be crossed by two dark lines of wavelengths 5890 and 5396 Å ; these dark lines constitute what is known as the absorption line spectrum of sodium. If the arc is removed, the continuous spectrum disappears and again two yellow lines are seen.

The temperature of the arc is much higher than that of the sodium flame. The arc emits out white light which produces a continuous emission spectrum consisting of all wavelengths from 4000 to 7600 Å. When the light emitted by the arc passes through the sodium flame the radiations corresponding to wavelengths 5890 and 5896 Å are absorbed by sodium vapours consequently two dark lines are noticed in the spectrum. It should be noted that sodium at lower temperature (flame temperature is lower than the arc temperature) absorbs those wavelengths, which it emits at higher temperature (when arc is absent the flame temperature should be regarded as a higher temperature) ; this is in accordance with the Kirchhoff's law. The existence of dark lines is due to the missing wavelengths.

15'A'4 SPECTRUM ANALYSIS

The process of resolution (separation) and study of different wavelengths present in a beam of radiations is termed spectrum analysis. So far we have been considering a beam of light but it does not mean that the term spectral analysis applies only to visible light. Any beam of electromagnetic radiations can be separated into its constituent wavelengths by a suitable apparatus. In visible region a glass prism or grating is employed as a dispersing device and a photographic plate is generally used to record the spectrum. While dealing with infrared radiations a prism made of salt (usually NaCl) is used and the resolved wavelengths are measured by means of a bolometer. For work in ultraviolet region a silica prism and photographic plates are used for studying the spectrum. Crystal gratings and photographic plates are used for studying the spectra of x-rays.

15·A·5. Origin of Spectra

Spectroscopic studies have played a tremendous role in the development of chemistry and physics. Besides, spectroscopic analysis has a very large number of applications both in qualitative and quantitative analysis. One of the most important aspects of spectroscopic studies is about the origin of spectral lines. A detailed study of this topic is beyond the scope of this book. However, an attempt is made here to give an elementary treatment regarding why atoms give spectra and why the spectrum of a particular atom contains wavelengths that are characteristic of that atom.

15·A·5·1 Quantum Theory

It is known that hot bodies emit out energy in the form of radiations. A hot piece of iron (at about 100°C-200°C) gives out energy in the form of thermal radiations, which have wavelengths greater than 7600 Å. As the temperature of the iron piece is raised it turns red and finally becomes white hot. At higher temperatures the emitted radiations have wavelengths between 4000 and 7600 Å also, that is why the iron piece looks white.

In 1900, M. Planck proposed that the emission of radiant energy is not continuous but is discontinuous in terms of energy packets called quanta of energy. Imagine a hot body which is emitting energy by means of a single radiation of wavelength λ. The frequency of this radiation will be :

$$\nu = \frac{C}{\lambda}$$

According to Planck's theory, the packet or quantum of energy E associated with this radiation is given by :

$$E = h \times \nu = \frac{h \times C}{\lambda} \quad [E \propto \nu] \quad \text{or} \quad \left[E \propto \frac{1}{\lambda} \right] \quad (...15·3)$$

where h is known as Planck's constant. It means that body will give out **energy** E or 2E or 3E.........or nE, where n is an integer. (The amount of energy equal to 0·1 E or 0·3 E will not be given out).

The same is true about the absorption of energy. Suppose we are supplying energy to a body by means of a single radiation of wavelength λ, then the body will take up either E or 2E .... or nE amount of energy. The magnitude of the quantum of energy E depends upon the wavelength of the radiation being emitted or absorbed. The greater the wavelength, the smaller is the associated energy quantum. For instance, the energy quantum associated with an electromagnetic wave of wavelength equal to 8000 Å (in the infrared region) will be much smaller than that of a wave of wavelength equal to 3000 Å (in the ultraviolet region).

15·A·5·2.   Excitation of Atoms

Bohr applied quantum theory to Rutherford atom model and concluded that in an atom there are different energy levels as shown in Fig. 15·3. Ordinarily the different electrons of an atom are in their normal energy levels. But when energy is supplied to the atom, the electrons jump to higher energy levels and thus the atom gets excited ; this process is known as *excitation*. Later the electrons return to their normal energy levels and the excess energy that they had absorbed is given out in the form of radiations, which on examination with a spectroscope show a spectrum.

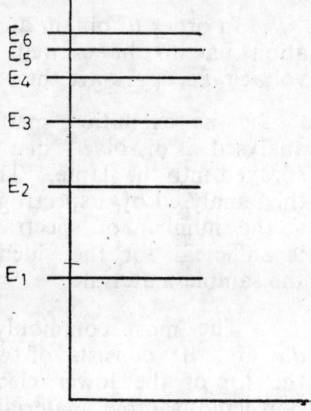

Fig. 15·3. Atomic energy level.

Consider an atom whose various energy levels are represented by E_1, E_2, E_3, E_4, etc. If energy is supplied to this atom, it will be excited, *i.e.*, its electrons will move to levels of higher energy. For example, an electron which is in energy level E_1 may absorb energy and jump to next higher energy level E_2 ; this excitation process will involve absorption of $(E_2 - E_1) = \Delta E$ amount of energy. When the electron returns from level E_2 to its original level E_1, the excess energy ΔE, which was absorbed during excitation will be emitted out in the form of a radiation. According to the quantum theory the energy of a radiation is proportional to its frequency ν [see equation (15·3)] so that :

$$(E_2 - E_1) = \Delta E$$

$$\left[\ \Delta E = h \times \nu = \frac{h \times c}{\lambda} \ \right] \qquad (\text{...}15\cdot4)$$

Since for a particular atom the values E_1 and E_2 are fixed, their difference $(E_2 - E_1) = \Delta E$ will also be fixed. Now, ΔE, h and c have fixed values, hence, the value of λ will also be definite. It means that the transition of an electron from level E_2 to E_1 in a particular atom will give rise to the radiation of a fixed wavelength. Similarly it can be shown that the transition E_3 to E_2 will produce a radiation of a definite wavelength. In this way each electronic transition will result in the emission of a radiation of fixed wavelength. This is the reason that a set of lines of fixed wavelengths is observed in an atomic spectrum. The measurement of wavelengths of spectral lines of an atom can therefore act as a basis for its identification. If a large number of atoms are present the number of electronic transitions will also be larger, consequently the spectral lines will be more intense. Thus the amount of material is related to the intensity of the spectral lines produced.

15·A·6   EXCITAITION METHODS

In order to obtain atomic spectrum the material under examination has to be excited. The flame, low voltage *d.c.* arc or high voltage *a.c.* spark are the common methods of excitation.

In the excitation method using a flame, the sample to be analysed is dissolved in a suitable solvent and the resultant soln is sprayed into the flame. The radiations given out by the flame are then analysed by a spectrograph. The flame is a low energy source so the number of spectral lines produced is small. However, this is sufficient for the identification of the elements present in the sample material.

The most commonly used excitation source is a low voltage *d.c.* arc. It consists of two electrodes made of pure graphite. On the top of the lower electrode there is a small cavity in which the powdered sample material is placed. A voltage in the range of 50 to 300 volts is applied to the electrodes in order to strike an arc. The temperature of the arc is very high (2000 to 5000°C) so the sample material vapourises, enters the arc and gets excited. The radiations from the arc are analysed by a spectrograph.

15·A·7   SPECTROGRAPHIC ANALYSIS

In order to detect the elements present in a sample its spectrum is obtained usually by excitation with a *d.c.* arc. The wavelengths of different lines observed in the spectrum are then compared with the wavelengths of known elements. From such a comparison, the elements present in the sample can be identified.

The quantitative spectrographic analysis is based on the fact that the intensity of a spectral line is proportional to the amount of an element present in the sample. For the determination of an element in the sample, the spectrum of the sample is first obtained and the intensity of its spectral lines are compared with those obtained in the spectrum produced under identical conditions by a known amount of the same element. Knowing the two intensity values and the amount of the element in the known sample, the quantity of the element present in the unknown sample can be calculated.

15·A·8. ADVANTAGES OF SPECTROGRAPHIC ANALYSIS

Since extremely small amounts of elements can be detected and determined by emission spectrography, the technique finds several analytical applications. Some of the advantages of this technique are :

(i) Rapid analysis of all the metallic constituents of a sample. This is very useful in the routine analysis of industrial samples.

(ii) Applicability for the analysis of minor constituents.

(iii) As a testing method for the purity of analytical reagents.

(iv) Detection of traces of metallic impurities in inorganic and organic substances.

15·B COLORIMETRY

Consider two solutions of $K_2Cr_2O_7$, of concentrations 1 per cent (soln A) and 5 per cent (soln B), placed into similar glass tubes. The colour of soln A will appear to be light yellow but that of soln B will be dark yellow. Thus simply by looking at the intensity of yellow colour in the two cases, we can know that soln B is more concentrated than soln A. It means that the colour intensity is related to the concentration of the substance producing the colour ; this is the basis of what is known as *colorimetric analysis.* If the substance to be determined is not coloured a suitable reagent which produces a coloured compound is added. For example, Fe^{3+} ions form a red coloured complex when treated with an excess of KCNS. The intensity of the red colour is proportional to the concentration of Fe^{3+} ions.

15·B·1. THEORY OF COLORIMETRIC ANALYSIS

When a beam of light falls upon a homogeneous medium, a part of the incident light is reflected, a part is absorbed and the remainder is transmitted, so that :

$$I_o = I_r + I_a + I_t \qquad (15·5)$$

where I_o is the intensity of the incident beam, I_r is, that of the reflected light, I_a is, that of the absorbed light and I_t is that of the transmitted light. If I_r is neglected (or eliminated by a comparison method) we can write :

$$I_o = I_a + I_t \qquad (15·6)$$

15·B·1·1 Lambert's Law

The change of absorption of light with the thickness of the medium is given by Lambert's law. This law states that the intensity of the transmitted light decreases exponentially as the thickness of the absorbing medium increases arithmatically. It means that the given thickness of the medium absorbs the same fraction of the light incident upon it. For example, consider a homogeneous medium of length 3 cm. The intensity of a beam of monochromatic light entering at one end of the medium is 1000 units and it falls to 100 units after travelling a distance of 1 cm through the medium, *i.e.*, it reduces to 1/10th of its original value. According to Lambert's law, when the light travels through another centimeter, its intensity will again be reduced by a factor of 1/10, *i.e.*, the intensity after the second centimeter will be $100 \times 1/10 = 10$ units. Similarly, after the third centimeter, the intensity of the transmitted light will be $10 \times 1/10 = 1$ unit as shown in Fig. 15.4.

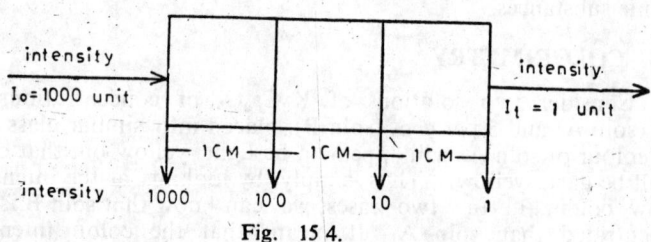

intensity
$I_0 = 1000$ unit

intensity
$I_t = 1$ unit

— 1CM — 1CM — 1CM—

intensity   1000   100   10   1

Fig. 15.4.

Lambert's law can be mathematically expressed as :

$$-\frac{dI}{dl} = KI \qquad \qquad ...(15.7)$$

where I is the intensity of the incident light of wavelength λ, l is the thickness of the medium and K is a proportionality constant. $\left(-\frac{dI}{dl}\right.$ represents the rate of *decrease* of intensity with the thickness of the medium. $\left.\right)$ Equation (15.7) can be written as :

$$-\frac{dI}{I} = Kdl$$

or, $\dfrac{dI}{I} = -Kdl$

or, $d \log I = -Kdl$ ...(15.8)

multiplying both sides by -1.

$$\frac{dx}{x} = d \log x$$

$$\frac{dI}{I} = d \log I$$

On integrating equation (15.8)

$$\int d \log I = -\int K \, dl$$

$$\log\ I = -Kl + C \quad ...(15\text{·}9)$$
when $\ l=0,\ I=I_o$,
$$\log I_o = K \times 0 + C$$
$$\log I_o = 0 + C$$
$$\log I_o = C \quad ...(15\text{·}10)$$

$C =$ integration constant
When the incident beam is just entering the medium, the thickness travelled by light is zero hence the intensity is equal to I_o, *i.e.* the intensity of incident light.

Substituting the value of C from (15·10) into (15·9) :

$$\log\ I = -Kl + \log\ I_o$$
or, $\ -\log I_o + \log\ I = -Kl$
$$\log I_o - \log I = +Kl$$
or, $\quad \log \dfrac{I_o}{I_t} = Kl \quad (15\text{·}11)$
or, $I_t = I_o . 10^{-Kl} \quad ...(15\text{·}12)$

multiplying both sides by -1. I_t is the intensity after the thickness l.

K is known as the *absorption coefficient*. Suppose after travelling l cms, the intensity is reduced to 1/10th of its original value, *i.e.*, $I_t = I_0/10$ or, $I_0 = 10\ I_t$. Substituting these values in equation (15·11), we get :

$$\log\ \frac{I_0}{I_t} =\ \log\ \frac{10}{1} = \log\ 10 = Kl$$

or, $\qquad Kl = 1 \qquad\qquad\qquad (\log\ 10 = 1)$
or, $\qquad\quad K = 1/l$

Thus, the absorption coefficient is equal to the reciprocal of the length l, required to reduce the light to 1/10 of its intensity. The ratio I_t/I_0 (the fraction of the incident light transmitted by a thickness l of the absorbing medium) is known as *transmittance* and is represented by T. The reciprocal of transmittance, *i.e.*, I_0/I_t is called the *opacity*. The absorbance A of the medium is defined as :

$$A = \log\ I_0/I_t \qquad\qquad\qquad ...(15\text{·}13)$$

If a medium transmits 10 per cent of the incident light $(I_0 = 10\ I_t)$, its absorbance will be 1.

15·B·1·2 Beer's Law

In quantitative analysis we mostly deal with solutions. Beer studied the absorption of light by coloured solutions and found the same relation between transmission and concentration which Lambert had discovered between transmission and thickness of absorbing medium. Thus the intensity of a beam of monochromatic light decreases exponentially as the concentration of the absorbing substance increase arithmatically. Hence we can write :

$$I_t = I_0 . 10^{-K'o} \quad ...(15.14)$$ [Compare with equation (15.12)] where c is the concentration and K' is a constant. By combining equations (15.12) and (15.14) we get :

$$I_t = I_0 . 10^{-acl} \qquad\qquad ...(15.15)$$

$$\text{or,} \quad \log \frac{I_0}{I_t} = acl \quad ...(15.16) \qquad \text{[Compare with equation (15.11)]}$$

where a is a constant. Equation (15.16) is the fundamental equation for colorimetry and spectrophotometry. If concentration of the soln is expressed in moles per litre and l in cms, a is replaced by ε which is known as *molar absorption coefficient* or *molar absorptivity*. If we have a molar soln of a substance, the absorption by 1 cm thickness of this soln will be called specific absorption coefficient represented by E_s. Now,

$$\log \frac{I_0}{I_t} = A \qquad\qquad \text{...[see equation (15.13)]}$$

$$\text{also,} \quad \log \frac{I_0}{I_t} = \varepsilon cl \qquad\qquad \text{...[see equation (15.16)]}$$

$$\therefore \quad A = \varepsilon.c.l. \qquad\qquad\qquad ...(15.17)$$

15.B.1.3. Application of Beer's Law

When radiant energy such as light passes through a soln, a part of it is absorbed. The absorption process involves a transfer of energy to the soln. The extent of absorption depends upon the concentration of the soln. A more concentrated soln will absorb more of radiant energy as compared to that absorbed by a dilute soln of the same substance. Consider two solutions of a substance whose concentrations are c_1 and c_2 and suppose their thickness can be changed. If the light of the same intensity is passed through these solutions and the thickness of these solutions are so adjusted that in the two cases the intensity of the transmitted light is the same then we can write,

$$I_{t1} = I_0 . 10^{-\varepsilon c_1 l_1}$$

and $$I_{t2} = I_0 . 10^{-\varepsilon c_2 l_2}$$

Since $$I_{t1} = I_{t2},$$

$$I_0 10^{-\varepsilon c_1 l_1} = I_0 . 10^{-\varepsilon c_2 l_2}$$

or, $$c_1 l_1 = c_2 l_2 \qquad\qquad ...(15.18)$$

If we know the thickness of layers of two solutions, and concentration (c_1) of one of the solutions, the concentration (c_2) of the other soln can be calculated.

15.B.2. COLORIMETRIC METHODS

A large number of substances can be determined by colorimetric methods. These methods are based on the comparison of the colour intensity of the unknown soln with that of a soln of known concentration. This comparison can be done by means of different instruments. Some of these involve a visual comparison while in some others a photocell is used for measuring the intensity of the transmitted light. Visual comparison methods are simple and do not require costly equipment but are not accurate. If a photoelectric colorimeter is used fairly accurate results can be obtained.

15·B·2·1 Visual Colorimetric Methods

These methods are not accurate and so are not used much in the colorimetric determinations. Hence, only two visual methods will be described here.

(*i*) *Standard series method.* In this method a series of known solutions of the substance to be determined are prepared, and their colour compared visually with that of the given unknown soln. The concentration of the unknown soln will be equal to the concentration of that known soln whose colour matches exactly with that of the unknown soln. This method may give 3 to 8 per cent error.

(*ii*) *Balancing method.* This method is based on the relationship :

$$c_1 l_1 = c_2 l_2 \ [\text{See equation (15·18)}].$$

A Duboscq colorimeter makes use of this relationship. This colorimeter consists of two cylindrical cups A and B. Cup A contains a known soln (of concentration c_1) of the substance to be determined and the unknown soln is taken in cup B. Two cylindrical glass rods C and D, which can move (on a scale) in upward and downward direction, are dipped in cups A and B as shown in Fig. 15·5. A beam of light from the source L is divided into two beams H and I which pass through the two cups. The emergent transmitted beams J and K are brought closer by means of an optical arrangement F. The two beams are viewed in G. The cylindrical glass rods are adjusted to such heights that the intensities of beams J and K are equal. The two heights l_1 and l_2 are measured, c_1 is known, hence the value of c_2, the concentration of unknown soln can be calculated using the equation :

$$c_1 \times l_1 = c_2 \times l_2$$

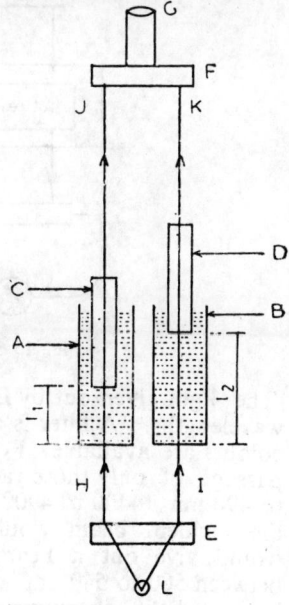

Fig. 15·5. Duboscq colorimeter.

15·B·2·2 Photoelectric Colorimeter

We have so far considered instruments in which there is a visual comparison of intensity of colours ; this involves a considerable error. If human eye is replaced by a photoelectric cell, much more accurate results are obtained. A photoelectric cell consists of a thin layer of cesium oxide and silver oxide, When light falls on this layer, electrons are emitted which cause a flow of current. The current after suitable amplification is fed to a galvanometer. The deflection in the galvanometer depends upon the intensity of light falling on the photocell. A colorimeter in which a photocell is used for the measurement of the transmitted light is called a *photoelectric colorimeter*.

The essential components of a photoelectric colorimeter have been shown in Fig. 15·6. Light from a tungsten filament lamp (L) after passing through a collimating lens (C) falls on a filter (F).

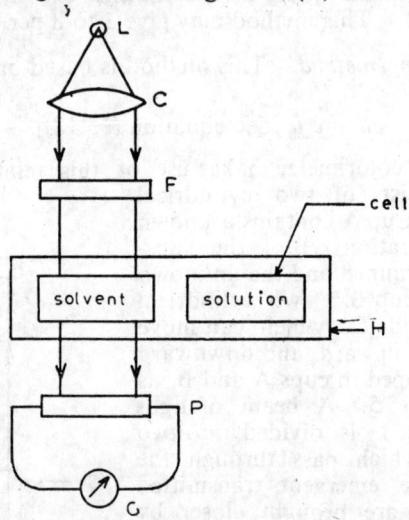

Fig. 15·6. Photoelectric colorimeter.

[The light given out by L contains radiations having a wide range of wavelengths. A filter is a piece of coloured glass. Filters of different colours are available. For example, a blue filter will permit the passage of only those radiations whose wavelengths are between 440 to 490 nm (4400 to 4900Å), all the other wavelengths present in the incident beam would be absorbed by the filter. A green filter would give out a beam consisting of radiations of wavelengths between 500 to 540 nm. The purpose of using a filter is to obtain a beam of light containing radiations within a small wavelength range.] The radiations coming out from the filter enter a small rectangular glass vessel called a cell. Two identical cells are used ; one for the solution of the substance to be determined and other for the solvent used which serves as a reference. The two cells are kept side by side in a cell holder (H). The cell holder can be moved in such a way that either the cell containing the soln or the cell containing the solvent can be brought into the path of the incident radiations. [It should be noted that the amount of light reflected from the walls of the two cells will be almost equal, hence we need consider only the absorbed and the transmitted light.] The light transmitted by the soln or the solvent is allowed to fall on a photocell (P) connected to a galvanometer (G) to record the current. The deflection in G is proportional to the intensity of light falling on the photocell.

15'B'3 COLORIMETRIC DETERMINATION METHOD

Suppose the concentration of a given $K_2Cr_2O_7$ soln is to be determined with the help of a photoelectric colorimeter, then the procedure is :

(i) Prepare several solutions of $K_2Cr_2O_7$ of known concentration in water. The range of concentration selected should be such so as to include that of the soln whose concentration is to be determined.

(ii) Fill one of the cells kept in the cell holder with water. Move the cell holder to bring it in the path of the light beam. Keep the measuring knob at zero absorbance.

(iii) Switch on the galvanometer and set its needle to zero by means of an adjusting knob provided for this purpose. Do not disturb this knob after it has been adjusted.

(iv) Now, switch on the lamp and wait for atleast 5 minutes so that the light intensity becomes constant.

(v) Again set the galvanometer needle to zero by another knob known as zero adjuster. Do not disturb this knob after this adjustment.

(vi) Fill the other cell with the soln to be determined and move the cell holder in order to bring the soln in the light path.

(vii) Once again set galvanometer needle to zero by means of a knob (measuring knob) moving on a graduated scale which gives the absorbance.

(viii) Measure the absorbance of different known solutions and plot a graph between absorbance and concentration. This is known as the calibration plot (See Fig. 15'9).

(ix) Measure the absorbance of the sample soln and find out its concentration with the help of the calibration graph. A blue filter should be used during all the absorbance measurements.

Notes :

(*a*) The absorbance-concentration plot gives a straight line only in a particular concentration range for a given substance. For accurate determination it is necessary that the concentration of the unknown soln should be in this concentration range.

(*b*) A suitable filter can be selected by measuring the absorbance of a soln of the given substance using filters of different colours. The filter which gives maximum absorbance is the appropriate filter. It has been observed that absorption is maximum when the colour of the filter is complementary to that of the soln. For example, if the soln is yellow, a blue filter is suitable. In the colorimetric determination of $K_2Cr_2O_7$ soln, a blue filter should be used. For a red soln ($KMnO_4$ soln) a green filter is the proper choice. A yellow filter should be used for a blue soln.

15'C   FLUORIMETRY

There are certain substances which absorb light and then emit out a part of it, this phenomenon is known as *fluorescence* and the substance having this property is said to be *fluorescent*. The wavelength of the emitted light is always greater than that of the incident light. The emitted radiation is called *fluorescent radiation*. It has been found that the intensity of the fluorescent radiation is practically proportional to the concentration of the fluorescent substance ; this forms the basis of fluorimetric analysis.

15'C'1   Fluorimeter

The essential parts of a fluorimeter are shown in Fig. 15'7. The light from a mercury vapour lamp L (a source of ultraviolet

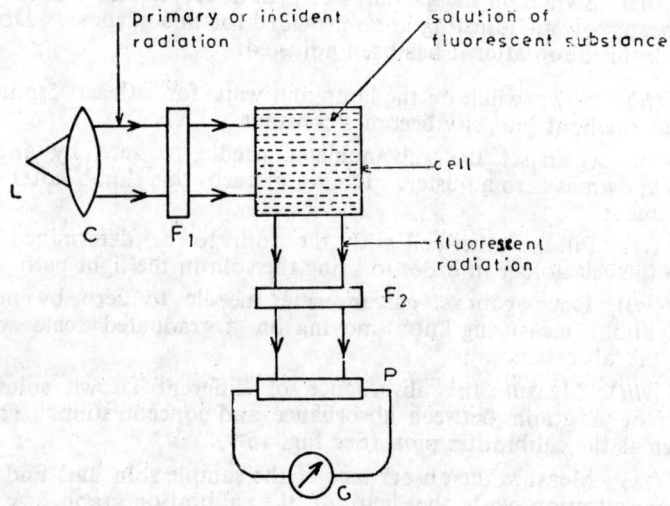

Fig. 15·7.   Fluorimeter.

light) is passed through a collimating lens C to obtain a parallel beam of light. This light, through a suitable filter F_1, falls on a cell containing the soln of fluorescent substance. Another filter F_2 is placed at right angles to the direction of the incident radiation (called primary radiation). The purpose of the secondary filter F_2 is to absorb the primary radiations and permit only the fluorescent radiations which are then allowed to fall on a photocell P, connected to a galvanometer G. The deflection in G is a measure of the intensity of the fluorescent radiation. [It should be remembered that the fluorescent intensity is proportional to that of the incident radiation hence the light source must be stable.]

15·C·2. Fluorimetric Method

A fluorimetric method involves the measurement of the intensity of fluorescent radiation, from several solutions of known concentration, by means of a fluorimeter. A graph between the intensity of fluorescent radiation and concentration gives the calibration curve. The fluorescent intensity of unknown soln is then measured and its concentration found out with the help of the calibration curve.

The great advantage of fluorimetric method is its applicability to the determination of a fluorescent substance at very low concentration level.

15·D TURBIDIMETRY AND NEPHELOMETRY

Consider a biphasic system consisting of fine particles of an insoluble substance (called dispersed phase) suspended in water to form a stable suspension. (The suspended particles should be fine so that they do not settle rapidly under the influence of gravity). When light falls on such a suspension, a part of it is reflected, a part is absorbed, a part is scattered and the remainder is transmitted. It has been found that the extent of absorption depends upon the concentration of the dispersed phase, *i.e.*, the greater the amount of the suspended particles, greater is the quantity of light absorbed ; this is the basis of *turbidimetric analysis*.

When the suspension is viewed from a direction at right angles to the direction of the incident beam of light, we observe the light scattered by the suspended particles. The intensity of the scattered light depends upon the concentration of the dispersed phase ; this is the basis of a *nephelometric determination*.

15·D·1 Construction of Calibration Curves for Turbidimetric and Nephelometric Determinations

The relation between the concentration of a suspension and the light absorbed or scattered by it is only empirical. A calibration curve has, therefore, first to be constructed with the help of suspensions of known concentrations. These known suspensions should be prepared under carefully controlled conditions.

A photoelectric colorimeter can be used as a turbidimeter. A blue filter is generally used. The transmitted intensities for different known suspension are measured and plotted against corresponding concentrations of suspensions to obtain a calibration curve. The intensity of transmitted beam from the sample suspension is then measured and its concentration determined from the calibration curve.

A fluorimeter can be used as a nephelometer. First a calibration curve is prepared with known suspensions which is then used for finding out the concentration of the sample suspension.

It should be noted that in a fluorimeter or in a nephelometer, the intensity of light is measured in a direction at right angles to that of the incident beam.

15·E SPECTROPHOTOMETRY

In some types of colorimeters, quantitative determinations are made using directly white light from a tungsten filament lamp. This light is called *polychromatic* because it contains radiation of different wavelengths. The selectivity and sensitivity of a colorimetric determination can be greatly increased by using *monochromatic radiations*, *i.e.*, radiations having similar wavelengths. In a photoelectric colorimeter described in 15·B·2·2, a light filter has been placed after the source of white light. The radiations emerging from the filter have wavelengths within a small range. If the light filter is replaced by a ·device known as a *monochromator*, we can have a beam of radiations of a particular wavelength, *i.e.*, a beam of monochromatic radiations. Such an instrument is then known as a *spectrophotometer*, because it is a combination of a spectrometer and a photometer. The function of the spectrometer is to provide a beam of radiations of a selected wavelength and that of the photometer is to measure the intensity of the transmitted radiation.

15·E·1 Dependence of Absorbance on the Wavelength

A particular substance selectively absorbs radiation of a particular wavelength. This wavelength which depends upon its nature is known as λ_{max} for that substance. The radiations of other wavelengths present in the incident beam are mostly transmitted by the substance.

Consider a substance (A) which absorbs blue light and transmits yellow and red. Suppose a beam of light (incident beam)·

containing blue, yellow and red light is passed through a soln of the substance. The substance (A) does not absorb yellow and red light so these will be transmitted by the soln and will then fall on to a photocell. A part of the blue light will be absorbed by the substance and remaining portion will be transmitted along with yellow and red light. The part of the blue light absorbed will depend upon the concentration of the substance in the soln. It is thus seen that most of the current generated (photocurrent) in the photocell is due to the transmitted yellow and red light which are not absorbed and hence are not related to the concentration of the substance. In other words, a very small fraction of the incident light will be absorbed which depends upon the concentration of the substance. [Now, if a quantity measured is small, the error in the measurement is greater.] Since we are measuring absorption which is quite small, the observed error will be larger. Besides, there is one more disadvantage. Suppose a substance (B) which absorbs red light is also present along with substance (A) being determined. If the incident light contains blue, red and yellow light, a part of the blue light will be absorbed by (A) and a part of the red light will be absorbed by the substance (B). The colorimeter will measure the total absorption so we will not know how much is the absorption due to the substance (A). Now, the absorption of radiation by a substance is a measure of its concentration. Since we do not know how much absorption is due to the substance (A), we cannot calculate its concentration. Thus, the determination of (A) will be interferred by the substance (B).

The above difficulties can be removed by using blue light for the colorimetric determination of the substance (A). The substance (B) does not absorb blue light, hence, the entire absorption, measured, is due to the substance (A), and because it depends upon the amount of (A) present in the soln, the concentration of (A) can be calculated. Thus, the interference due to the substance (B) can be eliminated. Another advantage is that since only blue light is being used as the incident light, the fraction of the light absorbed will now be greater. Hence, even with very dilute solutions of (A), the absorption, measured, will be considerable. It means that the sensitivity of the colorimetric determination would be greatly increased, i.e., it would be applicable to the quantitative analysis of extremely dilute solutions of the substance (A).

In the above discussion, blue, red or yellow light has been used. A beam of blue light consists of several radiations of differing wavelengths in the range 435-480 mm. For more precise work, a device is used which can provide radiation of a particular wavelength, corresponding to λ_{max} of the substance under consideration. This arrangement is available in a spectrophotometer. A photoelectriccolorimeter generally employs light filter to have blue, red, green or yellow light.

15·E·2 Spectrophotometric Determination

Suppose we have to determine the amount of a substance in its soln by spectrophotometric method, then the procedure will be as follows :

(*i*) Place the soln in a cell. Put the cell in the cell holder and move it into a position so that the soln comes in the light path.

(*ii*) Go on changing the wavelength of the incident radiation and note the absorbance for each value of the wavelength. Plot a graph between the absorbance and wavelength and find out the value of λ_{max} (see Fig. 15·8). This wavelength is used in the measurement of absorbance throughout the experiment.

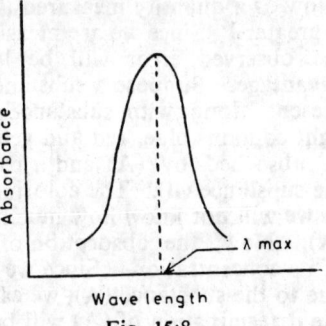

(*iii*) Prepare a series of solutions of the substance of known concentrations. Measure the absorbance of each of the solutions at the wavelength determined in step (*ii*).

(*iv*) Plot a graph between the different values of absorbances and corresponding concentrations. This is the calibration graph.

Fig. 15·8.

(*v*) Measure the absorbance of the given soln under identical conditions, and find out its concentration with the help of the calibration graph as shown in Fig. 15·9.

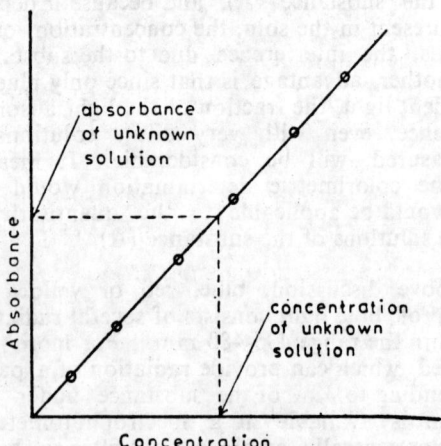

Fig. 15·9. Calibration plot.

15'E'3   Different Types of Spectrophotometers

A photoelectric colorimeter uses a tungsten filament lamp as a source which gives radiations in the visible region, *i.e.*, 400-760 nm. In a spectrophotometer such energy sources can be used which give out radiations in visible as well as in infrared and ultraviolet region. If an infrared source is used, the instrument is known as an I.R. spectrophotometer. An instrument in which there is a provision for visible and ultraviolet radiation sources, is called an U.V. spectrophotometer.

(A) *Infrared Spectrophotometer.* In this instrument, the source of radiant energy is the Nernst glower. It consists of a mixture of zirconium and yttrium oxides in the shape of a tube which is electrically heated to 1500-2000°C. Because infrared rays are not transmitted by glass, a prism made of salt (such as NaCl) is used as a monochromator. The radiations from the Nernst glower are polychromatic when these are passed through the salt prism the different wavelengths get separated. A slit is placed in the path of radiations emerging from the prism so that only radiant energy of the desired wavelength passes through and falls on to the soln under examination. The radient energy transmitted by the soln is then allowed to fall on a detector. Thermal detectors are used for measuring the intensity of the transmitted infrared radiations. The absorption pattern, obtained by measuring the absorption as a function of wavelength, is characteristic of a substance. An I.R. spectrophotometer can give the absorption spectrum of a substance. By analysing this spectrum, information regarding the structure of the substance can be obtained.

(B) *U.V. Spectrophotometer.* This type of spectrophotometer covers the range 220-1000 nm, *i.e.*, the ultraviolet, visible and near infrared region. The source of radiant energy is a tungsten lamp (for visible region) and a deuterium arc lamp (for ultraviolet region). A prism made of silica is used as a monochromator. The intensity of the beam transmitted by the sample soln is measured by means of a photocell. (A glass prism cannot be used because glass does not transmit ultraviolet light. A silica prism is suitable for both, visible and ultraviolet radiations.)

15'E'4   Photometric Titrations

The measurement of a property which shows a sudden change at the equivalence point can act as a basis of a titrimetric method. For example, the potential of an indicator electrode shows a sudden variation at the end point ; this is the basis of potentiometric titration method.

The measurement of absorbance can be employed to follow the progress of a titration and the end point can be located by means of a spectrophotometer. Such types of titrations are known as *photometric titrations*.

Suppose we have a soln of a substance A (titrand soln) whose λ_{max} is λ_A. Another soln of a substance B, whose λ_{max} is λ_B, acts as the titrant. The product of the reaction is C with a λ_{max} equal to λ_C. A known volume of the titrand is taken in the cell of a spectrophotometer in which the wavelength of the incident radiation is set to be equal to λ_A. The measured absorbance will be proportional to the amount of A. If to this soln, a small volume of the titrant is added, a part of A will react with B, hence the concentration of A will decrease and so the value of the absorbance. As we go on adding the titrant, the absorbance will go on decreasing. At the equivalence point, substance A has completely reacted so the absorbance will reach a minimum. On adding the titrant beyond the equivalence point, the absorbance will not show any change because neither B (titrant) nor C (product) absorb radiation of wavelength λ_A. Hence, if absorbance is plotted against the volume of the titrant, a graph as shown in Fig. 15·10(a) will be obtained. The point of intersection of the two straight lines in the graph will give the end point.

Let us consider what will happen if the above titration is carried out in a spectrophotometer set at a wavelength λ_B (the λ_{max} for the titrant). Since the substance A does not absorb λ_B, the absorbance will not show any change up to the equivalence point. The addition of the titrant after the equivalence point will cause an increase in the absorbance as shown in Fig. 15·10 (b).

A third case can be to carry out the titration with wavelength set equal to λ_C. Now, the titrand and titrant will not absorb but the product C will. As the titration progresses, more and more product is formed so the absorbance will go on increasing. After the equivalence point, the formation of the product will stop and the absorbance will become constant [see Fig. 15·10(c)].

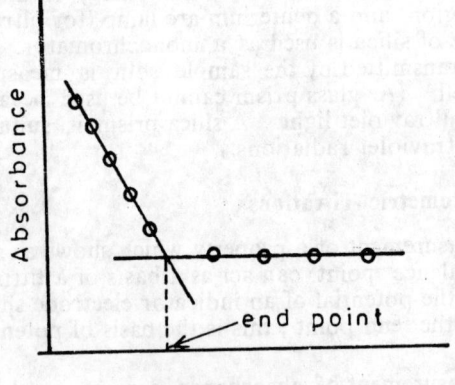

Vol. of titrant

Fig. 15·10(a).

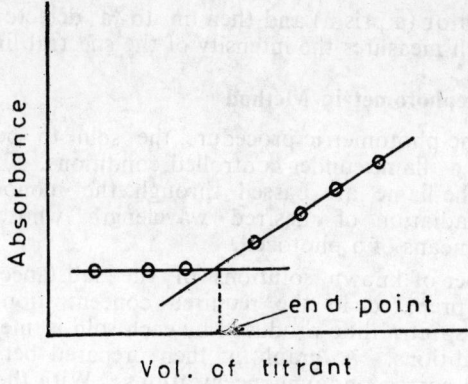

Fig. 15·10(b).

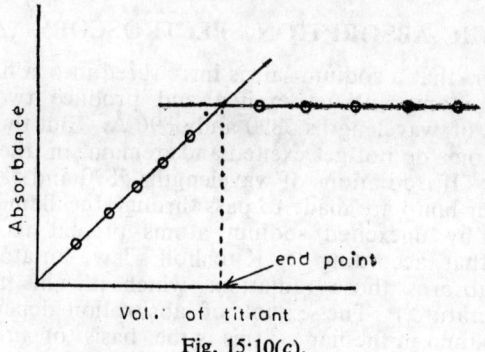

Fig. 15·10(c).

15·F FLAME PHOTOMETRY

It has been mentioned in 15·A that when a sodium salt is introduced into a flame, a yellow light is emitted by the flame. If this light is passed through a dispersing device, such as a prism, lines of characteristic wavelengths are observed. The intensity of these lines are related to the quantity of sodium introduced into the flame—this is the basic principle of *flame emission spectroscopy* (FES) or *flame photometry*.

15·F1 Flame Photometer

A flame photometer consists of a flame whose temperature is around 2000°C. The flow rate of the fuel and the oxidant gas (generally acetylene and oxygen) is properly controlled. An atomiser is used to obtain fine drops of sample soln which is sent into the flame. The radiations emitted by the flame are made to pass through a monochromator (a prism) and then on to a detector, such as a photocell which measures the intensity of the spectral line.

15'F'2. Flamephotometric Method

In a flame-photometric procedure, the soln to be analysed is sprayed into a flame under controlled conditions. The radiations given out by the flame are passed through the monochromator to isolate the radiation of desired wavelength whose intensity is measured by means of a photocell.

A number of known solutions of the substance being determined are prepared in the required concentration range. The intensity of a spectral line produced by each soln is measured under identical conditions. A graph is then prepared between different intensities and corresponding concentrations. With the help of this curve the concentration of the sample soln can be calculated. (The intensity measurements are done under identical conditions.)

15'G. ATOMIC ABSORPTION SPECTROSCOPY (A.A.S.)

Consider that a sodium salt is introduced into a flame. Some of the sodium atoms will get excited and produce two prominent spectral lines of wavelengths 5890 and 5896 Å. But the majority of the sodium atoms do not get excited and remain in the ground or normal state. If radiations of wavelengths 5890 and 5896 Å from a sodium vapour lamp are made to pass through the flame, these will be absorbed by unexcited sodium atoms present in the flame. (Remember that according to Kirchhoff's law, an atom at a lower temperature absorbs those radiations which it will itself emit at higher temperature.) The extent of absorption depends upon the amount of sodium in the flame ; this is the basis of *atomic absorption spectroscopy*. The absorption of the sample soln is compared with that of a known soln under identical conditions. From such a comparison, the concentration of the substance in test soln can be found out.

15'H. POLARIMETRY

Ordinary light consists of a very large number of electromagnetic waves vibrating in all possible planes. If by some means we can select only those waves which vibrate only in one plane ; we will have what is known as *plane polarized light*. A plane polarized light can be obtained in a number of ways. One of the most convenient method is to use a Nicol prism, which consists of a calcite crystal that has been properly cut. When light passes through the Nicol prism it gets polarized. This Nicol prism is, therefore, called a *polarizer*.

If the beam of light coming out from one Nicol prism (polarizer) is passed through another Nicol prism (analyzer) kept in an identical position as the first prism, the light will pass through the analyzer. But if the analyzer is turned so that it is at 90° to the polarizer, no light will pass through the analyzer.

Consider that a polarizer and an analyzer are at right angles, to each other so that no light is passing through the analyzer. A total darkness will be observed in an eyepiece kept on the other side of the analyzer. If an aqueous soln of cane sugar is placed between the polarizer and analyzer, the view will not be completely dark but some brightness will be visible. It means that cane sugar has the capacity to rotate the plane of polarization. This phenomenon is called *optical activity* and substances which possess this property are known as *optically active*. Certain substances rotate the plane of polarization of light to the right, (as seen from the viewer's end) ; these are called *dextro-rotatory*. Others rotate it to the left and are known as *laevo-rotatory*.

15'H'1.   Polarimeter

An instrument used to measure optical rotation is called a polarimeter. It consists of the following basic parts :

1. A light source (usually a sodium vapour lamp).
2. A polarizer (Nicol prism—fixed).
3. An analyzer (Nicol prism—can be rotated on a graduated circular scale).
4. A circular scale to measure the angle of rotation.
5. Tubes to hold the sample soln.
6. An eyepiece to view the emergent light.

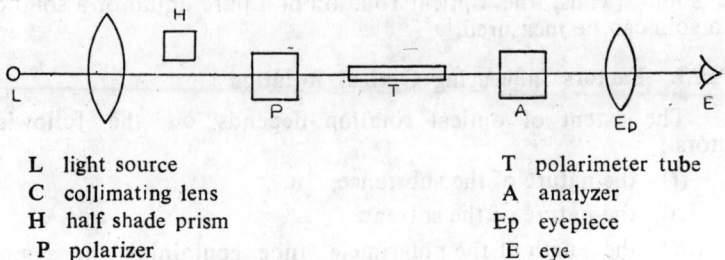

L light source	T polarimeter tube
C collimating lens	A analyzer
H half shade prism	Ep eyepiece
P polarizer	E eye

Fig. 15 11. Polarimeter

15.H.2   Measurement of Optical Rotation

The apparatus is set up as shown in Fig. 15'11. The tube T is filled with distilled water, analyzer is turned on a circular graduated scale to obtain total darkness and the reading on the scale is noted. The tube containing a soln of an optically active material is then. placed between the polarizer and analyzer. On looking through the analyzer, the field would appear to be bright, because the soln has rotated the plane of polarization. The analyzer is again turned to obtain the total darkness, and the angle through which it has been turned is found out from the two scale readings. This angle is equal to the angle of rotation of the given soln.

The problem in the above measurement is the difficulty in finding out when the view is exactly as dark as it was without the soln. In order to solve this problem, a small Nicol prism (known

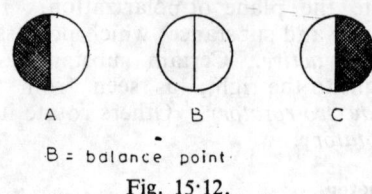

B = balance point

Fig. 15·12.

as half-shed prism) is placed in between the polarizer and light source. The view is now divided into two halves whose brightness can be more conveniently compared. On rotating the analyzer, different positions shown in Fig. 15·12 are observed. The position B, when the two halves are equally illuminated is the balance point. The balance point is first observed with distilled water in the tube, by rotating the analyzer on the circular graduated scale. The scale reading is noted. The tube containing the sample soln is then placed between the polarizer and analyzer. Analyzer is again rotated to obtain the balance point. The scale reading is again recorded ; the difference between the two readings gives the optical rotation of the soln. [Thus, the optical rotation of a pure liquid or a solid or of a soln can be measured.]

15·H·3. Factors Influencing Optical Rotation

The extent of optical rotation depends on the following factors :

(i)   the nature of the substance,

(ii) the nature of the solvent,

(iii) the length of the polarimeter tube containing the sample soln,

(iv) the temperature, and

(v)   the wavelength of the light used.

In order to compare the angle of rotation of different substances it is necessary that their optical rotations are measured under standard conditions. The length employed as standard is 10 cm (1 decimeter) for solutions, and 1 mm for solids. The standard wavelength is usually that of sodium doublet (5890 and 5896 Å). The standard temperature is 20°C. If α is the observed rotation at 20°C, for light of the sodium D line, l is the length of the polarimeter tube in decimeters and C is the concentration of the sample soln in g per 100 ml, then the specific rotatory power $[\alpha]$ is given by :

$$[\alpha]_D^t = \frac{100 \times \alpha}{C \times l}$$

The molecular rotation is given by :

$$[M]_D^t = \frac{M\,[\alpha]}{100}$$

where M is the molecular weight.

Example 15·H(i)

A 10% soln of pure cane sugar kept in a polarimeter tube of length 20 cms gave an optical rotation of 13·34°. The measurement was done at 20°C using sodium lamp as the light source. Calculate the specific rotation of cane sugar.

(i)   The observed rotation α
$$= 13·34°$$

(ii)   Because a 10% soln was used,

100 ml soln contains 10 g cane sugar
$$C = 10$$

(iii)   Length of the tube is 20 cms = 2 decimeters
$$l = 2$$

Substituting the values of α, C and l, we get :

$$[\alpha]_D^t = \frac{100 \times \alpha}{C \times l} = \frac{100 \times 13·34}{10 \times 2} = 66·7°$$

[Alternatively,

Specific rotation is the rotation when path length is 1 decimeter and soln is 100%.

For 2 decimeter path, rotation is 13·34°

∴ for 1 decimeter path, rotation is $\dfrac{13·34}{2} = 6·67°$

A 10% soln gives a rotation of 6·67° (for 1 decimeter path length)

∴ 100% soln gives a rotation of 6·67 × 10 = 66·7°].

15'H'4. Applications of Optical Rotation Measurement

In this section two examples will be given to illustrate how the measurement of optical rotation can be used in the quantitative analysis of optically active material.

Example 15'H (ii)

A pure soln of cane sugar kept in a polarimeter tube of length 1 decimeter gave an optical rotation of 13·34° at 20°C with a sodium lamp as the light source. Find out the concentration of sugar in the soln.

First, the specific rotation of pure cane sugar will be determined by the method described in Example 15'H(i). The value will come out to be 66·7°.

$$[\alpha] = 66·7° \qquad\qquad l = 1 \text{ decimeter}$$
$$\alpha = 13·34° \qquad\qquad C = ?$$

$$[\alpha] = \frac{100 \times \alpha}{C \times l} \qquad \text{or, } C = \frac{100 \times \alpha}{l \times [\alpha]}$$

$$C = \frac{100 \times 13·34}{1 \times 66·7} = 20$$

The amount of sugar will be 20 g per 100 ml i.e., it will be a 20% soln.

Example 15'H(iii)

A 10% soln of an impure sugar sample kept in a polarimeter tube of length 2 decimeter has an optical rotation equal to 12·5°. The specific rotation of pure sugar is 66·7°. Calculate the percentage purity of the sample.

$$[\alpha] = 66·7° \qquad\qquad l = 2 \text{ decimeter}$$
$$\alpha = 12·5° \qquad\qquad C = ?$$

where C is the amount of pure sugar in 100 ml of sample soln.

$$[\alpha] = \frac{100 \times \alpha}{C \times l} \qquad \text{or, } C = \frac{100 \times \alpha}{[\alpha] \times l}$$

$$C = \frac{100 \times 12·5}{66·7 \times 2} = 9·37$$

The amount of impure sugar in 100 ml = 10·00 g.
The amount of pure sugar in 100 ml = 9·37 g.
10 g of sample contains 9·37 g pure sugar

$$\therefore \quad 100 \text{ g of sample contains } \frac{100}{10} \times 9·37 = 93·7\%$$

The percentage purity of the sample is 93·7%.

15·I. LABORATORY EXERCISES

Experiment 15·1

Verification of Beer's Law for $KMnO_4$ soln and determination of the concentration of $KMnO_4$ in a given soln by colorimetric method.

Discussion

It has been seen in section 15·B.1·2 that :

$$\log \frac{I_o}{I_t} = \varepsilon \, cl \quad \text{and} \quad \log \frac{I_o}{I_t} = A$$

$$A = \varepsilon cl$$

where, I_o = intensity of the incident radiation

I_t = intensity of the transmitted radiation

ε = molar absorption coefficient or molar absorptivity

l = path length (length through which light travels in the soln)

A = absorbance

The value of ε is constant for a given substance, if path length l is also kept fixed, then :

$$A \propto c$$

Thus, according to Beer's law the absorbance of a soln is proportional to its concentration. The scales of many colorimeters and spectrophotometers are often calibrated so that the absorbance can be directly read.

In order to verify Beer's law a spectrophotometer is needed because it applies to monochromatic light. However, the law can be verified even with a photoelectric colorimeter, such as a Klett-Summerson Colorimeter.

Apparatus and Materials

A Klett-Summerson Colorimeter, a standard $KMnO_4$ soln and the soln of $KMnO_4$ whose concentration is to be determined.

[a] Verification of Beer's law

Procedure

(i) Insert a light filter in the filter holder and put back the filter holder into its position.

(ii) Set the galvanometer needle to zero by means of knob provided at the top of the galvanometer. The position of this knob should not be disturbed during the experiment.

(*iii*) Clean the cells provided with the colorimeter. Take $KMnO_4$ soln in one cell and distilled water in the other.

(*iv*) Insert the cell containing water in the light path and put the measuring knob at the zero of the absorbance scale.

(*v*) Swith on the light source and the galvanometer.

(*vi*) Set the deflection in the galvanometer to zero by means of an adjustment knob.

(*vii*) Remove the cell containing water and insert the cell containing $KMnO_4$ soln. Move the measuring knob on the scale in order to have no deflection in the galvanometer. The reading on the scale gives the absorbance of the sample soln.

(*viii*) Change the filter and again measure the absorbance of the soln (while filter is being changed the light source should be switched off). Go on changing the filter and recording the absorbance. The filter which gives the maximum absorbance is the suitable filter for the absorbance measurement. (If a spectrophotometer is used that wavelength will be suitable which gives the maximum absorbance.)

(*ix*) Prepare 0.1 N soln of $KMnO_4$ by standardisation with oxalic acid (see expt. 10.1). Dilute this solution to obtain 0.01, 0.005, 0.0025, 0.001, 0.0005, 0.00025 and 0.0001 N etc., solutions.

(*x*) Measure the absorbance of different solutions prepared in step (*ix*). Plot the absorbance against concentration of $KMnO_4$ (in $\mu g/ml$) as shown in Fig. 15.9. A straight line graph verifies the Beer's low.

[It should be noted that the absorbance-concentration plot will not give a straight line at all concentrations. There is a concentration range for which the law is applicable. Beyond this concentration range, deviations from Beer's law are observed. The straight line part of the graph can serve as a calibration curve for the colorimetric determination of $KMnO_4$.]

[*b*] Determination of concentration of $KMnO_4$ in a given soln

Discussion

A calibration curve is first constructed by plotting absorbance against concentration for known solutions. The concentration of the sample soln is then found out from this curve.

Procedure

(*i*) Prepare several solutions of $KMnO_4$ of known concentration. The concentration range, selected, should be such for which the Beer's law is applicable. Moreover, the concentration of the unknown soln should be within this concentration range.

(*ii*) Measure the absorbance of the known solutions using the suitable filter (a green filter). Obtain a graph between measured absorbance and the corresponding concentration of $KMnO_4$ soln. This is the calibration graph.

(*iii*) Measure the absorbance of the unknown soln under identical condition and find out its concentration with the help of calibration graph. (If the sample soln is concentrated and is beyond the concentration limits in which Beer's law is applicable, the soln should be suitably diluted.)

Experiment 15'2

Colorimetric determination of iron (III) with potassium thiocyanate reagent.

Discussion

A dilute soln containing Fe^{3+} ions is practically colourless. On adding KCNS soln, Fe^{3+} ions form an intensely red coloured compound which remains in soln (Fe^{2+} ions do not react). The red soln contains a mixture of complexes, most important of them being $[Fe(CNS)]^{2+}$:

$$Fe^{3+} + CNS^- \rightleftharpoons [Fe(CNS)]^{2+}$$

It has been observed that a large excess of KCNS increases the colour intensity. Nitric acid should also be present to prevent the hydrolysis :

$$Fe^{3+} + 3H_2O \rightleftharpoons Fe(OH)_3 + 3H^+$$

Several solutions containing known quantities of Fe^{3+} are prepared. To a portion of such a soln, add HCl or HNO_3 and then KCNS soln. The absorbance of the resultant soln is measured by means of a colorimeter. In this way absorbance with all the known solution is measured and a absorbance-concentration plot is obtained which acts as a calibration graph. The absorbance of the coloured soln obtained with the sample soln is then measured under identical conditions and its concentration determined from the calibration graph.

Procedure

(*i*) Prepare a 40% soln of KCNS.

(*ii*) Dissolve 2'0000 g of A.R. ferric ammonium sulphate in water, add 10 ml of concentrated HCl and dilute to 1 litre. Prepare several known solutions by suitably diluting this soln.

(*iii*) Take 10 ml distilled water in the test tube provided with the Klette-Summerson colorimeter and add 1 ml of 4N HCl and

1 ml of KCNS soln. Insert the tube in the light path, use a green filter, put the measuring knob at zero absorbance and adjust the galvanometer needle to zero by means of the adjustment knob provided in the colorimeter. The instrument is now set to measure the absorbance.

(*iv*) Take 10 ml of iron (III) soln of known concentration and add 1 ml of 4N HCl and 1 ml of KCNS soln. Measure the absorbance. Record the absorbance with other known solutions also in a similar manner and construct the calibration plot.

(*v*) Take 10 ml of the given iron (III) soln and add 1 ml of 4N HCl and 1 ml KCNS soln. Measure the absorbance of the resultant soln and then find out the concentration of the sample soln by means of the calibration plot.

16

Radiochemical Methods of Analysis

16'1. NATURAL AND ARTIFICIAL RADIOACTIVITY

The atoms of certain elements, such as uranium and radium, are unstable' and spontaneously (without any external help) disintegrate giving out radiations called *radioactive radiations*. The elements possessing this property are said to be *radioactive* and this phenomenon is known as *natural radioactivity*.

Certain non-radioactive elements on bombardment with α particles start behaving like a radioactive element; this phenomennon is known as *artificial* or *induced radioactivity*. The radioactive variety of the element so prepared is known as its *radio-isotope*. More than 500 radio-isotopes have been prepared by bombarding non-radioactive elements with fast moving particles, called projectiles. Radio-isotopes of all the elements, in the periodic table, have been obtained which find several applications in various branches of Physics, Chemistry, Agriculture, Medicine etc.

16'2. RADIOACTIVE RADIATIONS

On studying the nature of radioactive rays it was found that they are of the following three type.

(*i*) **α-rays.** These consist of α particles (He^{2+}, *i.e.*, doubly ionised helium atoms). These particles are positively charged, hence get deflected by electric or magnetic field. They cause extensive ionisation in the medium through which they pass but have relatively smaller penetrating power.

(*ii*) **β-rays.** These consist of fast moving β particles (electrons). These particles carry negetive charge and are deflected by electric or magnetic field in a direction opposite to that of α particles. The mass of a beta particle is much smaller than that of an α particle, hence β rays have a greater penetrating power but smaller ionising capacity.

(*iii*) γ-**rays**. They are not deflected by electric or magnetic field because they do not carry any charge. These are electromagnetic radiations of very short wavelength (smaller than that of x-rays). They produce little ionisation in the medium through which they travel but have the greatest penetrating power.

A radioactive element gives out either α or β particles (both the particles are not emitted out simultaneously), and this may or may not be accompanied by the emission of γ-rays. A radioactive element giving out α particles is called α emitter or α active, α particles are shot out from such an element with a high velocity, about one tenth that of light. A β emitter emits out β particles with speed almost equal to that of the light.

16·3. EXCITATION AND IONISATION CAUSED BY RADIOACTIVE RADIATIONS

Consider that an α particle, coming out from a radioactive element, passes through a gas. Since the emitted α particle is moving with a high velocity it will have considerable kinetic energy, *i.e.*, it will be energetic. When this energetic particle collides with an atom or a molecule present in the gas, it transfers a part of its energy to the atom. Consequently, the electrons of the atom jump to higher energy levels ; this process is known as *excitation*.

As the electrons return to their ground level, they emit a visible light flash. Thus the entry of an α particle can be detected and by counting the light flashes we can know the number of α particles.

If a greater energy is transferred by the α particle to the atom with which it is colliding, some of the electrons of the atom are knocked out of the atom resulting in the formation of a positive ion. (Remember that if an electron is detached from an atom, which is electrically neutral, a positive ion is formed). The detached electron soon attaches itself to a neutral atom or molecule giving rise to a negative ion. In this way, the passage of an α particle through a gas will result in the formation of positive and negetive ions, *i.e.*, there would be *ionisation*.

16·4. DETECTION AND MEASUREMENT OF RADIOACTIVE RADIATIONS

Radioactive radiations (α, β and γ rays) produce excitation and ionisation in the medium (gas, liquid or solid) through which they pass. This fact is utilised in developing instruments for the detection and measurement of radioactivity ; a few of them have been described below.

1. Spinthariscope. It consists of a layer of zinc **sulphide** coated on a glass plate. Each α particle striking the layer produces a flash of light which can be seen under a magnifying glass. This simple instrument can be used only for detecting α particles.

2. Scintillation counter. The light flashes (Scintillations) produced in a spinthariscope are quite weak. Besides, it is not possible to count more than 60 scintillations per minute. Certain substances known as phosphors (such as potassium iodide containing a trace of thallium) are sensitive to α, β and γ rays. The scintillations produced by a phosphor due to α, β or γ rays are allowed to fall on a photoelectric cell. Each scintillation generates an electric pulse which is suitably amplified and recorded by a recording system. Such electronic systems have been developed which can measure energy of the incident particles by measuring the height of the pulse. The modern scintillation counter can detect and record millions of flashes per second.

3. Electroscope. It consists of a glass chamber containing a vertical metal rod. At the end of the rod two gold foils are attached which are given the charge of the same sign so that they repel each other, forming an inverted V. When radioactive rays enter the chamber, the air between the gold leaves gets ionised and the leaves collapse. The rate of collapse of the gold leaves is a measure of the intensity of the incident radioactive radiations.

4. Geiger-Muller counter (also known as Geiger or G-M counter). It consists of a fine tungsten wire W mounted along the axis of a metal tube T which contains a mixture of argon and ethyl alcohol vapour at low pressure. A potential difference of 1000 to

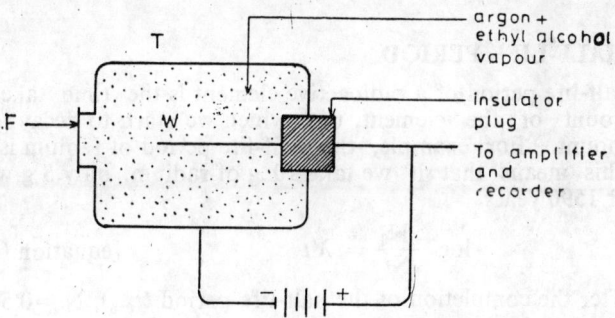

Fig. 16·1. Geiger Muller Counter.

2000 volts is applied between the central wire W (anode) and the tube T (cathode). The tube has a thin foil window F through which radioactive radiations can enter. These radiations cause ionisation in the gas present in the tube T. Each incident particle gives rise to a pulse of current which is amplified and recorded. The G-M counter can record counts up to 100,000 per second. The magnitude of the pulse is a measure of the energy of the incident particle.

16˙5. RATE OF DISINTEGRATION AND DECAY CONSTANT

Suppose that at a given instant there are N atoms of a particular radioactive element and, in a small interval of time dt, the number of atoms which integrate is dN. The rate of disintegration is proportional to the total number of atoms present :

$$-\frac{dN}{dt} \propto N \text{ or } -\frac{dN}{dt} = \lambda N \qquad (16˙1)$$

where λ is a constant called *radioactive constant* or *disintegration constant* or *decay coustant* of the element under consideration. The negetive sign in (16˙1) is necessary because the number of atoms of the radioactive element decreases with time, and hence the rate dN/dt is a negetive quantity. We can rearrange (16˙1) as :

$$\frac{dN}{N} = -\lambda \, dt \qquad (16˙2)$$

On integrating (16˙2), the result is

$$\log \frac{No}{Nt} = \lambda't \qquad (16˙3)$$

Notes :

(1) In (16˙3) $\log_e$ has been replaced by $\log_{10}$, that is why a new constant λ' has been used in place of λ.

(2) Integration of (16˙2) can be carried out in a manner similar to that described in 15˙B˙1˙1 in connection with Lambert's law.

16˙6. HALF-LIFE PERIOD

Half-life period of a radioactive element is the time taken for the amount of the element, with which we start, to decay to half that amount. For example, the half-life period of radium is 1590 years, this means that if we take 10 g of radium, only 5 g will be left after 1590 years.

$$\log \frac{N_0}{Nt} = \lambda't \qquad \text{[equation (16˙3)]}$$

After the completion of the half-life period $(t_{0.5})$, $N_t = 0˙5 \times N_0$, so that we can write :

$$\log \frac{N_0}{N_0 \times 0˙5} = \log 2 = \lambda' t_{0.5}$$

or,

$$t_{0.5} = \frac{\log 2}{\lambda'} \qquad (16˙4)$$

[N_0 = no. of atoms at time zero, and
N_t = no. of atoms at time t.]

Because log 2 and λ' are constant, hence $t_{0.5}$ will also be a constant for a given radioactive element. Thus a radioactive element can be recognised by measuring its half-life period. For instance, we are given a radioactive element whose half-life period is found to be 1590 years. Since the half-life period of radium is known to be 1590 years, we can conclude that the given radioactive element will be radium.

16·7. APPLICATIONS OF MEASUREMENT OF RADIOACTIVITY IN QUANTITATIVE ANALYSIS

The strength of a radioactive substance is generally expressed in term of a unit, called curie. The curie is defined as an activity of $3·7 \times 10^{10}$ disintegrations per second. This term is applicable to disintegrations resulting in the emission of α as well as β particles. A millicurie is 1/1000th part of a curie ; a microcurie is equal to 10^{-6} of a curie.

The radioactive isotopes of all the elements can be prepared, hence the measurement of radioactivity finds several applications in chemical analysis. Some radioanalytical techniques have been briefly described below.

1. **Neutron activation analysis.** This technique can be used in qualitative as well as in quantitative analysis. Suppose an element present in a sample is to be identified by means of neutron activation analysis. The sample will be bombarded with neutrons or other charged particles (slow neutrons are more effective). As a result of this bombardment the non-radioactive element present in the sample is converted into its radioactive isotope which will decay giving out its characteristic radioactive radiations. From half-life period measurement, it is possible to identify the element from which the radioisotope has resulted.

The activation technique can also be used for determining the amount of an element present in a given sample. The given sample is bombarded with neutrons and the radioactivity of the resultant radioisotope is measured. A known amount of the element in question is then bombarded with neutrons under identical conditions and the radioactivity of the radioisotope formed is measured. By comparing the radioactivity in the two cases, the quantity of the element present in the given sample can be calculated.

2. **Isotope dilution analysis.** There are certain cases when quantitative analysis for a component of a mixture is desired but there is no method available for the quantitative separation of the component from the mixture. In the case of some complex organic mixtures it may be possible to isolate the desired compound in pure form but the separation is not quantitative. In such cases the technique of isotope dilution is very useful. In this technique

radioactive variety of the compound in question is prepared by using radioisotope of the element present in the compound. (For example, if we have to determine $FeCl_3$, we will prepare radioactive variety of $FeCl_3$ by using a radioactive isotope of iron). The radioactivity of a known weight of the radioactive compound is measured. To the unknown mixture is added a known weight of the radioactive compound which mixes thoroughly with its non-radioactive variety. (Note that radioactive and the non-radioactive varieties of the same compound have identical chemical properties.) The compound is then separated from the mixture. (The separated product contains both radioactive and non-radioactive compound.) The activity of a known weight of the separated compound is recorded. The extent of dilution of radioactive compound shows the amount of inactive compound present in the original mixture.

Example 16(i)

Suppose a mixture contains 900 mg of a compound A. There is no method for the quantitative separation of the compound A from the mixture. Hence we cannot find out the quantity of A present in the mixture. In such a case the isotope dilution method can be applied in the following manner.

1. Prepare the radiactive variety of the compound A. Let us represent it by A*. Note that the composition and chemical properties of A and A* are similar.

2. Find out the radioactivity of a known amount (say 100 mg) of A*. Suppose it comes out to be x.

3. Add 100 mg of A* to the given mixture containing the compound A that is to be determined and mix them thoroughly.

4. Separate compound A by some suitable chemical method say by precipitation.

5. Weigh the purified precipitate (Suppose it corresponds to 500 mg of A) find out its activity (Suppose it comes out to be $0.5 x$).

Since the radioactivity has reduced to half of its original value, the separated ppt must contain only 50 mg of A*. (Note that 100 mg of A* had activity equal to x). It means that the amount of A in the separated ppt is $(500-50)=450$ mg.

Now, because only half of A* has been precipitated and A and A* have identical chemical properties, it is reasonable to conclude that the separated ppt contains only half of the amount of A present in the mixture. Since the separated ppt contains 450 mg of A, the quantity of A in the mixture must be $450 \times 2 = 900$ mg.

3. **Radiometric analysis.** We can prepare radioactive variety of KI by using radioisotope of iodine. The variety of KI so produced

will be tagged or labelled with radioactive iodine. Such *labelled* or *tagged compounds* find several applications in quantitative analysis.

Suppose we have to find out the amount of silver in a given soln or $AgNO_3$ by radiometric method. The steps will be :

(*i*) Prepare radioactive variety of KI using a radioisotope of iodine.

(*ii*) Prepare several known solutions of $AgNO_3$ and in each case precipitate silver as AgI by adding an excess of radioactive KI soln. Measure the radioactivity of AgI obtained from different known solutions. Plot a graph between the quantity of AgI and radioactivity. This is the calibration graph.

(*iii*) Take a known volume of the given $AgNO_3$ soln and precipitate AgI by adding an excess of radioactive KI soln. Measure the radioactivity of the precipitated AgI and find out its quantity with the help of the calibration graph. Knowing the weight of AgI, the quantity of Ag present in the sample soln can be calculated.

4. Radiometric titrations. Consider the titration of a chloride soln with labelled $AgNO_3$ soln taken in the burette. When a small volume of $AgNO_3$ is added it is converted into AgCl which carries the radioactive silver. Since the radioactivity is in AgCl which settles down, the supernatant liquid does not show any activity. After the equivalence point, the addition of radioactive $AgNO_3$ soln will be detected in the supernatant liquid. The point at which the supernatant liquid shows radioactivity will be the end point of the titration.

17

Quantitative Analytical Methods Based on Some Other Physical Properties

Any physical property which is related to the concentration of a substance can be made use of in its quantitative analysis. Several quantitative analytical methods have been developed based on the measurement of some physical properties, such as density, viscosity, refractive index, surface tension etc. A few of these will be briefly discussed here.

17·A METHOD INVOLVING VISCOSITY MEASUREMENT

17·A·1 Theory

Consider a liquid flowing over a horizontal plane as shown in Fig. 17·1. The liquid may be regarded as being made up of different layers l_1, l_2, l_3, l_4 etc. The lowest layer has the smallest velocity and as we move up, the layer velocity goes on increasing. For example, l_3 is faster than l_2 but slower than l_4. Because different layers have different flow rates, there is an internal friction between

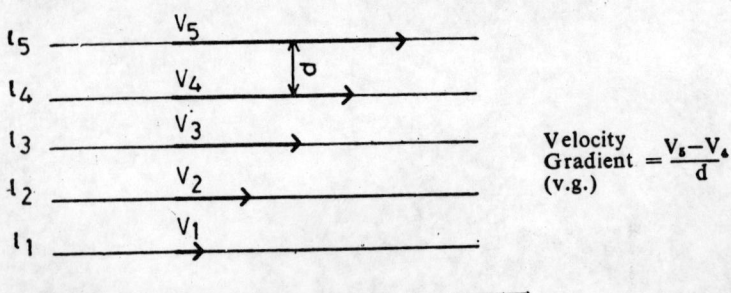

$$\text{Velocity Gradient} = \frac{V_s - V_t}{d}$$
(v.g.)

Fig. 17·1. Flow of a liquid over a horizontal plane.

them. These internal frictional forces constitute what are known as *viscous forces*.

Suppose the velocity of the fifth layer is V_5 and that of the fourth is V_4 and the distance between then is d cms. The velocity gradient for these layers will then be given as :

$$\text{Velocity gradient} = \frac{V_5 - V_4}{d}$$

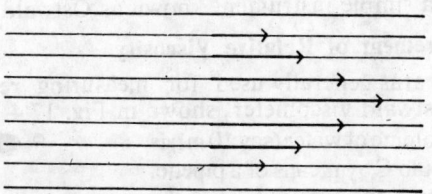

Fig. 17·2. Flow of a liquid through a tube.

17`A`1`1 Coefficient of Viscosity

The viscous forces in a liquid oppose its movement, hence a force has to be constantly applied in order to maintain the flow of a liquid. For a more viscous liquid a greater force has to be applied to keep it moving. In order to compare the viscosity of various liquids, a term viscosity coefficient represented by Greek letter η is used. It is defined as the force per unit area which must be applied tangentially to maintain unit velocity gradient between two parallel layers unit distance apart (see Fig. 17·3). The smaller the value of coefficient of viscosity of a liquid more rapidly it can flow.

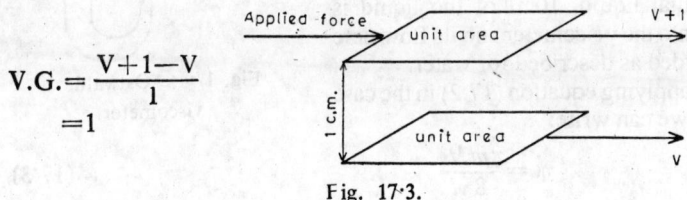

$$V.G. = \frac{V+1-V}{1}$$
$$= 1$$

Fig. 17·3.

17`A`1`2 Poiseuille Equation

When a liquid flows through a capillary tube of radius 'r' for time 't', under a constant pressure 'p', the volume 'v' of liquid coming out from the tube is given by poiseuille equation :

$$v = \frac{\pi p r^4 t}{8 \eta l} \qquad \qquad ...(17·1)$$

where l is the length of the capillary tube and η is the coefficient of viscosity of the liquid. This is the fundamental equation for measuring viscosity. The unit of viscosity is poise, after the name of Poiseuille who first made systematic study of flow of liquids through a capillary tube. Equation (17.1) can also be written in the following form :

$$\eta=\frac{\pi pr^4t}{8vl} \qquad \qquad ...(17.2)$$

Equation (17.2) can be readily applied for measuring relative viscosity using a simple instrument known as Ostwald viscometer.

17.A.2 Measurement of Relative Viscosity

The apparatus generally used for measuring relative viscosity of a liquid is Ostwald viscometer, shown in Fig. 17.4.

A known volume of water (say 10 ml) is introduced into bulb C by means of a pipette. By sucking through the rubber tube R the liquid is forced up through the capillary BD until the water level rises above the mark A. The liquid is then allowed to flow down through the capillary and stop watch is started the moment the lower maniscus of the liquid crosses the mark A and stopped as soon as it passes the lower mark B. The time duration is recorded. This step is repeated four or five times. If the time values differ much from each other, the viscometer should be cleaned and the experiment repeated. The flow time t_w for water is thus found out.

The viscometer is then rinsed with the experimental liquid, 10 ml of the liquid is pipetted into the viscometer and its flow time t_l is recorded as described for water.

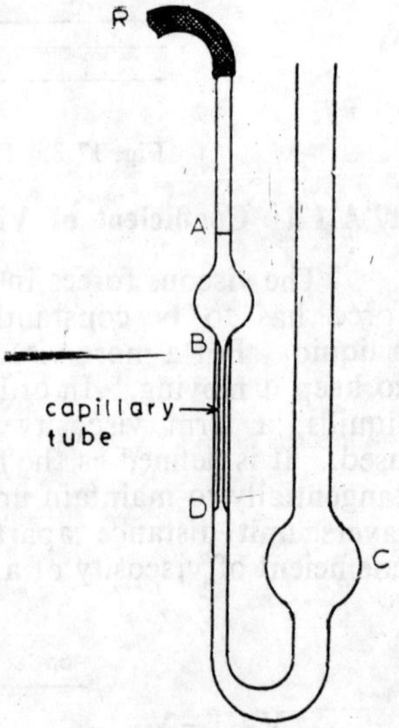

By applying equation (17.2) in the case of water, we can write:

Fig. 17.4. Ostwald viscometer.

$$\eta w=\frac{\pi pr^4 t_w}{8\,vl} \qquad \qquad ...(17.3)$$

where ηw is the coefficient of viscosity of water. Now, the driving force 'p' is given as :

$$p=\text{h.d.g.}$$

where h=difference in the height of liquid in the two columns of the viscometer

d=density of the liquid

g=acceleration due to gravity.

Suppose the density of water at experimental temperature is d_w, substituting for p in equation (17.3), the result is :

$$\eta_w = \frac{\pi h \, d_w \, g r^4 \, t_w}{8vl} \qquad \qquad ...(17\cdot 4)$$

Similarly, if d_l is the density of the liquid at the experimental temperature and η_l its coefficient of viscosity, it is possible to write :

$$\eta_l = \frac{\pi h \, d_l \, g \, r^4 \, t_l}{8vl} \qquad \qquad ...(17\cdot 5)$$

Dividing equation (17·5) by (17·4) :

$$\frac{\eta_l}{\eta_w} = \frac{\pi h d_l g r^4 t_l}{8vl} \times \frac{8vl}{\pi h d_w g r^4 t_w}$$

or,
$$\frac{\eta_l}{\eta_w} = \frac{d_l t_l}{d_w t_w}$$

or,
$$\eta_l = \eta_w \times \frac{d_l t_l}{d_w t_w} \qquad \qquad ...(17\cdot 6)$$

Expression (17·6) gives the coefficient of viscosity of the liquid relative to that of water. If we know the absolute viscosity of water that of the given liquid can be calculated.

17·A·3. Application of Viscosity Measurement to Quantitative Analysis

As an example, let us consider how the composition of a given mixture of ethyl and methyl alcohol can be determined by viscosity measurement.

Discussion

We must note that ethyl and methyl alcohol belong to the same class of organic compounds so they have practically similar chemical properties. It is, therefore, very difficult to find out a chemical method by which CH_3OH can be determined in the presence of C_2H_5OH or C_2H_5OH can be determined in the presence of CH_3OH. The only way left is to isolate CH_3OH from C_2H_5OH and then determine them separately by suitable chemical methods. This approach will obviously be quite tedious and time consuming.

Ethyl and methyl alcohol are the members of a homologous series so though their chemical properties will be similar but physical properties will show a difference, hence in such cases the measurement of a physical property can act as a basis of a method for their quantitative analysis. For example, the viscosity of ethyl and methyl alcohol is different ; this fact can be used for quantitatively analysing a given mixture of these compounds. First, a number of mixtures of CH_3OH and C_2H_5OH of known concentrations are prepared and their flow times recorded by means of an Ostwald viscometer. A graph is then plotted between flow time and composition of the mixture ; this is the calibration curve. Now, the flow time of the given mixture of CH_3OH and C_2H_5OH is determined using the same viscometer and the composition of the mixture found out with the help of the calibration curve.

Procedure

(i) Thoroughly clean nine glass bottles with glass stoppers.

Dry them and prepare the following nine known mixtures of CH_3OH and C_2H_5OH in these bottles. Shake well and close the bottles properly so that there is no loss due to volatalisation.

Volume (ml) CH_3OH 18 ; 16 ; 14 ; 12 ; 10 ; 8 ; 6 ; 4 ; 2

C_2H_5OH 2 ; 4 ; 6 ; 8 ; 10 ; 12 ; 14 ; 16 : 18.

(ii) Clean an Ostwald viscometer. Dry and rinse it with a known mixture. Introduce 10 ml of the mixture into the viscometer and find out its flow time. In this way record the flow time for each known soln prepared in step (i). Plot a graph between the different flow times and corresponding composition of the mixture to obtain a calibration curve.

(iii) Rinse the same viscometer with the given mixture of CH_3OH and C_2H_5OH, and find out its flow time using 10 ml of the mixture under the similar conditions.

(iv) Find out the composition of the given alcohol mixture with the help of the calibration curve as shown in Fig. 17.5.

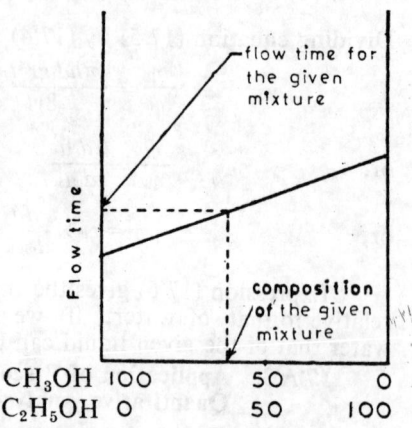

Fig. 17·5.

Notes

1. The viscometer should be thoroughly cleaned with chromic acid or soap water and then washed several times with distilled water.

2. The viscometer should be first rinsed two or three times with the liquid whose flow time is to be measured.

3. The viscometer should be held in a vertical position with the help of a clamp and a stand and its position must remain the same throughout the measurements.

4. Since viscosity depends upon temperature, the viscometer should be kept in a thermostat during the measurements of flow times.

17`B. METHOD INVOLVING SURFACE TENSION MEASUREMENTS

17`B`1. Theory

A molecule situated inside the body of a liquid is equally attracted in all directions by the surrounding molcules. Hence, there is no net force acting on it. On the other hand, a molecule of the liquid at its surface is pulled sideways and downwards but there is no molecules above it to balance the downward pull. As a result the molecules at the surface are subject to a force acting inwards at right angles to the surface. This is the reason why the surface of a liquid is always in tension and behaves like a stretched membrane. This property of liquids is known as surface tension. (If a slit is cut in a stretched rubber sheet, there would be a force on each side of the slit tending to open it.) The surface tension γ of a liquid is defined as the force in dynes acting upon a line of 1 cm length in the surface of the liquid. Thus, its unit is dyne per cm.

The surface tension of a liquid depends upon its nature. On increasing the temperature the surface tension of a liquid decreases.

17·B·2. Measurement of Surface Tension

The relative surface tension of a liquid can be conveniently measured by means of a stalagmometer (Fig. 17·6).

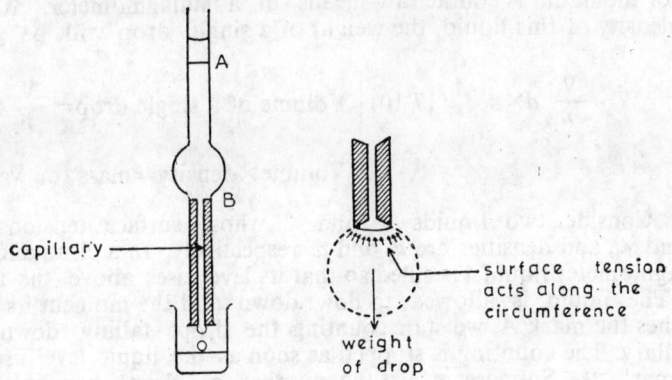

Fig. 17·6. Stalagmometer.   Fig. 17·7.

Consider a liquid flowing down a capillary tube as shown in Fig. 17·7. A drop formed at the end of the capillary grows in size up to a particular point and then falls down. If the radius of the capillary tube is 'r', the surface tension acting along the circumference of the tube is $2\pi r\gamma$. This force which acts in upward direction is responsible for holding the drop and this is the reason why the drop does not fall initially. As the size of the drop grows, its weight increases and so the force acting in downward direction and the moment it equals the upward force due to the surface tension, the drop falls. So we can write :

$$2\pi r\gamma = W \qquad \qquad ...(17·7)$$

where W is the weight of the drop and γ is the surface tension of the liquid. Now, the weight W of the drop is given by

$$W = v.d.g \qquad \qquad ...(17·8)$$

where v =volume of the drop, and

d =density of the liquid.

Substituting the value of W from (17.8) into (17.7) the result is :

$$2\pi r . \gamma = v.d.g$$

or,

$$\gamma = \frac{v.d.g}{2\pi r} \qquad \qquad ...(17.9)$$

Knowing the density of the liquid, the volume of a single drop and the radius of the capillary tube, the surface tension of the liquid can be calculated.

Now, it is not very convenient to determine the volume of a single drop, hence, number of drops (n) formed by a known volume (V) of the liquid is counted by means of a stalagmometer. If d is the density of this liquid, the weight of a single drop will be given by :

$$W = \frac{V}{n} . d \times g \qquad (17.10) \quad \bigg| \quad \text{Volume of a single drop} = \frac{V}{n} = v$$

$$\text{Volume} \times \text{density} = \text{mass (or weight)}$$

Consider two liquids 1 and 2 whose surface tensions are γ_1 and γ_2, and densities are d_1 and d_2 respectively. In a clean and dry stalagmometer liquid 1 is filled so that its level rises above the mark A. The liquid is allowed to flow down and the moment its level reaches the mark A, we start counting the drops falling down the capillary. The counting is stopped as soon as the liquid level crosses the mark B. Suppose n_1 is the number of drops counted with liquid 1 and n_2 is that with liquid 2. The volume of the liquid V in both the cases will be the same. By making use of equation (17.10) we can write :

$$W_1 = \frac{V}{n_1} \times d_1 \times g$$

and

$$W_2 = \frac{V}{n_2} \times d_2 \times g$$

where W_1 and W_2 are weights of a drop of liquids 1 and 2 respectively.

From equation (17.7) it is possible to write :

$$2\pi r \gamma_1 = \frac{V}{n_1} \times d_1 \times g \qquad ...(17.11)$$

and

$$2\pi r \gamma_2 = \frac{V}{n_2} \times d_2 \times g \qquad ...(17.12)$$

Dividing (17·11) by (17·12), the result is :

$$\frac{2\pi r \gamma_1}{2\pi r \gamma_2} = \frac{V \times d_1 g}{n_1} \Big/ \frac{V \times d_2 g}{n_2}$$

$$= \frac{V \times d_1 g}{n_1} \times \frac{n_2}{V \times d_2 g}$$

or,

$$\frac{\gamma_1}{\gamma_2} = \frac{d_1 \times n_2}{d_2 \times n_1}$$

or,

$$\gamma_1 = \gamma_2 \times \frac{d_1 \times n_2}{d_2 \times n_1} \qquad \qquad ...(17·13)$$

Thus, with the help of equation (17·13) it is possible to calculate the surface tension of liquid 1 relative to that of liquid 2.

If the value of surface tension of liquid 2 is known that of the liquid 1 can be found out.

17·B·3   Application of Surface Tension Measurement to Quantitative Analysis

Suppose we are given a soln of glycol in water and we want to find out the concentration of glycol. Since the surface tension of water and glycol are quite different, the glycol-water mixture can be quantitatively analysed from surface tension measurement as described below (the procedure is quite similar to one involving viscocity measurement described in 17·A·3).

Procedure

(i) Prepare several known solutions of glycol in water in the following manner :

Volume(ml)

Glycol 16 ; 12 ; 10 ; 8 ; 6 ; 4 ; 2

Water 4 ; 8 ; 10 ; 12 ; 14 ; 16 ; 18.

(ii) Clean a stalagmometer and fill it with a known soln of glycol and count the number of drops during the flow of the soln from the higher to the lower mark. Similarly find out the number of drops with each known soln.

(iii) Draw a graph between number of drops and concentration of glycol and thus obtain the calibration curve.

(iv) Count the number of drops for the given soln using the same stalagmometer.

(v) Find out the concentration of glycol in the unknown soln with the help of the calibration curve.

17·C. METHOD INVOLVING MEASUREMENT OF REFRACTIVE INDEX

When a ray of light moves from air into a denser medium (say water or some other liquid or solution) it is deviated or bent or refracted (see Fig. 17·8). If i is the angle of incidence and r that of the refraction, the refractive index μ of the liquid is given by :

$$\mu = \frac{\sin i}{\sin r} \qquad (17\cdot14)$$

For a given liquid the value of refractive index is constant and it is characteristic of that liquid.

The refractive index of a liquid can be very conveniently and rapidly measured by means of an Abbe refractometer.

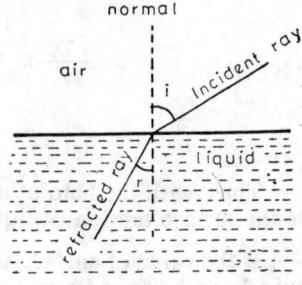

Fig. 17·8.

17·C·1. Refractometric Titrations

The measurement of refractive index can be applied to quantitative analysis as illustrated by the titration of oxalic acid with lead acetate.

A known volume of an unknown oxalic acid soln is titrated with a standard lead acetate soln. The refractive index of the titration liquid is measured at different stages of the titration. A graph is then plotted between the different values of refractive indices and the corresponding volumes of the titrant added. A break is noticeable in the curve which gives the end point of the titration.

17·D. METHODS BASED ON MEASUREMENT OF THERMAL PROPERTIES

Thermoanalytical methods include thermogravimetric analysis (TGA), differential thermal analysis (DTA) and thermometric titrations.

In thermogravimetry the weight of a compound is recorded at different temperatures. From the weight-temperature graph, the thermal stability of a compound, in a given range of temperature, can be studied. Such an information is essential in igniting a precipitate in gravimetric analysis.

17·D·1. Thermometric Titrations

In these titrations the temperature of the titration liquid is recorded as the unknown soln is being titrated. The temperature is then plotted against the volume of the titrant added. A sharp break in the curve marks the end point of the titration.

Experiment 17·1

Determination of the heat neutralisation of a strong acid and a strong base.

Chemicals required. Hydrochloric acid, sodium hydroxide and phenolphthalein indicator.

Apparatus required. Calorimeter, thermometer that can read up to $0·1°C$, burette, pipette, conical flasks and measuring flasks.

Discussion

Heat of neutralisation is defined as the quantity of heat, in calories, liberated when 1 g eq of an acid completely reacts with 1 g eq of a base at such a great dilution that further dilution does not cause any heat change. This definition incorporates three conditions :

(a) the quantities of acid and base taken should be 1 g eq. each,

(b) the reaction between the acid and the base should be complete, and

(c) the solutions of the acid and base used should be so dilute that on further diluting them no heat change should take place.

It should be noted that if an acid, for example H_2SO_4, is diluted a lot of heat known as heat of dilution is produced. If we go on diluting this soln, ultimately we will obtain a very dilute soln which on further dilution will not liberate any heat. If concentrated solutions of an acid and a base are mixed the heat generated will be due to neutralisation and also as a result of dilution. The purpose of using very dilute solutions is to eliminate the heat of dilution so that the quantity of heat produced gives only the heat of neutralisation. But if solutions taken are very dilute (say 100 ml 0·01 N acid and 100 ml 0·01 N alkali), the temperature rise is so small that it cannot be accurately measured. Hence, in practice the solutions used are neither too dilute nor too concentrated.

Another point to be noted is that the heat of neutralisation of a strong acid and a strong base has a constant value of 13·67 Kcal. The reason for this constant value is that strong acids and strong bases, in dilute soln, completely dissociate giving H^+ and OH^- ions respectively. Hence, when they are mixed the common reaction in all such cases is :

$$H^+ + OH^- \longrightarrow H_2O + 13·67 \text{ Kcal}$$

Thus the heat of neutralisation for strong acids and bases is essentially the heat of formation of water from H^+ and OH^- ions.

If a weak acid, such as CH_3COOH, is taken, it does not dissociate completely. When such an acid reacts with a base, a part of the heat of neutralisation is consumed in dissociating the weak acid into its ions. Hence, the heat of neutralisation recorded is less than that observed in the case of a strong acid and a strong base, i.e., 13.67 Kcal. Suppose with acetic acid and sodium hydroxide, the heat of neutralisation comes out to be 12.53 Kcal. Then $(13.67 - 12.53) = 1.14$ Kcal is the quantity of heat used up in the dissociation of 1 g eq of acetic acid. Thus 1.14 Kcal will be known as the *heat of dissociation* of acetic acid. If the acid and base both are weak, the value of heat of neutralisation will be still smaller because now some heat will be required for the dissociation of weak base also. Suppose in the case of acetic acid and ammonium hydroxide, the heat of neutralisation is found to be 11.41 Kcal, the value for the heat of dissociation for 1 g eq of ammonium hydroxide will be $(12.53 - 11.41) = 1.12$ Kcal.

Preparation of Solution

Prepare exactly 1 N HCl and 1N NaOH solutions as described in Experiments 8.1 and 8.2.

Procedure

(i) Weigh the calorimetric vessel (made of copper) along with the stirrer.

(ii) Take x ml (60-70 ml) of water and 10 ml of 1 N NaOH soln into the calorimetric vessel.

(iii) Insert a thermometer into the calorimeter.

(iv) Stir the contents of the calorimeter slowly and go on observing the temperature. When the temperature becomes constant, record it. It is the initial temperature $T_1 °C$.

(v) Open the lid of the calorimeter, quickly add 10 ml of 1 N HCl and immediately close the lid.

(vi) Go on slowly stirring the contents of the calorimeter and at the same time observe the temperature. When the temperature reaches a maximum and then begins to fall, note the maximum temperature. This is the final temperature $T_2 °C$.

Calculations

(a) Suppose the weight of the calorimeter and the stirrer (both made of copper) = 150.0 g. As the specific heat of copper is 0.1, the water equivalent of the calorimeter will be :

$$150 \times 0.1 = 15 \text{ g}$$

That is for heat transfer calculations, 150 g of copper can be regarded as equivalent to 15 g of water.

(b) Suppose 65 ml of water, 10 ml of acid and 10 ml of alkali solutions are taken in the calorimeter. Then the total volume of water can be taken as :

$$65+10+10+15 \text{ (water equivalent of calorimeter)} = 100 \text{ ml.}$$

(c) Suppose the initial temperature is 25.1°C and the final temperature is 26.5°C.

The difference in temperature is (26.5−25.1)=1.4°C.

(d) The heat received by the calorimeter and its contents is therefore equal to :

$$100 \times 1.4 = 140 \text{ calories}$$

(e) 1000 ml of 1 N acid or base contains 1 g eq.

$$\therefore 10 \text{ ml of 1 N acid or base contains } \frac{1}{100} \text{ g eq.}$$

It means that in the experiment we have used 0.01 g eq of the acid and 0.01 g eq of the base. But for the calculation of the heat of neutralisation 1 g eq of the acid and 1 g eq of the base should be considered. Now 0.01 g eq of acid and 0.01 g eq of base liberate 140 calories, therefore when 1 g eq of the acid and 1 g eq of base are taken, the heat liberated will be

$$140 \times 100 = 14000 \text{ calories}$$
$$= 14.0 \text{ Kcal.}$$

Notes

1. The amount of water taken in the calorimeter (65 ml) is so adjusted that the total volume becomes 100 ml ; this simplifies the calculations.

2. For more accurate work, a thermometer with a least count of 0.01°C should be used and cooling curves are constructed to take into account the radiation losses.

Experiment 17.2.

Determination of the heat of dissociation of acetic acid.

Chemical required. Acetic acid, sodium hydroxide and phenolphthalein indicator.

Apparatus required. Calorimeter, thermometer that can read up to 0 1°C, burette, pipette, conical flsak and measuring flasks.

Discussion

Hydrochloric acid is a strong acid whereas acetic acid is a weak acid. In a soln of HCl, almost all the molecules of the acid are dissociated. But in a soln of acetic acid of the same concentration very few molecules would dissociate and most of the acid would be in the molecular form.

It has been seen in Expt 17·1 that the heat of neutralisation for all strong acids and strong bases has the same value i.e., 13·7 Kcal. This is because of the fact that in all cases the common reaction is

$$H^+ + OH^- \longrightarrow H_2O + 13.7 \text{ Kcal}$$

If we find out the heat of neutralisation for CH_3COOH and NaOH, it would not be 13 7 Kcal because a part of the heat energy is used up in causing the dissociation of CH_3COOH molecules into H^+ and CH_3COO^- ions. Suppose x Kcal of heat is used up in causing the dissociation of 1 g mole of CH_3COOH, then the heat of neutralisation of CH_3COOH and NaOH would be $(13·7-x)$ Kcal so that we can write.

$$\left(\begin{array}{l} \text{Heat of neutralisa-} \\ \text{tion of } CH_3COOH \\ \text{and NaOH)} \end{array} \right) = \left(\begin{array}{l} \text{Heat of nutralisa-} \\ \text{tion of HCl and} \\ \text{NaOH} \end{array} \right) - \left(\begin{array}{l} \text{Heat of disso-} \\ \text{ciation of} \\ CH_3COOH \end{array} \right)$$

      (A)   (B)   (C)

$\therefore \quad x = B - A.$

Knowing the values of B and A. the value of x can be calculated. The value of B is known to be 13·7 Kcal hence, if we experimentally determine the value of A, then the valve of x can be found out.

Preparation of Solution

Prepare exactly 1 N CH_3COOH and 1 N NaOH soln as described in Experiments 8·1 and 8·2.

Procedure

Follow exactly the same procedure as described in Experiment 17·3 for the determination of the heat of neutralisation of HCl and NaOH. (In this experiment 1N CH_3COOH should be used in place of 1N HCl.

Calculations

Calculate the heat of neutralisation of CH_3COOH and NaOH as described in Experiment 17·3, suppose it comes out to be A Kcal. Then the heat of dissociation of CH_3COOH would be $(13·7-A)$ Kcal.

PART VI

ELEMENTARY ORGANIC ANALYSIS

18

Qualitative and Quantitative Organic Analysis

In order to identify an organic compound it is essential to analyse it qualitatively ; this involves detection of various elements and functional groups present. After detecting various constituents, their amounts in a given quantity of the compound are determined. These studies are important in finding out the structure of the compound under examination. In elemental analysis the elements present in a compound are detected and their amounts determined. The functional group analysis involves qualitative and quantitative analysis of certain groupings of atoms, such as hydroxyl group (−OH), carboxyl group (−COOH), nitro group (−NO$_2$), amino group(−NH$_2$) etc.

18·A QUALITATIVE ELEMENTAL ANALYSIS

18·A·1 Detection of Carbon and Hydrogen

Carbon is present in all organic compounds so there is no need to test it. However, by means of the following experiment the presence of carbon and hydrogen in an organic compound can be detected.

(*i*) Mix one part by weight of the given organic substance (should be dry) with about ten times its weight of *dry* cupric oxide (CuO). Keep the mixture in a *dry* hard glass tube.

(*ii*) Arrange the apparatus as shown in Fig. 18·1.

(*iii*) Heat the mixture strongly. Carbon and hydrogen present in the organic compound are oxidised by CuO according to the equation :

$$C+2CuO \longrightarrow CO_2+2Cu$$
$$H_2+CuO \longrightarrow H_2O+Cu$$

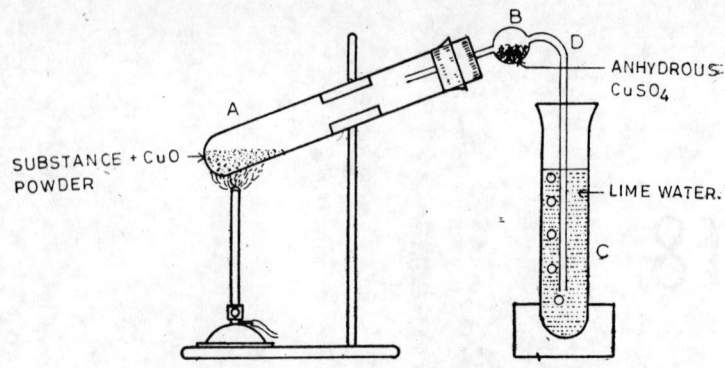

Fig. 18·1. Detection of carbon and hydrogen.

The water vapours formed in tube A pass out through delivery tube D and reach glass bulb B which contains anhydrous cupric sulphate. If the compound contains hydrogen, it will be oxidised to water which will convert anhydrous cupric sulphate (white) into hydrated cupric sulphate (blue). Thus if the white anhydrous $CuSO_4$ turns blue, it indicates the presence of hydrogen in the compound under test.

Carbon dioxide produced as a result of the oxidation of carbon is passed through a clear soln of lime water placed in a test tube C. If lime water turns milky the presence of carbon in the compound is indicated. The reaction involved is :

$$Ca(OH)_2 + CO_2 \longrightarrow \underset{\substack{\text{white} \\ \text{suspension}}}{CaCO_3} + H_2O$$

18·A·2 Detection of Oxygen

If a substance alone is heated strongly it may give water vapour (hydrogen is usually present in organic compounds, if oxygen is also present the two will combine to form water), which can be tested by means of anhydrous cupric sulphate. However, if the test is not given it is not sure that oxygen is absent. The presence of oxygen in organic compounds is found out by carrying out the quantitative analysis of different elements present. Suppose a compound is found to contain :

$$\begin{aligned} C &= 40\% \\ H &= 46\cdot 66\% \\ \hline \text{Total} &= 86\cdot 66\% \end{aligned}$$

Then it will be concluded that the rest, *i.e.*, $(100 - 86\cdot66) = 13\cdot34\%$ is the percentage of oxygen, provided no other element, except carbon and hydrogen, is detected.

18·A·3. Detection of Sulphur

(*i*) Take a small piece of sodium metal in an ignition tube **A** and add to it the compound under test. Heat the tube first gently and then strongly for about 2 minutes as shown in Fig. 18·2. Dip

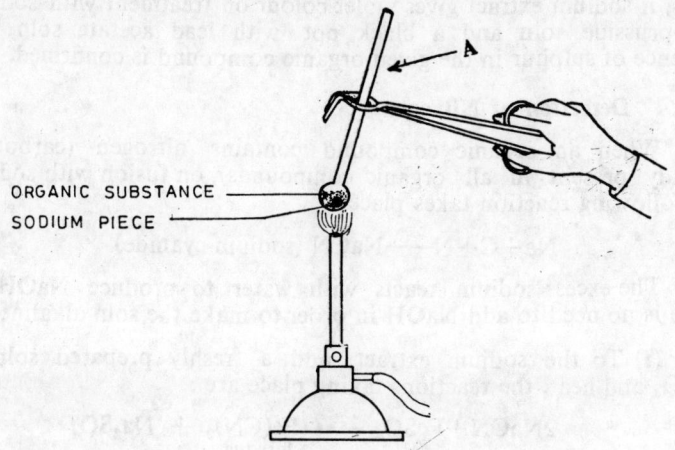

ORGANIC SUBSTANCE

SODIUM PIECE

Fig. 18 2. Fusion of organic substance with sodium.

the hot tube into about 10 ml of water taken in a porcelain dish. The tube breaks and its contents get mixed with water. Heat the procelain dish so that the water soluble portion of the product dissolves. Filter and collect the filtrate which is known as *sodium extract.*

[**Notes** : (1) Keep the mouth of the tube away from your face.

(2) Place sodium metal first and then add the compound to be fused with the metal. If metal is placed over the compound and heated strongly from the very beginning, the metal may start burning and may come out of the tube.]

If the organic compound being tested contains sulphur, the following reaction will take place on fusion with sodium :

$$2Na + S \longrightarrow Na_2S$$

(*ii*) Divide sodium extract into two parts.

(*iii*) To the first part, add a freshly prepared soln of sodium nitroprusside when a violet colour is seen due to the reaction :

$$Na_2S + Na_2[Fe(CN)_5NO] \longrightarrow Na_4[Fe(CN)_5NOS]$$
Sodium nitroprusside   (violet colour)
(colourless)

(*iv*) To the second part, add lead acetate soln when a black ppt is obtained due to the following reaction :

$$Na_2S+Pb(CH_3COO)_2 \longrightarrow PbS+2CH_3COONa$$

colourless   black
soln   ppt

Thus, if sodium extract gives violet colour on treatment with sodium nitroprusside soln and a black ppt with lead acetate soln, the presence of sulphur in the given organic compound is confirmed.

18'A'4   Detection of Nitrogen

When an organic compound contains nitrogen (carbon is already present in all organic compounds), on fusion with sodium the following reaction takes place :

$$Na+C+N \longrightarrow NaCN \text{ (sodium cyanide)}$$

The excess sodium reacts with water to produce NaOH so there is no need to add NaOH in order to make the soln alkaline.

(*i*) To the sodium extract, add a freshly prepared soln of $FeSO_4$ and heat, the reactions taking place are :

$$2NaCN+FeSO_4 \longrightarrow Fe(CN)_2 + Na_2SO_4$$

ferrous
cyanide

$$Fe(CN)_2+4NaCN \longrightarrow Na_4Fe(CN)_6$$

sodium ferrocyanide

(*ii*) Add HCl to dissolve $Fe(OH)_2$ formed due to reaction between excess $FeSO_4$ and NaOH.

(*iii*) Add $FeCl_3$ soln which will produce a blue colour or ppt confirming the presence of nitrogen.

$$3Na_4Fe(CN)_6+4FeCl_3 \longrightarrow 12NaCl+Fe_4[Fe(CN)_6]_3$$

ferric ferrocyanide
or prussian blue

18'A'5.   Detection of Nitrogen and Sulphur Present Together

(*i*) Fuse the given organic compound containing sulphur and nitrogen (Carbon is already present) with sodium. The following reaction occurs-:

$$Na+C+N+S \longrightarrow NaCNS$$

sodium thiocyanate

(*ii*) Acidify the sodium extract with HCl and add $FeCl_3$ soln. Formation of a blood red complex confirms the presence of nitrogen and sulphur in the given organic compound.

$$3NaCNS+FeCl_3 \longrightarrow 3NaCl+Fe(CNS)_3$$

red colour

18·A·6. Detection of Halogens

(i) Fuse the given organic compound containing chlorine, bromine or iodine with metallic sodium when the following reactions take place :

$$Na + Cl \longrightarrow NaCl$$
$$Na + Br \longrightarrow NaBr$$
$$Na + I \longrightarrow NaI$$

(ii) Acidify the sodium extract with an excess of HNO_3 and heat. Cool and add $AgNO_3$ soln : (If excess HNO_3 is not added then NaOH persent in sodium extract will give ppt of AgOH causing confusion) :

$$NaCl + AgNO_3 \longrightarrow NaNO_3 + AgCl \text{ (white ppt)}$$
$$NaBr + AgNO_3 \longrightarrow NaNO_3 + AgBr \text{ (yellow ppt)}$$
$$NaI + AgNO_3 \longrightarrow NaNO_3 + AgI \text{ (yellow ppt)}$$

The white ppt of AgCl is soluble in ammonium hydroxide. If yellow ppt is obtained it can be either of AgBr or of AgI ; these can be distinguished by the following test.

(iii) To the acidified sodium extract, add a few drops of CCl_4 and a few ml of chlorine water. Shake the mixture thoroughly. If CCl_4 layer turns violet, iodine is indicated while if it turns brown, bromine is present in the given organic compound. The chlorine water oxidises bromide ions (present in sodium extract) to bromine which dissolves in CCl_4 giving a brown soln. Similarly iodide ions are oxidised by chlorine to iodine which produces violet colour in the CCl_4 layer.

18·A·7 Detection of Phosphorus

Heat sodium extract with an excess of concentrated HNO_3 and add a few ml of ammonium molybdate soln—formation of a yellow ppt shows the presence of phosphorus.

18·A·8 Detection of Metals

Heat the given organic compound strongly on a piece ot porcelain if a residue is left it may be a metal. Dissolve the residue in dilute HCl and detect the metal by inorganic qualitative scheme discussed in Chapter 5.

18·B QUANTITATIVE ELEMENTAL ANALYSIS

After finding out the elements present in an organic compound, the next step involves the determination of amounts of these elements in a given quantity of the organic compound. These analytical data are necessary in the study of its structural determination.

18'B'1.   Determination of Carbon and Hydrogen (Liebig's Method) Theory

If an organic compound containing carbon and hydrogen is strongly heated with a large excess of CuO (acting as an oxidant) for sufficient time, carbon and hydrogen present in the compound are quantitatively oxidised to CO_2 and H_2O respectively. The water vapours and CO_2 so produced are passed through a U tube containing anhydrous $CaCl_2$ which absorbs H_2O but not CO_2. Knowing the weight of the U tube before and after the experiment, the quantity of water formed can be found out. The carbon dioxide coming out of the U tube is bubbled through a bulb containing KOH soln which absorbs CO_2. The increase in the weight of the bulb gives the amount of CO_2 formed.

Suppose 'x' g of an organic compound gives 'a' g of water and 'b' g of CO_2, then the percentage of hydrogen and carbon in the compound can be calculated as follows.

$$\underset{2\,g}{H_2} \;+\; \underset{16\,g}{O} \longrightarrow \underset{18\,g}{H_2O}$$

18 g of water is produced by 2 g of hydrogen

$\therefore$ 'a' g of water is produced by $\dfrac{a \times 2}{18}$ g hydrogen

Now, x g compound contains $\dfrac{a \times 2}{18}$ g hydrogen

$\therefore$ 100 g compound contains $\dfrac{100}{x} \times \dfrac{a \times 2}{18}$ g hydrogen

Thus, % of hydrogen in the compound is given by :

$$\frac{2}{18} \times \frac{\text{Weight of water}}{\text{weight of compound}} \times 100 \quad \cdots (18\text{-}A)$$

$$\underset{12\,g}{C} \;+\; \underset{32\,g}{O_2} \longrightarrow \underset{44\,g}{CO_2}$$

44 g of CO_2 is produced by 12 g carbon

$\therefore$ b g of CO_2 is produced by $\dfrac{b \times 12}{44}$ g carbon

Now, x g compound contains $\dfrac{b \times 12}{44}$ g carbon

$\therefore$ 100 g compound contains $\dfrac{100}{x} \times \dfrac{b \times 12}{44}$ g carbon

Thus, % of carbon in the compound is given by :

$$\frac{12}{44} \times \frac{\text{Weight of } CO_2}{\text{Weight of compound}} \times 100 \quad \text{...(18-B)}$$

Procedure

The quantitative determination of carbon and hydrogen in an organic compound is done in a single operation which consists of the following steps :

1. Filling up of the combustion tube,
2. Purification of air and oxygen used in combustion,
3. Combustion process,
4. Absorption of water and carbon dioxide and weighing them.

1. **Filling up of the Combustion Tube.** A weighed amount (about 0·2 g) of the given dry organic substance is heated with a large excess of dry cupric oxide in a current of pure oxygen gas. This is done in a dry hard glass tube called combustion tube which is about 85 cm long and about 1·5 cm in diameter. The filling of the tube has been shown in Fig. 18·3.

2. **Purification of Air and Oxygen.** Two reservoirs, one containing oxygen and the other air, are used. These are passed through two towers, one containing solid potassium hydroxide (to absorb CO_2) and the other containing fused calcium chloride (to absorb moisture). Thus air and oxygen become free of carbon dioxide and moisture. The purified oxygen and air are passed through a bubbler A (see Fig. 18·4) containing a small amount of concentrated sulphuric acid. The rate of bubble formation shows the rate at which air or oxygen is passed through the combustion tube.

3. **Combustion Process.** The apparatus is assembled as shown in Fig. 18·4. A small porcelain boat B is heated, cooled in a desiccator and weighed. This process is repeated until the weight of the boat is constant. About 0·2 g of the dry organic substance is then taken in the boat and it is weighed again. The difference in the two weighings gives the exact weight of the substance. The entire combustion tube C is then heated strongly. A slow stream of purified oxygen and air is passed through the tube when carbon is oxidised to carbon dioxide and hydrogen to water. After about an hour when the substance is completely oxidised, the heating is stopped, current of pure air is passed through the tube so that all the carbon dioxide and moisture are driven out of the combustion tube.

4. **Absorption of Water and Carbon Dioxide and Weighing Them.** The gaseous products coming out of the combustion tube are

Thus, % of carbon in the compound is given by :

$$\frac{12}{44} \times \frac{\text{Weight of } CO_2}{\text{Weight of substance}} \times 100 \quad \dots (18\text{-B})$$

Procedure

The quantitative determination of carbon and hydrogen in an organic compound is done in a single operation which consists of the following steps :

1. Filling up the combustion tube.
2. Purification of air and oxygen used in combustion.
3. Combustion process.
4. Absorption of water and carbon dioxide and weighing them.

1. Filling of the combustion Tube. A weighed amount (about 0.2 g) of the organic substance is heated with a large excess of oxide copper in a current of pure oxygen gas. This is done in a dry hard glass tube called combustion tube which is about 85 cm long and about 1.5 cm in diameter. The filling of the tube has been shown in Fig. 18·3.

2. Purification of Air and Oxygen. Two reservoirs, one containing oxygen and the other containing air are passed through two towers, one containing potassium hydroxide (to absorb CO_2) and the other containing calcium chloride (to absorb moisture). Thus air and oxygen become free of carbon dioxide and moisture. The purified oxygen and air are passed through a bubbler (containing some ...) having a small amount of concentrated sulphuric acid. The rate of bubble formation shows the rate at which air or oxygen is passed through the combustion tube.

3. Combustion Process. The apparatus is assembled as shown in Fig. ... . The ... porcelain boat is heated, cooled in a desiccator and weighed. This process is repeated until the weight of the boat is constant. About 0.2 g of the solid organic substance is then taken in the boat, and it is weighed again. The difference in the two weighings gives the exact weight of the substance. The entire combustion tube C is then heated. A slow stream of purified oxygen and air is passed over it. The oxide copper when carbon is oxidised to carbon dioxide and hydrogen to water. After about an hour when the substance is completely oxidised, the heating is stopped, current of pure air is passed through the tube so that all the carbon dioxide and moisture are driven out of the combustion tube.

4. Absorption of Water and Carbon Dioxide and Weighing Them. The gaseous products coming out of the combustion tube are

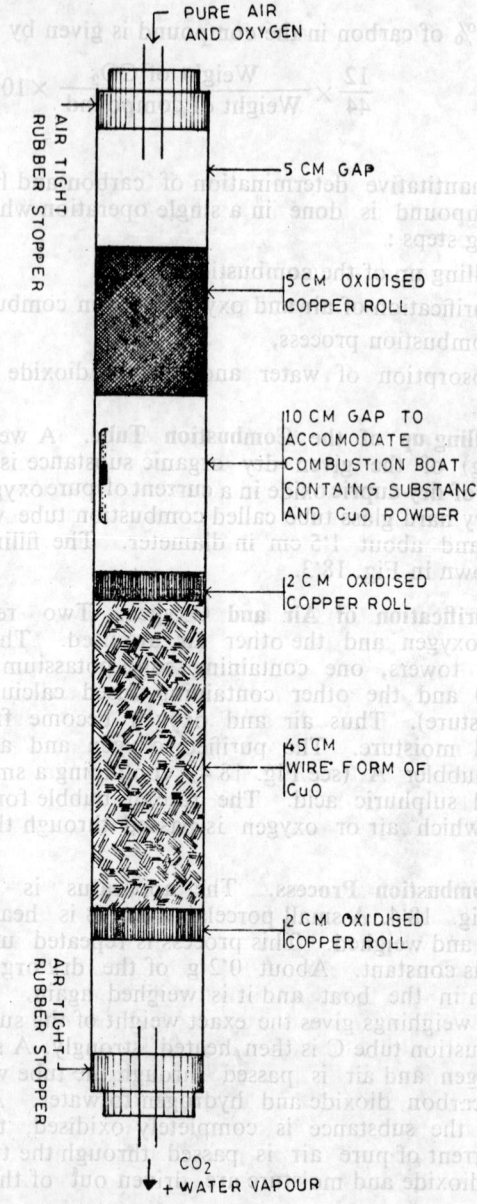

PURE AIR AND OXYGEN

AIR TIGHT RUBBER STOPPER

5 CM GAP

5 CM OXIDISED COPPER ROLL

10 CM GAP TO ACCOMODATE COMBUSTION BOAT CONTAINING SUBSTANCE AND CuO POWDER

2 CM OXIDISED COPPER ROLL

45 CM WIRE FORM OF CuO

2 CM OXIDISED COPPER ROLL

AIR TIGHT RUBBER STOPPER

CO_2 + WATER VAPOUR

Fig. 18·3. Filling up of the combustion tube.

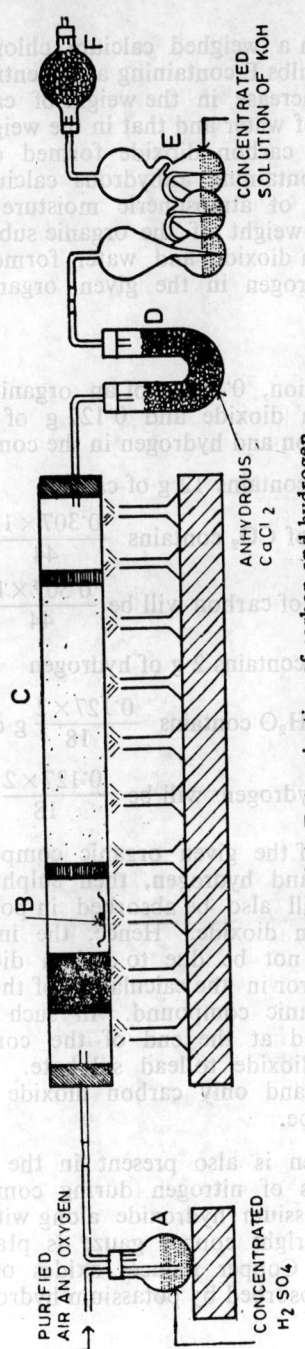

Fig. 18.4. Determination of carbon and hydrogen

passed first through a weighed calcium chloride tube D and then through weighed bulbs E containing a concentrated soln of potassium hydroxide. The increase in the weight of calcium chloride U tube gives the amount of water and that in the weight of potassium bulbs gives the weight of carbon dioxide formed during the combustion. A guard-tube F containing anhydrous calcium chloride is used to prevent the entry of atmospheric moisture into the combustion tube. From the weight of the organic substance taken, and the weights of carbon dioxide and water formed, the percentage of carbon and hydrogen in the given organic substance can be calculated.

Example 18(*i*)

On combustion, 0·210 g of an organic compound produced 0·307 g of carbon dioxide and 0·127 g of water. Calculate the percentage of carbon and hydrogen in the compound.

44 g of CO_2 contains 12 g of carbon

$$\therefore \quad 0\cdot307 \text{ g of } CO_2 \text{ contains } \frac{0\cdot307 \times 12}{44} \text{ g of carbon.}$$

The per cent of carbon will be $\dfrac{0\cdot307 \times 12}{44} \times \dfrac{100}{0\cdot210} = 39\cdot9$.

18 g of H_2O contains 2 g of hydrogen

$$\therefore \quad 0\cdot127 \text{ g } H_2O \text{ contains } \frac{0\cdot127 \times 2}{18} \text{ g of hydrogen.}$$

The % of hydrogen will be $\dfrac{0\cdot127 \times 2}{18} \times \dfrac{100}{0\cdot210} = 6\cdot7$

Notes : (1) If the given organic compound contains sulphur also with carbon and hydrogen, then sulphur dioxide will also be formed and it will also be absorbed in potassium hydroxide soln along with carbon dioxide. Hence, the increase in the weight of potash bulb will not be due to carbon dioxide alone. This will therefore cause error in the calculation of the percentage of carbon in the given organic compound. In such a case, some lead chromate is placed at the end of the combustion tube, which converts sulphur dioxide to lead sulphate. The sulphur dioxide is thus captured and only carbon dioxide is permitted to leave the combustion tube.

(2) If nitrogen is also present in the organic compound, it will produce oxides of nitrogen during combustion which are also absorbed by potassium hydroxide along with carbon dioxide. In such a case, a bright copper gauze is placed at the end of the combustion tube. Copper reduces oxides of nitrogen to nitrogen gas which is not absorbed by potassium hydroxide soln.

18·B·2 Determination of Nitrogen

Two methods are used for the determination of nitrogen in organic compounds.

18·B·2·1 Duma's Method

Theory

In this method a known weight of the given organic compound is strongly heated with cupric oxide in a combustion tube in a current of carbon dioxide gas. (Air or oxygen is not used because air contains nitrogen and oxygen is not absorbed by potassium hydroxide soln). The products are carbon dioxide, water vapour, nitrogen and some oxides of nitrogen. A bright metallic copper foil is placed at the end of the combustion tube which reduces oxides of nitrogen to nitrogen gas. The resultant mixture of gases (CO_2 and N_2) passes through a concentrated soln of potassium hydroxide which absorbs CO_2 but not N_2 which is collected over this soln. The volume of nitrogen obtained is measured and its volume at normal temperature and pressure is calculated, knowing which the percentage of nitrogen in the given organic compound is determined.

Suppose V c.c. of nitrogen is obtained from w g of the organic substance at $t°C$ and P' mm pressure. If p mm is the vapour pressure at $t°C$, the pressure due to gas alone would be $(P'-p)=P$ mm. Let V_0 be the volume of the gas at N.T.P. We know that :

$$\frac{P_0 V_0}{T_0} = \frac{PV}{T}$$

$$\therefore V_0 = \frac{P \times V \times T_0}{P_0 \times T}$$

$$V_0 = \frac{(P'-p) \times V \times 273}{760 \times (t+273)}$$

$P_0 = 760$ mm

$T_0 = 273°$

$T = (t+273)$

$P = (P'-p)$

Now, 22,400 c.c. of N_2 gas weighs 28 g

$\therefore$ V_0 c.c. of N_2 gas weighs $\dfrac{V_0}{22,400} \times 28$ g

[Remember that according to Avogadro's law, 1 g mole of a gas at N.T.P. occupies 22,400 c.c. The mol. wt. of N_2 is 28, hence 28 g of N_2 will occupy 22,400 c.c. or 22,400 c.c. of N_2 will weigh 28 g.]

Since w g of the substance contains $\dfrac{V_0 \times 28}{22,400}$ g of N_2

∴ 100 g of the substance contains $\dfrac{100}{w} \times \dfrac{V_0 \times 28}{22,400}$ g of N_2.

By substituting for V_0 in the above expression we can obtain the formula for calculating percentage of nitrogen in a given organic compound :

$$\% \text{ of } N_2 = \dfrac{100}{w} \times \dfrac{V \times (P'-p) \times 273}{760 \times (t+273)} \times \dfrac{28}{22,400} \qquad \ldots(18\text{-}C)$$

Alternatively,

Wt. of 1 c.c. of N_2 at N.T.P. is $= 0\cdot00126$ g

∴ Wt. of V_0 c.c. of N_2 at N.T.P. is $= V_0 \times 0\cdot00126$ g

Now, w g of substance contains $V_0 \times 0\cdot00126$ g N_2

∴ 100 g of substance contains $\dfrac{100}{w} \times V_0 \times 0\cdot00126$ g N_2

$$\text{Per cent of } N_2 = \dfrac{100}{w} \times \dfrac{V \times (P'-p) \times 273}{760 \times (t+273)} \times 0\cdot00126 \ldots(18\text{-}D)$$

$$\left[\text{Remember that } V_0 = \dfrac{V \times (P'-p) \times 273}{760 \times (t+273)} \right]$$

Procedure

The Duma's method for determining nitrogen in an organic compound involves the following steps :

1. Filling up of the combustion tube.
2. Preparation of CO_2 gas.
3. Combustion process.
4. Collection and measurement of nitrogen gas.

1. Filling up of the Combustion Tube. The constant weight of a porcelain boat is determined. A weighed amount of the given organic substance is taken in the boat and it is kept in a combustion tube. The filling of the combustion tube is done as shown in Fig. 18·5.

2. Preparation of CO_2. Carbon dioxide is prepared in a Kipp's apparatus using marble pieces and dil HCl. [Corbon dioxide can also be obtained by heating sodium bicarbonate in a hard glass tube.] The gas is passed through a bubbler A containing a small amount of concentrated sulphuric acid to observe the rate at which gas is passing through the combustion tube B.

3. Combustion Process. The apparatus is assembled as shown in Fig. 18·5. Carbon dioxide gas is passed through the combustion tube for about 10 minutes to displace all the air present in the tube

and then the outlet of the combustion tube is connected to a nitrometer. The combustion tube should completely oxidise the
organic compound. When this is complete, heating is
stopped and CO_2 is passed through it to drive out nitrogen
gas from the tube ; this process is called sweeping.

4. Collection and Measurement of Nitrogen Gas. The nitrogen
gas coming out of the combustion tube is collected in a nitrometer
C over a concentrated soln of potassium hydroxide (remember that
CO_2 gas is soluble in KOH soln). The volume of nitrogen collected
in the nitrometer is noted, from which the percentage of nitrogen in
the given organic compound is calculated.

Example 18(B)

0·256 g of an organic substance gives 19·5 c.c. of nitrogen at
27°C and 748 mm pressure. The vapour tension at 27°C is
17·2 mm, calculate the %age of nitrogen in the substance.

First of all let us calculate the volume of nitrogen at N.T.P.
(0°C or 273 A.)

$$V_0 = \frac{V \times (P - p)}{273} \times \frac{273}{(273 + 27)}$$

$$V_0 = \frac{20 \cdot 5 \times (748 - 17 \cdot 2)}{760} \times \frac{273}{300} = 17 \cdot 94 \text{ c.c.}$$

Now, wt of 1 c.c. of N_2 at N.T.P. is 0·00126 g

wt of 17·94 c.c. of nitrogen is 17·94 × 0·00126
= 0·02260 g

0·256 g of the compound contains 0·02260 g of N_2

10 g of the compound contains $\frac{100 \times 0 \cdot 02260}{0 \cdot 256}$

= 8·8 g of N_2.

or, using the formula (18·C) derived in sec 18 B 2,

% of $N_2 = \frac{100}{R} \times \frac{V \times (P - p) \times 273}{(1 + 273) \times 760} \times \frac{28}{22400}$

$$= \frac{100}{0 \cdot 256} \times \frac{20 \cdot 5 \times (748 - 17 \cdot 2) \times 273}{(27 + 273) \times 760} \times \frac{28}{22400}$$

= 8·8

Thus, both the methods give identical result, i.e.,
the percentage of N_2 in the given organic compound is 8·8.

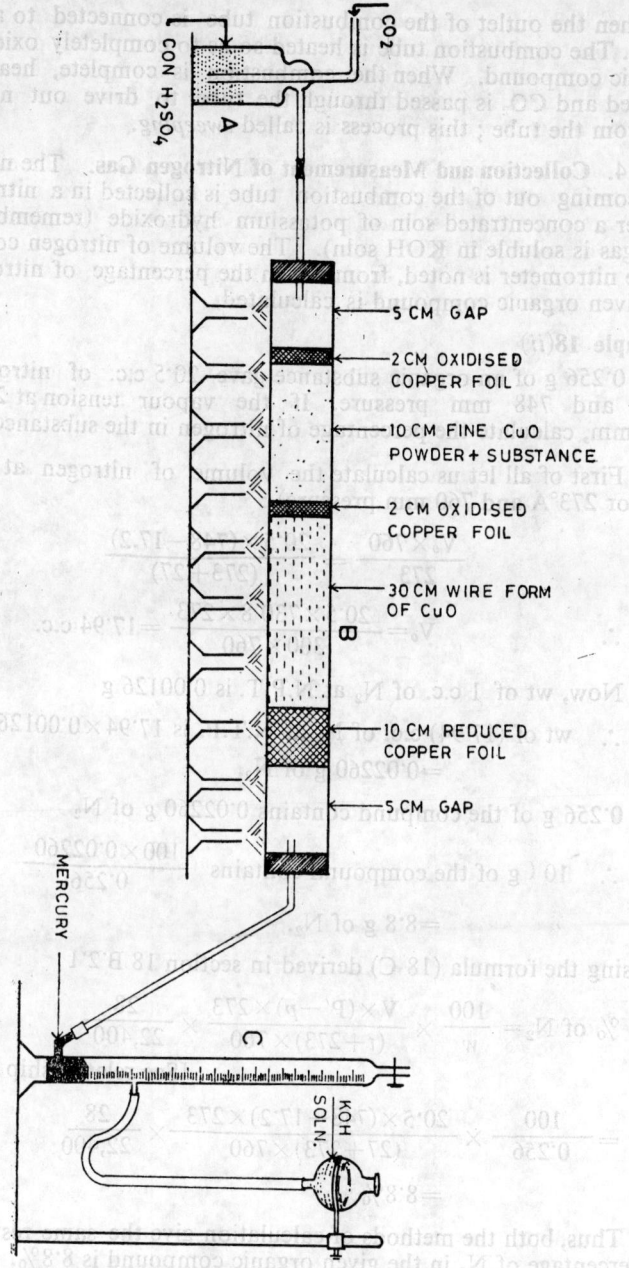

Fig. 18·5. Determination of nitrogen-Duma's method.

and then the outlet of the combustion tube is connected to a nitrometer. The combustion tube is heated so as to completely oxidise the organic compound. When the combustion is complete, heating is stopped and CO_2 is passed through the tube to drive out nitrogen gas from the tube ; this process is called *sweeping*.

4. **Collection and Measurement of Nitrogen Gas.** The nitrogen gas coming out of the combustion tube is collected in a nitrometer C over a concentrated soln of potassium hydroxide (remember that CO_2 gas is soluble in KOH soln). The volume of nitrogen collected in the nitrometer is noted, from which the percentage of nitrogen in the given organic compound is calculated.

Example 18(*ii*)

0·256 g of an organic substance gave 20·5 c.c. of nitrogen at 27°C and 748 mm pressure. If the vapour tension at 27°C is 17·2 mm, calculate the percentage of nitrogen in the substance.

First of all let us calculate the volume of nitrogen at N.T.P. (0°C or 273°A and 760 mm pressure) :

$$\frac{V_o \times 760}{273} = \frac{20·5 \times (748-17.2)}{(273+27)}$$

$$\therefore \qquad V_o = \frac{20·5 \times 730\ 8 \times 273}{300 \times 760} = 17·94 \text{ c.c.}$$

Now, wt of 1 c.c. of N_2 at N.P.T. is 0·00126 g

$\therefore$ wt of (17·94) c.c. of N_2 at N.T.P. is $17·94 \times 0·00126$
$\qquad = 0·02260$ g of N_2.

0·256 g of the compund contains 0·02260 g of N_2

$\therefore$ 10 (g of the compound contains $\dfrac{100 \times 0·02260}{0·256}$

$\qquad = 8·8$ g of N_2.

or, using the formula (18 C) derived in section 18 B·2·1

$$\% \text{ of } N_2 = \frac{100}{w} \times \frac{V \times (P'-p) \times 273}{(t+273) \times 760} \times \frac{28}{22,400}$$

[See relationship (18-C)]

$$= \frac{100}{0·256} \times \frac{20·5 \times (748-17·2) \times 273}{(27+273) \times 760} \times \frac{28}{22,400}$$

$$= 8·8\%.$$

Thus, both the methods of calculation give the same result, *i.e.*, the percentage of N_2 in the given organic compound is 8·8%.

18'B'2'2   Kjeldahl's Method

This method can also be used for determining nitrogen in organic compounds.

Theory

In this method a known weight (about 0'5 g) of the substance is heated with concentrated sulphuric acid and potassium sulphate or copper sulphate or potassium permanganate in a long-necked round-bottom flask made of hard glass : This flask is known as *Kjeldahl flask* (Fig. 18'6). In presence of potassium or copper sulphate, the carbon and hydrogen of the substance get oxidised to carbon dioxide and water respectively while the nitrogen is converted into ammonia which combines with excess of the acid present to

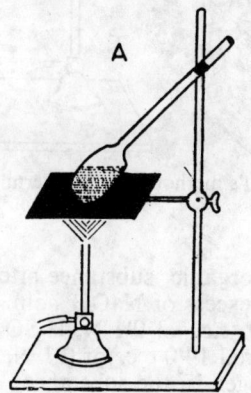

Fig. 18·6. Kjeldahl flask.

form ammonium sulphate. After the reaction is complete, the dark coloured mixture in the Kjeldahl flask becomes colourless. The heating is then stopped and the contents of the flask are distilled with an excess of sodium hydroxide soln when the following reaction takes place :

$$(NH_4)_2SO_4 + 2NaOH \longrightarrow Na_2SO_4 + 2H_2O + 2NH_3 \qquad ...(18'1)$$

The ammonia liberated in reaction (18'1) is absorbed in a known excess of sulphuric acid (Fig. 18'7). The reaction taking place is :

$$2NH_3 + H_2SO_4 \longrightarrow (NH_4)_2SO_4 \qquad ...(18'2)$$

The unused acid is then titrated with a standard alkali soln and so the amount of acid consumed in the reaction (18'2) becomes known, hence the quantity of ammonia liberated in the reaction (18'1) can be calculated. Knowing the amount of ammonia formed, the percentage of nitrogen in the given organic substance can be computed as shown in the following example.

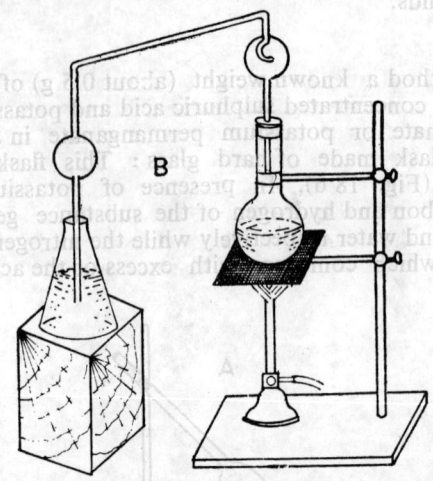

Fig. 18·7. Kjeldahl's method for the determination of nitrogen.

Example 18(iii)

0·442 g of an organic substance after digesting with H_2SO_4, was distilled with an excess of NaOH soln. The liberated NH_3 gas was absorbed in 50·0 c.c. of 0·1 N, H_2SO_4. The excess acid, left after absorption, required 14·0 c.c. of 0·1 N, NaOH soln. Calculate the percentage of nitrogen in the substance.

14·0 c.c. of 0·1 N, NaOH≡14·0 c.c. of 0·1 N, H_2SO_4.

∴ Volume of 0·1 N, H_2SO_4 used in the neutralisation of NH_3 will be (50·0−14·0)=36·0 c.c.

Weight of H_2SO_4 in 1000 c.c. of soln.

=normality×eq. wt.   [Eq. wt. of H_2SO_4=49]

=0·1×49=4·9 g

Now, 1000 c.c. of 0·1 N, H_2SO_4 soln contains 4·9 g of H_2SO_4

∴ 36·0 c.c. of 0·1 N, H_2SO_4 soln contains $\dfrac{36·0}{1000}$ ×4·9 g of H_2SO_4

=0·1764 g of H_2SO_4

$$2NH_3+H_2SO_4 \longrightarrow (NH_4)_2SO_4$$
$$34\text{ g} \qquad 98\text{ g}$$

Since, 98 g of H_2SO_4 absorbs 34 g of NH_3

$\therefore$ 0·1764 g of H_2SO_4 absorbs $\dfrac{0·1764 \times 34}{98}$ g of NH_3

$$= 0·061 \text{ g of } NH_3$$

$$\underset{28 \text{ g}}{N_2} + \underset{6 \text{ g}}{3H_2} \longrightarrow \underset{34 \text{ g}}{2NH_3}$$

Now, 34 g NH_3 contains 28 g N_2

$\therefore$ 0·061 g NH_3 contains $\dfrac{0·061 \times 28}{34}$ g of N_2

$$= 0·05 \text{ g of } N_2.$$

Since, 0·442 g of substance contains 0·05 g N_2

$\therefore$ 100 g of substance contains $\dfrac{100 \times 0·05}{0·442}$ g N_2

$$= 11·3 \text{ g of } N_2.$$

Thus, the percentage of nitrogen in the given organic compound is 11·3 per cent.

18·B·3 Determination of Halogens

Two methods can be used for the determination of halogens in organic compounds.

18·B·3·1 Carius Method

Theory

This method for determining halogens consists of heating the given organic compound with fuming nitric acid and a few crystals of silver nitrate in a sealed tube. Carbon and hydrogen are oxidised to carbon dioxide and water while the halogen will form insoluble silver halide which is filtered, washed, dried and weighed. From the weight of the silver halide, the percentage of halogen in the given organic compound can be calculated.

Procedure

This determination is carried out in a bomb tube which is made of special glass and has thick walls to withstand pressure. About 4 c.c. of pure fuming nitric acid and about 0·5 g of silver nitrate are placed in the bomb tube. An accurately weighed quantity (about 0·2 g) of the substance is taken in a small test tube which is allowed to slide down into the inclined bomb tube. The upper end of the bomb tube is sealed and it is kept in a bomb furnace (Fig. 18·8). The bomb tube is heated in this furnace at about 150–200°C for about six hours. The furnace is then cooled, bomb tube carefully

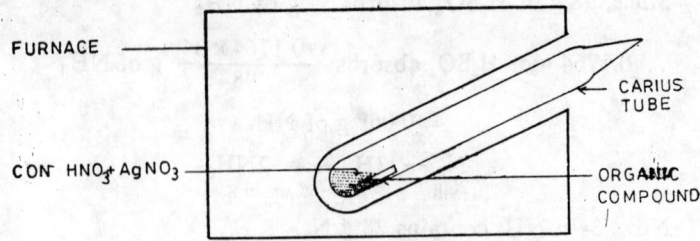

Fig. 18·8. Bomb furnace.

taken out and the upper narrow portion of the tube is cut open. The contents of the tube are washed out into a beaker. The ppt of silver halide is filtered, washed, dried and weighed.

Example 18(iv)

0·302 g of a compound containing bromine gave 0·268 g of silver bromide in a carius determination. Calculate the percentage of bromine in the given compound.

$$\underset{188\text{ g}}{AgBr} \equiv \underset{80\text{ g}}{Br}$$

Since, 188 g of AgBr contains 80 g of bromine.

$$\therefore\quad 0·268 \text{ g of AgBr contains } \frac{0·268 \times 80}{188} \text{ g of Br}_2$$

$$=0·1140 \text{ g of bromine.}$$

Now, 0·302 g substance contains 0·1140 g Br_2

$$\therefore\ 100 \text{ g substance contains } \frac{100 \times 0·1140}{0·302} \text{ g Br}_2$$

$$=37·7 \text{ g Br}_2.$$

The percentage of bromine in the given organic compound is 37·7.

18·B·3·2 Stepanow's Method

In this method an accurately weighed quantity of the given organic compound is refluxed (heated in a flask fitted with a condenser) with a very large excess of sodium metal in iso-amyl alcohol medium. The halogen present in the compound reacts with sodium to form sodium halide which is filtered, washed, dried and weighed. Knowing the weight of silver halide formed, the percentage of halogen in the organic compound can be calculated by the method given in example 18(iv).

18'B'4.   Determination of Sulphur

There are three methods that can be used for the determination of sulphur in organic compounds.

18'B'4'1   Carius Method

This method is quite similar to that described for halogens in 18'B'3'1. The only difference is that in place of silver nitrate, barium chloride is added. Sulphur present in the organic compound is oxidised and forms insoluble barium sulphate which is filtered, washed, dried and weighed. From the weight of barium sulphate, the percentage of sulphur in the organic compound is calculated as shown in the following example.

Example 18(v)

0·3386 g of an organic compound was heated in a sealed tube with an excess of fuming nitric acid and barium chloride. After the completion of the reaction, the weight of barium sulphate obtained was 0·3452 g. Calculate the percentage of sulphur in the compound.

$$\underset{233\cdot40 \text{ g}}{BaSO_4} \equiv \underset{32\cdot0 \text{ g}}{S}$$

233·40 g BaSO₄ contains 32·0 g of S

$$\therefore \quad 0\cdot3452 \text{ g BaSO}_4 \text{ contains } \frac{0\cdot3452 \times 32\cdot0}{233\cdot40} \text{ g of S}$$

$$= 0\cdot0473 \text{ g of S.}$$

Now, 0·3386 g of substance contains 0·0473 g of S

$$\therefore \quad 100 \text{ g of substance contains } \frac{100 \times 0\cdot0473}{0\cdot3386} \text{ g of S.}$$

$$= 13\cdot97 \text{ g of S.}$$

Thus the percentage of sulphur in the given compound is 13·97.

18'B'4'2   Na₂CO₃-KNO₃ Fusion Method

If the sulphur containing organic compound is non-volatile, its known weight is fused with potassium nitrate-sodium carbonate mixture. The sulphur present in the compound forms sulphate ions which can be determined gravimetrically with barium chloride. Knowing the weight of barium sulphate, the percentage of sulphur in the given compound can be calculated as shown in Example 18(v).

18'B'4'3.   Messenger's Method

In this method, an accurately weighed quantity of the given sulphur-containing organic substance is heated with an excess of sodium hydroxide and potassium permanganate for about six hours. During this heating sulphur is quantitatively oxidised to sulphate ions. Excess hydrochlroric acid is then added to the reaction mixture which reacts with unreacted potassium permanganate giving a colourless soln. The soln is filtered and an excess of barium chloride soln is added. The resultant ppt of barium sulphate is filtered, washed, dried and weighed. From the weight of barium sulphate, the percentage of sulphur in the given organic compound can be calculated as shown in example 18(v).

18·B·5 Determination of Phosphorus by Carius Method

In this method, an accurately weighed quantity of phosphorus-containing organic compound is heated with an excess of fuming nitric acid and ammonium molybdate in a sealed tube. The phosphorus present in the compound is oxidised to phosphate ion which can be determined gravimetrically as ammonium phosphomolybdate. The ppt is filtered, washed, dried and weighed ; knowing the weight of the ppt, the percentage of phosphorus in the organic compound can be calculated.

18·B·6 Determination of Oxygen

There is no definite method for the determination of oxygen. The procedure generally used is that the given organic compound is first qualitatively analysed, then the percentages of *all* the constituents detected are found out. If the total of these percentages does not come out to be 100, the difference is regarded as the percentage of oxygen. For example, an organic compound is found to contain 44% carbon, 7·4% hydrogen, 10·1% nitrogen and 26·2% chlorine and no other element is detected in the compound. Now, the total of these percentages comes out to be 87·7, hence, the remaining, i.e. (100—87·7)=12·3 is the percentage of oxygen.

18·B·7 Calculation of Empirical Formula from Quantitative Analytical Data

The ratio of different atoms present in the molecule of a compound gives the *empirical formula* of that compound. In order to find out the empirical formula of a given organic compound, first it is qualitatively analysed to know which elements are present in the compound. Then, from quantitative elemental analysis, the relative numbers of different atoms in a molecule (empirical formula) of the given compound is calculated as shown in the following example.

Example 18(vi)

An organic compound was found to contain only two elements namely carbon and hydrogen (no test for oxygen was done, hence, we do not know whether oxygen is present or not). The quantitative analysis of this compound gave the following results :

$$C=68\cdot84\% \text{ and } H=4\cdot92\%$$

Now, $(68\cdot84+4\cdot92)=73\cdot76$, hence, the rest, *i.e.*, $(100-73\cdot76)=26\cdot24$ must be the percentage of oxygen.

By dividing the percentage of each element by its atomic weight, we get the ratio of different atoms in the molecule of the compound that is its empirical formula. The calculations involved are :

$$C=\frac{68\cdot84}{12}=5\cdot74 \text{ (A)} \qquad\qquad \text{[At. wt. of C=12]}$$

$$H=\frac{4\cdot92}{1}=4\cdot92 \text{ (B)} \qquad\qquad \text{[At. wt. of H=1]}$$

$$O=\frac{26\cdot24}{16}=1\cdot64 \text{ (C)} \qquad\qquad \text{[At. wt. of O=16]}$$

Dividing (A), (B) and (C) by the smallest number, *i.e.*, $1\cdot64$, the result is :

$$C=\frac{5\cdot74}{1\cdot64}=3\cdot5 \qquad\qquad (3\cdot5\times2=7)$$

$$H=\frac{4\cdot92}{1\cdot64}=3\cdot0 \qquad\qquad (3\cdot0\times2=6)$$

$$O=\frac{1\cdot64}{1\cdot64}=1\cdot0 \qquad\qquad (1\cdot0\times2=2)$$

Since we want the ratio of atoms in whole numbers we will multiply the above values by 2, so that the atomic ratio comes out to be :

$$C : H : O : : 7 : 6 : 2$$

Thus the empirical formula of the compound under consideration would be $C_7H_6O_2$. The *empirical formula weight* of this compound can be calculated as given below :

At. wt. of C=12 ; 7 carbon atoms present $=12\times7=84$

At. wt. of H= 1 : 6 hydrogen atoms present $= 1\times6= 6$

At. wt. of O=16 ; 2 oxygen atoms present $=16\times2=32$

_____

The empirical-formula weight of the compund will be $=122$

18·B·8 Determination of the Molecular Weight and Molecular Formula

The molecular weight of a volatile organic compound can be determined by any one of the following methods :

1. Victor Meyer's method,
2. Duma's method, and
3. Hofmann's method.

For determining molecular weight of non-volatile substances, the methods used are based on :

1. Depression of freezing point.
2. Elevation of boiling point.

Suppose the molecular weight of a compound is found to be 244, its empirical formula is $C_7H_6O_2$ and empirical formula weight is 122, as in example 18(vi). Then,

$$\frac{\text{Molecular weight}}{\text{Empirical formula weight}} = \frac{244}{122} = 2$$

∴ Molecular formula of the compound under consideration will be $(C_7H_6O_2)_2 = C_{14}H_{12}O_4$.

18·C QUALITATIVE FUNCTIONAL GROUP ANALYSIS

The qualitative analysis of organic compounds is much more difficult and complicated than that of inorganic compounds for the following reasons.

1. Inorganic compounds are generally soluble in water. In aqueous soln, majority of these compounds dissociate giving ions which can be easily recognised by applying simple tests. Once these ions are known, the inorganic compound under examination can be identified. On the other hand, majority of organic compounds do not dissolve in water (which is a simple and easily available solvent ; also aqueous solutions are easiest to handle). Further, organic compounds, being covalent, do not dissociate in soln giving ions ; this makes the recognition of organic compounds more difficult.

2. The number of organic compounds is very much larger than that of inorganic compounds.

3. Several organic compounds contain the same functional group, such as $-COOH$, $-OH$ or $-NO_2$ etc. All such compounds are said to belong to a particular class of organic compounds (homologous series) ; these have similar chemical properties. For example, acetic acid, propionic acid and butyric acid belong to the same class because they contain the same functional group namely

carboxyl group (—COOH). All the three acids, therefore, have almost similar chemical properties and so it is very difficult to identify them by applying chemical tests. In such a case, physical properties like melting point, boiling point etc., are used to re-cognise the given organic compound.

Since organic compounds are very large in number, their analysis can be tedious and time-consuming if we do not proceed systematically step by step. This chapter does not describe a com-plete analysis scheme for the identification of various organic com-pounds, it simply indicates how we should proceed systematically to recognise organic compounds. In qualitative organic analysis we generally perform the following examinations.

18'C'1 Physical State

If the given compound is a solid, it cannot be ethyl alcohol, acetic acid, acetaldehyde, benzene etc., which are liquids. On the other hand if a liquid is given, it cannot be citric acid, α-napthol, acetamide etc., which are solids. In the case of a solid the study of the nature of the crystals of the solid can also be helpful in its identification. For instance, salicylic acid has shining needle shaped crystals. Benzoic acid has shining prismatic crystals. If it is a viscous colourless liquid it can be glycerol.

18'C'2 Colour

Most of the nitro compounds are yelleow in colour. Iodoform is in the form of a yellow powder.

18'C'3 Smell

Certain organic substances have peculiar smell by which they can be recognised. For instance, compounds like chloroform, iodo-form, formaldehyde, benzaldehyde etc., have characteristic smell. Esters, such as ethyl acetate, methyl salicylate have fruity smell. Alcohols have wine like smell.

18'C'4 Solubility

This property is also helpful in the identification. For example, aliphatic acids like formic acid, acetic acid are soluble in water whereas aromatic acids like salicylic and benzoic acid have poor solu-bility in water.

18'C'5 Heating on a Crucible Lid

Heat a small portion of the given organic compound on a piece of porcelain first gently and then strongly.

(i) If the substance burns with a clear flame, it may be an aliphatic compound like ethyl alcohol, methyl alcohol etc.

(*ii*) If it burns with a very smoky flame, it may be an aromatic compound like benzene, aniline etc.

(*iii*) Silver salts of organic acids leave a residue of silver.

(*iv*) Cane sugar melts, darkens, chars and then burns giving odour of burning sugar. Tartaric acid, tartrates and citrates also char on heating, giving out odours similar to that of burnt sugar.

18·C·6   Action of Sodium Hydroxide Solution

Take about 0·1 g of the compound in a boiling tube and add about 5 ml of 10% aqueous NaOH soln. If ammonia evolves in the cold, the compound may be an ammonium salt such as CH_3COONH_4. Acetamide would give ammonia on heating with NaOH soln. Acetaldehyde would give a yellow resin with bad smell.

18·C·7   Action of Concentrated Sulphuric Acid

Take about 0·1 g of the substance in a clean and dry test tube, add about 1 ml of concentrated H_2SO_4 and warm. Cane sugar and starch would turn black and give out CO, CO_2 and SO_2. In the case of citric acid, there is evolution of CO and CO_2 but no charring takes place, whereas tartaric acid would char and produce CO and CO_2. Resorcinol would turn black but no gas would be formed. Sodium formate will produce CO and oxalic acid will form CO_2 and in both the cases there would be no blackening and the soln will remain colourless.

18·C·8   Colouration with Aqueous Ferric Chloride Solution

Ferric chloride soln provided in the laboratory is quite acidic. To this $FeCl_3$ soln, add dil NH_4OH soln drop by drop with shaking until a ppt appears. Filter and collect the filtrate which contains almost neutral $FeCl_3$ soln ; this soln gives colourations or coloured ppt with various organic compounds, hence, $FeCl_3$ soln can be used as a reagent for the identification of these compounds.

Neutral salt solutions of lower fatty acids, such as formic and acetic acid, give a deep red colour with $FeCl_3$ soln which turns brown on boiling. [If free acid is given, add ammonia soln gradually until the soln becomes just alkaline as shown by a litmus paper.] Oxalic acid gives a faint yellow colour. Succinic acid forms a buff-coloured ppt which is soluble in dil H_2SO_4. Benzoic acid also gives a buff-coloured ppt in the cold which dissolves in dil H_2SO_4 but at the same time a white ppt of benzoic acid is produced. Salicylic acid gives a violet colouration with $FeCl_3$ soln. Phenol also produces violet colour when $FeCl_3$ soln is added to it. (Note that the test is done with neutral salt solutions of these acids and $FeCl_3$ soln used should also be neutral).

18·C·9   Detection of Elements

The examinations or tests described under sections 18·C·1 to 18·C·8 only roughly indicate the type to which the given compound can possibly belong. The next important step involved in the qualitative organic analysis is the detection of the elements present in the given compound which has been discussed in section 18·A.

It is extremely necessary to know the elements that are present in the compound under examination because by knowing these, we can find out the possible classes to which that componnd can belong. Since organic compounds are very large in number, it is very essential that we know the possible classes of organic compounds in which the compound under test can be placed. For instance, if by analysis we come to know that a particular substance contains only carbon and hydrogen then it can be nothing but a hydrocarbon (a class of organic compounds that contains carbon and hydrogen only). Now, by finding out the melting or boiling point or by other specific tests we can find out which particular hydrocarbon the given compound is. If the given compound contains only three elements namely carbon, hydrogen and nitrogen, then it cannot be an alcohol or a carboxylic acid or an amide or an aldehyde etc., but will belong to the class such as amines, cyanides or isocyanides. This information will save a lot of our time and energy because our attention now will be limited only to those classes of organic compounds to which the given compound can possibly belong.

18·C·10   Detection of Functional Group

A *function* or a *functional group* is defined as a reactive atom or group of atoms in an organic molecule. Thus a nitro compound contains the nitro group $(-NO_2)$ and an alkene, the unsaturated $-CH=CH-$ grouping, both of which can be detected by proper chemical reactions. After detecting the elements, the next important step in organic qualitative analysis is to detect the functional group present in the compound being examined. Suppose the given organic compound has been found to contain only three elements namely carbon, hydrogen and nitrogen. Now, this compound can have an amino group or a cyanide group or an isocyanide group. At this stage, appropriate chemical tests are made to find out which of the functional groups is present. If the compound does not give test for cyanide and isocyanide but gives the test for amino group then we are sure that the compound is an amine. Now, by determining melting point or boiling point or by using specific tests we can find out which particular amine the given compound is. The tests for some of the important functional groups have been described in the following sub-sections. (These tests will generally be for those compounds which have been mentioned in the beginning of the sub-section.)

18·C·10·1 Alcohols [—OH]

The common alcohols with which we have to deal are metha-nol, ethanol, propanol, isopropanol, butanol, glycol, glycerol, benzyl alcohol etc. All of these are colourless liquids soluble in water but for benzyl alcohol which has poor solubility in water. Pure glycol and glycerol are odourless and viscous, hence can be recognised by observing their rate of flow. Other alcohols have a faint typical smell. Alcoholic group can be detected by the follow-ing tests.

(*i*) On adding a small piece of sodium metal to about 1 ml of alcohol taken in a test tube there is evolution of hydrogen.

(*ii*) Primary alcohols like methanol, ethanol, propanol and butanol on oxidation give aldehydes which on further oxidation produce the corresponding carboxylic acid. Methanol on refluxing with potassium dichromate and sulphuric acid gives the characteris-tic pungent odour of formaldehyde. If the oxidation is continued further we get formic acid which can be distilled and collected in a separate flask. The liquid so collected will turn blue litmus red. On oxidation, ethanol will give acetaldehyde, propanol will form propanaldehyde and butanol will produce butyraldehyde. Isopro-panol is a secondary alcohol, hence, on oxidation it would produce a ketone namely acetone.

Another test for alcohols is that they form crystalline esters with 3, 5-dinitrobenzoyl chloride.

Special Tests

1. **For Methanol (CH_3OH).** Heat about 1 ml of methanol with about 0·5 g of sodium salicylate and a few drops of concen-trated sulphuric acid—a pleasant odour of methyl salicylate is observed.

2. **For Ethanol (C_2H_5OH).** Heat 1 ml of ethanol with 0·5 g of sodium acetate and a few drops of concentrated sulphuric acid— a fruity smell of ethyl acetate is noted.

Another test for ethanol is iodoform test. Warm a small quantity of ethanol with a crystal of iodine, and then add KOH soln drop by drop until the yellow colour of iodine just disappears. A yellow ppt of iodoform possessing a characteristic odour is obtained. (Isopropanol gives this test in the cold but methanol and other alcohols mentioned in this sub-section do not give iodoform test.)

3. **For glycerol ($CH_2OH.CHOH : CH_2OH$).** Heat 0·5 ml of glycerol with about 1 g of finely powdered potassium hydrogen sulphate—an irritating odour of acrolein is noticed.

18·C·10·2 Phenols [—OH]

Phenols generally given for identification are phenol, resorcinol, hydroquinone and 1- and 2-naphthol.

All the phenols listed above are solids (difference from alcohols which also contain —OH as the functional group). Phenols have a typical smell. 1- and 2-naphthol are sparingly soluble in water but phenol, resorcinol and hydroquinone are soluble in water. All phenols are soluble in NaOH soln. The important reactions of phenols are :

(i) Though they are acidic in nature but do not liberate CO_2 from Na_2CO_3 soln (difference from carboxylic acids).

(ii) Phenols give characteristic colouration with $FeCl_3$ soln. Phenol, resorcinol, o-, m- and p-cresol give violet or blue colour. Hydroquinone gives a green colouration and on adding more $FeCl_3$, a yellow soln is obtained.

(iii) Phenols on treatment with benzoyl chloride in presence of NaOH form derivatives with characteristic melting points. The melting points of the derivatives of some of the phenols are given below.

Benzoates of	Melting point
Phenol	69°
Resorcinol	117°
Hydroquinone	204°
1-Naphthol	56°
2-Naphthol	107°

Thus by preparing the benzoate of the given phenol and finding out the melting point of the purified derivative, we can recognise which particular phenol is given to us. Derivatives of phenols with other reagents can also be prepared.

18·C·10·3 Aldehydes [—CHO]

Formaldehyde, acetaldehyde, chloral hydrate and benzaldehyde —all these are colourless. Formaldehyde is a gas and so generally its aqueous soln is given which has a characteristic odour. Acetaldehyde is also given in the form of its aqueous soln and it too has got a characteristic odour. Chloral, CCl_3CHO, is a liquid but it is given in the form of $CCl_3C(OH)_2$ called chloral hydrate which is a solid. Benzaldehyde is a liquid with characteristic odour of bitter almond and is insoluble in water. Some of the general reactions of the aldehyde group are :

(i) Give pink colour with Schiff's reagent in the cold. With benzaldehyde the colour develops slowly. [Schiff's reagent is prepared by dissolving magenta in water and then passing SO_2 gas through it until the soln becomes colourless. The test with this reagent should be done in the cold because on heating, the reagent alone gives pink colour.]

(*ii*) Aldehydes form mirror with ammonical silver nitrate soln. With benzaldehyde the mirror is obtained on warming. [To prepare ammonical silver nitrate—take about 5 ml of $AgNO_3$ soln in a clean test tube, add 2-3 drops of dil NaOH when a ppt is formed. Add ammonia soln drop by drop with shaking until the ppt dissolves. To this clear soln, a few drops of aldehyde are added when a shining deposit of silver on the inside wall of the test tube is seen.]

(*iii*) Aldehydes react with NaOH soln in the following manner.

(*a*) Warm 1 ml of CH_3CHO with about 2-3 ml of 30% NaOH soln—a yellow resin with a bad characteristic smell is noticed.

(*b*) Warm 0·5 ml of benzaldehyde with 2 ml of 30% NaOH with shaking. Dilute with water and add concentrated HCl when a white ppt of benzoic acid is formed. Salicylaldehyde forms salicylic acid.

18·C·10·4. Ketones [>C=O]

Acetone, acetophenone and benzophenone are colourless. Acetone is soluble in water, it has a characteristic odour, its boiling point is 56°C. The melting point of acetophenone is 20°C and it is sparingly sobule in water. Benzophenone is a solid insoluble in water.

Acetone gives pink colour with Schiff's reagent and forms iodoform when treated with I_2 and NaOH soln. Acetophenone also gives iodoform test but benzophenone does not. On shaking acetone with a saturated soln of $NaHSO_3$, a white addition product is precipitated. Acetophenone and benzophenone do not give this test.

18·C·10·5 Carboxylic acids [—COOH]

The common carboxylic acids which we are generally required to test are formic, acetic, oxalic, succinic, tataric, citric, lactic, benzoic, salicylic, phthalic and cinnamic acid.

Formic and acetic acids are colourless liquids having characteristic pungent odour. Lactic acid is also a liquid. Other acids mentioned above are crystalline solids. The aliphatic acids are soluble in water but benzoic and salicylic acids are only sparingly soluble in water ; phthalic acid is relatively more soluble. The general reactions of carboxylic acids have been given below.

(*i*) Carboxylic acids turn blue litmus red and are soluble in NaOH soln forming their sodlim salts.

(*ii*) Carboxylic acids on treatment with Na_2CO_3 soln liberate CO_2 (difference from phenols).

(*iii*) When carboxylic acids are heated with ethanol and concentrated H_2SO_4, esters with fruity smell are formed.

(*iv*) The neutral salt solutions of several carboxylic acids produce colouration with neutral $FeCl_3$ soln. Formates and acetates give a deep red colour which turns into a reddish brown ppt on heating. Succinate, benzoate, phthalate and cinnamate give a buff-coloured ppt. On adding dil H_2SO_4, the ppt obtained with succinate dissolves giving a clear soln. In other cases, the ppt dissolves but simultaneously a white ppt of the free acid is produced.

Special Tests

1. **For formic acid** (HCOOH) :—Heat with concentrated H_2SO_4 when CO is given out which burns with blue flame.

When formic acid is heated with $HgCl_2$ soln, a white ppt of Hg_2Cl_2 insoluble in acids is produced (difference from acetic acid). Formic acid decolourises $KMnO_4$ soln in acidic or in alkaline medium. It also forms a mirror with ammonical silver nitrate soln.

2. **For acetic acid** (CH$_3$COOH) :—It does not reduce $KMnO_4$ or $HgCl_2$ or ammonical $AgNO_3$ soln (difference from formic acid). On heating acetic acid with C_2H_5OH and concentrated H_2SO_4—a fruity smell of ethyl acetate is observed.

3. **For oxalic acid** [(COOH)$_2$]. On heating oxalic acid with concentrated H_2SO_4, CO and CO_2 (difference from formic acid—which evolves only CO) are evolved. The liberated CO_2 can be detected by lime-water test.

Oxalic acid decolourises acidic $KMnO_4$. Neutral soln of an oxalate forms a white ppt of CaC_2O_4 on adding a neutral soln of $CaCl_2$. The ppt dissolves in dil H_2SO_4 and the resultant soln decolourises acidic $KMnO_4$ soln.

4. **For succinic acid** [(CH$_2$COOH)$_2$] :—Fuse a small amount of resorcinol with equal quantity of succinic acid or a succinate and a few drops of concentrated H_2SO_4 in a porcelain basin. Cool, dissolve the contents in water and add NaOH soln in excess—a red colour is produced which shows green fluorescence.

5. **For lactic acid** [CH$_3$ CH (OH) COOH] :—Warm 0·5 ml of lactic acid or 0·5 g of a lactate with 1 ml of concentrated H_2SO_4—there is evolution of CO and CO_2 at the same time soln turns black (difference from formic and oxalic acids) but no charring takes place (difference from tartaric acid).

6. **For tartaric acid** [(CH (OH)COOH)$_2$] Warm 0·5 g of tartaric acid or a tartrate with 1 ml of concentrated H_2SO_4—there is evolution of CO and CO_2 gases and charring takes place (difference from lactic, formic and oxalic acids). Tartaric acid gives mirror test on warming with ammonical $AgNO_3$ soln.

7. **For citric acid** [(HOOC.CH$_2$.C(OH) (COOH) CH$_2$. (COOH).] Warm 0·5 g of citric acid or a citrate with 1 ml of concentrated H_2SO_4—there is evolution of CO and CO_2 and the soln turns *yellow* (difference from tartaric, lactic, formic and oxalic acids). Citric acid does not give mirror test (difference from tartaric acid).

8. **For cinnamic acid** [C$_6$H$_5$CH=CH. COOH]. This acid decolourises alkaline $KMnO_4$ (difference from benzoic acid).

Take 0·2 g of cinnamic acid or a cinnamate in a boiling tube, add little Na_2CO_3 and $KMnO_4$ soln and boil—a characteristic odour of benzaldehyde can be noted.

9. **For phthalic acid** [C$_6$H$_4$(COOH)$_2$]. In a dry test tube, fuse a few crystals of phthalic acid or a phthalate, an equal quantity of phenol and a few drops of concentrated H_2SO_4. Cool, dissolve in water and add an excess of NaOH soln—a red colour is produced (which is due to phenolphthalein).

10. **For salicylic acid** [HOC$_6$H$_4$COOH]. Warm 0·5 g of salicylic acid with little CH_3OH and concentrated H_2SO_4—a pleasant characteristic smell of methyl salicylate is observed.

11. **For benzoic acid** [C$_6$H$_4$COOH]. Does not decolourise alkaline $KMnO_4$ (difference from cinnamic acid). Does not form phenolphthalein (difference from phthalic acid). Gives buff-coloured ppt with neutral $FeCl_3$ soln.

18·C·10·6 Ammonium Salts and Amides [−CONH$_2$]

Ammonium salts of carboxylic acids such as formic, acetic, oxalic, succinic, tartaric, citric, benzoic acid etc., evolve NH_3 on treatment with NaOH soln. Ammonium salts of these acids produce colouration with $FeCl_3$ soln.

Amides produce NH_3 when *boiled* with NaOH soln but do not give colouration with $FeCl_3$ soln (difference from ammonium salts).

Formamide alone on boiling gives ammonia. Acetamide on treatment with bromine and NaOH (Sodium hypobromite) liberates N_2 and CO_2.

Urea (NH$_2$CONH$_2$) on heating just above its melting point melts and gives out NH_3, the liquid then solidifies. Dissolve the solid in warm 10% NaOH soln and add a drop of very dilute $CuSO_4$ soln—a purple colouration is obtained.

18·C·10·7. Carbohydrates [Cx(H₂O)y]

Glucose, sucrose and starch are colourless solids which decompose on heating therefore have no definite melting points. Glucose and surcose are soluble in water giving a soln which has a sweet taste. Ordinary starch is insoluble in water.

These substances on heating with concentrated H_2SO_4 on a small flame turn black. On increasing the temperatare there is evolution of CO, CO_2 and SO_2.

Molisch's test. Dissolve 0·1 g of carbohydrate in 2 ml of water in a test tube and add 2—3 drops of 1% alcoholic soln of 1-naphthol.

Pour down the side of the test tube about 2 ml of concentrated H_2SO_4. A deep violet colour is produced.

Special tests

1. **For glucose** [$C_6H_{12}O_6$]. Warm 0·2 g of glucose with 5 ml of 10% NaOH soln—the soln turns yellow and then brown. Starch and sucrose do not give such colourations. Glucose gives mirror test with ammonical $AgNO_3$ soln and reduces Fehling's soln.

2. **For sucrose (cane sugar)** [$C_{12}H_{22}O_{11}$]. It does not reduce ammonical $AgNO_3$ or Fehling's soln (difference from glucose). But on warming sucrose with dil H_2SO_4, it hydrolyses and the resultant soln possesses reducing properties.

3. **For starch** [$(C_6H_{10}O_5)n$]. It does not reduce ammonical $AgNO_3$ or Fehling's soln. Starch produces deep blue colouration with iodine soln.

18·C·10·8. Amines [—NH₂]

The lower aliphatic amines, such as methyl amine, ethyl amine etc., are gases or liquids with low melting points.

Aniline, an aromatic amine, is a liquid which is sparingly soluble in water but with acids such as, HCl, forms a colourless crystalline salt aniline hydrochloride ($C_6H_5NH_2.HCl$) which is soluble in water.

Warm a mixture of aniline, chloroform and alcoholic soln of NaOH—a very bad smell of isocyanide is observed (carbylamine test).

Dissolve 0·2 g aniline in 1 ml concentrated HCl, dilute with about 3 ml of water, cool in ice and add a few drops of $NaNO_2$ soln. Add this soln to a cold soln of 2-naphthol prepared in an excess of NaOH soln—a brilliant red dye is formed.

18·C·10·9 Nitro Compounds [—NO₂]

Nitrobenzene and m-dinitrobenzene are nitro derivatives of the hydrocarbon benzene.

Nitrobenzene is a pale yellow liquid, insoluble in and heavier than water, it has a smell of bitter almonds (similar to that of benzaldehyde). Nitrobenzene can be reduced by tin and HCl to aniline which can be tested by dye test.

Warm nitrobenzene with concentrated HNO_3 and concentrated H_2SO_4—on pouring the resultant soln in ice-cold water, there is separation of solid m-dinitrobenzene whose melting point is 90°C.

Test for m-dinitrobenzene. Dissolve a few crystals of m-dinitrobenzene in 1-2 ml of acetone and add a few drops of aqueous NaOH soln—a deep violet colouration is produced which turns red on adding acetic acid.

18·C·10·10 Halogen Derivatives

Chloroform, iodoform and carbon tetrachloride are halogen derivative of methane, an aliphatic hydrocarbon.

Chloroform is a liquid with a characteristic smell. It is insoluble in and heavier than water. On warming with aniline and alcoholic NaOH soln it gives a foul smell of phenyl isocyanide (carbylamine test).

Dissolve 0·2 g of resorcinol in 1 ml of 30% NaOH, add 1 ml of chloroform and warm—a red colour is formed.

Iodoform is a yellow solid with a characteristic smell. On heating iodoform, violet vapours of iodine are formed. It also gives carbylamine test.

Carbon tetrachloride is a liquid with sweetish smell. It is insoluble in and heavier than water. It gives carbylamine test, but does not give colouration with alkaline soln of resorcinol (difference from chloroform).

18·C·10·11 Hydrocarbons [$C_X H_Y$]

Benzene and naphthalene are aromatic hydrocarbons. Benzene is a colourless liquid with a typical odour. It is insoluble in and lighter than water.

Benzene on heating with concentrated HNO_3 and concentrated H_2SO_4 produces nitrobenzene that can be recognised by its odour which is similar to that of bitter almonds.

Naphthalene is a solid with a characteristic odour. It is insoluble in water but dissolves in alcohol. Dissolve 1 g of naphthalene in 5 ml of glacial acetic acid by gentle warming. Cool, add 1 ml of concentrated HNO_3 and heat to about 80°C for about 1 minute—a clear yellow soln is obtained. Pour into cold water, the yellow-coloured solid nitro derivative is obtained whose melting point is 61°C.

18·D ORGANIC FUNCTIONAL GROUP DETERMINATION

A *functional group* means a reactive atom or group of atoms present in an organic molecule. If we consider compounds like methyl amine, ethyl amine, propyl amine and butyl amine, all of them are found to contain the amino group $[-NH_2]$. All of these compounds have been found to have similar chemical properties. As a matter of fact the chemical properties of amines are the chemical properties of the amino group. Now, suppose there is a chemical reaction in which amino group reacts rapidly and quantitatively, then this reaction can be used to determine amino group quantitatively. Since all amines have amino group as the functional group, by determining the amino group we can find the quantity of a particular amine present in a given sample.

Example 18(*vii*)

In a sample containing ethyl amine, the quantity of amino group was found to be 0·1298 g. Calculate the weight of ethyl amine in the given sample soln.

$$C_2H_5NH_2 \equiv -NH_2$$
$$45 \text{ g} \equiv 16 \text{ g}$$

Now, 16 g of amino group is present in 45 g of ethyl amine.

∴ 0·1298 g of amino aroup is present in $\dfrac{0·1298 \times 45}{16}$ g of ethyl amine = 0·365 g of ethyl amine.

It is thus seen that by determining the functional group in a given sample, we can find out the amount of the substance (present in the sample) containing that functional group. Hence, functional group determination is of very great importance in quantitative organic analysis. This section describes methods for determining some of the important functional groups.

18·D·1 Determination of Hydroxyl Group

Theory

A known weight of the given alcohol or phenol (in which hydroxyl group is to be determined) is refluxed with a mixture of acetic anhydride and pyridine until the following reaction is complete :

$$R(OH)_n + n \begin{bmatrix} CH_3 CO \\ CH_3 CO \end{bmatrix} O \longrightarrow (CH_3 COO)_n R + nCH_3COOH$$

...(18·3)

If we have ethanol which has only one hydroxyl group in its molecule, the reaction will be

$$C_2H_5OH + \begin{matrix} CH_3CO \\ CH_3CO \end{matrix} \Big\rangle O \longrightarrow CH_3COOC_2H_5 + CH_3COOH$$

For ethylene glycol which has two hydroxyl group in its molecule, the reaction will be

$$C_2H_4(OH)_2 + 2 \begin{matrix} CH_3CO \\ CH_3CO \end{matrix} \Big\rangle O \longrightarrow C_2H_4(CH_3COO)_2$$
$$+ 2CH_3COOH$$

It is seen that the number of molecules of acetic anhydride consumed is equal to the number of hydroxyl groups present in a molecule of the given hydroxy compound, that is :

$$R(OH)_n \equiv n \begin{matrix} CH_3CO \\ CH_3CO \end{matrix} \Big\rangle O$$

Thus, if we find out number of g moles of acetic anhydride consumed in reaction (18·3), we can calculate the number of hydroxyl group present in the given compound.

Procedure

The method of determining hydroxyl group consists of the following steps :

(i) Thoroughly clean and dry two 100 ml conical flasks marked A and B. .

(ii) Introduce an accurately weighed quantity (0·6 to 1·0 g) of the given hydroxy compound into flask B. (The flask A would remain empty in which a control or blank determination would be made).

(iii) Just before starting the experiment prepare acetylating mixture by adding one volume of pure acetic anhydride to four volumes of pure pyridine and then thoroughly shaking. Fill a burette with this acetylating mixture up to the zero mark. Introduce 10 ml of the mixture by means of the burette into flask A and the same volume, i.e., 10 ml into the flask B.

(iv) Attach water condensers to both the flasks A and B and circulate cold warer through the condensers. Heat the flasks by keeping them on a boiling water bath for 30 minutes.

(v) Then remove the water bath and add 20 ml of distilled water to each flask through the condenser. Thoroughly shake the contents of the flasks so that the unreacted acetic anhydride is hydrolysed to acetic acid.

(vi) Cool the flasks and titrate the contents of each flask by 0·5 N, NaOH soln using phenolphthalein as an indicator.

The difference in the volumes of NaOH soln required in the two cases gives the amount of acetic anhydride consumed (in terms of CH_3COOH) in the acetylation process. Thus,

1 g mole, NaOH $\equiv$ 1 g mole, CH_3COOH $\equiv$ 1 Hydroxyl group
or, 1000 ml, M NaOH $\equiv$ 1000 ml, M CH_3COOH $\equiv$ 1 Hydroxyl group

Example 18(*viii*)

0·953 g of phenol was refluxed with an excess of acetylating mixture. After the completion of the reaction, the unused acetic anhydride was hydrolysed and on titration was found to consume 33·9 ml of M NaOH soln. In the control experiment, the volume of NaOH required in the titration was 43·9 ml. The molecular weight of phenol is 94, calculate the number of hydroxyl groups in a molecule of phenol.

Difference in two titre values = (43·9 − 33·9) = 10·0 ml of M, NaOH.

Now, 1000 ml, M NaOH corresponds to 1 hydroxyl group.

∴ 10·0 ml, M NaOH corresponds to $\dfrac{10}{1000}$ hydroxyl group.

Since 0·953 g phenol contains $\dfrac{10}{1000}$ hydroxyl group

∴ 94 g (1 g mole) phenol contains $\dfrac{94 \times 10}{0·953 \times 1000}$

$$= 0·99 \text{ or } 1 \text{ hydroxyl group.}$$

Thus, 1 hydroxyl group will be present in a phenol molecule.

The method described above can be used for the determination of alcohols, phenols and also amines like aniline.

Example 18(*ix*)

1·009 g of aniline (mol. wt. = 93) was refluxed with acetylating agent. The blank or control titre was 32·6 ml, M NaOH and the experimental titre was found to be 21·7 ml, M NaOH soln. Calculate the number of amino groups in aniline molecule

Difference in the two titre values = (32·6 − 21·7)
$$= 10·9 \text{ ml, M NaOH}$$

1000 ml, M NaOH corresponds to 1 amino group

∴ 10·9 ml, M NaOH corresponds to $\dfrac{10·9}{1000}$ amino group.

Now, 1.009 g aniline contains $\dfrac{10.9}{1000}$ amino group.

$\therefore$ 93 g (1 g mole) aniline contains $\dfrac{93}{1.009} \times \dfrac{10.9}{1000}$

$$= 1.0 \text{ amino group.}$$

A molecule of aniline thus contains 1 amino group.

18·D·2. Bromometric Determination of Aniline and Phenol

Theory

When dil HCl is added to a mixture of potassium bromate and potassium bromide (called brominating mixture), there is liberation of bromine

$$\text{KBrO}_3 + 5\text{KBr} + 6\text{HCl} \longrightarrow 6\text{KCl} + 3\text{H}_2\text{O} + 3\text{Br}_2$$

When a known excess of brominating mixture is added to the given soln in which aniline is to be determined, there is formation of tribromoaniline. Then an excess of KI soln is added to the reaction mixture. The unreacted bromine reacts with KI as shown by the equation

$$\text{Br}_2 + 2\text{KI} \longrightarrow 2\text{KBr} + \text{I}_2$$

The liberated iodine is titrated with a standard thiosulphate soln ; this gives us the amount of unreacted bromine. Because we had taken known amount of brominating mixture, we can find out the quantity of bromine that has reacted with aniline, and from this the amount of aniline present in the given soln.

Procedure

The bromometric determination of aniline involves the following steps :

(i) Prepare a standard soln of brominating mixture. Dry some KBrO$_3$ at 120°C for about one hour and then cool it in a desiccator. Accurately weigh 0·696 g of the dried salt and transfer it to a 250 ml measuring flask. Introduce about 3 g of KBr also into the measuring flask. Add about 25 of water to dissolve KBrO$_3$ and KBr and then sufficient distilled water to make up the mark. Shake the soln thoroughly. (25 ml of this soln on acidifying would be equivalent to 25 ml of 0·1 N bromine soln).

(ii) Take a known volume of the given aniline soln into an iodine flask and add about 25 ml of dil HCl. Through a burette gradually add brominating soln [prepared in step (i)] with shaking until a permanent yellow colour is observed. Add 5 ml more of brominating soln as an excess. Shake the reaction mixture. Record the total volume (A ml) of brominating soln added.

(*iii*) Add about 5 ml of 20% KI soln and titrate the liberated iodine with a standard $Na_2S_2O_3$ soln. Note the titre (X ml) called the experimental titre.

(*iv*) In another iodine flask, take 25 ml dil HCl and A ml of brominating soln, add 5 ml of 20% KI soln and titrate the liberated iodine with $Na_2S_2O_3$ soln used in step (*iii*). Note the titre value (Y ml), *i.e.*, blank titre.

The difference between blank and experimental titre, *i.e.*, (Y−X) ml, gives the amount of bromine consumed by the aniline present in the given sample.

Example 18(x)

To 10 ml of a given soln containing aniline, 25 ml of brominating soln was added. After the completion of the reaction, an excess of KI was added and liberated iodine titrated with 0·1 M, $Na_2S_2O_3$ soln. The blank titre was 38·2 ml and experimental titre was found to be 25·9 ml. Calculate the amount of aniline present in the sample soln.

Difference between blank and experimental titre

$$=(38·2-25·9)=12·3 \text{ ml of } 0·1 \text{ M } Na_2S_2O_3 \text{ soln.}$$

$$6Na_2S_2O_3 \equiv 3I_2 \qquad \equiv 3 Br_2 \qquad \equiv C_6H_5NH_2$$
$$6000 \text{ ml, 1 M} \equiv 3000 \text{ ml, 1 M} \equiv 3000 \text{ ml, 1 M} \equiv 1000 \text{ ml, 1 M}$$
$$(\equiv 1 \text{ g mole aniline})$$

Now, 6000 ml 1 M, $Na_2S_2O_3$ corresponds to 93 g (1 g mole) aniline.

$$\therefore 12·3 \text{ ml } 0·1 \text{ M, } Na_2S_2O_3 \text{ corresponds to } \frac{12·3 \times 93}{6000} \times 0·1$$

$$=0·01906 \text{ g aniline.}$$

Thus, in 10 ml sample soln, the quantity of aniline will be 0·01906 g.

(**Note :** Phenol can also be determined by this bromometric method.)

18·D·3 Determination of Carboxyl Group

The number of carboxyl groups present in a molecule of an acid is equal to its basicity. For instance, acetic acid, CH_3COOH, is a monobasic acid, tartaric acid, $(CH.OH.COOH)_2$, is a dibasic acid and so on. Suppose we know the mol wt of a carboxylic acid then its basicity can be found out by the following relationship, if we determine its eq. wt :

$$\text{Basicity} = \text{no. of COOH group/molecule} = \frac{\text{mol. wt.}}{\text{eq. wt.}}$$

Thus, in order to determine the number of COOH groups in a molecule of the given carboxylic acid of known mol wt, it is necessary to find out its eq. wt. The eq. wt. of a carboxylic acid can be determined by the following three methods.

18·D·3·1 Silver Salt Method

Theory

In this method a soln (neutralised by NH_3) of the given carboxylic acid is treated with $AgNO_3$ soln when the silver salt of the carboxylic acid is formed. Since, the salt (RCOO Ag) is insoluble in water, it is precipitated. The ppt of the salt is filtered, washed, dried and weighed. The known weight (x g) of the salt is ignited at a proper temperature for a sufficient period of time so that the salt is *completely* decomposed leaving metallic silver which is weighed (y g). The eq. wt. of the silver salt ($E_{Ag.salt}$) is then calculated by using the following relationship :

$$\frac{\text{Eq. wt. of RCOOAg}}{\text{Eq. wt. of Ag}} = \frac{\text{wt. of RCOOAg}}{\text{wt. of Ag}} = \frac{x}{y}$$

Now, the eq. wt. of silver is known to be 108.

$\therefore$ Eq. wt. of RCOOAg=Eq. wt. of Ag$\times \dfrac{x}{y}$

or, $E_{Ag.\ salt}=108\times \dfrac{x}{y}$ ...(18-E)

When a carboxylic acid is converted into its silver salt, one hydrogen atom of the carboxyl group is replaced by a silver atom. The atomic weight of hydrogen is 1 and that of silver is 108. Hence, eq. wt. of silver salt will be equal to eq. wt. of the acid$+108$ (for Ag atom)-1 (for H atom). Thus,

eq. wt. of Ag salt=eq. wt. of acid$+108-1$

or, eq. wt. of Ag salt=eq. wt. of acid$+107$

or, eq. wt. of acid=eq. wt. of Ag salt-107 (18-F)

The eq. wt. of acid is calculated by the above method, the mol. wt. of the acid is also determined. Then, the number of carboxyl groups in a molecule of the acid is given by :

no. of carboxyl groups/molecule$=\dfrac{\text{Mol wt.}}{\text{Eq. wt.}}$ (18-G)

Example 18(xi)

0·3520 g of the silver salt of a carboxylic acid (mol wt.=60) on ignition gave 0·2271 g of silver. Calculate the number of carboxyl groups in a molecule of the acid.

$$E_{Ag.salt} = 108 \times \frac{x}{y} \qquad \left[\text{See relation (18-E)} \right]$$

$$E_{Ag.salt} = 108 \times \frac{0.3520}{0.2271} = 167.4$$

eq. wt. of acid $= E_{Ag.salt} - 107$ [See relation (18-F)]

$\therefore$ eq. wt. of acid $= 167.4 - 107 = 60.4$.

no. of COOH groups/molecule $= \dfrac{\text{mol. wt.}}{\text{eq. wt.}} = \dfrac{60}{60.4} = 0.99$

It means that one carboxyl group will be present in a molecule of the acid.

18·D·3·2   Alkalimetric Titration Method

In this method a soln of the given carboxylic acid is titrated with a standard soln of NaOH. Then by calculation we find out what amount of the acid would be equivalent to 1000 ml of 1 M' NaOH soln ; this amount of the acid is equal to its equivalent weight.

Example 18(xii)

0·48 g of an acid was dissolved in water to give 100 ml of soln. On titrating, 25·0 ml of this soln required 20·0 ml of 0·1 M NaOH soln. Calculate the eq. wt. of the acid.

25·0 ml of acid $\equiv$ 20·0 ml of 0·1 M NaOH

$\therefore$ $(25 \times 4) = 100$ ml acid $\equiv (20 \times 4) = 80$ ml of 0·1 M NaOH

or,   0·48 g of acid $\equiv$ 8·0 ml of 1 M NaOH soln

(Remember that 100 ml of acid soln contains 0·48 g of the acid).

Now, 8·0 ml of 1 M NaOH $\equiv$ 0·48 g of the acid

$\therefore$ 1000 ml of 1 M NaOH $\equiv \dfrac{1000 \times 0.48}{8.0} = 60$ g acid.

The eq. wt. of the given acid is 60.

18·D·3·3   Iodometric Method

In this method a soln of given carboxylic acid is prepared. Ten ml of this soln is pipetted out into an iodine flask and treated with 3 g each of KIO_3 and KI. The flask is stoppered and kept for 10 minutes with occasional shaking. The liberated iodine is titrated with a standard $Na_2S_2O_3$ soln using starch as indicator. Then by calculation we find out what amount of the acid would be equivalent to 1000 ml of 1 M, $Na_2S_2O_3$ soln ; this amount is the eq. wt. of the given carboxylic acid.

$$6RCOOH+5KI+KIO_3 \longrightarrow 6RCOOK+3H_2O+3I_2$$

and,
$$3I_2+6Na_2S_2O_3 \longrightarrow 3 Na_2S_4O_6+6NaI$$

$$6RCOOH \equiv 3I_2 \equiv 6Na_2S_2O_3$$

or,
$$Na_2S_2O_3 \equiv RCOOH$$

$$1000 \text{ ml, } 1 \text{ M } Na_2S_2O_3 \equiv 1 \text{ g eq. of the acid}$$

Example 18(xiii)

0·48 g of a carboxylic acid was dissolved in water to give 100 ml of soln. To 10 ml of this soln, 3 g of KIO_3 and 3 g of KI were added. After 10 minutes, the liberated iodine was titrated with 0·05 M, $Na_2S_2O_3$ soln. The volume of $Na_2S_2O_3$ soln required in the titration was 16·0 ml. Calculate the eq.wt. of the acid.

$$10 \text{ ml of the acid} \equiv 16·0 \text{ ml of } 0·05 \text{ M } Na_2S_2O_3$$

$$\therefore \quad 100 \text{ ml of the acid} \equiv 160·0 \text{ ml of } 0·05 \text{ M } Na_2S_2O_3$$

$$\therefore \quad 0·48 \text{ g of the acid} \equiv 80·0 \text{ ml of } 0·1 \text{ M } Na_2S_2O_3$$

or, $0·48$ g of the acid $\quad = 8·0$ ml of 1 M $Na_2S_2O_3$

Now, 8·0 ml of 1 M $Na_2S_2O_3$ corresponds to 0·48 g of acid

$$\therefore \quad 1000 \text{ ml of } 1 \text{ M } Na_2S_2O_3 \text{ correspond to } \frac{1000 \times 0·48}{8·0}$$

$$= 60 \text{ g of the acid}$$

The eq. wt. of the given acid will be 60.

[If mol. wt. of the acid is also 60, the number of COOH groups.

in a molecule of the acid will be $\dfrac{\text{mol.wt.}}{\text{eq.wt.}} = \dfrac{60}{60} = 1.$

18·D·4. Determination of Glucose

The determination of glucose is based on its reaction with Fehling's soln at elevated temperature. The determination of a given soln of glucose by this method involves the following steps :

(i) *Preparation of a standard soln of glucose.* Accurately weigh 1·25 g of pure anhydrous glucose, dissolve in water and make up the soln to 250 ml in a measuring flask. This standard soln is used for the standardisation of the Fehling's soln.

(ii) *Preparation and standardisation of Fehling's soln.*

Solution (A) Dissolve 6·93 g of pure $CuSO_4·5H_2O$ in water and make up the soln to 100 ml in a measuring flask.

Solution (B). Dissolve 34·6 g of crystalline sodium potassium tartrate (Rochelle salt, $C_4H_4O_6NaK·4H_2O$) in warm water. Dissolve 12 g of NaOH in water. Mix the two solutions and make up the volume to 100 ml in a measuring flask.

Just before the experiment, mix equal volumes of soln (A) and soln (B) and shake throughly ; this is the *Fehling's* soln which is standardised by the following procedure :

Pipette out 25 ml of Fehling's soln into a conical flask, add about the same volume of distilled water and heat to boiling. Place the conical flask on a white paper, and add gradually glucose soln [prepared in step (*i*)] through a burette. After each addition allow some time for the red coloured cuprous oxide to settle down and observe the disappearance of blue colour in the supernatant liquid. The temperature of the titration liquid will decrease during the observation of the colour, hence the contents of the flask should be again heated. The end point of the titration is shown by the just disappearance of the blue colour in the supernatant liquid. Repeat the titration until the titre values are consistent *i.e.*, do not differ by more than 0·1 ml.

(*iii*) *Determination of concentration of given glucose soln.* Take 25 ml of the Fehling's soln prepared in step (*ii*) and titrate it with the given soln of glucose in a manner similar to that described for the standardisation of Fehling's soln. Suppose,

25·0 ml of Fehling's soln ≡ 24·5 ml of standard glucose soln

and, 25·0 ml of Fehling's soln ≡ 26·7 ml of the given glucose soln

Then the strength of the given glucose soln will be = strength of the standard glucose soln × $\dfrac{24·5}{26·7}$

Now, 250 ml of standard glucose soln contains 1·25 g glucose

∴ 1000 ml of standard glucose soln contains $\dfrac{1000 \times 1·25}{250}$

= 5·0 g glucose/litre

∴ the strength of the given glucose soln will be

$$5·0 \times \frac{24·5}{26·7} = 4·59 \text{ g/l}$$

[Note : This method can also be used for determining sucrose or cane sugar. Sucrose is first hydrolysed by acid and the resultant glucose and fructose can be estimated by Fehling's soln. cane sugar can also be determined by means of a polarimeter (see chapter 15).]

18·D·5   Determination of Aldehydes and Ketones

The following two methods can be used for the determination of aldehydes and ketones.

18·D·5·1   Method Using Hydroxylamine Hydrochloride

In this method, a known volume of a given soln of an aldehyde or a ketone is treated with an excess of hydroxylamine hydrochloride in presence of pyridine :

$$\frac{R}{R'}\!\!\diagdown C=O+H_2NOH.HCl+C_6H_5N \rightleftharpoons$$

$$\frac{R}{R'}\!\!\diagdown C=NOH+H_2O+C_6H_5N.HCl \qquad (18·3)$$

Pyridine hydrochloride formed during the reaction can be titrated with standard sodium hydroxide soln using bromophenol blue as indicator. [The purpose of adding pyrine is to make the reaction (18·3) quantitative.]   A carbonyl group $\diagup C=0$ consumes a molecule of hydroxylamine hydrochloride to produce a molecule of HCl.

$$R.R'C=O \equiv NH_2OH\,HCl \equiv HCl$$

∴ 1 g mole of ketone or aldehyde [containing one carbonyl group in its molecule.]

$$\equiv 1000 \text{ ml, 1 M soln of HCl}$$

Knowing the amount of HCl produced, the quantity of aldehyde or ketone present in the sample soln can be calculated. [Note that for the reaction (18.3) eq. wt. of hydroxylamine hydrochloride is equal to its mol.wt.   Also, eq. wt. of aldehyde or ketone will be equal to its mol. wt.]

Procedure

(i) Dissolve 8·75 g of pure hydroxylamine hydrochloride in about 40 ml of water and dilute to 250 ml in a measuring flask with 95% alcohol.

(ii) Dissolve 5 g of NaOH in about 25 ml of the water and dilute to 250 ml with methanol.

(iii) Mix 0·25 ml of 1% bromophenol blue in alcohol with 5 ml of pure pyridine and dilute to 250 ml with 95% alcohol.

(iv) Pipette 30 ml of hydroxylamine hydrochloride reagent soln into an iodine flask and add a known volume (V_2) of a soln containing not more than 10 milli-equivalents of an aldehyde or ketone. Stopper the flask and keep it at room temperature for about 30 minutes.

(v) Meanwhile carry out a blank determination without adding the sample soln of aldehyde or ketone by titrating with methanolic NaOH soln of normality N_1 to a blue-green colour. Keep this soln for the comparison of colour while titrating the experimental soln prepared in step (iv).

(vi) Titrate the experimental soln with methanolic NaOH (normality N_1) to obtain the same colour that was obtained in the blank determination. Note the volume (V_1) of the NaOH soln required in this titration.

Calculations

$$V_1 \times N_1 = V_2 \times N_2$$

where, $V_1 =$ volume of alkali required for titration (blank—expt.titre)

$N_1 =$ normality of alkali used for titration

$V_2 =$ volume of aldehyde or ketone soln taken

$N_2 =$ normality of aldehyde or ketone soln taken

$$\therefore \quad N_2 = \frac{V_1 \times N_1}{V_2}$$

The weight of aldehyde or ketone in g present per litre of the soln

$$= \frac{V_1 \times N_1}{V_2} \times M$$

where M is the molecular weight of the given aldehyde or ketone.

18·D·5·2 Method Using 2 : 4 - Dinitrophenylhydrazine

In this method the given soln of the carbonyl compound (aldehyde or ketone) is taken in an iodine flask and treated with an excess of a saturated soln of 2 : 4 - dinitrophenylhydrazine prepared in 2 N HCl. The reaction mixture is allowed to stand for one hour on an ice-bath. The ppt formed is filtered and washed once with 2N HCl. It is then transferred to a weighed sintered crucible and again washed, first with 2N HCl and then by water. The crucible containing the ppt is dried at 100-105°C until it shows a constant weight. Knowing the weight of the ppt, the amount of carbonyl compound present in the given soln can be calculated.

18.D.5.3 Determination of Aldehydes by Sodium Bisulphite Method

Aldehydes react with sodium bisulphite in accordance with the equation.

$$RCHO + NaHSO_3 \rightleftharpoons RCH(OH)SO_3Na$$

A known weight of aldehyde sample is treated with a known excess of $NaHSO_3$ and the residual bisulphite is determined iodimetrically. Knowing the amount of $NaHSO_3$ consumed, the quantity of the aldehyde present in the sample can be calculated on the basis of the above equation. This procedure involves error due to the reversibility of the reaction and the instability of sodium bisulphite soultion.

18.D.5.4 Determination of Aldehydes by Sodium Sulphite Method

This procedure is based on the following reaction

$$RCHO + Na_2SO_3 + H_2O \rightleftharpoons RCH(OH)SO_3Na + NaOH$$

The aldehyde sample is treated with an excess of Na_2SO_3 solution and the NaOH formed is titrated with standard mineral acid. Knowing the amount of NaOH produced, the quantity of the aldehyde in the sample can be calculated. This procedure suffers due to the reversibility and slow rate of the reaction moreover, the end point is not sharp.

18.D.5.5 Determination of Aldehydes by Sodium Sulphide-Sulphuric Acid Procedure

The difficulties encountered in the procedures described in 18.D.5.3 and 18.D.5.4 can be solved by adding a known excess of H_2SO_4 to a large excess of Na_2SO_3 solution, just before adding the aldehyde sample. Sodium bisulphite generated in situ (within the system : $Na_2SO_3 + H_2SO_4 \rightarrow NaHSO_3 + NaHSO_4$) reacts with the aldehyde and the remaining acid is titrated potentiometrically with a standard alkali solution.

Reagents

1. **Na_2SO_3 Solution, 1 M.** Dissolve 126 g Na_2SO_3 in 1 litre distilled water and adjust its pH to 9.1 by the dropwise addition of 1 M sodium hydroxide solution. Use a pH meter with glass-calomel electrode combination for this pH adjustment.

2. **H_2SO_4 Solution 1 N.**

3. **NaOH Solution 1 N.**

Procedure

(i) Take 250 c.c. of 1 M Na_2SO_3 solution in a 500 c.c, glass-stoppered flask and gradually add 50.0 c.c. of 1 N H_2SO_4 with constant swirling of the flask. Immediately add a weighed quantity of the sample into the flask.

(ii) Shake the mixture vigorously for about 15 minutes and then quantitatively transfer the mixture into a 600 c.c. beaker.

(iii) Potentiometrically titrate the contents of the beaker with 1 N NaOH solution using the pH meter. Obtain the end-point graphically by plotting pH as ordinates and alkali added as abscissae.

Observations and Calculations

$y = $ c c. of 1 N NaOH required for the titration of 50 c.c. of H_2SO_4 added (blank titre)

$x = $ c c. of 1 N NaOH required for the titration of the mixture containing the sample (sample titre).

$M = $ mot wt of the aldehyde taken.

$w = $ wt of the aldehyde taken.

Now $RCHO \equiv NaHSO_3 \equiv NaOH$

∴   1000 c.c. 1 N NaOH $\equiv M$ g aldehyde

∴ $(y-x)$ c.c. 1 N NaOH $\equiv \dfrac{(y-x)}{1000} \times M$ g aldehyde

Now, w g sample contains $\dfrac{(y-x)}{1000} \times M$ g aldehyde

∴   100 g ... ... $\dfrac{(y-x) \times M \times 100}{1000 \times w}$ g aldeyde

∴   % of aldehyde $= \dfrac{(y-x) \times M}{w \times 10}$

The above expression is applicable when the normality of NaOH used is 1 N. If the normalty of NaOH isN_1 then % purity

$$= \dfrac{(y-x) \times N_1 \times M}{w \times 10}$$

18.D.5.6 Determination of Formaldehyde (Romijn's iodometric Method)

Formaldehyde is generally used in the form of its aqueous solution called *formalin* which contains about 35% by weight of formaldehyde. This method consists of treating a known weight of formaldehyde sample with a known excess of I_2 solution in alkaline medium when HCHO in oxidized to HCOOH in accordance with the equation

$$I_2 + 2NaOH = NaOI + NaI + H_2O$$
$$\underline{HCHO + NaOI + NaOH = HCOONa + NaI + H_2O}$$
$$HCHO + I_2 + 3NaOH = HCOONa + 2NaI + 2H_2O$$

Sodium hypoiodite is supposed to oxidize HCHO to HCOOH. After the completion of the reaction the unused NaOI is determined iodometrically. The raction mixture is acidified when the following reaction takes place

$$NaOI + NaI + 2HCl = 2NaCl + H_2O + I_2$$

The liberated iodine is titrated with a standard $Na_2S_2O_3$ solution; this gives sample titre.

$$2Na_2S_2O_3 + I_2 = 2NaI + Na_2S_4O_6$$

A blank is also run to obtain the value of blank titre. The difference between the blank and the sample titre gives the amount of I_2 that has reacted with the formaldehyde present in the sample. Knowing the amount of I_2 consumed, the qauntity of HCHO in the sample is calculated Using the following relationship

$$2Na_2S_2O_3 \equiv I_2 \equiv HCHO \ (= 30 \text{ g HCHO})$$

Remember that mol wt of HCHO is 30.

∴ $Na_2S_2O_3 \equiv \tfrac{1}{2}I_2 \equiv \tfrac{1}{2}HCHO \ (= 15 \text{ g HCHO})$

or,   1000 cc N $Na_2S_2O_3 \equiv 15$ g HCHO

or,   1000 cc 0.1 N $Na_2S_2O_3 \equiv 1.5$ g HCHO

or,   1 cc 0.1 N $Na_2S_2O_3 \equiv 0.0015$ g HCHO (= 1.5 mg HCHO)

Reagents

1. $Na_2S_2O_3$ Solution, 0.1 N
2. I_2 Solution, 0.1 N
3. NaOH Solution, 2 N
4. HCl Solution, 4 N
5. Starch Solution, 1% aqueous.

Procedure

(i) Accurately weigh about 1.0 g of given formalin into a 250 c.c. measuring flask and dilute with distilled water to the mark. Mix thoroughly. Take 25 c.c. of this solution into a 250 c.c. iodine flask and and 50.0 c.c. of 0.1 N I_2 solution. Immediately thereafter, add 2N NaOH *dropwise* with constant swirling until the solution becomes pale yellow.

(ii) In another iodine flask, place the same volumes of I_2 and NaOH solutions and 25 c.c. of distilled water in place of the sample solution. This is the blank.

(iii) After 10 minutes, acidify the contents of both the flasks by adding an excess of 4N HCl. Titrate the liberated I_2 with 0.1 N $Na_2S_2O_3$ solution using starch indicator and thus record the blank and the sample titre.

Observations and Calculations

Blank titre		y c.c.
Sample titre		x c.c.
Normality of $Na_2S_2O_3$ solution		0.1 N
Weight of formalin in 25 c.c. of the sample solution		w g

The amount of I_2 consumed by the sample in terms of 0.1 N $Na_2S_2O_3$ solution is given by $(y-x)$ c.c.

Now, 1 c.c. of 0.1 N $Na_2S_2O_3 \equiv 0.0015$ g HCHO

$\therefore$ $(y-x)$ c.c. of 0.1 N $Na_2S_2O_3 \equiv (y-x) \times 0.0015$ g HCHO

Since w g of of the sample contains $(y-x) \times 0.0015$ g HCHO

$\therefore$ 100 g ... ... $\dfrac{(y-x) \times 0.0015 \times 100}{w}$ g HCHO

Thus % HCHO $= \dfrac{(y-x) \times 0.0015 \times 100}{w}$

Alternatively,

$Na_2S_2O_3 \equiv \frac{1}{2} I_2 \equiv \frac{1}{2} HCHO$ (M/2 g of HCHO)

[where M = mol wt of HCHO]

. 1000 c.c. 1 N $Na_2S_2O_3 \equiv M/2$ g HCHO

or, $(y-x)$ c.c. 1 N $Na_2S_2O_3 \equiv \dfrac{(y-x) \times M}{2 \times 1000}$ g HCHO

Now, w g of the sample contains $\dfrac{(y-x) \times M}{2 \times 1000}$ g HCHO

$\therefore$ 100 g $\quad \ldots \quad \ldots \dfrac{(y-x) \times M \times 100}{2 \times 1000 \times w}$ g HCHO

If the normality of $Na_2S_2O_3$ solution used is N_1, then % HCHO

$$= \dfrac{(y-x) \times N_1 \times M \times 100}{2 \times 1000 \times w}$$

[Note. 1. This iodometric method is applicable only to dilute solutions of formaldehyde whose concentration is less than 1 %.

2. The presence of other aldehydes interfere with this method.]

18.D.5.7 Determination of Acetone (Messinger's iodometric method)

Acetone reacts with I_2 in presence of alkali according to the following equation

$$CH_3COCH_3 + 3I_2 + 4NaOH = CHI_3 + CH_3COONa + 3NaI + 3H_2O$$

From the above equation it is obvious that

$$CH_3COCH_3 \equiv 3I_2$$

Now, $\qquad\qquad I_2 \equiv 2Na_2S_2O_3$

So, $\qquad\qquad 6Na_2S_2O_3 \equiv 3I_2 \equiv CH_3COCH_3$

or, $\qquad Na_2S_2O_3 \equiv \dfrac{1}{2} I_2 \equiv \dfrac{1}{6} CH_3COCH_3$

The mol wt of CH_3COCH_3 is 58.081, hence

$$1000 \text{ c.c. of 1 N } Na_2S_2O_3 \equiv \dfrac{1}{6} \times 58.081 (= 9.680 \text{ g acetone})$$

or $\quad$ 1 c.c. of 0.1 N $Na_2S_2O_3 \equiv 0.9680$ mg acetone

Reagents

1. **Iodine Solution**, 0.1 N.
2. **NaOH Solution**, 1 N.
3. **H_2SO_4 Solution**, 1 N.
4. **Starch Solution**, 1 %.

Procedure

(i) Take a known volume of aqueous solution of the sample containing 0.01 to 0.025 g of acetone in a 500 c.c. iodine flask and add about 200 c.c. of distilled water. Add 25.0 of 1 N NaOH solution, shake well and allow to stand for 5 minutes. Then introduce 50.0 c.c. of 0.1 N I_2 solution through a burette while constantly swirling the flask.

(ii) In another iodine flask place the same volumes of water, I_2 and NaOH omitting the sample. This is the blank.

(iii) Acidify the contents of both the flasks by adding an excess of HCl and titrate the liberated I_2 with a standard $Na_2S_2O_3$ solution. The difference in the blank and sample titre gives the amount of iodine consumed by the acetone sample.

Observations and Calculations

   (i) Blank titre   ...   .   *y* c.c.

   (ii) Sample titre   ...   .   *x* c.c.

   (iii) Normality of $Na_2S_2O_3$ solution   ...   0-1

The amount of iodine consumed will be $(y-x)$ c.c. of 0.1 N $Na_2S_2O_3$ solution. Now,

$$1 \text{ c.c. of } 0.1 \text{ N } Na_2S_2O_3 \text{ soln} \equiv 0.9680 \text{ mg acetone}$$

$\therefore$ $(y-x)$ c.c. 0.1 N $Na_2S_2O_3$ soln $\equiv (y-x) \times 0.9680$ mg acetone

The sample will contain $(y-x) \times 0.9680$ mg of acetone.

[Note. This iodometric procedure can be applied for the determination of acetaldehyde and chloral hydrate also but in these cases, for obtaining satisfactory results, a large excess of I_2 solution should be used and then the alkali solution should be added *dropwise at a very slow rate* with constant swirling of the iodine flask containing the reaction mixture.]

18.D.6   DETERMINATION OF NITRO GROUP

Titanous salts reduce nitro groups to amines as shown by the equation

$$RNO_2 + 6\ Ti^{3+} + 6H^+ \rightarrow RNH_2 + 6\ Ti^{4+} + 2H_2O$$

A known weight of the nitro compound, dissolved in water, alcohol or acetic acid, is treated with a known excess of titanous salt solution. The reaction mixture is boiled in a current of hydrogen. Later the unused titanous is titrated back with a standard ferric ammonium sulphate solution using NH_4 CNS as indicator. Knowing the amount of the titanous salt consumed, the NO_2 content in the sample can be calculated.

$$NO_2 \equiv 6Ti^{3+} \equiv 6Fe^{3+}$$

6000 c.c. of N Ti^{3+} salt solution $\equiv 6000$ c.c. of N Fe^{3+} salt solution
$$\equiv 46 \text{ g of } NO_2$$

or,   1000 c.c. N Fe^{3+} salt solution $\equiv \dfrac{46}{6} = 7.667$ g NO_2

or,   1000 c.c. 0.1 N Fe^{3+} salt solution $\equiv 0.7667$ g NO_2

or,   1 c.c. 0.1 N Fe^{3+} salt solution $\equiv 0.7667$ mg NO_2

Reagents

1. *Ferric ammonium sulphate solution, 0.1 N.*—Dissolve 48.22 g of the A.R. salt in 500 c.c. distilled water (that has been freshly boiled and then cooled) containing 5 c.c. of 50% (w/w) H_2SO_4 and then dilute to 1 litre with boiled-out distilled water.

2. *Ammonium thiocyanate indicator solution, 10%.*

3. *Titanous sulphate solution*, *0.1 N*. Mix 12 g of titanium metal with 1200 c.c. of 1 : 3 (v/v) H_2SO_4 and warm on a water bath for 7 hours when all or most of the metal dissolves. Cool in a stream of H_2 or CO_2 gas and dilute to 2 litres with freshly boiled and then cooled distilled water.

Storage of Solution of Titanous Salt

A solution of titanous salt is oxidised on exposure to atmosphere hence it has to be stored under such conditions that it does not undergo airoxidation. A 2 litre capacity bottle is filled with titanous salt solution up to the neck of the bottle. Stopcock C is turned in such a way that the burette is filled with the solution. The stop cock is then opened until all the air in the bottle A and the burette is replaced by H_2 generated in Kipp's apparatus (see Fig. 18.9).

Standardisation of Titanous Salt Solution

[The problem with a titanous salt solution is that it is unstable as it is oxidized by atmospheric oxygen. Hence, the solution should be protected from atmospheric oxygen during its-storage and also when it is being used in titration process. The titration involving titanous salt solution is therefore performed in a special titration flask. This conical flask is fitted with a rubber stopper having two holes. Through one hole the burette tip is introduced while through the other a glass tube is inserted which touches the bottom of the flask [(see Fig. 18.10).]

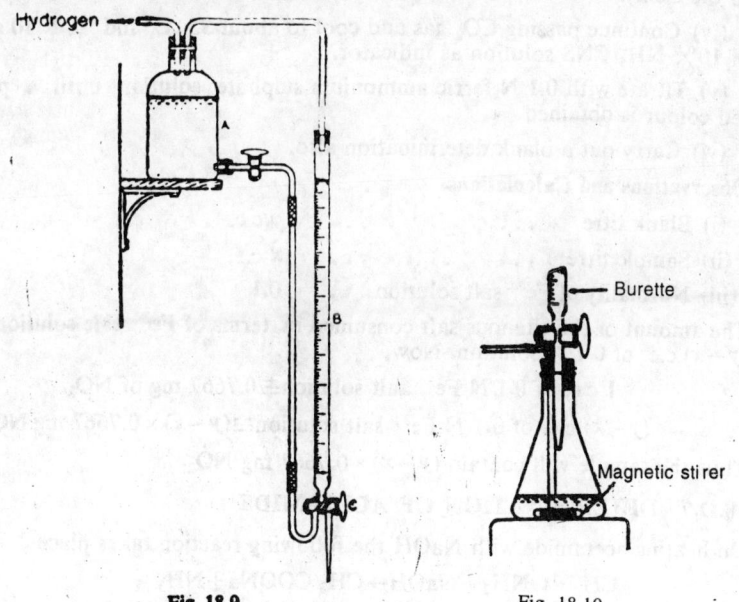

Hydrogen

Burette

Magnetic stirer

Fig. 18.9   Fig. 18.10

Take 25.0 c.c. of the standard ferric ammonium sulphate solution into a special titration flask (see Fig. 18.10), and add 25 c.c. of 15 N H_2SO_4. Pass CO_2 gas through the solution to expel air. Continue passing CO_2 and gradually add titanous salt solution from the burette until the yellow colour of the ferric salt solution almost disappears. At this stage add 10 c.c. of 10% NH_4CNS solution, a red colour will be produced due to the formation of ferric thiocyanate. Continue titration until the red colour disappears. The reaction tends to slow down near the end point at room temperature. Hence, the titration mixture is heated to boiling (with CO_2 flowing), then cooled down to 35 °C and titration is carried out with titanous salt solution. the reaction involved is

$$Ti^{3+}+Fe^{3+}\rightarrow Ti^{4+}+Fe^{2+}$$

Thus, knowing the normality of the ferric salt solution, the normality of the titanous salt can be calculated.

Procedure

(i) Weigh out accurately a dry sample containing about 0.015 g of nitro group into the special titration flask (see Fig. 18.10) and dissolve it in water or a dilute mineral acid or alcohol or acetic acid. Then add 25 c.c. of 14 N H_2SO_4 solution.

(ii) Pass CO_2 gas through the flask for 5 minutes to remove oxygen.

(iii) Add 50.0 c.c. of 0.1 N titanous sulphate solution and boil for 5 to 10 minutes. (If the sample is volatile a water condenser should be attached to the flask).

(iv) Continue passing CO_2 gas and cool to about 35 °C, and add 10 c.c. of 10% NH_4 CNS solution as indicator.

(v) Titrate with 0.1 N ferric ammonium sulphate solution until a pale red colour is obtained.

(vi) Carry out a blank determination also.

Observations and Calculations

(i) Blank titre . . .   . y c.c.

(ii) Sample titre . . .   . x c.c.

(iii) Normality of Fe^{3+} salt solution . . .   0.1

The amount of the titanous salt consumed in terms of Fe^{3+} salt solution is $(y-x)$ c.c. of 0.1 N solution. Now,

$$1 \text{ c.c. of } 0.1 \text{ N } Fe^{3+} \text{ salt solution} \equiv 0.7667 \text{ mg of } NO_2$$

∴ $(y-x)$ c.c. of 0.1 N Fe^{3+} salt solution $\equiv (y-x) \times 0.7667$ mg NO_2

Thus the sample will contain $(y-x) \times 0.7667$ mg NO_2.

18.D.7 DETERMINATION OF ACETAMIDE

On heating acetamide with NaOH the following reaction takes place

$$CH_3 CONH_2 + NaOH \rightarrow CH_3 COONa + NH_3$$

This reaction can be used for determining acetamide in two ways.

1. Method Based on the Determination of Liberated Ammonia (Amminometric method)

In this method a measured volume of the acetamide sample solution is heated with NaOH solution. The liberated NH_3 is absorbed in a known excess of HCl solution. After completion of the reaction the remaining acid is titrated with a standard alkali solution. Knowing the amount of the acid consumed, the quantity of NH_3 produced and hence the amount of acetamide in the sample solution can be calculated.

$$(NaOH\equiv) \ HCl\equiv NH_3\equiv CH_3CONH_2 (Mol \ wt=59)$$

$$1000 \ c.c. \ of \ N \ HCl\equiv 59 \ g \ CH_3 \ CONH_2$$

or, $\qquad$ 1 c.c. of N HCl$\equiv$59 mg CH_3CONH_2

Example 18 (xiv)

In a flask 10 c.c. of acetamide sample was heated with NaOH solution. The liberated NH_3 was absorbed in 50 c.c. of N HCl solution. The remaining acid was titrated with N NaOH. The blank and sample titres were found to be 50.0 and 28.0 c.c. respectively. Calculate the amount of acetamide in the sample.

$$\text{blank titre}=50.0$$
$$\text{Sample titre}=28.0$$
$$\text{Difference}=22.0 \ c.c. \ of \ N \ NaOH \ solution$$

Now, NaOH$\equiv$HCl, hence the acid consumed in neutralizing NH_3 gas= 22.0 c.c. of N HCl. Now,

$$1 \ c.c. \ N \ HCl\equiv 59 \ mg \ CH_3 \ CONH_2$$
$$\therefore \qquad 22.0 \ c.c. \ N \ HCl\equiv(22\times59)=1298 \ mg \ CH_3CONH_2$$
$$=1.298 \ g \ CH_3 \ CONH_2$$

The sample solution contains 1.298 g acetamide per 10 c.c. of sample solution.

2. Method Based on the Determination of Unreacted Alkali

In this method a measured volume of the amide sample solution is taken in a 250 c.c. conical flask and treated with a known excess of NaOH solution. The reaction mixture is heated until all the NH_3 gas is expelled (if all the NH_3 gas has been removed, a red limus paper kept at the mouth of the conical flask will not turn blue). The contents of the flask are then cooled and the unused NaOH is titrated with 0.5 N oxalic acid solution using phenolphthalein indicator. Knowing the amount of NaOH used up, the quantity of acetamide in the sample solution can be calculated.

$$NaOH\equiv CH_3 \ CONH_2 \ (Mol \ wt=59)$$

$$1000 \ c.c. \ of \ N \ NaOH\equiv 59 \ g \ CH_3CONH_2$$

$$1 \ c.c. \ of \ N \ NaOH\equiv 59 \ mg \ CH_3CONH_2$$

[A blank is also run. The difference between the blank and sample titres gives the amount of the alkali consumed in terms of the concentration of the acid used for the titration.]

18.D.8 DETERMINATION OF UREA

Urea on treatment with sodium hypobromite decomposes giving out N_2 gas according to the equation

$$CO(NH_2)_2 + 3NaOBr + 2NaOH \rightarrow N_2 + Na_2CO_3 + 3NaBr + 3H_2O$$

Thus, $\quad N_2$ (Mol wt$=28$)$\equiv$CO (NH$_2$)$_2$ (Mol wt$=60.06$)

The volume of 28 g of N_2 at N.T.P. is 22.415 litres, so if the volume of the liberated N_2 is measured, the quantity of urea in the sample solution can be calculated. Thus this is a *gasometric method* (see p. 7); it can also be called an *azotometric method* as it is based on the measurement of the volume of N_2 gas. The above reaction, however, is not stoichiometric because of a side reaction in which a part (about 4.3%) of urea is converted into ammonium cyanate. Hence, the calculation of the quantity of urea is done by assuming that the above reaction goes only up to 95.7%. It can be shown theoretically that 1 g of urea should yield 373.2 c.c. of N_2 but due to incomplete reaction only 357.0 c.c. of the gas is produced at S T.P.

Reagents

1. Sodium hypobromite solution

Dissolve 50 g of NaOH in 250 c.c. of water and cool the solution in an ice bath to 0—5 °C. Then slowly add 12.5 c.c. of A.R. bromine with constant stirring.

Procedure

(i) Place 60 c.c. of hypobromite solution in a conical flask A.

(ii) Weigh accurately about 100 mg of urea sample in a small test tube B and put B in A as shown in Fig. 18.11.

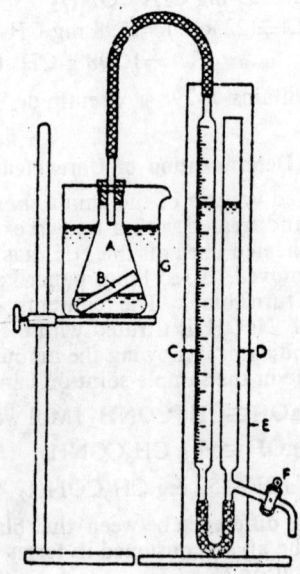

Fig. 18.11

(iii) Close A with a tight-fitting rubber stopper having a hole through which A can be connected to a gas measuring tube C. Connect C to another tube D called the levelling tube as shown in Fig. 18.11. Tubes C and D are clipped to a wooden board E. Tube D is provided with a stop cock F through which water can be removed.

(iv) Place A in a large beaker G containing water at room temperature. Wait for about 30 minutes for the attainment of thermal equilibrium and then make the levels of water in C and D equal either by pouring water into D or removing water from D through F.

(v) Tilt A so that urea and hypobromite get mixed.

(vi) Make water levels equal in C and D. Note the volume of N_2 gas collected in C, temperature of water in G and barometric pressure.

Observations and Calculations

(i) Weight of urea sample ... ... 0.125 g
(ii) Volume of N_2 liberated ... ... 48.7 c.c.
(iii) Barometric pressure ... ... 756.7 mm
(iv) Temperature ... ... 27 °C
(v) Vapour pressure at 27 °C ... ... 26.7 mm

We know that

$$\frac{P_0 V_0}{T_0} = \frac{P_1 V_1}{T_1}$$

or,

$$V_0 = \frac{P_1 V_1}{T_1} \times \frac{T_0}{P_0}$$

$$P_1 = (756.7 - 26.7) = 730 \text{ mm}$$

$$V_1 = 48.7 \text{ c.c.}$$

$$T_1 = (273 + 27) = 300 \text{ °C}$$

$$T_0 = 273 \text{ °C}$$

$$P_0 = 760 \text{ mm}$$

∴

$$V_0 = \frac{730 \times 48.7 \times 273}{300 \times 760} = 42.6 \text{ c.c.}$$

Now, 357 c.c. N_2 gas is produced by 1 g urea

∴   42.6 c.c. ... ... $\dfrac{42.6 \times 1}{357}$

$$= 0.119 \text{ g urea}$$

0.125 g Urea sample contains 0.119 g urea

∴   100 g ... ... $\dfrac{0.119 \times 100}{0.125}$ g urea

$$= 95.2 \text{ g urea}$$

Thus the purity of the given urea sample is 95.2%.

19

Analysis of Some Commercial and Biological Samples

The approach to analysis of the commercial products is slightly different from that adopted for chemical analysis in theoretical analytical chemistry. Usually a commercial sample given for analysis has a history i.e., some general preliminary information about its probable composition, which provides a hint as to how to plan its analysis. But this information is not always sufficient and the analytical chemist carrying out the analysis has to depend on his experience to work out a plan for analysing the given sample.

19.1 FACTORS DECIDING THE PLAN OF ANALYSIS OF A COMMERCIAL SAMPLE

The following factors are generally taken into consideration while planing the analysis of a commercial sample.

1. The first consideration is the amount of the sample available for analysis. Sometimes the sample is costly or is available in small quantity. In such cases non-destructible methods are chosen so that two, three or more constituents can be determined in the same portion of the sample. To analyze such a sample, micro-methods are employed which require much smaller amounts of the sample.

2. Different constituents of a given sample are found out, if these are not already known. Sometimes, it is desired to know the amounts of only a few constituents. In such a case, the complete quantitative analysis is quite unnecessary and only partial analysis pertaining to the constituents of interest is done. However, the knowledge of the qualitative composition of the sample is essential in order to properly plan its quantitative analysis. The method for determining a particular constituent is so selected that it is not interfered by the other constituents present in the sample. If such a methods is not available, the interfering material has to be removed by some separative technique.

3. Before starting the analysis, it should be known that what degree of accuracy is desired by the agency that has supplied the sample for analysis.

For example, suppose a manufacturer wants to keep the amount of a parti-cular constituent, in a product, in the range of 20 to 22%, then it is mean-ingless to spend time and energy to obtain results up to the second place of decimal such as 20.29 or 21.56%. Attempts should be made to obtain very accurate results only when such a high degree of accuracy is desired.

4. Economy of time and money are of great consideration in commer-cial analysis. In many cases several samples are to be analyzed in a day hence, the method selected should be rapid and should not involve very costly chemicals unless it is a must.

5. After taking into account the above mentioned points, a sequence is decided for determining various constituents of a given sample.

19.2 GENERAL APPARATUS USED IN COMMERCIAL ANALYSIS

The tools required for commercial analysis are quite similar to those used in various analytical procedures. Some of the important tools that are commonly used will be described here. A good analytical chemist should have knowledge about their utility and limitations.

19.3 THE ANALYTICAL BALANCE

This is one of the most important tools of an analytical chemist and the principle underlying its construction should be properly understood. It should be carefully handled and well maintained. A good analytical balance should have the following properties.

(i) It should give reproducible results.

(ii) The beam of the balance must return to the horizontal position after swinging.

(iii) It should be sensitive enough so that even a change of weight by 0.1 mg is detectable.

Balances of different weighing capacities and designs are now available which can be used for rapid and accurate weighing. In certain balances weights are suspended within the balance and these can be loaded by means of controlling dials; this facility eliminates the tedious process of transfer-ring the weights from the box to the pan of the balance. Such balances are preferred in commercial analysis. Rough balances should also be available for a rapid and approximate weighing.

19.4 DISTILLED WATER PLANT

In an analytical chemistry laboratory, ample supply of distilled water is essential. Hence, a laboratoy must have units for producing distilled water. For this purpose electrically operated distillation water plants are very use-ful which are convenient to operate and can generally produce 2 to 3 litres of distilled water per hour.

19.5 HEATING DEVICES

Several analytical operations require heating of solutions, precipitates or other substances. For this purpose the following devices are generally employed.

Bunsen Burner. It is widely used for obtaining moderately high temperatures. The temperature of the flame depends upon the quantity of air supplied to the flame (see Fig. 19.1). In certain burners, both the gas and air supply can be regulated by suitable devices (see Fig. 19.2). It is thus possible to have temperatures in the range of 600 to 1100 °C. Gas burners of various designs are commercially available.

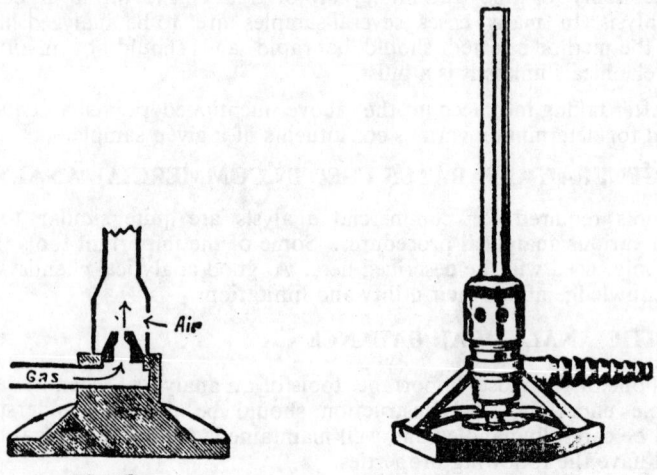

Fig. 19..1   Fig. 19.2

HOT PLATES. Electrically operated hot plates (see Fig. 19.3) with

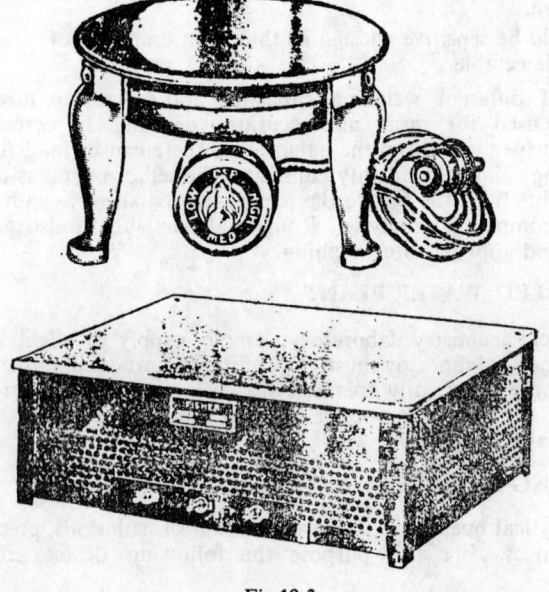

Fig 19.3

regulators to control the temprature are very convenient for heating solutions as compared to gas burners.

Electric ovens. These consist of closed boxes which are electrically heated (see Fig. 19.4). A controlling dial is provided for regulating the temperature of the oven. These ovens are generally used to dry precipitates or solids. The temperature of most ovens can be regulated from room temperature to 250-300° C within $\pm$ 1 to 2 °C.

Murffel furnace. These are used for heating precipitates or solids up to a temperature of about 1200°C. In these furnaces heating is done electrically. A thermo-couple, placed in the furnace, is attached to a calibrated ammeter which indicates the temperature of the furnace.

Infra-red lamps. These are very useful for evaporating solutions. The lamp is placed at the top of the liquid or solution to be heated.

Air baths. Certain substances on heating give out corrosive vapours; such substances should not be heated in an oven. Heating of these substances is done in an air bath which consists of a conical metallic vessel with a perforated bottom. The substance to be heated is kept in a crucible or a dish which is placed in the middle portion of the vessel on a loop made of copper wire (see Fig. 19.5.). The bottom of the vessel is heated by means of a gas burner.

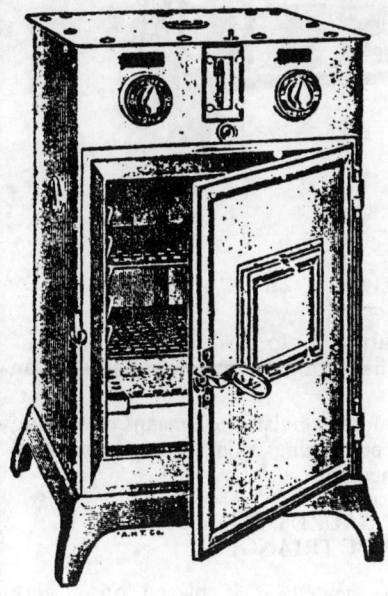

Fig. 19.4

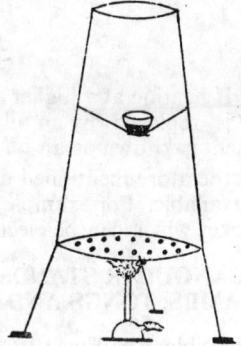

Fig. 19.5 Air bath

Water or steam bath. These can be used only when heating below 100 °C is required, such as for heating aqueous solutions just below boiling, for slow evaporation of liquids to reduce their volumes, for digestion of precipitates etc. A water bath consists of a copper vessel containing a number of concentric rings which act as its cover (see Fig. 19.6.). These rings are removable and also act as a base for beakers of different sizes. The vessel is filled with water and the beaker containing the solution is kept at the top. On heating the vessel elecrically or by means of a burner, water gets heated which in turn heats the solution taken in the beaker. The use of water bath ensures gradual heating without any danger of bumping. A multiple-unit water bath consists of a rectangular vessel with

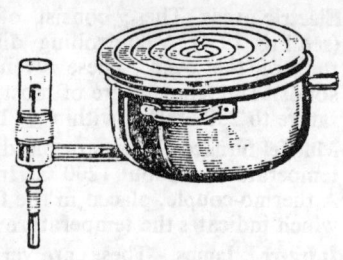

Fig. 19.6

a number of openings at the top where beakers of different sizes can be placed (see Fig. 19.7). A regular supply of water to these vessels must be made to compensate the loss of water due to evaporation.

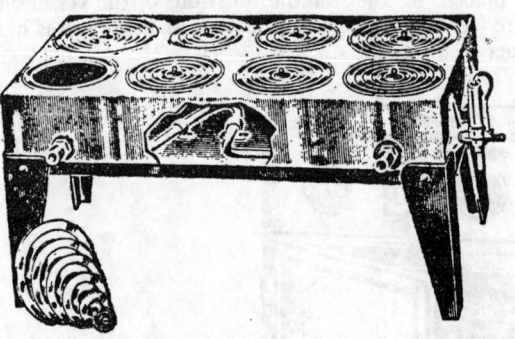

Fig. 19.7

Oil bath. If heating at a higher temperature is to be done, then water in the bath is replaced by an oil which has a higher boiling point; such an arrangement is known as an *oil bath.*

Besides the afore-mentioned devices, more sophisticated means of heating are now available. For example, a flask containing a liquid may be covered with a jacket which can be electrically heated.

19.6 TRIANGULAR STANDS, WIRE GAUZES IRON STANDS, CLAMPS, TONGS AND CLAYPIPE TRIANGLE

When a crucible (see Fig. 19.8) is to be heated, it is placed on a clay pipe triangle which is kept on a triangular stand (see Fig. 19.9.) A Bunsen burner is used to heat the crucible. Iron stand and clamps are used for keeping beakers, flasks, thermometers etc.. in proper position (see Fig. 19.10 and 19.11). When a glass vessel is heated, a wire gauze is placed between the vessel and the burner (see Fig. 19.10). A wire gauze is made of iron wire mesh square in shape with a circular asbestos coating in the central area.

Tongs (see Fig. 19.12) made of metals are used to handle hot crucibles, basins etc.

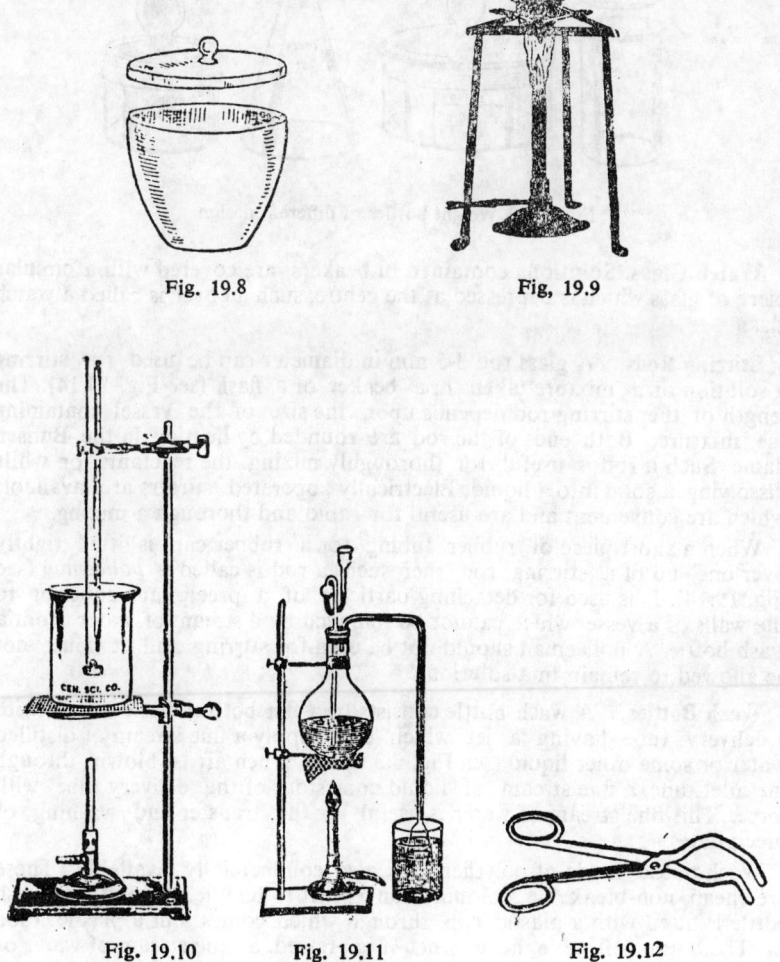

Fig. 19.8　　　　　　　　　　Fig, 19.9

Fig. 19.10　　　Fig. 19.11　　　　　Fig. 19.12

19.7 GLASSWARE

Following glassware are commonly required for carrynig out various analytical operations.

Weighing Bottles.   Laboratory samples are weighed in weighing bottles.
Weighing bottles of different shapes and sizes are available (see Fig. 19.13).

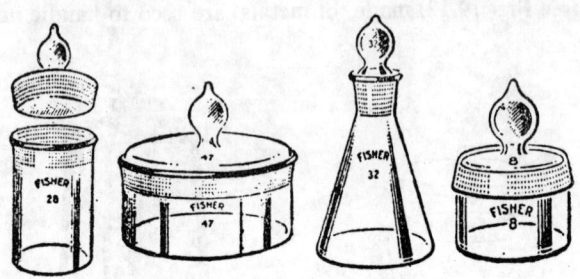

Fig. 19.13 Weight bottles of different design

Watch Glass. Solutions contained in beakers are covered with a circular
piece of glass which is depressed at the centre; such a cover is called a watch
glass.

Stirring Rods.   A glass rod 3-5 mm in diameter can be used for stirring
a solution or a mixture taken in a beaker or a flask (see Fig. 19.14). The
length of the stirring rod depends upon the size of the vessel containing
the mixture. Both ends of the rod are rounded by heating in the Bunsen
flame. Such a rod is useful for thoroughly mixing the reactants or while
dissolving a solid into a liquid. Electrically   operated stirrers are available
which are convenient and are useful for rapid and thorough a mixing.

When a short piece of rubber tubing (or a rubber cap) is fitted tightly
over one end of a stirring rod then such a rod is called a *policeman* (see
Fig. 19.14). It is used for detaching particles of a precipitate adhering to
the walls of a vessel which cannot be removed by a stream of water from a
wash bottle. A policeman should not be used for stirring and it must not
be allowed to remain in a solution.

Wash Bottles.   A wash bottle consists of a flat bottom flask fitted with
a delivery tube having a jet which can supply a fine stream of distilled
water or some other liquid (see Fig. 6.3 a, b). When air is blown through
the inlet tube, a fine stream of liquid comes out of the delivery tube with
force. This fine stream of water is useful for the transfer and washing of
precipitates.

Wash bottles made of polythene are also commercially available. These
are cheap, non-breakable and more convenient to handle. A polythene wash
bottle is fitted with a plastic cap through which comes out a plastic tube
jet. The bottle is flexible, hence when it is pressed, a fine stream of water or
some other liquid comes out with force. Such a wash bottle can be used
only for cool liquids. When the wash liquid is other than water, the wash
bottle should be cleaned with distilled water after a reasonable interval of
time.

Separatory Funnels.   These are used for separating immiscible liquids.
Separatory funnels of different shapes are available. The pear shape is

preferable when a small amount of lower layer is to be drawn off. Normally the sizes of the separatory funnels commonly needed are 250 and 500 c.c. (see Fig. 13.1).

Funnels. Whenever a liquid is transferred from one vessel to another with a narrow opening, a glass funnel is used. Funnels are also needed in the filtration process (see Fig. 19.15). Funnels enclose an angle of 60°. The most commonly used funnels are those with diameters 5.5, 7 and 9 cm. The internal diameter of the stem is about 4 mm and it is about 15 cm long. For filling burettes and transferring solids to volumetric flasks, a short-stem and wide-necked funnel is useful.

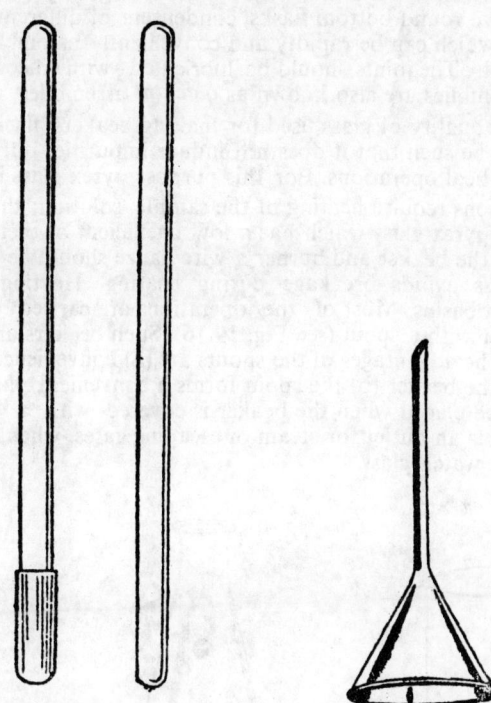

Fig. 19.14 Stirring rod and policeman   Fig. 19.15 Funnel

Desiccator. If a substance which has been dried by heating in an oven or by ignition, is to be cooled then it must be kept in a dry atmosphere. If the hot substance is cooled in open, it will absorb moisture from the atmosphere and the purpose of heating will be defeated. Hence, hot substances are cooled in a dry vessel which does not contain moisture. Such a device is called a desiccator (see Fig. 6.2).

A desiccator is a glass vessel which has an air-tight cover. The lower part of this vessel is filled with anhydrous calcium chloride, silica gel,.

alumina or anhydrous calcium sulphate. These substances, called dehydrating agents or desiccants, absorb the moisture from the air contained in the vessel so that the substance kept in the vessel cools down in a moisture free atmosphere. Silica gel, alumina or anhydrous calcium sulphate is mixed with a cobalt salt which gives a blue colour to the desiccant. When the desiccant absorbs sufficient moisture, it turns pink. At this stage the desiccant is no longer effective and should be replaced. In a vacuum desiccator, the desiccator is evacuated. In such a desiccator drying takes place more rapidly.

All Ground-Glass-Joint Assemblies. In quantitative organic analysis, sometime the sample is to be refluxed or distillation process is to be carried out. For these purposes, assemblies with all ground glass-joints are available. These involve round bottom flasks, condensers of different types and receiving vessels which can be rapidly and conveniently assembled through ground glass joints. The joints should be lubricated with silicone stopcock grease. Such assemblies are also known as *quick-fit* assemblies.

Beakers. The quality of glass used for making beakers, flasks and other glassware should be such that it does not induce impurities during their use in different analytical operations. For this purpose pyrex glass is preferred.

Several operations require heating of the sample solution; this is done in beakers made of pyrex glass which has a low coefficient of thermal expansion. In between the beaker and burner a wire gauze should be placed. The use of pyrex glass avoids breakage during heating. Heating can also be done in procelain basins. Most of the operations are carried out in a 250 or 450 c.c. beaker with a spout (see Fig. 19.16): Such beakers are known as *Griffin beakers*. The advantages of the spouts are (a) convenience of pouring a solution from the beaker (b) the spout forms a convenient place at which stirring rod can be placed when the beaker is covered with a watch glass (c) the spout forms an outlet for steam or escaping gases when the beaker is covered with a watch glass.

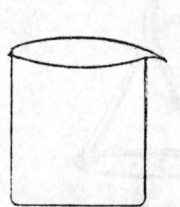

Fig. 19.16 Griffin beaker

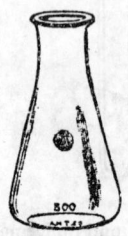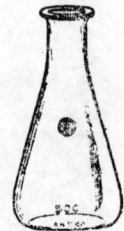

Fig. 19.17 Conical
(a) wide mouth   (b) narrow mouth

Conical Flasks. For titrations, 100 or 250 c.c. conical flasks with narrow or wide mouth are used; these are called *Erlenmeyer flasks* (see Fig. 19.17). In micro-analytical work flasks and beakers of much smaller size are employed. In certain cases a reaction mixture is allowed to stand for some time before titration and the reaction product may be volatile, such as, iodine or bromine etc. Such reaction mixtures are taken in a conical flasks with ground glass stoppers; these flasks are called *iodine flasks*.

Test Tubes. These are commonly used for performing qualitative tests of samples. If the sample is to be heated, a boiling test tube should be used.

19.8 GRADUATED GLASSWARE

In order to obtain reliable results in quantitative chemical analysis, burettes; pipettes and volumetric flasks certified by some standard agency should be used. If certified glassware are not available then these should be calibrated.

19.8.1 Volumetric or Measuring Flasks

A volumetric flask consists of a glass bulb with a flat bottom and a long neck. The neck has a mark. If a liquid is filled up to the mark then its volume will have a particular value as mentioned on the volumetric flask (see Fig. 7.1). Measuring flasks with different capacities such as 2000, 1000, 500, 250, 200, 100, 50, 25 and 10 c.c. etc., are available. These flasks should be cleaned after a reasonable interval of time. Soap and water containing little soda ash is satisfactory for cleaning glassware. Chromic acid can also be used as a "cleaning solution." Many commercially available detergents such as "Decon 90", Teepol etc., are suitable for cleaning glassware.

19.8.1.1 Calibration of a Volumetric Flask

The calibration of a volumetric flask requires determining the weight of water held by the flask when it is filled up to the mark. It should be noted that

1 litre of water weighs

$$997.18 \text{ g at } 20\ ^{\circ}C$$
$$996.17 \text{ g at } 25\ ^{\circ}C$$

A litre means the volume occupied by one kilogram of water at 4 °C, the temperature at which its density is maximum. It has been shown that

1 litre = 1000.028 c.c. (cm^3)

1 litre = 1.000028 dm^3 (1 dm = 10 cm)

1 ml = 1.000028 cm^3 (or c.c.)

It is thus seen that there is a very small difference between "ml" (millilitre) and "c.c. (cubic centimeter or cm^3). However, the term litre now means dm^3 i.e., cubic decimeter. The use of term "cm^3" is preferred to "ml", and dm^3 to litre.

Example 19 (i)

A dry graduated flask, marked "250 c.c. at 20 °C, weighed 128.3958 g. The flask was then filled up to the mark with distilled water at 20°C and was found to weigh 378.6930 g. Find out the exact volume of a liquid contained by the flask.

Weight of the water contained
by the flask at 20°C is

378.6930 g

−128.3958 g

250.2972 g

Now, 0.9972 g water at 20 °C occupies 1 c.c. volume

$$\therefore \quad 250.2972 \; ,, \quad ,, \quad ,, \quad \frac{250.2972}{0.9972} = 251.0 \text{ c.c.}$$

Thus the exact volume of a liquid contained by the volumetric flask (or graduated or measuring flask) at 20°C will be 251.0 cm³ and not 250 cm³ as marked on the flask.

[Note. Before weighing the flask filled with water, the outer surface should be wiped with a clean piece of cloth so that there is no water adhering to the outer surface of the flask.]

19.8.2 Pipettes

These are also called transfer pipettes because by means of these a fixed volume of a liquid or a solution can be transferred from one container to another. A transfer pipette consists of a cylindrical glass bulb joined at both the ends by narrow tubes (see Fig. 19.18). The upper tube has a mark while the end of the lower tube is drawn out to a tip. Pipettes of different capacities such as 100, 50, 25, 20, 10, 5, 2 c.c. are available. On the pipette, its capacity at a particular temperature is given such as 25 c.c. at 20 °C. The time required for the delivery of the liquid through the pipette is also given. For example, if on the pipette 15+13 seconds are mentioned (see Fig. 19.18), then it means that 15 sec. is the delivery time and the tip of the pipette should be touched for 13 sec. to the wall of the container in which liquid is being transferred, then only the pipette will deliver the volume mentioned on it at the given temperature. One should neither blow out the liquid from the pipette nor warm the bulbs of the pipette to expel the liquid.

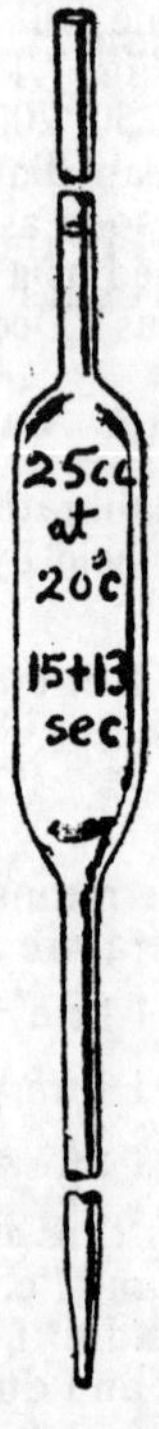

19.8.2.1 Calibration of Pipettes

If the quality of the pipette has not been certified by some standard agency then it should be calibrated as shown in the following example.

Example 19 (ii)

Fig.19.18

A pipette has the markings, 25 c.c. at 20 °C; 15+13 sec. This pipette was filled with distilled water up to the mark. A beaker was cleaned, dried and weighed. The weight of the beaker was found to be 35.2987 g. The water contained in the pipette was transferred to the beaker. (It should be checked that the delivery time is 15 seconds), Then the tip of the pipette was touched to the wall of the beaker for 13 seconds. The beaker along with the transferred water was found to weigh 60.0292 g. Find out the exact volume of the water delivered by this pipette.

Wt. of the beaker+water=60.0292 g

Wt. of empty beaker   =35.2987 g

Wt. of the volume of water

delivered by the pipette $=\overline{24.7305 \text{ g}}$

Now, 0.9972 g of water at 20 °C occupies 1 c.c.

∴   24.7305 g . . .   . . , $\dfrac{24.7305}{0.9972} = 24.80$ c.c.

The correct volume delivered by the piperte would be 24.8 c.c. and not 25.0 c.c. as marked on the pipette:

[Note. Pipettes are used for two purposes:

    (i) to deliver a definite volume of a liquid, and

    (ii) to withdraw a definite amount of a liquid.

For these two purposes different kinds of pipettes are used: these are to deliver and to contain type].

19.8.3 Graduated Pipettes

These consist of narrow tubes with no central bulb (Fig. 19.19). The tube has markings so that a desired volume of a liquid can be delivered through these pipettes.

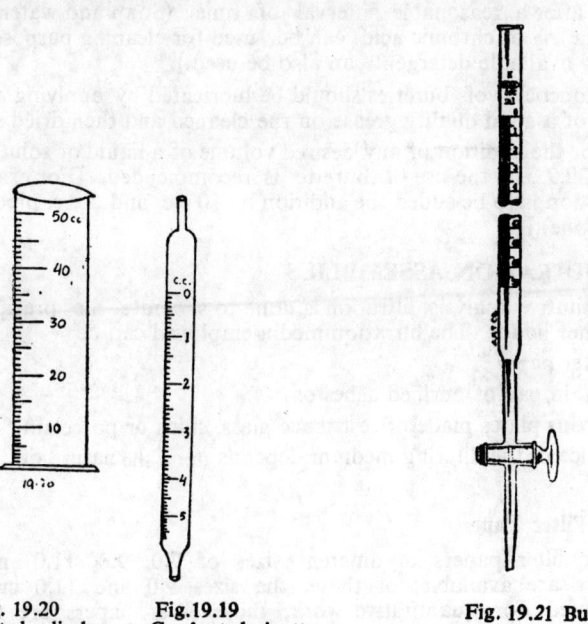

Fig. 19.20   Fig.19.19   Fig. 19.21 Burette
Graduated cylinder   Graduated pipette

[Note. If the liquid to be delivered is toxic or corrosive, it should not be sucked into the pipette by mouth. Rubber bulbs are available which can be fitted to the pipette and liquid can be sucked in by gradually expanding the bulb].

19.8.4 Graduated Cylinders, or Measuring Cylinders

These consist of cylindrical glass vessels which have been marked to measure volume (Fig. 19.20). Measuring cylinders of capacities from 2 to 2000 c.c. are available but these should be used only when a rough measurement is to be done.

19.8.5 Burettes

These consist of a rather wide glass tube of uniform cross-section having a stopcock at the end of the tube which is graduated in c.c. (Fig. 19.21). A burette is used to add a known volume of a liquid or a solution. Burettes of different capacities such as 50 c.c., 25 c.c. and 10 c.c. are available which read up to one tenth of a c.c. For adding smaller volumes microburettes can be used which can read up to one fiftieth of a c.c. (i.e. 0.02 c.c.).

[Note. (1) The tips of pipettes and burettes become clogged after sometime: These should be cleared with the help of a thin wire. (If this is not done the delivery time will be increased causing inconvenience, moreover then the volume of the liquid, delivered by the pipette, will not be in accordance with the volume marked on the ptpette).

(2) Graduated glasswares should be cleaned with a suitable cleaning solution after a reasonable interval of time. (Soap and water containing little soda ash or chromic acid can be used for cleaning purpose or a commercially available detergent can also be used.]

(3) Stopcocks of burettes should be lubricated by applying a very small amount of a good quality grease on the cleaned and then dried surface.

(4) For the addition of any desired volume of a liquid or solution say 5.9, 11.0 or 20.9 c.c., the use of burette is recommended. (For example, if 15 c.c. solution is to be added the addition by 10 c.c. and 5 c.c. pipettes should not be done).]

19.9 FILTRATION ASSEMBLIES

In quantitative analysis, filtration is done to separate the precipitate from the mother liquor. The filtration media employed can be

(a) Filter paper

(b) A thin pad of purified asbestos

(c) Porous plates made of resistance glass, silica or porcelain

The choice of the filtering medium depends upon the nature of the precipitate.

19.9.1 Filter Paper

Circular filter papers of different sizes of 7.0, 9.0, 11.0 and 12.5 cm diameter are available; of these, the sizes 9.0 and 11.0 cm are most widely used. For quantitative work, those filter papers are used which on burning give an ash content not exceeding 1 mg. Filter papers are made of different porosity. When the precipitate consists of very small particles a filter paper with small porosity is used. Whatman quantitative filter paper no. 541 permits fast filtration but can retain only coarse particles: Number 542 is suitable for filtering medium-sized particles and no. 543 should be used for the filtration of fine particles. The bulk of the ppt to be handled decides the size of the filter paper as well as the funnel.

The filter paper is carefully fitted into a funnel so that the outer surface of the paper tightly sticks against the funnel surface. During filtration, the funnel containing the properly fitted filter paper is placed in a funnel stand and a clean beaker is placed below in such a way that the stem of the funnel just touches the side of the beaker (see Fig. 6.6). The liquid to be filtered is slowly poured down a glass rod into the filter paper fitted in the funnel. The filter paper cone should never be completely filled; the level of the liquid in the cone should be about 1 cm below the top of the paper. Filter paper is suitable for separating gelatinous precipitates. In ordinary filtration no suction is applied to accelerate the process of filtration.

The ordinary filtration process using a funnel and a filter paper has two disadvantages. One, the process is slow as no suction is applied. Hence, in filtration and then repeated washing of the ppt much time is needed. Secondly, the washed ppt. along with the filter paper is transferred to a crucible where the ppt. is ignited and filter paper is completely burnt. This procedure is quite cumbursome. In order to overcome these difficulties, filter crucibles are used in which filtration under suction is carried out and then the washed ppt. is dried or ignited (see Fig. 6.4) in the crucible itself.

19.9.2 Buchner Funnel

A Buchner funnel is used when large quantities of material is to be filtered. It consists of a cylindrical porcelain vessel with holes in the bottom which ends into a stem (similar to a funnel). The holes of the bottom are covered with a circular filter paper. In another kind of Buchner funnel a sintered glass plate is used for the purpose of filtation (see Fig. 19.22).

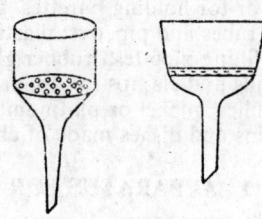

Fig. 19.22

19 9.3 Sintered Glass Crucible

These are made of resistance glass and their bottom consists of a porous disc of sintered ground glass which acts as a filtering device (Fig. 6.4a). A suction is applied to accelerate the filtration process. Another advantage with such crucibles is that the use of filter paper is eliminated. Sintered glass crucibles of different porosities are available. There are very convenient to use but cannot be heated to higher temperatures. Crucible fitted with permanent porous plates are cleaned by removing the solid and then using a suitable solvent for dissolving out the remainder solid.

19.9.4 Gooch Crucibles.

A Gooch crucible consists of a tall crucible whose base has a number of holes. These holes are covered with a pad of purified asbestos fibres. These fibres are mixed with distilled water and this mixture is poured into the crucible. Thus a layer of asbestos gets set which acts as a filtering medium. A Gooch funnel is used to hold the crucible (see Fig. 19.23). The funnel is fitted into a filter flask which is connected to a filter pump. The Gooch crucible can be heated upto 200° C.

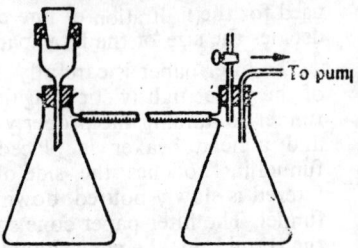

[Note. When a precipitate is to be heated to a high temperature, crucibles made of platinum, silica or porcelain are used.]

Fig. 19.23

19.9.5 Centrifuge

A centrifuge can be used for a rapid separation of a solid from a liquid. Hand driven centrifuge as well as electrically operated centrifuges are available.

19.10. MISCELLANEOUS ITEMS

Besides the items mentioned in the earlier sections, a number of other articles made of wood, rubber, plastic or of different metals are also used in a chemical laboratory. For example, wooden stands for filtration assembly or for holding burettes, pipettes and test tubes; plastic racks for holding test tubes and pipettes; plastic wash bottles and reagent bottles; ruber bulbs for filling pipettes; rubber gloves when handling corrosive substances; iron stands and clamps for apparatus assembly of different types; crucibles made of silica, nickel or platinum; pestle and mortar made of porcelain or agate; basins and dishes made of china clay etc.

19.11 APPARATUS FOR MICRO ANALYSIS

For performing analysis at micro level we need micro-burettes, micro-pipettes, beakers, conical flasks etc., of relatively smaller capacity.

19.12 MEASURING INSTRUMENTS

In last 50 years or so there has been a growing tendency to make use of instrumental methods of analysis. The instrumental methods are very valuable for commercial analysis due to their high sensitivity, rapidity and convenience in operation. The following instrument are generally used in qualitative and quantitative analysis.

Colorimeter, turbidimeter, nephelometer, fluorometers, flame photometer, spectrophotometer U.V. and I.R., polarimeter, x-ray spectrometer, refractometer, potentiometer, conductivitimeter, polorograph, various types of chromatographs.

Data on the strength of aqueous solutions of some common acids and aqueous ammonia have been shown in Table 19.1.

TABLE 19.1

Acid/Alkali	Per cent by weight	Specific gravity	Normality
Hydrochoric acid	35	1.18	11.3
Nitric acid	70	1 42	16.0
Sulphuric acid	96	1.84	36.0
Hydrofluoric acid	46	1.15	26.5
Perchloric acid	70	1.66	11.6
Phosphoric acid	85	1.69	41.1
Acetic acid	99.5	1.05	17.4
Ammonia	27	0 90	14.3

19.A ANALYSIS OF WATER

Like air, water is also essential for the existence of all kinds of life on the earth. But as a result of activities of human beings and animals, air and water are adversely affected and many unwanted and harmful substances enter into our atmosphere; in other words, air and water get polluted. This process of pollution has been continuously taking place since the existence of life but now it has assumed dangerous proportions due to the population explosion and rapid growth of industries. The pollutants present in the air in the industrial areas also ultimately contaminate water of rivers, lake, spirings etc., through rains. Previously it was thought that rivers had the capacity to purify their water. This is true to some extert but when huge quantities of domestic and industrial wastes are dumped into rivers, they are no longer capable of self-purification.

Unpolluted natural water contains some organic as well inorganic matter to such a small extent that it does not affect human bealth. The cause of water pollution is the discharge of domestic and industrial wastes into different sources of water such as rivers, lakes etc. If this waste is discharged on land surface, it percolates down the earth surface and contaminates groundwater. The disposal of industrial waste is one of the most important causes of water pollution. There are various industries such as those related to dairy products, distilleries, fruit and vegetable products, tanneries, textiles, pulp and paper, drugs, organic chemicals, explosives, pesticides, fertilizers, steel mills, oil refineries, thermal power plants etc. These industries produce a variety of pollutants such as carbon dioxide, carbon monoxide, sulphur dioxide, ammonia, organic matter of different kinds, colloidal material, suspended solids, acidic and basic substances, mineral oils, variety of inorganic substances, some toxic material and heat which are discharged into receiving waters. Some of these pollutants are highly toxic. Hence water pollution is responsible for a large variety of diseases. Polluted water affects irrigated land and leads to decline in fisheries. Due to rapid industrialization the availability of water is becoming increasingly difficult. People have now become aware of the hazards of water pollution and steps are being taken to minimize it. The waste water flow from factories is analyzed and is subjected to suitable treatment before it is allowed to be discharged in receiving waters such as a river or a lake, so that it does not cause pollution.

19A.1 MAJOR WATER POLLUTANTS

There are the following major types of water pollutants. Out of these any one or more may be present in a water sample.

1. Organic material
2. Dissolved gases
3. Inorganic dissolved solids
4. Suspended solids
5. Fertilizing elements
6. Pathogenic organisms
7. Heat

1. Organic Material

Many organic pollutants undergo biochemical oxidation in receiving waters; this decreases the level of dissolved oxygen which has an adverse effect on aquatic life. The pollutants that do not undergo oxidation, escape removal by treatment process and get accumulated in receiving waters. The type of organic pollutant present depends upon the nature of the industry which has produced it. Some of the organic pollutants are acetone, amines, aniline, benzene and its derivatives, dichloraethane, formal dehyde, hydroquinone. lactose, naphthalene, nitrobenzene, oils and greases, proteins, pyridine, sugar, tar, turpentine etc.

2. Dissolved Gases

These can also come from air pollution through rains. Many industries produce gases such as carbon monoxide, carbon dioxide, oxides of nitrogen, sulphur dioxide, ammonia etc., which pollute the receiving waters into which the industrial wastes are discharged.

3. Inorganic Dissolved Solids

Even natural water contains dissolved solids such as salts of calcuim, magnesium, sodium, potassium, iron and traces of heavy metals. This is mainly due to the minerals present in the rocks and soils. But the amount of dissolved inorganic solids is considerably increased as a result of discharge from industries.

4. Suspended Solids

The presence of extremely small particles of insoluble substances is the cause of turbidity in water. The turbidity is due to clay, silt, organic matter and microscopic organisms. Such waters are unsuitable for use in domestic purposes, food and beverage industry and in many other industries. When suspended material is present in excessive quantities, it causes sedimentation and thus affects the ecology of rivers, lakes and streams. Turbidity can be removed by filtration or by the process of coagulation.

5. Fertilizing Elements

Sometimes industrial wastewaters bring in nitrates and phosphates into receiving waters which result in abundant growth of aquatic plants.

6. Pathogenic Organisms

Viral and bacterial pollution usually results from the discharge of domestic, agricultural and food-processing wastewaters. Advances in the technology for the purification of drinking water have greately reduced the incidence of human disease resulting from bacterial pollution. But still water-borne diseases occur frequently since the conventional water purification processes are not very effective in completely removing water-borne viruses.

7. Heat

Increase in temperature of receving waters may be due to the heat generated during chemical and biological reactions. This heat can disturb the ecological balance.

19.A.2 DESIGN OF ANALYTICAL SCHEME FOR WATER ANALYSIS

Analysis of industrial wastewaters presents challanging problems to analytical chemists. This work requires considerable knowledge of the application of standard analytical methods, instruments, idea regarding the nature of likely interferences and other problems that may come up during analysis of different types of water samples.

In order to design an overall analytical scheme for water analysis, the following factors are generally taken into consideration.

1. The history of the wastewater
2. The aim or objective of the analysis
3. The choice of parameters for analysis
4. The choice of method for analysis.

1. The History of the Wastewater

Before planning the analysis one must know the history of the water sample under consideration. For example, wastewaters from oil refineries can contain oils and greases, pyridine. quinoline, acridine etc., dairy wastewaters can contain lactose. Formaldehyde will be the pollutant produced by plastic industrry and so on.

2. The Objective of Analysis

The purpose and aim of the analysis is an important step in designing water analysis. Some the objectives can be

(i) Estimation of possible harmful effects due to ingridients present in waste effluent on the quality of receiving waters.

(ii) Determination of quality standards for reuse of water or its disposal into municipal sewers.

(iii) Deciding the treatment of polluted water for its reuse or disposal in sewers.

(iv) Recovery of valuable by-products from the wastewaters.

The aim of the analysis decides the designing of analysis programme.

The analysis of fresh water is necessary to ascertain its suitability for use as drinking water or for irrigation or for the growth of aquatic animals. The purpose of study will decide the type of analysis to be carried out.

3. The Choice of Parameters for Analysis

After knowing the purpose of anaylsis the parameters for analysis are decided. The choice of the properties to be studied are decided by the type of information required about the water sample.

4. The Choice of the Method for Analysis

The selection of a particular method for determining a particular pollutant present in the given water sample usually depends upon

    (i) the nature of the other substances present in the sample

    (ii) the required degree of accuracy

    (iii) the amount the pollutant

    (iv) the frequency of analysis

19.A.3 INSITU ANALYSIS

This type of analysis is rapid, avoids sample collection and its subsequent transfer to a laboratory for analysis. Following are the examples of insitu analysis.

    (i) Placing a flow conductivity meter in a stream of water which can monitor the quantity of ionic substances present from time to time.

    (ii) Putting a fixed number of fishes in a cage placed in water and then finding out the number of dead fishes after a fixed interval of time: This number will be proportional to the quantity of toxic substances present in water.

19.A.4 STUDY OF PROPERTIES OF POLLUTED WATER

The study of polluted water consists of its qualitative and quantitative analysis. Several parameters related to the quality of water have been proposed. The properties of water have been divided into the following three categories.

    A. Physical Parameters. These involve the measurement of parameters such as colour, odour taste, density, viscoity, surface tension, temperature, turbidity, foam and froth, conductivity, dissolved solids, pH, redox potential, radioactivity etc.

    B. Chemical Paramcters These include measurement of acidity, alkalinity, dissolved oxygen, biochemical oxygen demand (B.O.D), chemical oxygen demand (C.O.D), ammonia, nitrite, nitrate, phosphorus, sulphur, sulphides, chlorides, silica, calcium, magnesium, sodium, potassium, iron, copper, cobalt, zinc, cadmuim, mercury etc. Besides inorganic matter organic material such as detergents, pesticides, oils and greases, benzene, pyridine, tar, sugars, formaldehyde, turpentine, proteins, lactose, nitrobenzene, chloroderivaties of benzene, hydroquinone, aniline etc., are also determined depending upon the history of the water sample and objective of analysis.

    C. Biological Parameters These are of great importance from public health point of view. All natural waters contain a variety of organisms both plant and animal. Sewage, domestic and industrial wastewaters also contain various organisms. These can cause a number of water-borne diseases like cholera, typhoid, fever, dysentry etc.

19.A.5 COLLECTION OF THE SAMPLE

The objective of the programme decides the selection of the sites for sample collection. For example, if one is interested in studying the pollution caused by a particular waste discharge then the sample would be collected from the site where the wastewater is being discharged. Sampling points must be located to provide an accurate understanding of the existing water quality. The selection of sampling location also depends on the character of the waterbody. In a lake or in a wide river many sampling sites should be selected at various corners to have a more complete understanding of the type and extent of pollution. In a narrow and fast moving stream a single selection site may be sufficient.

One of the problems in sample collection is that of the aceessibility. Bridges often provide good sample collection centres. Samples should never be collected from disturbed areas like *ghats* as samples from such sites cannot be representative. Samples are collected in glass or polythene bottles. Surface water can be collected readily but special type of equipment is needed for collecting a sample from a depth. The analysis of rain water gives an idea about the air pollution in a particular area.

19.A.6 MEASUREMENT OF PHYSICAL PARAMETERS

1. Temperature The temperature of surface water can be readily measured by means of a mercury thermometer. For the measurement of depth temperature special devices are used.

2. Colour The colour of water sample is compared with known colour standards. If the sample is turbid, the turbidity should be removed as it may interfere with the colour judgement. Since pH influences colour, the pH of the sample at which colour judgement is done, should be mentioned.

3. Odour. The sample is diluted with odour free water until a least perceptible odour is detected. The extent of dilution is a parameter for odour.

4. Turbidity This is due to the presence of fine particles in the sample. This property is measured by means of a nephelometer. The turbid sample is illuminated by means of light and the light scattered by the particles is measured in a direction at right angles to that of the incident light. The intensity of the scattered light is proportional to the turbidity. The turbidity of the sample is compared with that of a standard turbidity suspension.

5. Density, viscosity and surface tension. In certain samples the measurement of these properties is also useful.

6. Conductivity. The conductivity of water sample is due to the presence of various kinds of ions. Hence the measurement of conductance is a measure of the amount of different kinds of ions present in the sample.

7. pH This terms is defined as

$$pH = -\log [H^+]$$

where $[H^+]$ represents the concentration of H^+ ions in g ions per litre of sample solution. If for the sample

$$pH = 7 \text{ , sample is neutral}$$

pH$>$7 , sample is alkaline

pH$<$7 , sample is acidic,

The pH value of the given water sample can be conveniently and rapidly measured by means of a pH meter having glass-calomel electrode combination.

8. Redox Potential If a system contains an oxidant and also its reduced form such as MnO_4^-, Mn^{2+} or Cl_2, Cl^-, then it is called a *redox system*. If an inert electrode is dipped in a redox system, the electrode acquires certain potential which is called the *redox potential*. The sign and the magnitude of the redox potential provides information about the oxidizing or reducing capacity of the sample under investigation.

9. Total Solids (T.S.) A silica crucible is heated to about 550 to 600 °C for about half an hour, cooled in a desiccator and then weighed. This process of heating, cooling and weighing is repeated until a constant weight is obtained. Then V c.c. of the *unfiltered* water sample is taken in the crucible and evaporated on a water bath. The solid residue is heated, cooled in a desiccator and then weighed. This process is repeated until a constant weight is obtained. The difference in two weights gives the weight of solid (W g) obtained from the evaporation of V c.c. of sample.

V c.c. of sample contains $W \times 1000$ mg residue

$\therefore$ 1000 c.c. $\ldots$ $\ldots$ $\ldots$ $\ldots$ $\dfrac{W \times 1000 \times 1000}{V}$ mg.

Thus weight of the total solid in mg/litre=$\dfrac{W \times 1000 \times 1000}{V}$

[Note. The volume of the sample solution taken should be such that we get sufficient amount of residual solid so that there is no significant weighing error. If a large volume of sample solution is to be taken, it can be first evaporated in a beaker and when the volume is reduced to about 10 c.c. then it can be tradsferred into a 20 c.c. crucible. The evaporation process is then continued.]

10. Total dissolved solids. (T.D.S.). This is determined by a similar method as described for the determination of total solids. The only difference is that in this case we take V c.c. of *filtered* water sample.

11. Total Suspended Solid. (T.S.S) The amount of suspended solid or particulate matter can be obtained by subtracting total dissolved solid from total solids, that is

T.S.S.=T.S.$-$T.D.S.

19.A.7. MEASUREMENT OF CHEMICAL PARAMETERS

19.A.7.1 The Determination of Total Alkalinity

The water sample may be alkaline due to the presence of free OH^- ions and also certain salts like carbonates, bicarbonates, borates and silicates which produce alkalinity as a result of hydrolysis. However, the contribution of carbonates and bicarbonates is a major source of alkalinity. The total alkalinity indicates the capacity of water to neutralize acids. Total alkalinity can be determined by titration with a standard HCl solution.

Theory. When the sample is titrated with a standard solution of HCl using phenolphthalein as the indicator, the colour change at the end point is pink to colourless and this change occurs at pH 8.3. In this titration hydroxyl ions are completely and the carbonate ions are half neutralized, as shown by the following equations

$$OH^- + H^+ \rightarrow H_2O \quad \ldots \quad \ldots \quad \ldots \quad (19.1)$$

$$[NaOH + HCl \rightarrow NaCl + H_2O]$$

$$CO_3^{2-} + H^+ \rightarrow HCO_3^- \quad \ldots \quad \ldots \quad \ldots \quad (19.2)$$

$$[Na_2 CO_3 + HCl \rightarrow NaCl + NaHCO_3]$$

The titre obtained with phenolphthalein is known as *phenolphalein alkalinity* which is denoted by PA or P. After this first stage of titration, 2-3 drops of methyl orange solution is added. The solution turns yellow because it is still alkaline due to the presence of bicarbonate. The addition of HCl solution is continued until colour changes from yellow to red at pH 3.5. The reaction involved in the second stage of the titration is

$$HCO_3^- + H^+ \rightarrow H_2O + CO_2 \quad \ldots \quad \ldots \quad (19.3)$$

$$[NaHCO_3 + HCl \rightarrow NaCl + H_2O + CO_2]$$

The *total volume* of the acid required is called the *total alkalinity* which is denoted by T.A. or T.

Reagents

1. 0.1N, NaOH; standardized with 0.1N, oxalic acid
2. 0.1N, HCl; standardized with 0.1N, NaOH.
3. 0.05% aqueous methyl orange solution.
4. 0.5% phenolphthalein solution; (1 g of the indicator dissolved in about 100 c.c. of rectified spirit and diluted to 200 c.c. with distilled water.)

Pocedure

(i) Introduce 100 c.c. of sample into a 250 c.c. conical flask and add 2 drops of phenolphthalein solution.

(ii) If the solution does not turn pink, the P value is zero indicating that OH^- and CO_3^{2-} ions are absent. Add 2 drops of methyl orange indicator solution. If the solution becomes yellow the presence of bicarbonate ion is indicated. Add HCl from a burette until the solution turns red. Record the burette reading. This titre will give the total alkalinity i.e., the T value. (Note that the P value in this case will be zero.)

(iii) If on adding phenolphthalein indicator, the sample turns pink, the presence of OH^- and/or CO_3^{2-} is indicated. Titrate with HCl until the solution becomes colourless. The titre so obtained in the first stage of the titration gives the P value. After recording this value, add 2 drops of methyl orange indicator. The solution will turn yellow due to its alkaline nature (this is due to the hydrolysis of the bicarbonate which may be present in the sample and also due to the bicarbonate produced in the first stage of titration). Add HCl from a burette while swirling the conical flask until the solution becomes red. The combined titre value is the total alkalinity or T value.

Observation and calculation

Suppose the volume of the sample taken is V c.c. The P value is A c.c. and T value is B c.c.. Since HCl is 0.1N, we can write
1000 c.c. of HCl solution contains 0.1 g eq of acid

$$\therefore \quad A \text{ c.c.} \quad \cdots \quad \cdots \quad \cdots \quad \cdots \quad \frac{A \times 0.1}{1000} \text{ g eq of acid}$$

The reaction between calcium carbonate and hydrochloric acid is given by

$$CaCO_3 + 2HCl \rightarrow CaCl_2 + H_2O + CO_2$$

[Mol wt of $CaCO_3$ is 100 and $2HCl \equiv CaCO_3$]
Thus 2 g eq of HCl are equivalent to 100 g of $CaCO_3$

$$\therefore \quad \frac{A \times 0.1}{1000} \text{ g eq} \quad \cdots \quad \cdots \quad \cdots \quad \cdots \quad \frac{A \times 0.1}{1000 \times 2} \times 100 \text{ g } CaCO_3$$

$$= \frac{A \times 0.1 \times 100 \times 1000}{1000 \times 2} \text{ mg of } CaCO_3$$

$$= (A \times 0.1) \times 50 \text{ mg of } CaCO_3$$

Now, V c.c. of sample is equivalent to $(A \times 0.1) \times 50$ mg $CaCO_3$

$$\therefore \quad 1000 \text{ c.c.} \quad \cdots \quad \cdots \quad \cdots \quad \cdots \quad \frac{(A \times 0.1) \times 50 \times 1000}{V} \text{ mg } CaCO_3$$

Hence
P value in terms of $CaCO_3$, mg/litre

$$= \frac{(A \times \text{Normality of HCl}) \times 1000 \times 50}{V}$$

and T value in terms of $CaCO_3$, mg/litre

$$= \frac{(B \times \text{Normality of HCl}) \times 1000 \times 50}{V}$$

where A = c.c. of HCl required with phenolphthalein

B = c.c. of HCl required with phenolphthalein and methyl orange

P (or P.A) = phenolphthalein alkalinity

T (or T.A) = total alkalinity.

19.A.7.1.1 Determination of OH^- and CO_3^{2-} ions present in the sample

Suppose a water sample contains OH^- and CO_3^{2-} ions and HCO_3^- ions are *absent*. Then, in the sample the concentrations of OH^- and CO_3^{2-} ions can be determined by means of the following procedure.

(i) A known volume (say 100 c.c.) of the sample is titrated with a standard solution of HCl (say 0.1N) using phenolphthalein as indicator. The titre so obtained is the P value.

(ii) After recording the P value, methyl orange indicator is added and titration with 0.1N HCl is continued until colour changes from yellow to red. The combined titre value is the T value.

If OH^- ions are reported as NaOH and CO_3^{2-} ions as Na_2CO_3, we can write

$$P \equiv NaOH + \tfrac{1}{2} Na_2CO_3$$

$$T \equiv NaOH + \tfrac{1}{2} Na_2CO_3 + \tfrac{1}{2} Na_2CO_3 \equiv NaOH + Na_2CO_3$$

$\therefore \qquad (T-P) \equiv \tfrac{1}{2} Na_2CO_3$

or, $\qquad 2(T-P) \equiv Na_2CO_3$

and, $\quad T - 2(T-P) \equiv NaOH$

Thus the quantitities of OH^- and CO_3^{2-} ions can be calculated in term of P and T values.

Example 19 (iii)

A water sample contains OH^- and CO_3^{2-} ions but not HCO_3^- ions. On titrating 100 c.c. of the sample with 0.1N HCl, P and T values were found to be 9.8 and 13.2 c.c. respectively. Calculate the amount of NaOH and Na_2CO_3 present per litre of the sample. Also calculate the concentrations of OH^- and CO_3^{2-} ions in term of mg of $CaCO_3$ per litre.

Now, $\qquad P \equiv NaOH + \tfrac{1}{2} Na_2CO_3 = 9.8$ c.c. of 0.1N HCl

and, $\qquad T \equiv NaOH + Na_2CO_3 = 13.2$ c.c. of 0.1N HCl

$\therefore \qquad NaOH \equiv T - 2(T-P) \equiv [13.2 - 2(13.2 - 9.8)]$

$$\equiv 13.2 - 2 \times 3.4$$

$$\equiv 13.2 - 6.8 = 6.4 \text{ c.c.}$$

and $\quad Na_2CO_3 \equiv 2(T-P) \equiv 2(13.2 - 9.8)$

$$\equiv 2 \times 3.4 = 6.8 \text{ c.c.}$$

Calculation of the amount of NaOH

Now, $\qquad OH^- \equiv HCl \equiv NaOH$

$\therefore \qquad$ 1000 c.c. 1M HCl $\equiv$ NaOH

[Since mol wt of HCl = eq wt of HCl]

$\qquad$ 1000 c.c. 1N HCl $\equiv$ 40 g NaOH [Mol wt of NaOH = 40]

or, $\qquad$ 1000 c.c. 0.1N HCl $\equiv$ 4.0 g NaOH

or, $\qquad$ 1 c.c. 0.1N HCl $\equiv$ 4.0 mg NaOH

$\therefore \qquad$ 6.4 c.c. 0.1N HCl $\equiv 6.4 \times 4.0 = 25.6$ mg NaOH

Now, 100 c.c. of the sample contains 25.6 mg NaOH

$$\therefore \quad 1000 \text{ c.c.} \quad \ldots \quad \ldots \quad \ldots \quad \frac{1000}{100} \times 25.6$$

$$= 256.0 \text{ mg NaOH/litre}$$

Calculation of the amount of Na_2CO_3

$$Na_2CO_3 + 2 \text{ HCl} \rightarrow 2 \text{ NaCl} + H_2O + CO_2$$

$$\therefore \qquad 2 \text{ HCl} \equiv Na_2CO_3$$

or, $\qquad \qquad \text{HCl} \equiv \frac{1}{2} Na_2CO_3$

The mol wt of Na_2CO_3 is 106, hence we can write

$$1000 \text{ c.c. 1N HCl} \equiv 53 \text{ g } Na_2CO_3$$

or, $\qquad 1000 \text{ c.c. 0.1N HCl} \equiv 5.3 \text{ g } Na_2CO_3$

or, $\qquad 1 \text{ c.c. 0.1. HCl} \quad \equiv 5.3 \text{ mg } Na_2CO_3$

$\therefore \qquad 6.8 \text{ c.c. 0.1N HCl} \quad \equiv 6.8 \times 5.3 = 36.04 \text{ mg } Na_2 CO_3$

Now, 100 c.c. of the sample contains 36.04 mg Na_2CO_3

$$\therefore \quad 1000 \text{ c.c.} \quad \ldots \quad \ldots \quad \ldots \quad \ldots \quad \frac{1000}{100} \times 36.04$$

$$= 360.4 \text{ mg } Na_2CO_3/\text{litre}$$

Calculation of OH^- and CO_3^{2-} ion concentrations in term of mg of $CaCO_3$ per litre

$$2HCl \equiv 2NaOH \equiv Na_2CO_3 \equiv CaCO_3$$

$\therefore \qquad HCl \equiv \frac{1}{2} CaCO_3 \qquad [\text{Mol. wt. of } CaCO_3 = 100]$

$$1000 \text{ c.c. 1N HCl} \equiv 50 \text{ g } CaCO_3$$

$$1000 \text{ c.c. 0.1N HCl} \equiv 5.0 \text{ g } CaCO_3$$

$$1 \text{ c.c. of 0.1N HCl} \equiv 5.0 \text{ mg } CaCO_3$$

$\therefore \qquad 6.4 \text{ c.c. 0.1N HCl} \equiv 6.4 \times 5.0 = 32.0 \text{ mg } CaCO_3$

Now $\qquad 100 \text{ c.c. of the sample} \equiv 32.0 \text{ mg } CaCO_3$

$\therefore \qquad 1000 \text{ c.c. of the sample} \equiv 320.0 \text{ mg } CaCO_3$

Thus OH^- ion concentration in term of $CaCO_3$ will be 320.0 mg $CaCO_3$ per litre.

$$1 \text{ c.c. of 0.1N HCl} \equiv 5.0 \text{ mg } CaCO_3$$

$\therefore \qquad 6.8 \text{ c.c. of 0.1N HCl} \equiv 6.8 \times 5 = 34.0 \text{ mg } CaCO_3$

Now, $\qquad 100 \text{ c.c. of water sample} \equiv 34.0 \text{ mg } CaCO_3$

$\therefore \qquad 1000 \text{ c.c. of water sample} \equiv 340.0 \text{ mg } CaCO_3$

Thus CO_3^{2-} ion concentration in term of $CaCO_3$ will be 340.0 mg $CaCO_3$ per litre.

Result

1. The concentration of OH^- ions in the sample
   (a) in term of NaOH is 256 mg NaOH/litre
   (b) in term of $CaCO_3$ is 320 mg $CaCO_3$/litre
2. The concentration of CO_3^{2-} ions in the sample
   (a) in term of Na_2CO_3 is 360.4 mg Na_2CO_3/litre
   (b) in term of $CaCO_3$ is 340.0 mg $CaCO_3$/litre.

19.A.7.1.2 Determination of CO_3^{2-} and HCO_3^- ions present in the sample

Suppose a water sample contains CO_3^{2-} and HCO_3^- ions and OH^- ions are absent. The concentrations of CO_3^{2-} and HCO_3^- ions can be determined by means of the following procedure.

(i) A known volume (say 50 c.c.) of the sample is titrated with a standard solution (say 0.05N) of HCl using phenolphthalein as indicator. The titre value so obtained is the P value.

(ii) After noting the P value, methyl orange is added and the titration is completed so as to obtain the T value.

If CO_3^{2-} and HCO_3^- ions are reported as Na_2CO_3 and $NaHCO_3$ respectively, we can write

$$P \equiv \tfrac{1}{2} Na_2CO_3 \qquad [\because OH^- \text{ ions are absent}]$$
$$T \equiv NaHCO_3 + \tfrac{1}{2}Na_2CO_3 + \tfrac{1}{2}Na_2CO_3 \equiv NaHCO_3 + Na_2CO_3$$
$$\therefore \qquad 2P \equiv Na_2CO_3$$
and $(T-2P) \equiv NaHCO_3$

Example 19 (iv)

A water sample contains CO_3^{2-} and HCO_3^- ions and OH^- ions are absent. On titrating 50 c.c. of the sample with 0.05N HCl, the P and T values were found to be 10.3 and 28.8 c.c. respectively. Calculate the amounts of CO_3^{2-} and HCO_3^- ions in term of mg of $CaCO_3$ per litre.

$$P \equiv \tfrac{1}{2}Na_2CO_3 \qquad = 10.3 \text{ c.c}$$
$$T \equiv NaHCO_3 + Na_2CO_3 = 28.8 \text{ c.c.}$$
$$\therefore \qquad Na_2CO_3 \equiv 2P = 2 \times 10.3 = 20.6 \text{ c.c. of 0.05N HCl}$$
and $NaHCO_3 \equiv (T-2P) = (28.8 - 20.6) = 8.2$ c.c. 0.05 N HCl

Calculation of the amounts of CO_3^{2-} and HCO_3^- ions present per litre in term of mg of $CaCO_3$

$$2HCl \equiv Na_2CO_3 \equiv CO_3^{2-}$$
$$HCl \equiv \tfrac{1}{2}Na_2CO_3 \equiv \tfrac{1}{2}CO_3^{2-}$$

1 c.c. of 0.1N $HCl \equiv 5.3$ mg $Na_2CO_3 \equiv 3.0$ mg of CO_3^{2-} ions
[Remember that ionic wt of CO_3^{2-} ion is $12+48=60$]

1 c.c. of 0.05N $HCl \equiv 1.5$ mg of CO_3^{2-} ions

$\therefore$ 20.6 c.c. of 0.05N $HCl \equiv 1.5 \times 20.6 = 30.9$ mg CO_3^{2-} ions

Now 50 c.c. of the sample contains 30.9 mg of CO_3^{2-} ions

$$\therefore \quad 1000 \text{ c.c.} \quad \cdots \quad \cdots \quad \cdots \quad \cdots \quad \frac{1000}{50} \times 30.9$$

$$= 618.0 \text{ mg } CO_3^{2-} \text{ ions/litre.}$$

We know that $\quad CO_3^{2-} \equiv Na_2CO_3 \equiv CaCO_3$

Ionic wt of $\quad CO_3^{2-}$ ion $= (12+48) = 60$

Mol wt of $\quad CaCO_3 = (40+12+48) = 100$

Hence we can write

$$60 \text{ mg } CO_3^{2-} \text{ ions} \equiv 100 \text{ mg } CaCO_3$$

Now, $\quad 60 \text{ mg } CO_3^{2-} \text{ ions} \equiv 100 \text{ mg } CaCO_3$

$$\therefore \quad 618 \text{ mg } CO_3^{2-} \text{ ions} \equiv \frac{618 \times 100}{60}$$

$$= 1030.0 \text{ mg } CaCO_3/\text{litre}$$

Calculation of the amount of HCO_3^- ions in term of mg of $CaCO_3$ per litre

$$NaHCO_3 + HCl \longrightarrow NaCl + H_2O + CO_2$$

$$\therefore \quad HCl \equiv NaHCO_3 \equiv HCO_3^-$$

1000 c.c. of 1N $HCl \equiv 84$ g $NaHCO_3 \equiv 61$ g HCO_3^- ions

[Remember. (i) Mol wt $NaHCO_3 = 84$ and

(ii) Ionic wt of $HCO_3^- = 61$]

$\therefore \quad$ 1000 c.c. 0.1 N $HCl \equiv 6.1$ g HCO_3^- ions

or, $\quad$ 1000 c.c. 0.05N $HCl \equiv 3.05$ g HCO_3^- ions

or, $\quad$ 1 c.c. 0.05N $HCl \equiv 3.05$ mg HCO_3^- ions

$\therefore \quad$ 8.2 c.c. 0.05N $HCl \equiv 8.2 \times 3.05 = 25.01$ mg HCO_3^- ions

Now, 50 c.c. of the sample contains 25.01 mg of HCO_3^- ions

$$\therefore \quad 1000 \text{ c.c.} \quad \cdots \quad \cdots \quad \cdots \quad \cdots \quad \frac{1000}{50} \times 25.01$$

$$= 500.2 \text{ mg } HCO_3^-/\text{litre}$$

$$2HCl \equiv 2NaHCO_3 \equiv CaCO_3$$

$$\therefore \quad 2HCO_3^- \equiv CaCO_3$$

$$122 \text{ g } HCO_3^- \equiv 100 \text{ g } CaCO_3$$

or, $\quad 122 \text{ mg } HCO_3^- \equiv 100 \text{ mg } CaCO_3$

Now, $\quad 122 \text{ mg } HCO_3^- \equiv 100 \text{ mg } CaCO_3$

$$\therefore \quad 500.2 \text{ mg } HCO_3^- \equiv \frac{500.2 \times 100}{122} = 410 \text{ mg } CaCO_3/\text{litre}$$

Result

1. $[CO_3^{2-}] = 618.0$ mg/l
2. $[HCO_3^-] = 500.2$ mg/l
3. $[CO_3^{2-}]$ in term of $CaCO_3 = 1030.0$ mg $CaCO_3$/litre
4. $[HCO_3^-]$ in term of $CaCO_3 = 410.0$ mg $CaCO_3$/litre.

[Note. The concentration of the acid used in the alkalinity determination should be such that the titre values are more than 10 c.c. If the titre value is less, an appreciable error will be caused owing to measurement of a small volume. If the titre value is less than 10 c.c., then the concentration of the acid should be decreased or/and the volume of the water sample should be increased.]

19.A.7.1.3 Determination of total alkalinity of a water sample

In a water sample, the alkalinity may be due to the presence of

(a) Hydroxides alone
(b) Carbonates alone
(c) Bicarbonates alone
(d) Hydroxides and Carbonates
(e) Carbonates and Bicarbonates.

The combination "hydroxides and bicarbonates" has not been included in the above list because they combine to produce carbonate and water according to the equation

$$OH^- + HCO_3^- \rightarrow CO_3^{2-} + H_2O$$

Thus whenever OH^- ions are present, HCO_3^- ions will not be present as they are converted into carbonate ions.

In order to determine the total alkalinity in a water sample, the following procedure is used.

(i) A known volume of the water sample is taken in a conical flask and is titrated with a standard HCl solution using phenolphthalein indicator. The colour change at the end point is pink to colourless. The titre value so obtained is called the P value. The reactions involved in this stage of titration are

$$OH^- + H^+ \rightarrow H_2O \quad \ldots \quad \ldots \quad (19.4)$$
$$CO_3^{2-} + H^+ \rightarrow HCO_3^- \quad \ldots \quad \ldots \quad (19.5)$$

(ii) After recording the P value, methyl orange indicator is added when the titration mixture becomes yellow. The addition of HCl from the burette is continued until the solution turns red. The total burette reading is noted which gives the T value. The reaction taking placed in this stage of titration is

$$HCO_3^- + H^+ \rightarrow H_2O + CO_2 \quad \ldots \quad \ldots \quad (19.6)$$

Thus in the second stage of titration only HCO_3^- ions are titrated; this includes HCO_3^- formed in the first stage of the titration [see equation (19.5)] and also HCO_3^- originally present in the sample.

The concentrations of OH^-, CO_3^{2-} and HCO_3^- ions in the sample can be calculated from P and T values as shown in Table 19.2.

TABLE 19.2

Result of titration	OH^- alkalinity	CO_3^{2-} alkalinity	HCO_3^- alkalinity
1. $P=0$	O	O	T
2. $P=T$	P or T	O	O
3. $P=\frac{1}{2}T$	O	$2P$ or T	O
4. $P<\frac{1}{2}T$	O	$2P$	$T-2P$
5. $P>\frac{1}{2}T$	$2P-T$	$2(T-P)$	O

Example 19 (v)

On titrating 100 c.c. of a water sample with 0.05N HCl, the P value was zero and T value was 10 c.c. Calculate the concentrations of OH^-, CO_3^{2-} and HCO_3^- ions in term of 0.05N HCl. [Case 1: $P=0$].

When phenolphthalein indicator is used then OH^- and half the carbonate is titrated. Since P value is zero, OH^- and CO_3^{2-} ions are absent. The T value will therefore the equivalent to the HCO_3^- ion concentration. Thus,

$$[OH^-]=0$$
$$[CO_3^{2-}]=0$$

and $\qquad [HCO_3^-] \equiv 10$ c.c. 0.05N HCl/100 c.c. of sample.

Example 19 (vi)

On titrating 100 c.c. of a water sample with 0.1N HCl, the P value was 10 c.c. and T value remained the same. Calculate the concentrations of OH^-, CO_3^{2-} and HCO_3^- ions in term of 0.1N HCl. [Case 2 : $P = T$]

On titrating to phenolphthalein end point the titre was 10 c.c. After this end point, methyl orange was added and on adding a drop of HCl, the solution turned red. It follows that no acid is required in the second stage of titration. Since the second stage of the titration involves the neutralization of bicarbonate alone, it is obvious that bicarbonate is not present in the sample. Further, if carbonate ions were present in the sample they would have produced bicarbonate ions in the first stage of the titration which would have been neutralized in the second stage. Since no acid is consumed in the second stage of titration, it is evident that the sample does not contain carbonate and bicarbonate ions. Hence, the alkalinity of the sample is entirely due to OH^- ions. Thus we can write that in the sample

$$[OH^-] \equiv P = 10 \text{ c.c. of 0.1 N HCl/100 c.c. of sample}$$
$$[CO_3^{2-}]=O$$

and $[HCO_3^-]=O$

Example 19 (vii)

On titrating 50 c.c. of a water sample with 0.05 N HCl, the P value was found to be 10 c.c. and T value was 20 c.c. Find out the concentrations of OH^-, CO_3^{2-} and HCO_3^- ions in term of 0.05 N HCl. [Case 3: $P=\frac{1}{2}T$].

The reaction between carbonate and HCl is given by

$$CO_3^{2-} + H^+ \rightarrow HCO_3^-$$

or,

$$Na_2CO_3 + HCl \rightarrow NaHCO_3 + NaCl$$

Thus every carbonate ion consumes a molecule of HCl to produce a bicarbonate ion (as shown in the titration with phenolphthalein indicator). Each bicarbonate ion so produced reacts with a molecule of HCl (as shown in the titration with methyl orange indicator) according to the equation

$$HCO_3^- + H^+ \rightarrow H_2O + CO_2$$

or,

$$NaHCO_3 + HCl \rightarrow NaCl + H_2O + CO_2$$

From the above equations it is evident that the amount of the acid required for the conversion of carbonate to bicarbonate (in the first stage of the titration) is equal to the amount of the acid consumed in the neutralization of the resultant bicarbonate (in the second stage of the titration). In the given problem P value is 10 c.c. and the volume of the acid required with methyl orange indicator is also 10 c.c. Thus in all 20 c.c. of 0.05 N HCl is used up. Hence, in the given sample

$$[OH^-] = 0$$

$$[CO_3^{2-}] \equiv 2P = 2 \times 10 = 20 \text{ c.c. } 0.05 \text{ N HCl per 100 c.c. of sample}$$

and, $[HCO_3^-] = 0$

Example 19 (viii)

On titrating 100 c.c. of a water sample with 0.05 N HCl, the P and T values were 8.0 and 20.0 c.c. respectively, Calculate the concentrations of OH^-, CO_3^{2-} and HCO_3^- ions in term of 0.05 N HCl. [Case 4: $P < \frac{1}{2}T$].

Since. $P < \frac{1}{2}T$, it can be reasoned out that OH^- ions are absent. Hence, the P value i.e., 8.0 c.c. of 0.05 N HCl is needed for the conversion of CO_3^{2-} to HCO_3^- ions and then another 8.0 c.c. acid is used up in the neutralization of the bicarbonate formed. Thus $8.0 + 8.0 = 16.0$ c.c. of the acid is used up in the neutralization of the carbonate and the remaining $(20 - 16) = 4.0$ c.c. of the acid is consumed for the neutralization of HCO_3^- ions originally present in the sample. Thus in term of 0.05 N HCl, the concentration of different ions in 100 c.c. of the sample will be

$$[OH^-] = 0$$

$$[CO_3^{2-}] \equiv 2P = 2 \times 8.0 = 16.0 \text{ c.c. of 0.05 N HCl}$$

and, $[HCO_3^-] = (T - 2P) = (20 - 16) = 4.0$ c.c. of 0.5 N HCl

Example 19 (ix)

On titrating 100 c.c. of a water sample with 0.02 N HCl, the P value was 12.0 c.c. and T value was 20.0 c.c. Calculate the concentrations of OH^-, CO_3^{2-} and HCO_3^- ions in the sample in term of 0.02 N HCl. [Case 5: $P > \frac{1}{2}T$].

It can be reasoned out that when $P > \frac{1}{2}T$ then OH^- ions are present in the sample. And it has been shown in 19.A.7.1.3. that HCO_3^- ions react with OH^- ions to form CO_3^{2-} ions and water. Hence, in this water sample we will have only OH^- and CO_3^{2-} ions.

The difference between T and P is $(20.0-12.0)=8.0$ c.c. and this volume is needed for the neutralization of bicarbonate produced in the first stage of the titration [see equation (19.2)]. The acid used up for the conversion of carbonate into bicarbonate in the first stage will also be 8.0 c.c. Thus in all $(8.0+8.0)=16.0$ c.c. acid would be required for the neutralization of the carbonate; this is double the difference between T and P i.e., $2(T-P)$. The remaining acid i.e., $(20.0-16.0)=4.0$ c.c. would be used up in the neutralization of OH^- ions in the first stage of the titration. This is the reason that $(8.0+4.0)=12.0$ c.c. of the acid is used in the first stage. The second stage of the titration requires 8.0 c.c. of the acid which is used up for the neutralization of the bicarbonate produced in the first stage. Thus in term of 0.02 N HCl, the concentrations of different ions per 100 c.c. of the water sample will be

$$
\begin{array}{l|l}
[OH^-] \equiv 4.0 \text{ c.c.} & [2P-T = (24-20)=4.0 \text{ c.c.}] \\
[CO_3^{2-}] \equiv 16.0 \text{ c.c.} & [2(T-P)=2(20-12)=16.0 \text{ c.c.}] \\
[HCO_3^-] \equiv 0.0 \text{ c.c.} & \text{in term of 0.02 N HCl/100 c.c. of the sample.}
\end{array}
$$

[Note. Once the quantities of these ions are known in term of acid concentration, then these can be converted in term of amount of mg of $CaCO_3$/litre by using the following formula

$$
\text{Amount of } CaCO_3 : \text{mg/litre } \left. \frac{\text{Vol of acid} \times \text{Normality of acid} \times 1000 \times 50}{\text{Vol. of the sample}} \right]
$$

Example 19 (x)

In 50 c.c. of a water sample, the concentration of CO_3^{2-} ion is equivalent to 20.6 c.c. of 0.05 N HCl. Calculate the concentration of CO_3^{2-} ion in term of mg of $CaCO_3$ per litre.

Concentration of CO_3^{2-} ion in term of mg of $CaCO_3$ per litre

$$
= \frac{\text{Vol. of acid} \times \text{Nor. of acid} \times 1000 \times 50}{\text{Vol. of the sample}}
$$

$[CO_3^{2-}]$ as $CaCO_3$ mg/litre

$$
= \frac{20.6 \times 0.05 \times 1000 \times 50}{50}
$$

$$
= 1030.0 \text{ mg } CaCO_3/\text{litre}
$$

Thus the $[CO_3^{2-}]$ in the sample in term of mg of $CaCO_3$ per litre will be 1030.0 mg. [Compare this result with that obtained in example 19 (iv)].

19.A.7.2 The Determination of Acidity

Acidity of water is its capacity to neutralize a strong base to a particular pH. Acidity in water samples is due to the presence of mineral acids, weak acids and hydroylysis of salts of strong acids and weak bases. In natural unpolluted water the main source of acidity is the dissolved carbon dioxide.

Theory. A known volume of water sample is first titrated with a standard solution of NaOH using methyl orange as indicator so that the pH at the end point is 3.7; this titre gives the amount of strong acids and their salts formed with weak bases. This titre is called *methyl orange acidity*.

If the sample is directly titrated using phenolphthalein as indicator, the pH at the end point is 8.3; the titre value in this case gives the total acidity. The titrimetric method for determining the acidity is applicable to colourless samples only which do not interfere with the judgement of colour change at the end point. For coloured samples, conductometric or potentiometric titration methods can be used.

Reagents

1. 0.05N NaOH, standardized with a standard oxalic acid solution.

2. Methyl orange indicator (0.05%).

3. Phenolphthalein indicator solution (0.5%).

Procedure

(i) Take 100 c.c. (V) of a colourless sample in a conical flask and add 2-3 drops of methyl orange indicator solution.

(ii) If the solution turns yellow, the methyl orange acidity is absent (mineral acids and their salts are absent). If the solution turns pink, titrate with 0.05 N NaOH solution until colour changes from pink to yellow. Note the titre value (A); this is known as *methyl orange acidity*.

(iii) Now add 2-3 drops of phenolphthalein indicator solution to the same titration mixture and continue titration with 0.05 N NaOH until the colour becomes pink. Record this titre value (B); this is known as *phenolphthalein acidity*.

Calculation

Methyl orange acidity in mg of $CaCO_3$/litre

$$= \frac{A \times N \text{ of NaOH} \times 1000 \times 50}{V}$$

Phenolphthalein acidity in mg of $CaCO_3$/litre

$$= \frac{B \times N \text{ of NaOH} \times 1000 \times 50}{V}$$

Total acidity in mg of $CaCO_3$/litre

$$= \frac{(A+B) \times N \text{ of NaOH} \times 1000 \times 50}{V}$$

where

A = volume in c.c. of NaOH required with methyl orange indicator

B = volume in c.c. of NaOH required with phenolphthalein indicator

N = normality of NaOH

V = volume in c.c. of water sample

[NaOH solution used is 0.05 N, hence
1000 c.c. of NaOH solution will contain 0.05 g eq of alkali

$\therefore$ A c.c. „ „ „ „ $\dfrac{A \times 0.05}{1000}$ g eq of alkali

$\dfrac{A \times 0.05}{1000}$ g eq of alkali $\equiv \dfrac{A \times 0.05}{1000}$ g eq of acid

Now, 2g eq of acid $\equiv$ 1g mole (= 100 g) of $CaCO_3$

$\therefore \dfrac{A \times 0.05}{1000}$ g of eq of acid $\equiv \dfrac{A \times 0.05}{1000} \times \dfrac{100}{2}$ g $CaCO_3$

$\equiv \dfrac{A \times 0.05}{1000} \times \dfrac{100}{2} \times 1000$ mg $CaCO_3$

$\equiv A \times 0.05 \times 50$ mg $CaCO_3$

Now, V c.c. sample of water $\equiv A \times 0.05 \times 50$ mg $CaCO_3$

$\therefore$ 1000 c.c. sample of water $\equiv \dfrac{(A \times 0.05) \times 50 \times 1000}{V}$ mg $CaCO_3$]

19.A.7.4 Determination of Dissolved Carbon dioxide

Theory. Dissolved carbon dioxide in a water sample can be determined by titration with a standard solution of NaOH using phenolphthalein as indicator. The pH at the end-point is 8.3.

Reagents

1. 0.05 N NaOH solution. Dissolve 22−25 g NaOH in, boiled and then cooled, 1 litre of water (this water would be CO_2 free). Standardize this solution with a standard oxalic acid solution, and then dilute suitably to obtain 0.05 N NaOH solution.
2. 0.5% phenolphthalein indicator solution.

Procedure

(i) Take 100 c.c. (V) of the sample in a 250 c.c. conical flask and add 2-3 drops of phenolphthalein indicator solution.

(ii) If the colour turns pink, free CO_2 is absent. But if the sample remains colourless, titrate with 0.05 N NaOH solution until a pink colour appears. Record the titre (A c.c.).

Calculation

Free CO_2, mg/lite $= \dfrac{A \times N \text{ of NaOH} \times 1000 \times 44}{2 \times V \text{c.c.}}$

where N is the normality of NaOH.

19.A.7.5 Determination of Dissolved Oxygen (by Winkler's Method)

Theory : Manganous sulphate reacts with alkali to form $Mn(OH)_2$ which in the presence of oxygen gets oxidized into a brown coloured compound of manganese in trivalent state. In a strong acidic medium, manganic ions (which are trivalent) oxidize iodide to iodine which can be titrated with a standard thiosulphate solution. The liberated iodine is equivalent to the amount of oxygen present in the water sample. Thus by knowing the amount of liberated iodine, the amount of oxygen present in the given sample can be calculated.

Reagents

1. **0.025 N sodium thiosulphate solution.** Dissolve about 26 g of $Na_2S_2O_3$. $5H_2O$ in 1 litre of previously boiled and then cooled distilled water. Add 0.4 g of borax or a pallet of NaOH as stabilizer. Dilute this solution four times. Standardize this diluted solution with a standard KIO_3 solution and dilute suitably to obtain 0.025 N thiosulphate solution.

2. **Alkaline KI solution.** Dissolve 10 g of KOH and 5 g of KI in 20 c.c. of previously boiled distilled water and filter.

3. **Manganous sulphate solution.** Dissolve 10 g of $MnSO_4.4H_2O$ in 20 c.c. of previously boiled distilled water and add a few drops of formaldehyde.

4. **1% starch solution.** Make a paste of 1 g of soluble starch and pour it in 100 c.c. of boiling water. Stir and cool. Add a few drops of formaldehyde solution.

5. **Concentrated sulphuric acid.** (sp. gravity 1.84).

Procedure

(i) Fill the given water sample in a glass-stoppered conical flask (iodine flask) of known volume (100 − 300 c.c.), carefully avoiding any kind of bubbling and trapping of the air bubbles in the bottle after placing the stopper (see Fig. 19.24).

(ii) Introduce 1 c.c. each of alkaline KI and $MnSO_4$ solution, if the volume of the flask is 100 c.c. (If the volume of the flask is 300 c.c., then 2 c.c. each of the reagents should be added). The reagents should be added by means of two seperate pipettes well below the surface of water so that there is through mixing (see Fig. 19.24).

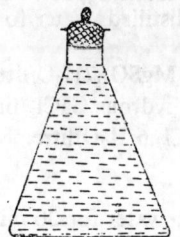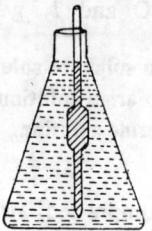

Fig. 19.24

(iii) Place the stopper and shake the contents well by inverting the flask repeatedly. Keep the bottle for sometime so that the ppt settles.

(iv) Add 1-2 c.c. of concentrated H_2SO_4 and shake well to dissolve the ppt.

(v) Po**u**r carefully the whole content (or 50 or 100 c.c. portion) into another conical flask.

(vi) Titrate with $Na_2S_2O_3$ solution using starch as indicator until the blue colour di**s**appears.

Calculation

When th**e** whole content has been titrated

$$\text{Dissolved oxygen in mg/litre} = \frac{\text{(c.c.} \times \text{N) of the titrant} \times 8 \times 1000}{V_1 - V}$$

where,

V_1=Volume of the sample bottle after placing the stopper

V=Volume of $MnSO_4$ and KI solution added.

[Hints : $Mn^{2+} \equiv \frac{1}{2}O \equiv KI \equiv \frac{1}{2}I_2 \equiv Na_2S_2O_3$

∴   1000 c.c. N $Na_2S_2O_3 \equiv 8$ g of oxygen.]

Note. The above method is interfered by the presence of oxidizing or reducing **s**ubstances as these can oxidize iodide to iodine or reduce iodine to iodide.

19.A.7.6 Determination of Biochemical Oxygen Demand (B.O.D)

This term means the amount of oxygen required by the microorganisms in stabilizing the biologically degradable organic matter under aerobic conditions. The determination of B.O.D. involves the measurement of the oxygen concentration of the sample immediately and that after incubating it for 5 days.

Apparatus and Reagent

1. **B.O.D. bottles** (glass-stoppered bottles).
2. **B.O.D incubator** having temperature control at 20 °C.
3. **Phosphate buffer.** Dissolve 8.5 g KH_2PO_4, 21.75 g K_2HPO_4, 33.4 g. Na_2HPO_4. 7 H_2O and 1.7 g NH_4Cl in distilled water to prepare 1 litre solution.
4. **Magnesium sulphate solution** 82.5 g $MgSO_4.7H_2O$/litre.
5. **Calcium chloride solution.** 27.5 g anhydrous $CaCl_2$/litre.
6. **Ferric chloride solution.** 0.25 g $FeCl_3.6 H_2O$/litre.

Procedure

(i) Bubble compressed air in distilled water for 30 minutes—this water is then called *dilution water*.

(ii) In a litre of dilution water add 1 c.c. each of phosphate buffer, $MgSO_4$, $CaCl_2$ and $FeCl_3$ solution and mix well.

(iii) Neutralize the water sample to pH 7.

(iv) The dissolved oxygen of the sample may not be sufficient for the oxidation of biologically degradable organic matter so that the sample is mixed with a known volume of dilution water whlch is rich in oxygen.

(v) Carry out dilution in a large trough or bucket and mix well.

(vi) Fill two sets I and II of B.O.D. bottles.

(vii) Determine the dissolved oxygen in the sample bottles of set I immediately as described in 19.A.7.5.

(viii) Determine the dissolved oxygen in the sample bottles of set II after keeping the bottles in a B.O.D. incubator at 20 °C for 5 days.

[For blank determination, take 2 B.O.D. bottles and fill them with dilution water. In one bottle determine the dissolved oxygen immediately and in the other, make the determination after incubation for 5 days.]

Calculation

B.O.D., mg/litre $= (D_0 - D_5) \times$ dilution factor

where, $D_0 =$ concentration of the dissolved oxygen in the sample.

$D_5 =$ concentration of the disolved oxygen after 5 days.

19.A.7.7 Determination of Chemical Oxygen Demand (C.O.D)

This term means amount of oxygen required for the oxidation of oxidizable organic matter by a strong oxidizing agent. For C.O.D. determination, potassium dichromate in presence of H_2SO_4 is generally used as an oxidizing agent. The water sample is refluxed with $K_2Cr_2O_7$ and concentrated H_2SO_4 in presence of $HgSO_4$ and Ag_2SO_4 (catalysts). The residual dichromate is titrated back with a standard solution of ferrous ammonium sulphate using ferroin as indicator.

Regents

1. 0.25 N $K_2C_2O_7$. Dissolve 12.25 g of dried $K_2Cr_2O_7$ in distilled water and make up the volume to 1 titre.

2. 0.1 N ferrous ammonium sulphate. The solution is standardized with standard $K_2Cr_2O_7$ solution.

3. Ferroin indicator solution. Dissolve 1.485 g of 1, 10—phenanthroline and 0.695 g of ferrous sulphate in distilled water and dilute to make 100 c.c. solution.

4. Concentrated H_2SO_4 (sp. gr. 1.84).

5. Solid $HgSO_4$ and Ag_2SO_4 .

Procedure

(i) Introduce 20 c.c. of the water sample in a 250 c.c. round bottom flask with ground glass joint for fixing a reflux condenser.

(ii) Add 10 c.c. of 0.25 N $K_2Cr_2O_7$, a pinch of Ag_2SO_4 and $HgSO_4$ and 20 c.c. of H_2SO_4. Reflux for 2-3 hours (see Fig. 19.25).

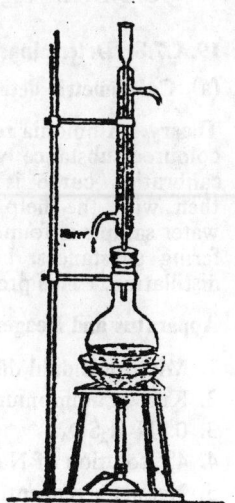

Fig. 19.25

(iii) Cool, dilute and titrate with 0.1 N (or 0.05 N if titre is small) ferrous ammonium sulphate solution using ferroin as indicator until colour changes from blue to red.

(iv) Run a blank also.

Calculation

$$\text{C.O.D. in mg/litre} = \frac{(b-a) \times \text{N of Fe-Am-SO}_4 \times 1000 \times 8}{\text{c.c. of sample } (V)}$$

where,　　　　　a=c.c. of the titrant with the sample

b=blank titre in c.c.

N=Normality of FeAmSO$_4$ used.

V=c.c. of the sample taken.

[Hint : 1 N K$_2$Cr$_2$O$_7$≡1 N FeAmSO$_4$≡$\frac{1}{2}$O≡8000 mg of O$_2$

1000 c.c. of 1 N FeAmSO$_4$≡8000 mg of oxygen

∴ $(b-a)$ c.c. of 1 N FeAmSO$_4$≡$\dfrac{(b-a) \times 8 \times 1000}{1000}$ mg of O$_2$

Now, V c.c. of the sample contains $(b-a) \times 8$ mg of O$_2$

∴ 1000 c.c. ...　　　...　　　...　　$\dfrac{(b-a) \times 8 \times 1000}{V}$ mg of O$_2$

If the normality of FeAmSO$_4$ is N then

$$\text{C.O.D. in mg/litre} = \frac{(b-a) \times N \times 1000 \times 8}{V} \quad \Big]$$

19.A.7.8 Determination of Ammonia

(a) Colorimetric determination

Theory. Ammonia reacts with Nessler's reagent (K$_2$HgI$_4$) to form a brown coloured substance which can be determined colorimetrically. First, a calibration curve is constructed by using known ammonia solutions and then with the help of this curve the quantity of ammonia in the given water sample is found out. Natural and wastewaters generally have interfering substances, hence ammonia is obtained from the sample by steam distillation. This process eliminates non-volatile interfering substances.

Apparatus and Reagents

1. Micro Kjeldahl distillation unit.
2. Known ammonium chloride solutions.
3. 0.1N H$_2$SO$_4$.
4. 4% solution of Na$_2$B$_4$O$_7$.10H$_2$O (buffer solution).
5. Nessler's reagent.
   (a) Dissolve 25 g of HgI$_2$ and 20 g of KI in 500 c.c. distilled water.
   (b) Dissolve 100 g NaOH in 500 c.c. distilled water.

Store solutions (a) and (b) in brown glass air-tight stoppered bottles, Mix 1:1 of these solutions just before use. This is Nessler's reagent.

7. Ammonia free distilled water can be obtained by redistilling distilled water with little $KMnO_4$ and Na_2CO_3. All the above solutions should be prepared in ammonia free distilled water.

Procedure

(i) Take 50 c.c. of the water sample, add 1 c.c. of borax buffer and pass steam through it.

(ii) Collect the distillate in about 10 c.c. of 0.1N sulphuric acid for about 40 minutes when the ammonia, distilled out, forms ammonium sulphate.

(iii) Make up the volume of the distillate to 50 c.c. and 1 c.c. of Nessler's reagent, a brown colour will develop. Measure the absorbance at 425 nm by means of a spectrophotometer.

(iv) Prepare a calibration curve using known solutions of NH_4Cl and find out the concentration of ammonia in the sample with the help of this curve.

(b) Titrimetric Method

Ammonia after distillation is mixed with boric acid and titrated with a standard solution of HCl using bromocresol green and methyl red as mixed indicator. At the end point the colour changes from pink to brown.

19.A.7.9 Determination of Nitrate

Theory. Nitrate and brucine react to produce a yellow colour whose intensity can be measured at 410 nm.

A known volume of water sample is treated with NaCl, H_2SO_4 and brucine-sulphanilic acid solution. The mixture is then dipped in boiling water for 20 minutes and its absorbance measured at 410 nm. A calibration curve using known nitrate solutions is prepared which is then utilized for knowing the amount of nitrate in the given water sample.

19.A.7.10 Determination of Nitrite

Theory. Nitrite forms a diazonium salt with sulphanilic acid in acid medium, which combines with α-napthylamine hydrochloride to form a red coloured dye. This reaction underlies the colorimetric determination of nitrites.

If the water sample is colured, its colour is removed by treatment with animal charcoal. A known volume of the sample is treated with suitable amounts of EDTA, sulphanilic acid, α-napthylamine hydrochloride and sodium acetate when a wine red colour is produced whose absorbance is measured at 520 nm. The amount of nitrite in the sample is found out with the help of a calibration curve.

19.A.7.11 Determination of Total Nitrogen (Organic nitrogen + ammonia nitrogen)

Theory. On digesting the water sample with concentrated H_2SO_4 and K_2SO_4, the organic nitrogen is converted into ammonium salt, $(NH_4)_2SO_4$.

The digested solution contains the ammonium salt that is produced from nitrogeneous organic matter and also the ammonium salts originally present in the sample. The digested solution is then treated with NaOH and distilled. The librated NH_3 is collected in a known volume of standard HCl solution. The residual acid is then titrated with a standard alkali solution. Knowing the amount of the acid consumed, the quantity of NH_3 formed can be calculated : This gives the total nitrogen i.e., that present in the form of organic compounds (organic-nitrogen) and also that in the ammonium salts (ammonia-nitrogen).

If the nitrogen determination is done without digestion then we will get the amount of nitrogen present in the form of ammonium salts alone. Thus

Organic N=Total N—Ammonia N

19.A.7.12 Determination of Inorganic Phosphorus

The phosphates present in a water sample on treatment with ammonium molybdate form a complex. This complex with stannous chloride produces a blue colour whose absorbance can be measured at 690 nm. Thus phosphates in water can be colorimetrically determined. A calibration curve is constructed with known phosphate solutions and later the amount of phosphate (or phosphorus) in a water sample is found out with the help of this curve. This colorimetric method gives the phosphorus present as phosphates i.e., inorganic phosphorus.

19.A.7.13 Determination of Total Phosphorus

All the forms of phosphorus are converted into inorganic form when the sample is digested with concentrated H_2SO_4 and HNO_3 in presence of $CuSO_4$ and K_2SO_4. After digestion, the solution is neutralized with NaOH using phenolphthalein indicator. If the solution is coloured, its colour is removed by adding animal charcoal. The colourless solution is then treated with ammonium molybdate and stannous chloride solution and then allowed to stand for 5 minitus. A blue colour is developed whose absorbance at 690 nm is measured by means of a spectrophotometer. The amount of phosphorus in the sample is found out with the help of a calibration curve constructed by using known phosphate solutions. By subtracting inorganic phosphorus from total phosphorus, we can find out the amount of phosphorus present in organic compounds. Thus,

Organic P=Total P – Inorganic P

19.A.7.14 Determination of Reactive Silica

Silica reacts with ammonium molybdate to form molybdosilicic acid of yellow colour. This reaction underlies the colorimetric determination of silica in water sample.

19.A.7.15 Determination of Sulphate

Sulphate is precipitated as barium sulphate by adding an excess is barium chloride solution. The ppt is filtered, washed, dried, ignited and weighed.

Suspended matter and silica interfere with this gravimetric determination giving a positive error. For removing silica a known volume of water sample is evaporated to dryness. The residue is then treated with a small volume of HCl and again evaporated to dryness. This process is repeated 2 or 3 times when the silica is precipitated and can be separated by filtration.

If $BaSO_4$ is present in the form of small particles then it can be determined by means of a turbidimeter.

19.A.7.16 Determination of Hydrogen Sulphide

Sulphide is precipitated as cadmium sulphide which in acidic medium is treated with a known exces of iodine solution. The sulpide gets oxidized and the residual iodine is titrated with a standard solution of thiosulphate using starch as indicator. A blank is also carried out. The difference between the blank and experimental titre gives the amount of iodine used up in the oxidation of the sulphide. Knowing the quantity of iodine consumed, the amount of sulphide in the water sample can be calculated using the following relationship

$$H_2S, \text{ in mg/litre} = \frac{(b-a) \times N \text{ of titrant} \times 1000 \times 17}{V}$$

where, a=c.c. of the titrant thiosulphate with sample

b=c.c. of the titrant thiosulphate with blank

N= normality of thiosulphate solution, and

V=c.c. of the water sample taken.

19.A.7.17 Determination of Chloride

The given water sample is titrated with a standard solution of $AgNO_3$ using potassium chromate as indicator (Mohr's titration). At the end point a reddish brown colour appears. The amount of chloride in the sample is calculated by the following relationship

$$\text{Chloride, mg/litre} = \frac{(\text{c.c.} \times N) \text{ of Ag } NO_3 \times 1000 \times 35.5}{V}$$

where, N=normality of $AgNO_3$

V=volume of the sample in c.c.

19.A.7.18 Determination of Hardness of Water

Hardness in water is mainly due to Ca^{2+} and Mg^{2+} ions. Although certain other ions like those of iron, strontium, aluminium and zinc also cause hardness but their concentrations are generally low. Hence, the hardness is generally measured as concentrations of calcium and mgnesium (in terms of $CaCO_3$ in mg present per litre) which are present in comparatively higher quantities.

Theory. Calcium and magnisium react with Eriochrome black T (indicator) at pH of about 10, to form a wine red coloured complex. However, this complex is not very stable and on adding EDTA, it is broken down and blue coloured indicator (HIn^{2-}) is produced so that at the end point the colour changes from red to blue.

Reagents

1. 0.01 M EDTA solution Dissolve 3.723 g of disodium   salt of EDTA in distilled water and make up the volume to 1 litre.
2. Buffer solution. Dissolve 7 g of NH_4Cl in 60 c.c. of concentrated (15 M) ammonia.
3. Indicator. Grind 0.40 g of Eriochrome black T with 100 g A.R. NaCl. (Alternatively 0.2 g of Eriochrome black T can be dissolved in 20 c.c. of ethanol).

Procedure

(i) Take 50 c.c. (V) of the water sample in a conical flask and add 1 c.c. of buffer solution.

(ii) Add 1 c.c. of 5% Na_2S solution if the sample contains higher concentration of heavy metals.

(iii) Add 100-200 mg of Eriochrome black T-NaCl mixture when the sample will turn wine red.

(vi) Titrate the contents with EDTA solution until the solution turns blue.

Calculation

$$\text{Hardness, mg of } CaCO_3/\text{litre} = \frac{\text{c.c. of 0.01 M EDTA used} \times 1000}{V}$$

[Hint   1000 c.c. 1M EDTA$\equiv$100 g $CaCO_3$

1 c.c. 0.01 M EDTA$\equiv$1 mg of $CaCO_3$]

19.A.7.19 Determination of Calcium

Ammonium purpurate forms a complex with Ca^{2+} ions but not with Mg^{2+} ions at higher pH. This fact is used for the determination of calcium in presence of magnesium by titration with EDTA solution.

19.A.7.20 Determination of Magnesium

First V c.c. of the given water sample is taken and the hardness determined by titration with 0.01 M EDTA solution as described in 19.A.7.18. This gives the amount of Ca^{2+} and Mg^{2+} ions present in the sample. Suppose the titre value is y c.c.

Then, again V c.c. of the sample is taken and calcium determined by titration with 0.01 M EDTA solution as described in 19.A.7.19. This gives only the amount of calcium present in the sample. Suppose the titre value in this case is x c.c. The amount of magnesium in the sample is then calculated on the basis of these two titre values.

19.A.7.21 Determination of Sodium

When the sample containing sodium is sprayed into a flame, radiations characteristic of sodium are emitted out. The intensity of this radiation is proportional to the concentration of sodium. A calibration curve is constructed using NaCl solutions of known concentrations. This curve is then used to determine the amount of sodium in the sample solution.

19.A.7.22 Determination of Potassium

Potassium in a water sample can also be determined using a flame photometer.

19.A.7.23 Determination of Residual Chlorine

Chlorine is added to water to destroy harmful microorganisms. But the presence of excess chlorine affects the taste and odour of drinking water. This excess chlorine is treated with KI in presence of acetic acid when iodine is liberated which is titrated with a standard thiosulphate solution. The liberated iodine is proportional the quantity of chlorine present in the water sample.

Residual chlorine in mg/litre

$$= \frac{(\text{c.c.} \times \text{N}) \text{ of thiosulphate} \times 1000 \times 35.5}{\text{c.c. of water sample}}$$

19.A.7.24 Determination of Oil and Grease

A known volume of water sample is shaken with H_2SO_4 and ether in a separatory funnel when oil and grease are transferred to the ether layer which can be separated from the aqueous layer. The etherial layer on evaporation leaves back oil and grease which can be weighed.

19.A.7.25 Determination of Volatile Acids

The given water sample is steam distilled. The distillate contains volatile acids which can be titrated with a standard solution of NaOH using phenolphthalein as indicator.

19.A.7.26 Determination of Iron

The given water sample is treated with hydroxylamine in presence of HCl when the iron present is reduced to the ferrous state. The ferrous iron so produced is treated with an excess of 1, 10-phenanthroline when a red colour is developed whose absorbance can be measured at 510 nm. A calibration curve is prepared using known solutions of ferrous iron and with the help of this curve the amount of iron in the water sample can be found out.

19.A.7.27 Determination of Arsenic

Arsenic in acid medium reacts with zinc to produce AsH_3. This gas is absorbed in glass wool soaked with lead acetate and then treated with silver diethyl-dithiocarbomate dissolved in pyridine, when a red complex is formed. This reaction forms the basis of colorimetric determination of arsenic.

19.A.7.28   Determination of Chromium

Colorimetric determination of chromium is based on the reaction between Cr (VI) and diphenylcarbazide in acidic medium. Total chromium (dissolved and particulate) can be determined after digestion with H_2SO_4 and HNO_3. For the determination of dissolved chromium, the trivalent chromium is oxidized to the hexavalent state with $KMnO_4$.

19.A.7.29   Determination of Cadmium

Cadmium ions react with dithiozone to produce a pink red colour. This coloured complex is extracted with chloroform and is determined colorimetrically.

19.A.7.30   Determination of Zinc

A blue coloured complex is formed by zinc with zincon which forms the basis of the colorimetric determination of zinc.

19.A.7.31   Determination of Mercury

The colorimetric determination of mercury with dithiozone is interfered by other metals. A satisfactory determination of mercury can be done by atomic absorption spectroscopy.

19.B.   Analysis of Soils

Soils are of great importance from agriculture view point. Due to dumping of wastes, sediments are formed. Hence analysis of soils and sediments is important.

The first important step in soil analysis is collecting a representative sample which depends upon the type of analysis to be performed. Special equipment is needed to collect samples from depths. There are certain properties such as pH, redox potential, amount of ions in the reduced state etc., which should be measured immediately after the collection of the sample, while for certain other properties, one can wait for sometime after the sample collection. Certain determinations are made after drying and grinding the soil sample. After grinding the sample is passed through 2 mm sieve. For some determinations more fine grinding has to be done. Moisture content of a fresh soil sample is determined by drying a known weight of the soil in an oven at 105 °C until constant weight is obtained. The difference in weight gives the moisture content.

19.B.1   Determination of pH

This property of a soil is a measure of its acidity or alkalinity. For the pH measurement, 20 g of ground soil is taken in a beaker, 100 c.c. of distilled water is added to it and the mixture is stirred at regular intervals for about an hour. The pH of this 1 : 5 soil solution is measured by means of a pH meter having glass-calomel electrode combination. While reporting the pH, the dilution of the soil sample must be mentioned e.g., 1 : 5 in the above case.

19.B.2   Determination of Conductivity

The determination of the specific conductance of a soil sample is a measure of the quantity of soluble salts present in the soil. Since, specific conductance depends upon the dilution, it is usual practice to prepare 1 : 5 soil suspension for conductivity measurement at 25 °C. This measurement should be made on a fresh soil sample.

19.B.3   Determination of Total Alkalinity

The procedure for determining total alkalinity (soluble hydroxides, carbonates and bicarbonates) of a soil sample involves titration with a standard solution of H_2SO_4 or HCl using phenolphthalein and methyl orange as indicators as described in 19.A.7.1. in the case of water sample. The reagents needed are also the same as mentioned in 19.A.7.1.

Fresh sample of soil is passed through a 2 mm sieve and to 20 g of this sample, 100 c.c. of water is added, and the mixture is stirred for one hour at regular intervals preferably using a magnetic stirrer. The suspension so obtained is filtered. The filtrate is known as 1 : 5 soil solution. The alkalinity of this solution is determined by titration with a standard solution of HCl.

Observations and Calculations

Suppose for the titration of 100 c.c. of soil solution, V_A c.c. of the acid solution is required when methyl orange is used as the indicator, and the normality of the acid is N_A. If the normality of the alkali in the soil solution is N_S, then we can write

$$N_S \times 100 = V_A \times N_A$$

or,
$$N_S = \frac{V_A \times N_A}{100}$$

Now, normality means the number of g eq per litre, hence
g eq of alkali per litre of soil solution

$$= \frac{V_A \times N_A}{100}$$

or,   g eq of alkali/100 c.c.

$$= \frac{V_A \times N_A}{100 \times 10}$$

Since 100 c.c. of the soil solution is prepared from 20 g of the soil, so we can write

g eq of alkali per 20 g soil

$$= \frac{V_A \times N_A}{100 \times 10}$$

or,   g eq of alkali per 100 g of soil

$$= \frac{V_A \times N_A \times 5}{100 \times 10}$$

or,   m eq of alkali per 100 g of soil

$$= \frac{V_A \times N_A \times 5 \times 1000}{\text{c.c. of sample} (=100 \text{ c.c.}) \times 10}$$

[∴   1 g eq=1000 m eq (milli-equivalent)]
or,   m eq of alkali per 100 g of soil

$$= \frac{V_A \times N_A \times 500}{\text{c.c. of the sample}}$$

In this way the total alkalinity of the soil sample can be calculated.

19.B.4   Determination of Chlorides

A 1 : 5 soil solution is prepared as described in 19.B.3. and 100 c.c. of this solution is transferred into a 250 c.c. conical flask by means of a pipette. The chloride content in this portion is determined by titration with a standard $AgNO_3$ solution using K_2CrO_4 indicator as described in 19.A.7.17 (Mohr's titration).

Observations and Calculations

Suppose for the titration of 100 c.c. of the soil solution V_1 c.c. of $AgNO_3$ solution of N_1 normality is required. If N_{Cl} is the normality of chloride in the soil solution, then

$$100 \times N_{Cl} = V_1 \times N_1$$

or,

$$N_{Cl} = \frac{V_1 \times N_1}{100}$$

Now,   (i) amount of substance per litre of a solution=normality × eq wt of the substance
         (ii) Eq wt of chloride ion is 35.5, so

wt of chloride per litre

$$= \frac{V_1 \times N_1 \times 35.5}{\text{c.c. of sample} (=100 \text{ c.c.})}$$

or,   wt of chloride per 100 c.c. of soil solution or per 20 g of soil

$$= \frac{V_1 \times N_1 \times 35.5}{\text{c.c. of sample} \times 10}$$

or,   wt of chloride per 100 g of soil

$$= \frac{V_1 \times N_1 \times 35.5 \times 5}{\text{c.c. of sample} \times 10}$$

or   % of chloride $= \dfrac{V_1 \times N_1 \times 35.5}{\text{c.c. of sample} \times 2}$

19.B.5   Determination of Sulphates

Soluble sulphates can be driectly determined in soil solution. A 1 : 5 soil solution is prepared and sulphate is this sample is determined gravimetrically as $BaSO_4$. Alternatively, sulphate can be converted into $BaSO_4$ by adding an excess of $BaCl_2$ solution and the resultant $BaSO_4$ can be determined by means of a turbidimeter.

19.B.6 Determination of Organic Matter

A known weight of the given sample is taken in a round bottom flask and treated with a known excess of $K_2Cr_2O_7$ solution and H_2SO_4. A water condenser is attached to the flask and its contents are refluxed for about an our. Later the residual $K_2Cr_2O_7$ is titrated back with a standard ferrous ammonium sulphate solution using ferroin indicator. Knowing the amount of $K_2Cr_2O_7$ consumed, the quantity of oxidizable organic matter present in the soil sample can be estimated in terms of oxidIzing equivalents (see 19.A.7.7). This method is not applicable to carbon present in the elementry form such as charcoal or graphite. It should be noted that even the carbon in the form of organic compounds is not fully oxidized. The recovery of organic carbon is to the extent of 60 to 90%.

19.B.7 Determination of Nitrogen

The nitrogen present in the soil in the form of organic compounds and ammonium salts can be determined by Kjeldahl's method (see 19.A.7.11).

About 10 g of accurately weighed soil sample is ground to 0.15 mm size, placed in a Kjeldahl flask and some water is added to moisten the soil. The soil is then treated with concentrated H_2SO_4 and $CuSO_4$, HgO, Se powder and K_2SO_4 which act as catalyst. The contents of the flask are then digested for about 2 hours. The digest is transferred to a distillation flask, NaOH solution is add to it and this mixture is subjected to distillation for about 40 minutes. The distillate is received in a known amount of acid. After the distillation, the remaining acid is titrated back with a standard alkali solution using suitable indicator. Knowing the amount of the acid consumed, the quantity of the liberated NH_3 and then the quantity of nitrogen in the given soil sample can be calculated.

19 B.8. Determination of Phosphorus

The phosphorus content of a soil sample can be expressed in terms of *available phosphorus* and also as *total phosphorus*.

(i) Determination of available phosphorus

Available phosphorus is extracted from the given soil sample with 0.002N H_2SO_4. The extracted phosphorus is then determined colorimetrically as described in 19.A.7.12. in the case of water sample.

(ii) Determination of total phosphorus

In order to determine total phosphorus, the given soil sample is heated with concentrated HNO_3 and $HClO_4$ on a hot plate to near dryness. The residue is then boiled with dilute H_2SO_4. The resultant solution is cooled, filtered and volume made up to 250 c.c. with distilled water. A 50 c.c. portion of this solution is taken and its phosphorus content is measured colorimetrically as described in 19.A.7.13 in the case of water.

19.B.9 Determination of Calcium and Magnesium

A cation present in a soil sample is determined (i) as present in exchangable form and (ii) as the total content.

(i) Determination of Exchangable Calcium and Magnesium

Calcium and magnesium present in the exchange complex of the soil can be determined by the following procedure.

For determining only exchangable calcium and magnesium, the soil sample is washed 4-5 times with 40% alcohol and finally with absolute alcohol to dry the soil; this process removes the soluble fraction. The soil so obtained is mixed with ammonium acetate solution and thoroughly stirred. The resultant suspension is kept overnight. Next day filtration is done through Whatman No. 42 filter paper using Buchner funnel and vacuum pump. The soil is thus leached 4-5 times more with ammonium acetate solution. The combined filtrates are collected and volume made up to 500 c.c. in a measuring flask. The concentration of calcium and magnesium in this solution is found out by titration with EDTA as described in 19.A.7.18 for water analysis.

(ii) Determination of Total Calcium and Magnesium

If the total calcium and magnesium content in a soil sample is to be determined, the washing with alcohol is not done. A known weight of the soil sample is leached with ammonium acetate solution. In this solution the amount of calcium and magnesium is determined by titration with EDTA as described in 19.A.7.18 for water analysis.

19.B.10. Determination of Sodium and Potassium

For the determination of exchangable sodium and potassium, the given soil is washed with alcohol. The washed soil is then leached with ammonium acetate solution as decribed in 19.B.9. The amounts of sodium and potassium in this solution are then determined by flame photometric method. If total sodium and potassium content is to be determined, washing with alcohol is not done. The soil extract with ammonium acetate solution is directly prepared and Na and K in this solution is estimated by flame photometry.

19.C Analysis of Coal

Coal is a fossil fuel found well below the earth's surface. Millions of years ago, forrests were buried deep under the earth's surface due to some geological activity. It is believed that under the conditions of high pressure and temperature, the plant material partially decayed and got converted into coal. Thus coal is dug out from well below the earth's crust. Coal is a very important fuel for industry as well as for domestic use. Coal obtained from different mines differ in composition, it is therefore necessary to analyse coal in order to know its suitability for different industrial utilization. The analysis of coal is of two types.

   (i) Proximate analysis
   (ii) Ultimate analysis

19.C.1 Proximate Analysis

This type of analysis involves determination of moisture, volatile matter, ash and carbon content of a coal sample. The advantage of this kind of analysis is that it is rapid and gives ideas regarding commercial classification and suitability of coal, under examination, for different purposes. For example, a coal sample with a high moisture content will have a lower price due to increased transport cost, because of increased weight moreover it will have a low calorific value.

It is important to note that in the determination of moisture, volalite matter or ash content, the results depend upon several factors such as size and shape of the crucibles used, the mode and period of heating etc. Hence, in order to get reproducible results experimental conditions have been specified and if the stipulated conditions are followed, fairly reproducible results can be obtained.

19.C.1.1. Determination of Moisture

Moisture is determined by heating a known weight of a coal sample at 105-110 °C for 1 hour and then finding the loss in the weight of the sample as described below.

Procedure

(i) Take a clean low-form porcelain crucible and heat it on a Bunsen burner for about 20 minutes. Cool in a desiccator and weigh. Again heat the crucible, cool and weigh. Repeat this process until a constant weight of the crucible is obtained (W_1 g).

(ii) Dry the powdered coal sample in air and transfer about 1 g of the sample into the crucible and weight the crucible with the sample (W_2 g).

(iii) Place the crucible (without lid) containing the sample in an air oven maintained at a temperature of 105 ± 5 °C for 1 hour. Cool the crucible in a desiccator and weigh (W_3g).

Calculations

Wt. of the sample before heating $=(W_2 - W_1)$ g

Wt. of the sample after heating $=(W_3 - W_1)$ g

$\therefore$ loss in Wt. $=(W_2 - W_1)-(W_3 - W_1)$

or Wt. of moisture $=(W_2 - W_3)$ g

Now, $(W_2 - W_1)$ g of the sample contains $(W_2 - W_3)$ g moisture

$\therefore$ 100 g   „   „   „ $\dfrac{(W_2 - W_3)}{(W_2 - W_1)} \times 100$ g moisture

Thus % moisture $= \dfrac{(W_2 - W_3)}{(W_2 - W_1)} \times 100$

19.C.1.2 Determination of Volatile Matter

This determination involves heating of a known weight of air-dried coal sample at 925 °C for exactly 7 minutes and then finding the loss in weight. Silica crucible of specified dimensions are used for this determination.

Procedure

(ii) Find out the constant weight of the crucible (W_4 g).

(ii) Transfer about 1 g of the powdered air-dried coal sample into the crucible and weigh the crucible with the sample (W_5 g).

(iii) Place the crucible (containing the sample) with the lid in a muffle furnace maintained at 925 ± 15 °C.

(iv) After exactly 7 minutes, take out the crucible, cool in a desiccator and weigh (W_6 g).

Calculations

$$\% \text{ (moisture} + \text{volatile matter)} = \frac{(W_5 - W_6)}{(W_5 - W_4)} \times 100$$

$$\% \text{ volatile matter} = \left[\frac{(W_5 - W_6)}{(W_5 - W_4)} \times 100 - \frac{(W_2 - W_3)}{(W_2 - W_1)} \times 100 \right]$$

19.C.1.3 Determination of Ash

A known weight of the powdered air-dried sample is completely oxidized and the residue is weighed.

Procedure

(i) Find out the constant weight of a shallow procelain crucible (W_7 g).

(ii) Transfer about 1g of powdered air-dried coal sample into the crucible and weigh (W_8 g).

(iii) Put the crucible containing the sample (without lid) in a muffle furnace and heat to 400-450 °C in a muffle furnace for 60 to 80 minutes.

(iv) Increase the temperature of the furnace to 925 ± 15 °C and heat the crucible without lid for 1 hour. Cool the crucible in a desiccator and weigh (W_9 g).

Calculation

Wt of the sample $= (W_8 - W_7)$g

Wt of the ash $= (W_9 - W_7)$g

Now, $(W_8 - W_7)$ g of the sample contains $(W_9 - W_7)$ g ash

$\therefore$ 100 g „   „   „ $\dfrac{(W_9 - W_7)}{(W_8 - W_7)} \times 100$ g

$\therefore$ % ash $= \dfrac{(W_9 - W_7)}{(W_8 - W_7)} \times 100$

19.C.1.4 Determination of Carbon Content

This is calculated in the following manner.

% carbon content$=100-[\%$ moisture$+\%$ volatile matter$+\%$ ash]

19.C.2 Ultimate Analysis

This is a more detailed analysis involving the determination of carbon, hydrogen, nitrogen, sulphur, ash and oxygen content of a coal sample.

19.C.2.1 Determination of Carbon and Hydrogen

This determination is important as it governs the calorific value of the given coal sample. Higher the percentage of C and H, greater is the calorific value and so better is the quality of the coal.

The percentage of C and H in a coal sample is determined by the procedure described in 18.B.1, employed for organic compounds. A known weight of the coal somple is heated in a current of pure oxygen gas when C and H_2 are completely oxidized to H_2O and CO_2 respectively; these are then absorbed separately in anhydrous calcium chloride and KOH solution. The increase in the weights of the absorbents give the amounts of CO_2 and H_2O formed, from which the percentage of C and H can be calculated using the relationship

$$\% \text{ carbon} = \frac{\text{wt of } CO_2 \text{ formed}}{\text{wt of the sample}} \times \frac{12}{44} \times 100$$

$$\% \text{ hydrogen} = \frac{\text{wt of } H_2O \text{ formed}}{\text{wt of the sample}} \times \frac{2}{18} \times 100$$

19.C.2.2 Determination of Nitrogen (Kjeldahl method)

This method involves heating a known weight of the ground coal sample with concentrated H_2SO_4 in persence of K_2SO_4 and $CuSO_4$ (or selenium powder) catalyst for about 4 hours. The nitrogen present in the sample is converted into NH_3 which combines with the excess acid present to form $(NH_4)_2SO_4$. The contents of the flask are then destilled with an excess of NaOH solution and the liberated NH_3 is absorbed in a known excess of H_2SO_4. The unused acid is then back titrated with a standard NaOH solution. The amount of the acid consumed thus becomes known hence the quantity of NH_3 liberated and so the amount of nitrogen present in the sample can be calculated (see 18.B.2.2.).

[Note: 1. About 1 g of coal sample is taken for analysis.
2. For coke, add about 0.1 g of Cr_2O_3 before boiling with H_2SO_4.
3. Bituminous coal samples require a total digestion period of 3 to 4 hours. Coke and anthracite coal require much longer period.
4. Selenium powder or $HgSO_4$ can also be used as catalyst.]

Calculations

See section 18.B.2.2.

19.C.2.3   Determination of Sulphur

Coal contains sulphur in organic as well as in inorganic form. In general, high sulphur content in coal is undesirable. In metallurgy and ceramic industry the use of coal with high sulphur content is particularly objectionable as this contaminates the metal. Thus the determination of sulphur in coal is of importance.

The procedures for the determination of sulphur in coal involves its oxidation to sulphate which is determined gravimetrically as $BaSO_4$ (see expt. 6.4).

For determining sulphur in coal, the method of Eschka is a standard one which is applicable to any organic compound that does not volatalise before heating. A known weight of finely ground coal sample is heated with a mixture of anhydrous MgO and Na_2CO_3. (This mixture is known as Eschka mixture). The resultant mass is dissolved in hot water and sulphate in this solution is determined gravimetrically as $BaSO_4$.

Procedure

(i) Eschka mixture is prepared by mixing 2 parts of porous calcined MgO with 1 part of anhydrous Na_2CO_3 (both should be sulphur free).

(ii) In a platinum or silica or porcelain crucible, 1g of the finely ground sample is thoroughly mixed with 3 g of Eschka mixture. This mixture is then covered with 2 g more of Eschka mixture.

(iii) The open crucible is gently heated when charring takes place. This mixture is frequently stirred with a platinum wire. After 30 minutes the mixture is heated to a dull redness (800 °C) for 1 hour, when the mixture becomes light brown or yellow. Heating is then stopped and crucible is cooled.

(iv) The crucible with its content is placed in a beaker containing 100 c.c. of water which is boiled for 30 minutes. The mixture is filtered and ppt is washed with water. The filtrate and combined washings are heated with 5 c.c. of saturated solution of bromine to oxidize any sulphites to sulphates. The solution is made acidic with 1 : 1 HCl. The excess bromine is boiled off and solution diluted to 200 c.c.

(v) The solution is neutralized with concentrated ammonia solution to methyl orange indicator (solution should become yellow), and then 4 c.c. of 1 : 1 HCl solution is added. The solution is boiled, and 10% $BaCl_2$ solution is added in slight excess to completely precipitate $BaSO_4$. Boiling is continued for 30 minutes and ppt is allowed to settle. The ppt is filtered through Whatman filter paper No. 40 and washed with hot water until the washings are free from chloride ions (by testing with $AgNO_3$ solution). The final washing is done with 10% NH_4NO_3 solution; this helps in the combustion of filter paper and oxidation of the ppt, The filter paper and ppt is ignited in a weighed crucible for about 30 minutes. The crucible with its content is cooled in a desiccator and weighed.

The process of heating and cooling is repeated until a constant weight is obtained.

Calculations

1. wt of the coal sample $= x$ g
2. wt of the empty crucible $= W_1$ g
3. wt of the crucible+ppt $= W_2$ g
   wt of the ppt$= (W_2 - W_1) = W_3$ g

Now, 233.4 g of BaSO₄ contains 32 g sulphur

$\therefore$ W_3 g   ...   . $\dfrac{W_3 \times 32}{233.4}$ g of sulphur

x g of the sample contains $\dfrac{W_3 \times 32}{233.4}$ g sulphur

$\therefore$ 100 g   ...   . $\dfrac{100 \times W_3 \times 32}{x \times 233.4}$ g sulphur

Thus % of sulphur $= \dfrac{\text{wt of BaSO}_4}{\text{wt of sample}} \times \dfrac{32}{233.4} \times 100$

19.C.2.4 Determination of Phosphorus

A known weight (5 g) of coal sample is converted into its ash as described in 19.C.1.3. The ash is taken in a 30 c.c. platinum crucible and is treated with 10 c.c. of concentrated HNO_3 and 5 c.c. of 48% hydrofluoric acid. The contents are evaporated to dryness. The residue is treated with 5 c.c. of concentrated HNO_3 and again evaporated to dryness, and residu heated to redness and then fused with Na_2CO_3. The melt is leached thoroughly with hot water and filtered. The filter paper and residue is ignited and fused with sodium carbonate. The melt is again leached with hot water. The two filtrates are combined and treated with ammonium molybdate solution when a complex is formed. This complex on treatment with stannous chloride produces a blue colour whose absorbance can be measured at 690 nm. A calibration curve is constructed with known phosphate solutions and later the amount of phosphorus in the sample solution is found out with the help of this calibration curve.

19.C.2.5 Determination of Oxygen

In ultimate analysis, the composition of coal is conventionally expressed in percentages of ash, sulphur, nitrogen, carbon, hydrogen and oxygen. The sum of these percentages is taken to be 100. Since there is no method to determine oxygen, its percentage is calculated by subtracting the sum of the percentages of ash, sulphur, nitrogen, carbon and hydrogen from 100. The disadvantage in this calculation is that sum of all the errors occurring in other determinations is included in the percentage of oxygen.

19.C.3 Determination of Calorific Value of a Coal Sample

The calorific value of coal means the quantity of heat evolved by complete combustion of a unit mass of the given coal sample. This property of coal is expressed in calorie/g or Kilocalorie/Kg. The calorific value is the most important property of a fuel; greater the calorific value, better is the quality of the fuel.

The calorific value of coal is determined by means of an oxygen bomb calorimeter. This determination involves the complete combustion of a known weight of a coal sample in a closed vessel called *bomb* containing oxygen gas at a pressure of 25 atmosphere. The ignition of the sample is done by electrical means. The bomb is kept in a calorimeter (whose water equivalent is known) containing a known amount of water at a known temperature. After the complete combustion of the coal sample, rise in temperature of water in the calorimeter is noted: This gives the quantity of the liberated heat, knowing which the calorific value of the coal sample is calculated.

19.C.3.1   Components of Oxygen Bomb Calorimeter

An oxygen bomb calorimeter consists of the following parts (see Fig. 19.26).

1. The Combustion bomb. This is a vessel (A) of capacity about 300 c.c. which is made of a special kind of steel that is resistant to acids. (Remember that coal contains N and S which produce HNO_3 and H_2SO_4 during the combustion process). This vessel has a cap with a screw (B) so that the bomb can be made air tight. Two stainless steel electrodes (C and D) pass through this cap into the bomb. One of the electrodes (C) is in the form of a tube through which oxygen can be introduced into the bomb. A ring (E) is attached to this electrode which holds a nickel or silica crucible (F) containing a known weight of the coal sample. Through platinum wires G and H the sample can be ignited electrically.

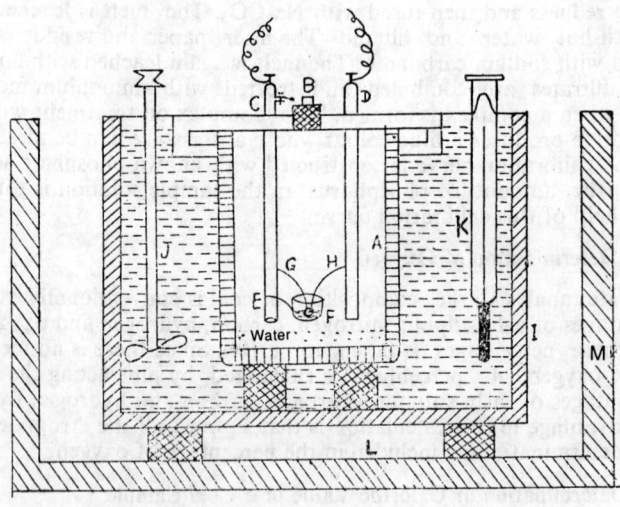

Fig. 19.26

Calorimeter. It is a cylindrical copper vessel (I) with a capacity of about 2500 c.c. A known weight of water is taken in this vessel which contains stirrer (J) and a Beckman thermometer (K). The bomb (A) is immersed in the calorimeter containing water as shown in Fig. 19.26. The calorimeter is surrounded by a water jacket (M) so that an air jacket (L) is formed in between the water jacket and the calorimeter.

The water equivalent of the calorimeter is found out by burning a known weight of benzoic acid and noting the rise in temperature of a known weight of water in the calorimeter. Since the calorific value of benzoic acid is known, the water equivalent of the calorimeter can be calculated.

[Note. In the case of a copper calorimeter the approximate value of the water equivalent is given by the product $m \times s$, where m is the mass of the calorimeter and s is the specific heat of copper ($=0.1$). If the water equivalent of a calorimeter is W g water then it means that the calorimeter is equivalent to Wg of water as far as heat receiving capacity is concerned.]

19.C.3.2 Procedure for Measuring the Calorific Value

About 1 g of the coal sample in pellet form is kept in the crucible (F) and 10 c.c. water is introduced into the bomb. Firing wires (G and H) are so arranged that the sample gets ignited on passing current through the electrodes (C and D). Oxygen gas is introduced into the bomb through the electrode (C) until the pressure inside the bomb rises to 25 atmosphere. The bomb is then made airtight by tightening the screw (B). The calorimeter is weighed and enough water is poured into it so that the bomb is submerged when placed in the calorimeter as shown in Fig. 19.26. The weight of the calorimeter and water is taken. The difference in the two weight readings gives the weight of water taken in the calorimeter. (The water equivalent of the calorimeter is previously determined). The initial temperature of the water in the calorimeter is noted. The bomb is placed in the calorimeter which is then surrounded by a water jacket (M) in such a way that an air jacket (L) is entrapped. The stirrer is switched on and current is passed through the electrodes so that the combustion of the sample begins. The temperature in the thermometer is observed and the maximum temperature reached is noted.

Observations and Calculations

(i) Wt of the coal sample	...	...	...	x g
(ii) Water equivalent of calorimeter	...	...		W_1 g
(iii) Wt of water taken in calorimeter	...	...		W_2 g
(iv) Initial temp. of water in calorimeter		...		T_1
(v) Final temp. of water in calorimeter		...		T_2

The heat gained by the calorimeter and water contained in it is given by
$$Q = (W_1 + W_2)(T_2 - T_1) \text{ cal}$$

obviously Q cal of heat is obtained by burning x g of coal,
Now, x g of coal on combustion produces $(W_1 + W_2)(T_2 - T_1)$ cal

$\therefore$ 1 g   , ... $\dfrac{(W_1 + W_2)(T_2 - T_1)}{x}$

Thus the calorific value of the given sample would be

$$\frac{(W_1+W_2)\,(T_2-T_1)}{x}$$

19.D Analysis of Fats and Oils

The fatty glycerides of animal and vegetable origin form an important class of organic compounds: Out of these, those which are solids at ordinary temperature are called *fats* and those that are liquids are known as *oils*. Both these categories are referred to as *saponifiable oils*. These are used in foods, manufacture of soap and medicine etc. Majority of fats and oils are composed of glycerides of fatty acids containing 16 to 18 carbon atoms such as oleic, stearic and palmitic acid. Normally the oil sample is extracted from a meal or cosmetics. The oil sample is filtered to remove suspended matter. The following properties of oils are generally studied.

19.D.1 DETERMINATION OF VOLATILE MATTER

A known weight of the sample, taken in a crucible, is heated in an oven around 100°C until constant weight is obtained. The loss in weight gives the amount of volatile matter.

Observations and Calculations

(i) Wt of the crucible ... ... W_1 g
(ii) Wt of the crucible+sample ... ... W_2 g (before heating)
(iii) Wt of the crucible+sample ... ... W_3 g (after heating)

Wt of the sample before heating $=(W_2-W_1)$ g

Wt of the sample after heating $=(W_3-W_1)$ g

$\therefore$ loss in wt $=(W_2-W_1)-(W_3-W_1)=(W_2-W_3)$ g

Now, (W_2-W_1) g sample contains (W_2-W_3) g volatile matter

$\therefore$ 100 g ... ... $\dfrac{(W_2-W_3)}{(W_2-W_1)}\times 100$ g

Thus % volatile matter $= \dfrac{(W_2-W_3)}{(W_2-W_1)}\times 100$

19.D.2 DETERMINATION OF ACID VALUE

The acid value or acid number gives the amount of free acid, present per g of the sample, which is determined by titration with a standard solution of potassium hydroxide.

Reagent

1. 0.1 N aqueous KOH solution.
2. Phenolphthalein indicator solution.

Procedure

(i) Weigh 20 g of oil into a flask and add 50 c.c. of 95% alcohol which has been neutralized to phenolphthalein end point with 0.1N alkali. Heat to boiling and swirl the flask.

(ii) Titrate the hot sample with 0.1 N KOH solution until colour persists for 30 seconds (after vigorous swirling).

[Note. (1) On treating oils with alkali soaps are formed which precipitate in the cold and occlude some of the solution. This is the reason that the titration is done in hot condition so that no precipitation of soaps takes place.

(2) Sometimes fugitive or fleeting end points are obtained i.e., the pink colour appears but on shaking the solution for 10-15 seconds, the colour disappears. In the above titration, the end point is supposed to have been reached when the pink colour persists for 30 seconds even after vigorous shaking of the titration solution.]

Observations and Calculations

The acid value or acid number is the number of mg of KOH required to neutralize the free fatty acid in 1 g oil.

$$\text{Mol. wt of KOH} = 56.1 = \text{eq wt of KOH}$$

$\therefore$ 1000 c.c. of 1 N KOH $\equiv$ 56.1 g KOH

or. 1000 c.c. of 0.1 N KOH $\equiv$ 5.61 g KOH

or, 1 c.c. of 0.1 N KOH $\equiv$ 5.61 mg KOH

If B c.c. of 0.1N KOH solution is required to neutralize A g of oil, then

$$\text{A g of oil} \equiv B \times 5.61 \text{ mg KOH}$$

$\therefore$ $$1 \text{ g of oil} \equiv \frac{B \times 5.61}{A} \text{ mg KOH}$$

In general, the acid number of an oil is given by

$$\text{Acid number} = \frac{\text{c.c. of 0.1N KOH} \times 5.61}{\text{weight of the sample}}$$

If 0.1N NaOH is used for the titration, then

$$\text{Acid number} = \frac{\text{c.c. of 0.1N NaOH} \times 4.0}{\text{weight of the sample}}$$

19.D.3 DETERMINATION OF SAPONIFICATION VALUE

This value is a measure of the amount of saponifiable matter present in the oil sample. It is also known as *saponification number* which is defined as the number of mg of KOH required to titrate 1 g of oil after its saponification (treatment with alkali). The saponification value generally exceeds the acid value because the saponification value includes

(i) alkali used in the neutralization of fatty acids

(i) alkali used for the saponification of glyceride.

Reagent

1. 0.5 N alcoholic KOH solution. About 28 g of KOH in 500 c.c. alcohol is warmed and the mixture is constantly stirred. The solution is allowed to stand overnight and then filtered. The filtrate is diluted to 1 litre. This will give approximately 0.5 N KOH solution.

2. Phenolphthalein indicator solution (1 % in 1 : 1 water-alcohol mixture).

3. 0.5 N HCl solution.

Procedure

(i) Weigh out accurately about 5 g of the oil sample into a 250 c.c. conical flask (1) and add 50 c.c. of 0.5 N alcoholic KOH solution by means of a pipette.

(ii) Introduce 50 c.c. of 0.5 N alcoholic KOH in another conical flask (2). [For blank determination.]

(iii) Attach air condensers to both the flasks and keep them dipped in boiling water for about 30 minutes.

(iv) Cool both the flasks and titrate their contents with 0.5 N HCl solution using phenolphthalein as indicator.

Observation and Calculations

Suppose c c. of the acid needed in flask $1 = x$ c.c.
    (experimental titre)

and, c.c. of the acid needed in flask $2 = y$ c.c.
    (blank titre)

Then,

$$\text{Saponification value} = \frac{(y - x) \times 56.1 \times \text{Normality of acid}}{\text{weight of the sample}}$$

If the normality of HCl used is 0.5, then

$$\text{Saponification value} = \frac{(y - x) \times 56.1 \times 0.5}{\text{weight of the sample}}$$

19.D.4 DETERMINATION OF ESTER VALUE

The ester value of an oil sample is a measure of the amount of esters present. This can be obtained by subtracting acid value from the saponification value.

19.D.5 DETERMNIATION OF IODINE VALUE

The iodine value of an oil sample is a measure of the unsaturated bonds present in the oil or fat. It is the percentage of halogen absorbed and this is calculated in terms of iodine. The reaction involves the addition of halogen to unsaturated bonds. Since the reaction may not be complete, it is necessary to mention the name of the method and the specified experimental condition must be strictly followed.

19.D.5.1 Hanus Method

This method consists of treating a known weight of oil sample with an excess of iodine bromide (IBr) solution. After 30 minutes the unused iodine bromide is determined iodometrically. A blank is also carried out, and thus the quantity of halogen used up in the reaction is calculated.

Reagent

1. **Hanus Solution.** (Iodine monobromide). Dissolve 13.62 g of iodine in 825 c.c. of glacial acetic acid by warming and stirring. Cool and pipet out 25 c.c. of this solution into a conical flask. dilute to 200 c.c. and titrate with 0.1 N thiosulphate using starch as indicator. (The pipetting should be done by suction bulb as the solution and its vapours are poisonous). Suppose the titre value is 'a' c.c.

Add 3 c.c. of bromine through a burette to 200 c.c. of glacial acetic acid and mix thoroughly. Take 5 c.c. of this solution and dilute to 150 c.c. with water, add 10 c.c. of 15% KI solution and titrate the liberated iodine with 0.1 N thiosulphate solution. Suppose the titre value is 'b' c.c. This titre will be approximately 80% of 'a'. Calculate the c.c. of bromine solution that should be added to 800 c.c. of iodine solution as follows

$$\frac{a}{25} \times \frac{5}{b} \times 800 = \text{c.c. of bromine solution to be added.}$$

For example, suppose

25 c.c. of iodine solution$\equiv$25.3 c.c. of 0.1 N $Na_2S_2O_3$,

and, 5 c.c. of bromine solution$\equiv$20.8 c.c. of 0.1 N $Na_2S_2O_3$, then

$$\frac{25.3}{25} \times \frac{5}{20.8} \times 800 = 193.9 \text{ c.c.}$$

Thus, to 800 c.c. of iodine solution, 193.9 c.c. of bromine solution should be added. The volume will be then 993.9 c.c.; to this solution 6.1 c.c. of acetic acid should be added so that the total volume of the iodine monobromide solution becomes 1 litre. This solution is stored in amber coloured glass-stoppered bottle. It is slightly more than 0.1 N IBr solution.

2. **Sodium Thiosulphate Solution, 0.1 N**

3. **Starch Solution 1%.**

Procedure

(i) Weigh out 0.3 to 0.5 g of oil or fat into a 250 c.c. iodine flask. Dissolve the sample in 10 c.c. of $CHCl_3$ or CCl_4 warming slightly if necessary. Cool and introduce 25 c.c. of Hanus solution into the flask. Also take 25 c.c. of Hanus solution in another iodine flask (this is blank solution which does not contain the oil sample). Shake each flask vigorously and set aside for 30 minutes, with occasional shaking. Then add about 70 c.c. of water and 10 c.c of 15% KI solution to both the flasks.

(ii) Titrate the solutions (blank and experimental) with 0.1 N $Na_2S_2O_3$ solution. (This titration is done by gradual addition of $Na_2S_2O_3$ solution with vigorous shaking after each addition because the iodine is in the non-aqueous layer.) Continue the gradual addition of $Na_2S_2O_3$ solution until the solution becomes pale yellow. At this stage add 1 c.c. of 1% starch indicator solution when the titration solution will become blue. Continue dropwise addition of $Na_2S_2O_3$ solution with thorough shaking until the disappearance of the blue colour.

[It should be noted that if the titre of the unreacted Hanus solution is not alteast 60% of the blank then the experiment should be repeated by taking a smaller amount of the oil sample. For example, consider an experiment in which

blank titre $= 24.8$ c.c.

and, experimental titre $= 12.4$ c.c.

The experimental titre corresponds to the unreacted Hanus solution. In this case unreacted Hanus solution is only 50% of the amount taken. Hence, this experiment should be discarded and another experiment should be carried out with a lesser amount of the oil sample so that more than 660% of the Hanus solution remains unreacted. For example, in another experiment

blank titre $= 24.8$ c.c.

and experimental titre $= 16.3$ c.c.

Since, 16.3 is 65% of 24.8, we can say that the excess of Hanus solution added was more than 60% hence the results obtained in this experiment will be accepted.]

Observation and Calculations

1. Wt of the oil sample   ...   ... w g
2. Blank titre   ...   ... y c.c.
3. Experimental titre   ...   ... x c.c.
4. Normality of thiosulphate solution   ... 0.1 N

We know that

$$IBr \equiv \tfrac{1}{2}Br_2 \equiv \tfrac{1}{2}I_2 \equiv Na_2S_2O_3$$

We had taken y c.c. of 0.1 N IBr solution and got back x c.c. solution, It means that w g of oil sample reacted with $(y-x)$ c.c. of 0.1 N IBr solution. Since, $(y-x)$ c.c. of 0.1 N IBr $\equiv (y-x)$ c.c. of 0.1 N I_2 solution, it follows that w g oil corresponds to $(y-x)$ c.c. of 0.1 N I_2 solution.

Now,   1000 c.c. 1 N I_2 solution $\equiv 127$ g I_2

$\therefore$ 1000 c.c. 0.1 N I_2 solution $\equiv 12.7$ g I_2

$\therefore$ $(y-x)$ c.c. 0.1 N I_2 solution $\equiv \dfrac{(y-x) \times 12.7}{1000}$ g I_2

Now, w g oil sample corresponds to $\dfrac{(y-x) \times 12.7}{1000}$ g I_2

$$\therefore \quad 100 \text{ g oil} \quad \ldots \quad \ldots \quad \frac{(y-x) \times 12.7 \times 100}{1000 \times w} \text{ g } I_2$$

$$\text{Iodine value} \quad = \frac{(y-x) \times 12.7 \times 0.1}{w}$$

In general iodine value is given by

$$\frac{(\text{blank titre} - \text{exptal titre}) \times 12.7 \times \text{Normality of Na}_2S_2O_3}{\text{wt of the sample}}$$

19.D.6 DETERMINATION OF BROMINE VALUE

Bromine value is a little used determination although it is a more accurate measure of the degree of unsaturation. This value is determined by the following procedure.

(i) Weigh out 0.2 to 1 g of oil sample and dissolve it in 10 c.c. of CCl_4 in a 250 c.c. iodine flask. Warm if necessary.

(ii) Dissolve 26.6 g Br_2 in CCl_4 and dilute with CCl_4 to 1 litre; this is approximately 0.33 N.

(iii) Introduce 2 c.c. of Br_2 solution into the flask containing the sample and the same volume in another iodine flask which contains 10 c.c. of CCl_4 but not the oil sample (blank).

(iv) After 2 minutes, add 25 c.c. of 25% KI solution to each flask and titrate the liberated iodine in each flask with 0.1 N $Na_2S_2O_3$ solution using starch as indicator.

The difference between the blank and the sample titration will give the amount of Br_2 consumed by the sample in terms of thiosulphate solution. The bromine consumed may be used up for

(i) addition at a double bond, and

(ii) substitution.

Now in the addition of Br_2 at a double bond there is no formation of HBr but whenever Br_2 is substituted in an organic molecule, then HBr is also produced. The HBr produced can be easily determined iodometrically and the equivalent thiosulphate can be subtracted from the total thiosulphates equivalents used up. Thus it is possible to calculate the amount of bromine consumed only in addition at double bonds : This is a more accurate measure of the degree of unsaturation. The determination of the HBr produced can be continued after step (iv).

(v) Record the titre value obtained in step (iv) and add 5 c.c. of 2% KIO_3 solution which will convert HBr, formed during the substitution of bromine, into the equivalent amount of iodine. Mix well and titrate the liberated I_2 with $Na_2S_2O_3$ in the second stage.

(vi) Treat blank also with the same quantity of KIO_3 and titrate with $Na_2S_2O_3$ solution.

Thus it is possible to know how much bromine is used for addition and how much for substitution.

19.E. Analysis of Urine

Normally fresh human urine is clear but may develop turbidity on keeping. It is yellow in colour having an aromatic odour. Fresh urine is normally acidic however, the pH can vary from 4.7 to 8.0. On standing urine becomes alkaline by the bacterial action on urea and formation of NH_3. The specific gravity of urine lies in the range 1.016 to 1.022. The chief chemical constituents of urine are urea, uric acid, amino acids, hippuric acid, creatinine, ammonia, chloride, phosphate, sulphate, calcium, sodium and potassium. In abnormal conditions glucose starts passing into urine. Some other substances such as ketone bodies (like acetone), bile, blood and albumen may also be found in urine.

19.E.1 QUALITATIVE ANALYSIS OF URINE

First of all the appearance, colour, specific gravity and pH of urine sample are noted. Then the following chemical tests are performed.

19.E.1.1 Test for Chlorides

Place about 5 c.c. of urine sample in a test tube, add a few drops of con. HNO_3 and then about 2 c.c. of 3% $AgNO_3$ solution. If a white ppt (soluble in NH_4OH) appears, the presence of chloride is indicated. [The white ppt formed is that of AgCl which readily dissolves in NH_4OH. If HNO_3 is not added prior to the addition of $AgNO_3$ solution, silver urates and phosphates will be precipitated causing interference with the chloride test.]

19 E.1.2 Test for Sulphates

Acidify 5 c.c. urine with 1 c.c. of con. HCl and then add 5 c.c. of 10% $BaCl_2$ solution. The appearance of a white ppt of $BaSO_4$ indicates the presence of sulphate (inorganic). Filter and boil the filtrate. On boiling free sulphate is released from the organic sulphate. Hence, if a white ppt appears on boiling the filtrate, the presence of organic sulphate is indicated.

19.E.1.3 Test for Phosphates and Calcium

Add a few drops of con. NH_4OH to 10 c.c. of urine. Boil the mixture and then cool. Filter the ppt formed and discard the filtrate. Dissolve the ppt in hot 10% acetic acid and divide the resultant solution to two parts.

   (i) Add ammonium molybdate solution and add a few drops of con. HNO_3 to one part and warm. The appearance of a yellow colour shows the presence of phosphates.

   (ii) Add 5 c.c. of 2% potassium oxalate solution to the second part of the solution. If a white ppt (of calcium oxalate) is observed, calcium is present in the urine sample.

   [Note. Ammonium molybdate reagent solution is prepared in the following manner

   Dissolve 100 g molybdic acid in 144 c.c. of NH_4OH of sp. gr. 0.9 and 271 c.c. water. Add this solution with constant stirring into a beaker containing 489 c.c. con HNO_3 and 1148 c.c. water, Mix well.]

19.E-1.4 Test for Ammonia

Take 10 c.c. of urine sample in a test tube, add 2 drops of phenolphthalein indicator solution and make it just alkaline by adding 0.1 N NaOH dropwise with constant shaking until the solution becomes just pink. Heat the test tube and put a paper dipped in phenolphthalein solution at the mouth of the tube. The indicator solution will turn pink if ammonia is present in urine.

19.E.1.5 Test for Urea

(A) Hypobromite Test Add 1 c.c. of freshly prepared sodium hypobromite solution to 5 c.c. urine, a brisk effervescence (due to the evolution of N_2 gas) indicates the presence of urea. The hypobromite reagent liberates N_2 gas from urea in accordance with the equation

$$CO(NH_2)_2 + 3NaOBr + 2NaOH \rightarrow 3NaBr + Na_2CO_3 + 3H_2O + N_2$$

[Notes 1. The above reaction is also used for the quantitative determination of urea (see 18.D.8).

2 Sodium hypobromite reagent is prepared by mixing 25 c.c. of liquid bromine with 250 c.c. of 40% NaOH. The solution should be cooled during the mixing. This reagent should be prepared just before use.]

B. Urease Test

This is a specific test for urea and is performed in the following manner.

(i) Place 5 c.c. of urine in a test tube. Check its pH. If it is acidic, neutralize the sample by dropwise addition of 2% Na_2CO_3.

(ii) Add 3-4 drops of phenolphthalein solution when the solution will turn pink due to slightly alkaline nature.

(iii) Add 1% CH_3COOH dropwise until the solution just becomes colourless. It means that the solution is now neutral.

(iv) Add a small amount of horse gram powder (which is a source of the enzyme urease) and mix thoroughly. If pink colour reappears the presence of urea is confirmed.

[Note. In presence of urease, urea changes into ammonium carbonate which makes the solution alkaline. This is the reason that the pink colour reappears.]

19.E.1.6 Test for Uric Acid

Place 5 c.c. of urine in a test tube and add 1 c.c. of 10% Na_2CO_3 and 1 c.c. of dilute phosphotungstic acid (Folin and Denis reagent). Formation of blue colour shows the presence of uric acid.

[Note. *Preparation of Phosphotungstic acid Reagent*. Dissolve 100 g of sodium tungstate in 800 c.c. water in a round bottom flask. Add 80 c.c. of 85% phosphoric acid and reflux the mixture for about 2 hours on a small flame. Cool, dilute to 1 litre and store in a brown bottle. Dilute 10 c.c. of this solution to 100 c.c. and then use it for testing uric acid].

19.E.1.7 Test for Creatinine (Jaffe's Test)

Place 5 c.c. of water in test tube A and 5 c.c. of urine in test tube B. To both A and B, add 1 c.c. of 1% picric acid solution and 1 c.c. of 10% NaOH. Mix and keep for a few minutes. The solution in tube B will become orange red due to the formation of creatinine picrate thereby indicating the presence of creatinine in the given urine sample. (Compare the color in tube B with that in tube A).

19.E.1.8 Test for Proteins

(i) Fill three-fourths of a test tube with urine and acidify with 2% acetic acid. Mix and heat the upper portion of the tube. As compared to the lower cooler part, coagulation will be observed in the upper part of the tube.

(ii) Add 1 c.c. of 20% sulphosalicyclic acid to 5 c.c. of urine. The appearance of a ppt indicates the presence of proteins.

(iii) Place 3 c.c. of con. HNO_3 in a test tube and gently introduce 3 c.c. of urine over the acid layer. The formation of a white ring indicates presence of proteins or albumin.

19.E 1.9 Test for Blood

(i) The presence of blood in urine can be examined by spectroscopic examination.

(ii) Take a small amount of benzidine powder in a dry tube and shake it with 1 c.c. of glacial acetic acid. Add 2 c.c, of urine sample and a few drops of a fresh H_2O_2 solution, a greenish colour is observed which on keeping for about 5 minutes turns purple or brown.

19.E.1.10 Test for Bile Salts

Dissolve a few crystals of canesugar in about 5 c.c. of urine sample taken in a test tube. Add about 5 c.c. of con. HNO_3 gently through the sides of the tube. The formation of a purple ring at the junction of two liquids indicates the presence of bile salts.

19.E.1.11 Test for Ketone Bodies (Rothera's Test)

This test is used for detecting acetone, acetoacetic acid or both in the given urine sample.

Add enough $(NH_4)_2SO_4$ to 5 c.c. of urine sample so as to reach saturation stage. Then add 5 drops of 2% freshly prepared sodium nitroprusside solution and shake. Now add about 1 c.c. of con. ammonia. A purple colour shows the presence of ketone bodies.

19.E.1.12 Test for Reducing Sugar (Benedicts Test)

[Benedict's Reagent (Qualitative)] (i) Dissolve 173 g sodium citrate and 100 g anhydrous sodium carbonate in about 600 c.c. of water taken in a beaker, by gentle warming.

(ii) In another beaker dissolve 17.3 g $CuSO_4.5H_2O$ in about 100 c.c. of water and add this solution to the first beaker slowly with constant stirring and make up the volume to 1 litre.]

Place 5 c.c. of Benedict reagent in a test tube and add 8 drops of urine and keep the tube in boiling water for 5 minutes and then cool observe the colour.

Colour of the preciptate	% glucose in urine sample
Green	0.5
Yellow	1.0
Orange	1.5
Red	2.0

19.E.2 QUANTITATIVE ANALYSIS OF URINE

19.E.2.1 Determination of Reducing Sugar (Bendict's Method)

In this method we find out the c.c. of urine sample required to completely reduce 25 c.c. of Benedict's solution of specified concentration. The concentration of Benedict's solution is so selected that 25 c.c. of the solution can be completely reduced by 50 mg of glucose. Knowing the titre value of urine the percentage of glucose in it can be calculated.

If the urine contains a large amount of reducing sugar. it must be diluted and calculations should be accordingly modified. If protein is present then proceed as follows-place a measured quantity of urine in a beaker, acidify with acetic acid and boil until all of the protein has coagulated. Cool, filter and add water to bring the volume of urine to its original value.]

Reagents

1. Benedict Quantitative Reagent

(i) Dissolve 200 g sodium citrate, 75 g anhydrous sodium carbonate and 125 g potassium thiocyanate in about 700 c.c. of water by warming. Cool and filter.

(ii) Weigh accurately 18 g of $CuSO_4$. $5H_2O$ and dissolve it in 100 c.c. of water.

Slowly add $CuSO_4$ solution gradually to the first solution with constant stirring. Add 5 c.c. of 5% potassium ferrocyanide solution and dilute to 1 litre.

2. Sodium Carbonate, Solid.

3. Pumice or Talc Podwer or Glass Beads

Procedure

Rough Titration

(i) Introduce 25 c.c. of Benedict's quantitative reagent by means of a pipette into a 250 c.c. pyrex beaker. Add 5-10 g Na_2CO_3 and a few glass beads.

(ii) Heat to boiling and while heating arrange a burette on a stand in such a manner that the tip of the burette is a few inches above the beaker. Fill the burette with the urine to be tested.

(iii) As the mixture in the beaker boils, add a few drops of urine at a time. The blue colour of the mixture will begin to fade. Add the urine more slowly now to the boiling mixture until the last trace of blue colour just disappears. This is the end-point. Note the volume of the urine-which is the approximate titre.

Final titration

(iv) Take 25 c.c. of Benedict solution in a beaker, add a few glass beads, 5 to 10 g Na_2CO_3 and heat to boiling. Add about 90% of the approximate titre rapidly to the boiling mixture. Then add urine slowly in a dropwise manner and complete the titration. Note the titre value (A c.c.).

Calculation

25 c.c. of Benedict solution $\equiv$ 50 mg of glucose

$\therefore$ A c.c. urine must contain 50 mg of glucose

$\therefore$ 1 ... ... $\dfrac{50}{A}$ mg of glucose

Thus mg of glucose/c.c. of urine sample

$$= \frac{50}{\text{c.c. of urine used in titration}}$$

[Notes 1. If the approximate titre value comes out to be less than 10 c.c., the urine should be diluted to such an extent that the titre would be more than 10 c.c. The final titration should be done with this diluted urine sample and allowance for this dilution should be made in the calculations. It should be remembered that if titre value is small, a considerable error will be caused owing to a measurement of small volume. Suppose the given urine sample is double diluted and then used in the final titration, then

mg of glucose per c.c. of urine sample $= \dfrac{50}{\text{c.c. of urine}} \times \dfrac{1}{2}$

2. The qualitative and quantitative Benedict's solutions have different composition. The quantitative reagent contains potassium thiocyanate and potassium ferrocyanide in addition to those present in the qualitative reagent (sodium citrate, sodium carbonate and copper sulphate). The purpose of adding thiocyanate is to convert the cuprous oxide formed into white cuprous thiocyanate which provides a white background against which the disappearance of blue colour can be seen and end point correctly located. Ferrocyanide keeps cuprous oxide in solution. Because of the addition of these two chemicals, it is not possible to add the required amount of sodium carbonate while preparing the quantitative reagent as it will make the reagent unstable. This is the reason that more Na_2CO_3 is added to the reagent just before performing the titration.

3. The reagent is kept boiling throughout the titration using a small flame so that boiling is not vigorous. The addition of talc powder or glass beads prevents bumping. The boiling itself will mix the reagent and urine added through the burette. The presence of steam over the titration solution prevents the auto-oxidation of cuprous oxide resulting from the reduction of copper sulphate by reducing sugar present in the urine sample.]

19.E.2.2. Determination of Urea

MacLean's hypobromite method is used for determining urea in urine. This procedure is similar to that described for the determination of urea in organic compounds (see 18.D.8). The only difference is that in place of a weighed amount of an oragnic compound, a measured volume of urine sample is taken in tube B. (See Fig. 18.11).

19.E.2.3 Determination of Chloride

A measured volume of urine is treated with a known excess of a standard $AgNO_3$ solution in presence of dilute HNO_3. The chloride present in urine is precipitated as AgCl. (Addition of HNO_3 prevents the precipitation of silver phosphate and silver urate as they are soluble in HNO_3). The unused $AgNO_3$ is then back titrated by a standard solution of NH_4CNS using ferric alum as indicator. Knowing the amount of $AgNO_3$ consumed, the quantity of chloride in urine can be calculated

$$1000 \text{ c.c. of } 0.1N \text{ } AgNO_3 \equiv 3.55 \text{ g of } Cl^-$$

or,   1 c.c. of 0.1N $AgNO_3 \equiv 3.55$ mg of Cl^-

Reagents

For the sake of convenience in calculation, the following solutions of given concentration are prepared.

1. Silver nitrate solution. Dissolve 29.07 g of pure $AgNO_3$ in distilled water and make up to 1 litre. Store in a dark coloured bottle; 1 c.c. of this solution is equivalent to 10 mg of NaCl.

2. Ammonium thioeyanate solution. Dilute 100 c.c. of N thiocyanate solution to 585 c.c. Standardize this solution against standard $AgNO_3$ solution and adjust its concentration such that 1 c.c. of this solution is equivalent to 1 c.c. of $AgNO_3$ solution prepared in 1.

3. Con. HNO_3

4. Indicator Solution. Prepare a cold saturated solution of A.R. ferric ammonium sulphate in water and add a few drops of 6M HNO_3.

Procedure

(i) Take 10 c.c. of urine into a 100 c.c. conical flask. Add 2 c.c. of con. HNO_3 and 2 c.c. of indicator solution and then 40 c.c. of $AgNO_3$ solution by means of a burette. Shake the contents of the flask and let it stand for 5 minutes.

(ii) Filter quantitatively (wash the ppt 3—4 times), collect the filtrate and washings in a 100 c.c. measuring flask and make up the volume to 100 c.c. by adding distilled water.

(iii) Pipette out 25 c.c. of the filtrate into a 100 c.c. conical flask and titrate with standard NH_4CNS solution until a light reddish brown colour is obtained (due to the formation of ferric thiocyanate). Repeat the titration with another 25 c.c. portion of the filtrate. Suppose the titre value is x c.c.

Calculation

$$\text{1 c.c. of } NH_4CNS \text{ solution} \equiv 1 \text{ c.c. of } AgNO_3 \text{ solution}$$

∴ x c.c. of NH_4CNS solutions $\equiv x$ c.c. of $AgNO_3$ solution

Now, in 25 c.c. of filtrate unused $AgNO_3 = x$ c.c.

∴ in 100 c.c. of filtrate unused $AgNO_3 = 4x$ c.c.

$$AgNO_3 \text{ solution added} = 40 \text{ c.c.}$$

∴ $AgNO_3$ solution consumed
by 10 c.c. of urine sample $= (40\text{-}4x)$ c.c.

Now, 1 c.c. of $AgNO_3$ solution $\equiv 10$ mg of NaCl

∴ $(40-4x)$ c.c. of $AgNO_3$ solution $\equiv (40-4x) \times 10$ mg NaCl

or, in 100 c.c. of urine sample, the amount of chloride as $NaCl = (40-4x) \times 100$ mg NaCl.

19.E.2.4. Determination of Acidity and Ammonia

The acidity in urine is measured by titration with 0.1 M (=0.1N) NaOH solution using phenolphthalein indicator in presence of potassium oxalate. The added oxalate precipitates calcium as calcium oxalate so that the interference due to the precipitation of calcium phosphate towards the end point is avoided.

After neutralizing the titrable acid in urine, an excess of neutral formalin (formaldehyde solution) is added when the following reaction takes place.

$$4NH_4Cl + 6HCHO \longrightarrow N_4(CH_2)_6 + 6H_2O + 4HCl$$

Thus the ammonium salt present in urine are decomposed liberating HCl which can be determined by titration with standard NaOH solution. Knowing the amount of acid liberated, the quantity of ammonia in urine can be calculated.

$$NH_3 \equiv NH_4Cl \equiv HCl$$

1000 c.c. of N HCl $\equiv 17$ g ammonia

or 1 c.c. of 0.1 N HCl $\equiv 1.7$ mg of ammonia

Reagents

1. Sodium hydroxide solution, 0.1N

2. Potassium oxalate, solid.

3. Phenolphthalein indicator solution.

4. **Neutral Formalin.** (Formalin is an aqueous solution containing about 33 to 37% by weight of formaldehyde). To formalin, 2-3 drops of phenolphthalein indicator solution is added and then a dilute NaOH solution is added dropwise with thorough shaking until a faint pink colour is obtained.

Procedure

Determination of Titrable Acidity

(i) Take 20 c.c. of urine sample into a 250 c.c. conical flask and shake it with 4 g potassium oxalate. Add 2-3 drops of phenolphthalein and titrate with 0.1N NaOH to light pink end point. Note the titre (A c.c.)

(ii) After the titration, add 10 c.c. of neutral formalin to the same titration mixture. The pink colour will disappear as a result of formation of acid. Titrate with 0.1N NaOH solution to light pink end point. Note the titre (B c.c.).

Calculation

$$NaOH \equiv HCl$$

So,   1000 c.c. N NaOH $\equiv$ 36.5 g HCl

or,   1 c.c. 0.1N NaOH $\equiv$ 3.65 mg HCl

$\therefore$ A c.c. 0.1N NaOH $\equiv (3.65 \times A)$ mg HCl

Thus, 20 c.c. of urine sample will contain $(3.65 \times A)$ mg of acid in terms of HCl.

For 100 c.c. urine the titrable acidity will be $(3.65 \times 5 \times A)$ mg of HCl.

Now, $4NH_4Cl \equiv 4NH_3 \equiv 4HCl \equiv 4NaOH$

or, $NaOH \equiv NH_3$ (mol. wt $= 17$)

or,   1000, c.c. N NaOH $\equiv 17$ g NH_3

or,   1 c.c. 0.1 N NaOH $\equiv 1.7$ mg NH_3

Hence, 100 c.c. of urine sample will contain $(1.7 \times 5 \times B)$ mg NH_3

19.E.2.5 Determination of Creatinine

The given urine sample is treated with picric acid in presence of NaOH solution when creatinine present in urine reacts with picric acid to produce an orange colour whose absorbance is measured at 520 nm. A calibration curve is constructed using standard solutions of creatinine. With the help of this curve the amount of creatinine in urine sample is found out.

Reagent

1. Picric acid solution. Dissolve 10 g picric acid in water and make up to 1 litre.

2. Sodium hydroxide solution. Dissolve 30 g NaOH in water and make up to 1 litre.

3. Creatinine solution

(a) *Stock solution.* Dissolve 100 mg of pure creatinine in 0.1N HCl and make up with acid to 100 c.c. so that 1 c.c. solution contains 1 mg creatinine.

(b) *Standard solution.* The stock solution can be suitably diluted to prepare a number of solutions of known concentration.

Procedure

(i) Dilute 1c.c. of urine to 100 c.c.

(ii) In six 200 c.c. volumetric flasks take 1 to 6 c.c. of creatinine stock solution. Add 20 c.c. of 0.1N HCl to each flask and make up to the mark with water. Shake the contents of each flask. Thus six known solutions of ceatinine will be obtained.

(iii) Take 5 c.c. each of solutions of different concentrations in test tubes. Add to each tube 1 c.c. 1% picric acid and 1 c.c. of NaOH solutions. Allow to stand for 15 minutes for colour development. Measure the absorbance in each case and plot a curve between absorbance and concentrations: this is the calibration plot.

(iv) Take 5 c.c. of diluted urine sample and treat it with 1 c.c. of 1% picric acid and 1 c.c. NaOH solution. Keep the mixture for 15 minutes and then measure the absorbance at 520 nm in a spectrophotometer.

(v) Find out the quantity of creatinine in the given volume of urine sample with the help of the calibration plot.

19.F. Analysis of Blood

Blood is a two-phase system of plasma and corpuscles. Thus blood is constituted of the cells which are present in the liquid fraction of the blood called plasma. The cell volume is 45% while that of plasma in 55% of the total volume of the blood. The normal pH of the blood is 7.4. The various chemical constituents of blood are proteins (albumin, globulin and fibrinogen), lipids, glucose, amino acids, urea, uric acid, creatinine, vitamines, hormones, ions of sodium, potassium, magnesium, calcium and chloride, bicarbonate and phosphate. The chemical composition of the blood may be altered by diet, therapy and disease. The concentration of any material in whole blood is an average of the concentrations of that substance in the plasma and in the corpuscles (or cells). Howerver, it is plasma or serum that is used for analysis.

19.F.1 COLLECTION OF BLOOD SAMPLE

Blood sample taken out in the morning before breakfast and after a fast of 12 to 14 hours is more representative. A blood sample is collected in a clean, sterile glass bottle with a plastic cap. The bottle should contain suitable amount of anticoagulant.

19.F.2 ANTICOAGULANTS AND PRESERVATIVES

In a 15 c.c. blood sample 30 mg of powdered potassium oxalate is added which is a good anticoagulant. It is quite soluble in blood but has little preserving power. The blood containing oxalate is called oxalated blood. [Sodium fluoride is both an anticoagulant and preservative. A mixture containing sodium fluoride, thymol and potassium oxalate in weight ratio 10 : 1 : 3 is prepared and 60 mg of this mixture is added to 15 c.c. of blood.]

19.F.3 SEPARATION OF PLASMA

The sample of oxalated blood is centrifugalized at about 2000 r.p.m. for 10 minutes when plasma separates out in the form of a pale yellow liquid. Plasma should be seperated from blood cells as soon as possible.

19.F.4 SEPARATION OF SERUM

To 10 c.c. of oxalated blood 0.5 c.c. of 2.5% $CaCl_2$ solution is added when the blood clots. Calcium ions precipitate oxalate ions as CaC_2O_4 and additional calcium ions cause clotting. The clotted blood is kept for an hour when a fluid separates which is transferred to a tube and centrifugalised. The supernatant liquid is the serum which is light yellow in colour. Plasma and serum are chemically the same, the only difference is that serum does not contain fibrinogen.

19.F.5 QUALITATIVE ANALYSIS OF SERUM

19.F.5.1 Test for Albumin

Add 2 c.c. of saturated $(NH_4)_2SO_4$ solution to 2 c.c. of serum when globulin precipitates out. After filtration, the filtrate is subjected to the biuret test as described below.

The filtrate is treated with 4 c.c. of 5% NaOH and then 3 to 4 dops of 1% $CuSO_4$ solution. On mixing a purple colour is obtained which shows the presence of albumin (which was not precipitated along with globulin).

19.F.5.2 Test for Fibrin

In a small beaker, take 0.5 c.c. plasma, 15 c.c. water and 0.5 c.c. 2.5% $CaCl_2$ solution. Allow to stand for 20 minutes at 37 °C in an incubator. Collect a transparent clot formed with the help of a glass rod by pressing it against the wall of the beaker. The clot is fibrin which is the insoluble form of fibrinogen. Place the fibrin in normal saline to remove the adhering proteins then dissolve it in 5 c.c. of 5% NaOH. Carry out biuret test as described in 19.F.5.1. It the test is positive, fibrin is present.

19.F.5.3 Deproteinisation of Serum

Proteins present in the blood interfere with many other determination hence proteins must be removed from the blood sample before performing further analysis.

The proteins of the blood are removed by precipitation with tungstic acid by means of the following method of Folin and Wu.

A solution of sodium tungstate ($Na_2WO_4.2H_2O$) is prepared by dissolving 100 g of the reagent in water. (This solution is made neutral to phenolphthalein indicator by adding suitable quantities of 0.1 N HCl or 0.1 N NaOH as the case may be). Finally the neutral solution is diluted to 1 litre. A solution of H_2SO_4 of normality 0.66 is also prepared.

One volume of serum is mixed with 8 volumes of water, 0.5 volume of 10% sodium tungstate and 0.5 volume of 0.66 N H_2SO_4. The proteins are precipitated which are filtered and the filtrate is collected which is then used for performing other tests.

19.F.5.4 Test for Chlorides

To 1 c.c. of the filtrate add 2 drops of con. HNO_3 and 2 drops of 3% $AgNO_3$ solution. The appearance of a white ppt shows the presence of chlorides.

19.F.5.5   Test for Phosphates

Take 2 c.c. of filtrate and add a few drops of con. HNO_3 and 2 c.c. of ammonium molybdate reagent. Warm the mixture. The formation of a canary yellow ppt indicates the presence of phosphates. [See 19.E.1.3. for the preparation of ammonium molybdate reagent.]

19.F.5.6   Test for Calcium

Place 2 c.c. filtrate in a test tube and add a few drops of a saturated solution of ammonium oxalate. If white ppt is produced, the presence of calcium is indicated.

19.F.5.7   Test for Glucose

To 0.5 c.c. filtrate add 1 c.c. Folin's alkaline $CuSO_4$ solution. Mix and keep the mixture dipped in boiling water for 5 minutes. Cool and add 1 c.c. of phosphomolybdic acid reagent. Appearance of a deep blue colour shows the presence of glucose.

[**Folin's Alkaline Copper Sulphate Reagent.** Dissolve 40 g anhydrous sodium carbonate in 400 c.c. water then add 7.5 g tartaric acid and dissolve. In another beaker dissolve 4.5 g $CuSO_4.5 H_2O$ in 100 c.c of water. Add this solution to the first solution gradually with constant stirring and make up the volume to 1 litre.

Phosphomolybdic Acid Reagent Dissove 35 g molybdic acid and 5 g sodium tungstate in 200 c.c. of 10% NaOH. Add 200 c.c. water and boil until the liberation of NH_3 ceases. Cool, transfer to a 500 c.c. measuring flask and dilute to 350 c.c. Add 125 c.c. 85% phosphoric acid, make up the volume to 500 c.c. and mix well.]

19.F.5.8   Test for Urea

Add 0.2 c.c. of horsegram suspension (10%) to 0.5 c.c. filtrate. (If the filtrate contains urea it is converted into ammonium carbonate by the enzyme urease present in horsegram). Warm and keep for 10 minutes. Add 5 c.c. water and filter. To the filtrate add 2 c.c. Nessler's reagent which gives a brownish yellow colour with ammonium salts. Thus the formation of brown colour indicates the presence of urea.

19.F.5.9   Test for Uric Acid

To 0.5 c.c. filtrate add 1 c.c. of 10% Na_2CO_3 solution and 1 c.c. of phosphotungstic acid. If a blue colour is developed, the presence of uric acid is indicated. [Sec 19.E.1.6. for the preparation of phosphotungstic acid reagent.]

19.F.5.10.   Test for Creatinine

Take 1 c.c. of filtrate and add 0.5 c.c. of 1% picric acid and then 0.5 c.c. of 10% NaOH. A change of colour from yellow to orange indicates the presence of creatinine.

19.F.6   QUANTITATIVE ANALYSIS OF BLOOD

This section describes method for the determination of certain important constituents of blood.

19 F.6.1 Determination of Blood Sugar (Folin and Wu method)

In this method, blood is deproteinised by tungstic acid when proteins. are precipitated and can be separated by filtration. The filtrate is heated with alkaline copper sulphate solution. The glucose present in the blood sample reduces copper sulphate to cuprous oxide which is then treated with phosphomolybdic reagent. Cuprous oxide reduces the reagent to blue coloured oxides of molybenum. The colour intensity is proportional to the quantity of glucose present in the blood sample and it can be measured at 680 nm by means of a photoelectric colorimeter or a spectrophotometer. A calibration curve is constructed using known solutions of glucose and with the help of this curve the amount of glucose in the given blood sample is found out.

Reagents

1. **Sodium Tungstate Solution. 10%**
2. **Sulphuric Acid, 0.66 N.**
3. **Alkaline CuSO$_4$ Solution.** Folin's alkaline copper reagent prepared as described in 19.F.5.7.
4. **Phosphomolybdic acid.** Prepared as described in 19.F.5.7.
5. **Glucose, Stock Solution, 0.1%.** Dissolve 100 mg of glucose in 100 c.c. of saturated benzoic acid solution.
6. **Glucose, Standard Solution, 0.01%.** Dilute 10 c.c. of the stock solution to 100 c.c. with water just before the measurement.

Procedure

(i) Take 7 c.c. of water in a dry test tube and introduce 1 c.c. of oxalated blood into the tube. Add 1 c.c. of 10% sodium tungstate and 1 c.c. of 0.66 N sulphuric acid so that the total volume becomes 10 c.c. Shake the tube vigorously and allow to stand for a few minutes. A ppt will be formed; it should be chocolate in colour, if not add a drop of 9 N H$_2$SO$_4$. Mix and keep the tube for a few more minutes. Filter and collect the filtrate in a dry test tube.

(ii) Take three Folin's tube (see Fig. 19.27) and mark them A, B, and C for standard (std), test and blank. Make the additions into these tubes as shown below.

	A (std) c.c.	B (test) c.c.	C (blank) c.c.
Glucose, 0.01%	2.0	—	—
Protein free filtrate	—	2.0	—
Water	—	—	2.0
Alkaline copper sulphate reagent	2.0	2.0	2.0
Total volume	4.0	4.0	4.0

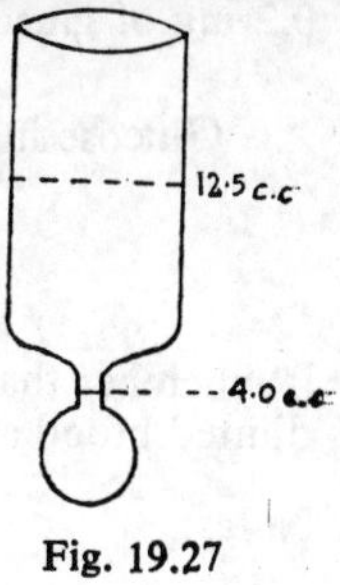

Fig. 19.27

(iii) Mix the contents of each tube and keep the tubes immersed in boiling water for 8 minutes so that glucose reduces CuSO$_4$ to Cu$_2$O.

(iv) After 8 minutes take out the tubes from boiling water, cool immediately under tap water for 1 minute and without delay add 2.0 c.c. phosphomolybdic acid reagent to each tube. Blue colour will appear in tubes A and B (remember the C is the blank). Mix the contents of the tubes until the effervescence cease (CO_2 will be liberated due to reaction between Na_2CO_3 present in alkaline $CuSO_4$ and acid). Keep the tubes again in boiling water for 1 minute. Cool, make up the volume to 12.5 c.c. in each tube and mix the contents thoroughly.

[The concentration is directly proportional to the absorbance. Hence the amount of glucose in the blood sample can be found out by measuring absorbance of test solution at 680 nm (using red filter) and comparing it with that of the standard glucose solution after identical treatment.

The colour comparison can be done by a visual colorimeter but the use of a photoelectric colorimeter or a spectrophotometer is preferred which gives more accurate results.]

(V) Place the tube (C) containing the blank in the sample holder of a photoelectric colorimeter and set transmission to 100% using red filter (680 mm). Read % transmission (T) for both std and test solution. Convert % T to absorbance (A).

Calculation

Since absorbance (A) $\propto$ concentration (C)

Absorbance of test solution (AT) $\propto$ con. of test solution (CT)

Abrorbance of std solution (AS) $\propto$ con. of std solution (CS)

$$\therefore \quad \frac{AT}{AS} = \frac{CT}{CS} \qquad \therefore \quad CT = \frac{AT}{AS} \times CS$$

Thus glucose in 0.2 c.c. blood $(CT) = \dfrac{AT}{AS} \times 0.2$ mg

[Standard glucose solution is 0.01% i.e., 100 c.c. solution contains 10 mg glucose $\therefore$ 1 c.c. solution will contain 0.1 mg or 2 c.c. solution will contain 0.2 mg of glucose.]

$$\therefore \quad \text{Glucose in 100 c.c. test solution} = \frac{100}{0.2} \times \frac{AT}{AS} \times 0.2 \text{ mg}$$

$$= \frac{AT}{AS} \times 100 \text{ mg}$$

[Remember that 1 c.c. of blood sample was diluted to 10 c.c. and 2 c.c. of diluted blood sample was used in colorimetric measurement.]

Notes:

1. A calibration curve can be constructed by taking several known solutions of glucose and measuring their absorbance. The absorbance of test solution is also measured and the amount of glucose in it can be found out with the help of the calibration. This procedure will give more accurate result.

2. When the volume of the reaction mixture is 4 c.c., its level in the Folin's tube is in the constriction area (see Fig. 19.27) which is the minimum. Now, the cuprous oxide formed is oxidized by atmospheric oxygen but because the area of the solution exposed to air is minimum the oxidation of cuprous oxide is negligible.

3. Glucose is rapidly oxidised in blood hence, to blood sample a preservative should be added. A mixture of sodium fluoride and potassium oxalate in 1 : 3 ratio acts as a preservative as well as anticoagulant.

4 It should be remembered that in the method of Folin and Wu the result includes the amount of glucose as well as the amounts of non-glucose reducing substances present in the blood. Hence, the values obtained do not represent true glucose and are higher. The value obtained by this method should therefore be termed *blood sugar*. The normal range of blood sugar by this method is 80-120 mg per 100 c.c.

5. In Nelson and Somogyi method for determining blood sugar deproteinisation is done by zinc hydroxide. The advantage of zinc hydroxide is that cuprous oxide is stable in its presence. The results obtained by this method are nearer to the glucose value hence are less than those obtained by the method of Folin and Wu. The normal range of blood sugar by this method is 70-100 mg per 100 c.c.

19.F.6.2 Determination of Blood Urea (Vanslyke's method)

In this method, urea present in blood is mixed with enzyme urease when urea is converted into ammonium carbonate. This salt is treated with K_2CO_3 to liberate NH_3 which is absorbed in a known excess of H_2SO_4 Later the unused acid is titrated back with standard alkali solution. Knowing the amount of the acid consumed, the amount of NH_3 liberated and hence the quantity of urea in the blood sample can be calculated. The reactions involved are

$$CO(NH_2)_2 \xrightarrow[\substack{H_2O}]{\text{Urease}} (NH_4)_2CO_3 \xrightarrow{K_2CO_3} 2NH_3 + 2KHCO_3$$

$$2NH_3 + H_2SO_4 \rightarrow (NH_4)_2SO_4$$

$$H_2SO_4 \equiv 2NH_3 \equiv CO(NH_2)_2 \qquad [\text{Mol wt} = 60]$$

1000 c.c. M $H_2SO_4 \equiv 60$ g Urea

1000 c.c. N $H_2SO_4 \equiv 30$ g Urea

$$\left[\text{For } H_2SO_4, \text{ eq wt} = \frac{\text{mol wt}}{2} \right]$$

1000 c.c. 0.01N $H_2SO_4 \equiv 0.3$ g Urea

1 c.c. 0.01N $H_2SO_4 \equiv 0.3$ mg Urea

Procedure

In a glass tube 3 c.c. of blood sample is taken and urease is added. Ammonia free air is drawn through the reaction mixture so that urea is converted to $(NH_4)_2CO_3$. Then K_2CO_3 is added and NH_3 free air is drawn through the tube to sweep out the liberated NH_3 gas. The swept out NH_3 is received in 20 c.c. of 0.01N H_2SO_4. After about 30 minutes the unused acid is titrated with 0.01N NaOH using methyl red as indicator.

Calculations

   (i) The volume of blood sample $=3.0$ c.c.

   (ii) The volume of 0.01N H_2SO_4 taken $=20.0$ c.c.

   (iii) The volume of 0.01N NaOH required $=x$ c.c. for titrating the unused acid

   (iv) The volume of 0.01N H_2SO_4 used $=(20-x)$ c.c. in neutralizing the liberated NH_3 gas

Now,   1 c.c. of 0.01N $H_2SO_4 \equiv 0.3$ mg Urea

$\therefore$ $(20-x)$ c.c. 0.01N $H_2SO_4 \equiv (20-x) \times 0.3$ mg Urea

       3 c.c. of blood contains $(20-x) \times 0.3$ mg Urea

$\therefore$ 100 c.c. of blood contains $\dfrac{(20-x) \times 0.3 \times 100}{3}$

$\therefore$ Blood urea $=(20-x)$ 10 mg/100 c.c.

19.F.6.3   Determination of Urea by Colorimetic Method

Urea present in blood is converted into ammonium carbonate by means of enzyme urease. The proteins present in blood and the enzyme are precipitated by adding a freshly prepared tungstic acid solution. The mixture is centrifuged. The supernatant liquid containing ammonium salt is treated with Nessler's reagent and the colour produced is measured at 480 mm. A calibration curve is constructed using known solutions of urea and with the help of this curve the amount of urea in blood sample is found out.

Reagent

1. *Blood sample,* which has been oxalated with NH_4^+ free potassium oxalate.

2. *Urease suspension,* 10% in phosphate buffer of pH 7.0.

3. *Sodium tungstate,* 10%.

4. *Sulphuric acid,* 0.66 N.

5. *Urea, stock solution,* 0.8% containing a few drops of $CHCl_3$.

6. *Urea, standard solution,* 0.04%. 1 c.c. of this solution will contain 0.4 mg of Urea.

7. *Nessler's reagent.* In a flask mix 150 g KI, 100 g I_2, 100 c.c. water and 150 g Hg and shake the contents vigorously. Cool the flask under tap water. Decant the solution and wash the mercury with water. Dilute the solution and washings to 2 litre. This is the stock solution.

Take 350 c.c. of 10% NaOH and add 75 c.c. of the stock solution and make up the volume to 1 litre. Shake well. This is the reagent solution.

Procedure

(i) Take three centrifuge tubes, mark them A, B and C and make the additions into theses tubes as shown below.

	A (std) c.c.	B (test) c.c.	C (blank) c.c.
Water	2.0	2.0	2.2
Blood	—	0.2	—
Urea, 0.04%	0.2	—	—
Buffered urease suspension	0.2	0.2	0.2
Total volume	2.4	2.4	2.4

(ii) Mix gently each tube and incubate in a water bath at 55 °C for 15 minutes. The urea present in blood is converted into ammonium carbonate. Add 0.3 c.c. of 10% sodium tungstate and 0.3 c.c. of 0.66 N H_2SO_4 to each tube. Mix well, allow to stand for a few minutes and add 5.0 c.c. water to each tube. (Note that the volume in each tube will be $2.4+0.3+0.3+5.0=8.0$ c.c.). Shake well and then centrifuge for 5 minutes.

(iii) Transfer 5.0 c.c. of supernatant liquid from each tube to three corresponding dry test tubes marked A, B and C. To each tube add 5.0 c.c. water and 2.0 c.c. Nessler's reagent. Mix well and immediately take the readings in a photoelectric colorimeter at 480 mm, after setting blank at 100% T.

Calculation

$$CT = \frac{AT}{AS} \times CS \quad \text{[See calculation in 19.F.6.1]}$$

CS = con. of urea in standard solution

Note that 1 c.c. of standard urea solution contains 0.4 mg urea, 0.2 c.c. of this solution was diluted to 8 c.c. in step (ii). Out of these 8 c.c., 5 c.c. were taken for measurement in step (iii).

Now, 1 c.c. standard solution contains 0.4 mg Urea

$$\therefore \quad 0.2 \text{ c.c.} \quad \ldots \quad \ldots \quad \ldots \quad \frac{0.2 \times 0.4}{1} = 0.08 \text{ mg Urea}$$

In step (ii) the volume became 8 c.c. hence, 8 c.c., solution contained 0.08 mg urea. Out of 8 c.c., 5 c.c. solution was taken for measurement.

Now, 8 c.c. solution contained 0.08 mg Urea

$$\therefore \quad 5 \text{ c.c. solution contained } \frac{0.08 \times 5}{8} = 0.05 \text{ mg Urea}$$

$\therefore$ Con. of Urea in standard solution (CS) = 0.05 mg

$$CT = \frac{AT}{AS} \times 0.05 \text{ mg}$$

It should be noted that 0.2 c.c. blood was diluted to 8 c.c. in step (ii) and out of this 5 c.c. solution was taken in step (iii), hence the volume of blood in the sample solution will become

$$\frac{0.2 \times 5}{8} = 0.125 \text{ c.c.}$$

Thus, urea in 0.125 c.c. blood $= \dfrac{AT}{AS} \times 0.05$ mg

$\therefore$ urea in 100 c.c. blood $= \dfrac{AT}{AS} \times \dfrac{0.05 \times 100}{0.125}$ mg

     % blood urea $= \dfrac{AT}{AS} \times 40$ mg.

A more accurate procedure is to prepare a calibration curve using known solutions of urea and then using this curve to determine the amount of urea in the given blood sample.

19.F.6.4 Determination of Serum Uric Acid

After deproteinisation, serum is treated with phosphotungstic acid and sodium carbonate when a blue colour is produced whose intensity is measured at 700 nm.

Reagent

1. *Serum.*
2. *Sodium tungstate*, 10%.
3. *Sulphuric acid*, 0.66N.
4. *Phosphotungstic acid* (for preparation, see 19.E.1.6).
5. *Uric acid, stock solution.* Dissolve 100 mg uric acid in 300 c.c. of 0.77% soudium tetraborate solution, add 0.9 c.c. of glacial acetic acid and make up the volume to 500 c.c.
6. *Uric acid, working standard solution.* Dilute 2.0 c.c. of stock solution to 100 c.c.; 1 c.c. of this solution will contain 0.004 mg of uric acid.

Procedure

(i) Take 7.0 c.c. water in a test tube, add 1.0 c.c. of serum and then 1 c.c. of tungstate and 1 c.c. of H_2SO_4. Mix, allow to stand for 5 minutes and then filter. Thus protein free filtrate is obtained which contains serum.

(ii) Mark three test tubes A, B and C. Make the following additions.

	A (std.) c.c.	B (test) c.c.	C (blank) c.c.
Uric acid, std. soln.	5.0	—	—
Protein free filtrate	—	5.0	—
Water	—	—	5.0

(iii) To each tube add 1.0 c.c. 10% Na_2CO_3 and 1.0 c.c. phosphotungstic reagent. Mix and allow to stand for 30 minutes. Set blank to 100% T and measure the transmittance of std and test solutions. Convert transmittance (T) to absorbance (A)

Calculation

$$CT = \frac{AT}{AS} \times CS$$

$$\left[\begin{array}{l} \text{1 c.c. std uric acid soln.} = 0.004 \text{ mg of acid} \\ \therefore \quad 5 \text{ c.c.} \quad \ldots \quad \ldots \quad 0.02 \text{ mg uric acid} \\ \therefore \quad CS = 0.02 \text{ mg} \end{array} \right]$$

Now, 1 c.c. of serum was diluted to 10 c.c. in step (i) and out of this 5 c.c. serum was taken for photometric measurement. It means that 0.5 c.c. serum was present in test solution hence $CT = 0.5$ c.c. Thus Uric acid in 0.5 c.c. serum

$$(CT) = \frac{AT}{AS} \times 0.02 \text{ mg}$$

$\therefore$ Uric acid in 100 c.c. serum

$$= \frac{AT}{AS} \times \frac{0.02}{0.5} \times 100 \text{ mg}$$

% uric acid $\qquad = \frac{AT}{AS} \times 4 \text{ mg}$

An alternative procedure is to construct a calibration curve with known uric acid solutions and use it for finding out the amount of uric acid in the given blood sample.

19.F.6.5 Determination of Serum Proteins

The serum sample is mixed with 28% Na_2S solution. A measured volume from this mixture is taken out in a test tube for determining the total proteins. The rest of the mixture is filtered and the filtrate is used for determining albumin.

A known volume of the filtrate is treated with biuret reagent and allowed to stand for 15 minutes at 37 °C. The colour developed is measured at 540 nm in a photoelectric colorimeter. A cabiration curve is constructed which is then used for determining albumin in the serum sample. A similar procedure is used for finding out total proteins.

19.F.6.6 Determination of Serum Cholesterol

The given serum sample is treated with ferric chloride-acetic acid reagent to precipitate proteins. The filtrate contains proteins free serum which is treated with con. H_2SO_4 and the intensity of purple colour developed is measured at 560 mm.

19.F.6.7 Determination of Serum Calcium

In serum, calcium is found as free ionic calcium as well as protein bound calcium. The total calcium is precipitated by adding ammonium oxalate solution. The resultant ppt of calcium oxalate is dissolved in H_2SO_4 when oxalic acid is formed which is titrated with a standard solution of $KMnO_4$. Knowing the amount of oxalic acid formed, the quantity of calcium in the serum sample is calculated.

$$5Ca^{2+} \equiv 5CaC_2O_4 \equiv 5H_2C_2O_4 \equiv 2KMnO_4$$

$$2KMnO_4 \equiv 200.5 \text{ g Ca}$$

1000 c.c. M $KMnO_4 \equiv 100.25$ g Ca

1000 c.c. N $KMnO_4 \equiv 20.05$ g Ca

1   c.c. N $KMnO_4 \equiv 20.05$ mg Ca

1 c.c. 0.1 N $KMnO_4 \equiv 2.005$ mg Ca.

19.F.6.8   Determination of Serum Phosphate

To the given serum sample, trichloroacetic acid is added to precipitate the proteins. The proteins-free filtrate is treated with molybdate reagent when phosphomolybdic acid is formed which on reduction gives a blue colour. The intensity of this colour is measured at 680 mm using a photoelectric colorimeter. The intensity of the colour is proportional to the amount of phosphorus. Thus the above reaction is used for the colorimetric determination of phosphorus.

20

Gas Analysis and Gasometric Methods

In section 1.3.7 a reference was made to *gas analysis* and *gasometric methods*. A brief description of these methods will be made in this chapter.

20.1 THE CLASSIFICATION OF METHODS OF GAS ANALYSIS

The methods of gas analysis are used to find out the composition of a gas mixture. These methods can be divided into three categories.

 A. Volumetric methods
 B. Titration methods
 C. Physical methods

20.1.A VOLUMETRIC METHODS

In these methods, a known volume of the given gas mixture is taken at a known temperature (T) and pressure (P). (Remember that the volume of a gas depends upon its T and P). By qualitative analysis the different constituent gases of the mixture are found out. Then for a particular constituent, say gas A, such a solution is selected which will absorb only A but not the other gases present in the mixture. When the entire gas mixture is shaken with the absorbent solution, only gas A is absorbed, hence there is a decrease in the volume of the gas mixture coming out of the absorbent solution. This decrease in the volume of the gas mixture is measured which is equal to the volume of the gas A present in the mixture. In a similar manner, the volumes of other component gases of the mixture are found out by using suitable absorbent solutions.

Example 20 (i)

A gas mixture is given whose composition is to be determined. The mixture was first analysed qualitatively and was found to contain only four gases N_2, O_2, CO and CO_2. The volumes of these gases present in the mixture can be determined by using the following procedure.

 (i) A known volume (100 c.c.) of the given gas mixture is taken at atmospheric pressure and room temperature (which can be readily measured).

 (ii) It is known that a solution of KOH absorbs only CO_2 but not N_2, O_2 and CO. The entire gas mixture is shaken throughly with a solution of KOH when all the CO_2 present in the gas mixture is absorbed but not N_2, O_2 and CO. The volume of the remaining gas mixture which contains

N_2, O_2 and CO_2 is measured at room temperature and atmospheric pressure; suppose this volume comes out to be 78 c.c. Then the volume of the CO_2 gas present in the gas mixture would be $(100-78)=22$ c.c.

(iii) The remaining gas mixture (78 c.c.) containing N_2, O_2 and CO is then shaken with an alkaline solution of pyrogallol whick absorbs only O_2 and not N_2 and CO. The volume of this remaining mixture containing N_2 and CO is measured, suppose it is found to be 58 c.c. Then $(78-58)=20$ c.c. is the volume of O_2 in the gas mixture.

(iv) The remaining gas mixture (58 c.c.) containing N_2 and CO is shaken with an ammonical solution of cuprous chloride when CO is absorbed leaving back N_2. Suppose the volume of the remaining gas is 23 c.c., then $(58-23)=35$ c.c. is the volume of CO in the gas mixture.

(v) The only remaining gas is now N_2 whose volume will obviously be equal to 23 c.c.

In this way, the gas mixture can be quantitatively analysed. Following are the results of the analysis : 100 c.c, of the gas mixture at room temperature (T) and atmospheric pressure (P) contains.

$$22 \text{ c.c. } CO_2$$
$$20 \text{ c.c. } O_2$$
$$35 \text{ c.c. } CO$$
and $$23 \text{ c.c. } N_2$$

The volume of N_2 is found out indirectly by subtracting the sum of the volumes of CO_2, O_2 and CO from the volume of the gas mixture taken for analysis i.e.,

$$[100-(22+20+35)]$$
$$= 100-77=23 \text{ c.c.}$$

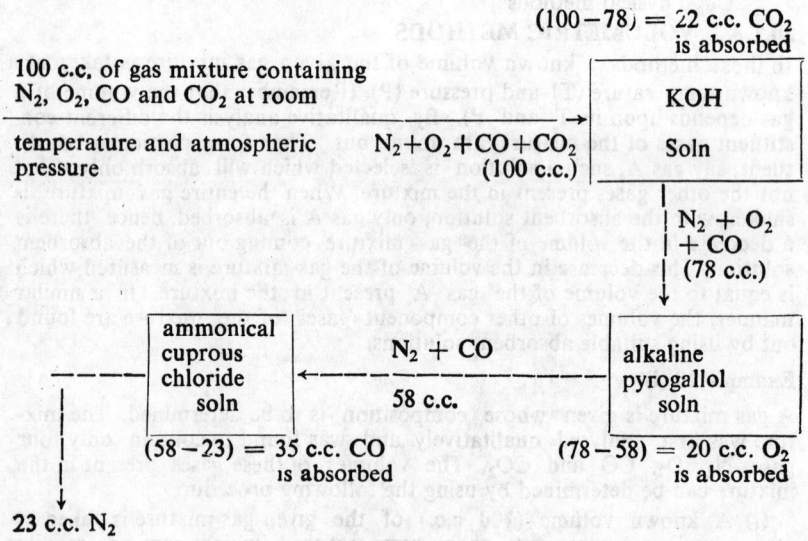

Note. In using the volumetric method of gas analysis the following points must be remembered.

1. The volume of a gas (or gas mixture) depends upon pressure (P) and temperature (T) to which it is subjected. Hence, whenever the volume (V) of a gas is reported it should be reduced to the corresponding value of volume (V_0) at 0°C and 760 mm of mercury; these are termed as standard conditions of temperature and pressure or in brief S.T.P. If we have a dry gas having volume V at t°C and at a pressure P', then its volume (V_0) at S.T.P. is given by

$$V_0 = \frac{PV}{T} \times \frac{T_0}{P_0}$$

or, $\quad V_0 = \frac{PV}{(273+t)} \times \frac{273}{760}$

Remember

For a given mass of a gas

$$\frac{P_0 V_0}{T_0} = \frac{PV}{T}$$

In the present case

P = P $\qquad$ P_0 = 760 mm

V = V $\qquad$ V_0 = to be found

T = (273 + t) T_0 = 273°A

If the gas measured is wet i.e., saturated with water vapour, the vapour pressure (p) of water at the experimental temperature must be deducted from the gas pressure. For such a case

$$V_0 = \frac{(P-p)V}{(273+t)} \times \frac{273}{760} \text{ c.c.}$$

where, p = vapour pressure of water at t°C.

It is extremly important to follow a proper-sequence (or order) for shaking the gas mixture with different absorbent solutions. In example 20 (i), the correct sequence is KOH, alkaline pyrogallol and ammonical cuprous chloride solution. If this order is changed the results obtained will be incorrect. If the order is changed to aqueous alkaline pyrogallol, KOH and ammonical cuprous chloride, then on shaking with alkaline aqueous pyrogallol solution both CO_2 and O_2 will be absorbed because CO_2 is soluble in water. Hence, the decrease in the volume of the gas mixture will be the sum of the volumes of CO_2 and O_2.

The proper sequence is so planned that the first absorbent absorbs only one constituent gas of the mixture but not others. The next absorbent solution then absorbs only one of the remaining constituents and so on.

20. 1.A 1 Apparatus used in Gas Analysis

In a volumetric method of gas analysis the only measurement involved is that of the volume of a gas or gas mixture. Hence, the accuracy of the method depends upon the accuracy with which the volumes of different gases are measured. For measuring gas volume different kinds of burettes are available. Here we will consider the simplest type known as *Hempel gas burette*. Fig. 20.1 shows a modified from of Hempel burette called *Hempel-Winckler burette*.

Hempel-Winckler Gas Burette

It consists of tubes A and B. Tube B has a capacity of more than 100 c.c. and it is graduated; this is the proper burette. In the modified form of Hempel burette Tube B has three-way tap E at the upper end. (In certain burettes there is a three-way tap at the lower end of the tube also). The graduated tube B (which is actually the burette) is connected to another ungraduated tube A by means of a long pressure rubber tubing. Both the tubes are mounted on heavy metallic stands C and D. Tube A is called the pressure or levelling tube. By adjusting the height of tube A. the air from the tube B can be driven out and the pressure of gas in B can be made equal to the atmospheric pressure (see Fig. 20.1).

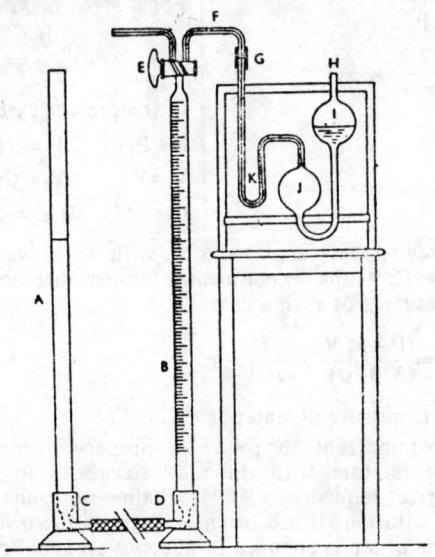

Fig. 20.1

Hempel Gas Pipette

The part of the apparatus on the right side of tube B in Fig. 20.1 is the *Hempel gas pipette*. It consists of two large bulbs I and J connected to each other. The capacity of bulb J is about 100 c.c. and that of I is about 150 c.c. The pipette is used to subject the gas mixture, taken in the burette, to the action of absorbent liquid taken in bulb J.

Manipulation of the Hempel Gas Apparatus

The experimental details for using Hempel gas analysis apparatus are given below.

(i) *Driving out air from the gas burette.* Since in the gas analysis we measure the volume of a gas or a gas mixture, it is important that the gas analysis apparatus must not contain any air otherwise the gas volume recorded will be incorrect. Hence, the first step of gas analysis is to drive out the air from the gas measuring apparatus. This is done in the following manner.

Saturate water with the given gas mixture. Open tap E and pour saturated water into tube A. Drive out air from the tube connecting A and B, by raising and lowering the tubes alternately. Then raise tube A until water begins to flow from open tap E so that all the air from the gas burette B is expelled. Then close the tap E.

(ii) *Introduction of 100 c.c. of gas mixture into the gas burette.* Connect tap E to the supply of gas mixture to be analysed. Lower the tube A so that little more than 100 c.c. of the gas mixture entres the tube B. Close the tap E. Adjust the height of the tubes and manipulate tap E in such a way that the volume of the gas mixture in B is exactly 100 c.c. when the levels of water in two tubes are the same.

(iii) *Absorption of one of the constituents of the gas mixture.* The absorbent solution is poured into bulb I through the opening H. The air is then sucked in through the capillary tube G so that the solution comes into the bulb J. The solution should reach the siphon bend of the capillary K and bulb I should become nearly empty. Blow air through H so that the liquid level rises to the top of the capillary tube K and then connect K and F through a rubber tube G. Open tap E and lower tube B and slowly raise the levelling tube A, thus drive the gas from the burrette into the pipette. Move the pipette stand forward and backward so that the constituent gas to be removed is completely absorbed. Open tap E, and lower the tube A to draw back the remaining gas mixture into the burette. Record the remaining volume of the gas mixture and subtract it from the original volume of the mixture taken; this will give the volume of the constituent gas that has been absorbed.

The absorption of a constituent may not be complete in one operation. Hence, it shupld be repeated until the reading for the volume of the mixture becomes constant i.e., there is no further decrease in the volume of the remaining gas mixture. Then another absorbent is taken in the gas pipette which absorbs only one of the constituents of the remaining mixture. In this way by taking different absorbent solutions successivelv, the volumes of different gases present in the gas mixture can be measured at room temperature and atmospheric pressure. Then these volumes are reduced to the corresponding values at S.T.P.

[Note: 1. A gas mixture may contain a gas like CO_2, SO_2 or NH_3 which is soluble in water. In such a case the levelling tube containing water cannot be used. The clean burette (tube B) is thoroughly dried by washing it successively with alcohol and ether or by acetone alone then drawing air through it. The dry burette is filled with 100 c.c. gas mixture and then connected to the levelling tube A containing water. The lower tap of the burette is opened so that water enters the burette and the soluble component of the gas mixture is dissolved. The decrease in the volume of the gas mixture can be read directly by the burette which is equal to the volume of the soluble gas present in he mixture.

2. In many burettes, mercury is used as confining liquid to contain the sample of the gas mixture. Mercury is a good containing liquid and can be used when more than one water soluble gas is present in the gas mixture

However, it cannot be used when chlorine, hydrogen sulphide, sulphur dioxide or nitrous oxide gas is present. The disadvantage with mercury is that it is expensive, poisonous and quite heavy so that is difficult to handle.

3.   Water is a good replacement for mercury as a confining liquid as it is readily available but the problem is that it is a good solvent for many gases. The solubility of gases in water is less if it contains sodium chloride and hydrochloric acid.]

20..1.A.2.   Absorbents for various Gases

The selection of suitable absorbents for various component gases of a mixture is an important step in the volumetric method of gas analysis. Another important point is to follow a proper order in which gas mixture is shaken with different absorbent solution. The constituents of a gas mixture are usually determined in the following order.

1.   **Carbon dioxide.** About 30% KOH solution is used for absorbing CO_2 gas. Sodium hydroxide solution is not recommended as its bicarbonate has a tendency to crystallise out, but potassium bicarbonate is more soluble. It should be remembered that acidic gases like H_2S, SO_2, HCl, oxides of nitrogen are also absorbed by KOH hence should be removed first by absorption with a suitable solution.

2.   **Unsaturated hydrocarbons.** (These are not absorbed by KOH solution). Con. H_2SO_4 containing silver sulphate or vanadium pentoxide is used as absorbent for unsaturated hydrocarbons. A five percent solution of KBr saturated with Br_2 can also be used. But both con. H_2SO_4 and bromine water attack mercury.

3.   **Oxygen.** Alkaline pyrogallol solution is generally used as an absorbent for oxygen. But it cannot be employed if the gas mixture contains acidic gases like CO_2 and SO_2, unless these are removed first by some suitable absorbent.

Chromous chloride in dilute HCl can also be used for absorbing O_2. This reagent reacts with oxygen in accordance with the equation

$$4Cr^{2+}+4H^++O_2 \rightarrow 4Cr^{3+}+2H_2O$$

Another absorbent for O_2 is sodium dithionite which reacts with O_2 according to the equation

$$Na_2S_2O_4 + O_2 + H_2O \rightarrow NaHSO_3 + NaHSO_4$$

Ammonical cuprous chloride solution also acts as an absorber for O_2 but CO must be absent (because CO is also absorbed by amm. CuCl).

Yellow phosphorus in the form of thin sticks can also be employed as a solid reagent for the absorption of O_2.

4.   **Carbon monoxide.** Cuprous chloride solution, both in acidic as well as in alkaline medium absorbs CO. In acidic medium this reagent, combines with CO according to the equation

$$CuCl + 2H_2O + CO \rightarrow CuCl.2H_2O\cdot CO$$

Cuprous chloride in ammonical medium also acts as an absorber of CO. The drawback of this reagent is that it absorbs CO slowly. A better reagent is cuprous sulphate-β-napthol.

5. Hydrogen. Hydrogen combines with O_2 at 100 °C in presence of palladinised asbestos catalyst. But any CO or methane present also gets partly oxidised.

6. Hydrogen and other hydrocarbons. For determining the volume of H_2, CO and hydrocarbons like CH_4, C_2H_6 etc., the gas mixture is subjected to combustion in presence of a known excess of O_2. The volume of CO_2 formed and that of the residual oxygen is recorded. From these measurements, the volume of H_2, CO or CH_4, C_2H_6 etc., can be calculated.

7. Nitrogen. Its volume in the gas mixture is calculated indirectly by subtracting the sum of the volumes of other constituent gases from the volume of the gas mixture taken for analysis.

The usual order of interaction with various absorbents is

(i) KOH solution for CO_2.

(ii) Con. H_2SO_4 in presence of V_2O_5 for unsaturated hydrocarbons.

(iii) Alkaline pyrogallol for O_2.

(iv) Ammonical cuprous chloride for CO.

(v) Oxidation in presence of palladium for H_2

(vi) Oxidation in presence of platinum for H_2 and saturated hydrocarbons

(vii) Nitrogen by difference.

20.1.B TITRATION METHODS OF GAS ANALYSIS

In these methods, the constitutent to be sought is absorbed in a known amount of reagent solution which reacts with the constituent (but not with the other components of the gas mixture). Later the remaining reagent is determined by a suitable titrimetric method. Knowing the amount of the reagent consumed, the quantity of the constituent under consideration can be calculated. For example, consider a mixture containing N_2, O_2 and NH_3 and its composition is to be found out. The gas mixture is passed through a known volume of a standard solution of H_2SO_4, when the following reaction takes place

$$2NH_3 + H_2SO_4 \longrightarrow (NH_4)_2SO_4$$

The unused acid is then titrated with a standard NaOH solution. The amount of acid consumed becomes known so that the amount of NH_3 present in the mixture can be calculated. It should be noted that N_2 and O_2 are not absorbed by H_2SO_4.

Example 20(ii)

A gas mixture containing N_2, O_2, CH_4 and NH_3 was passed through 50.0 c.c. of 0.01N H_2SO_4. Later the unreacted acid required 18.0 c.c. of 0.01N NaOH for neutralisation. Calculate the volume of NH_3 gas present in the mixture at S.T.P. (Given that 1 g mole of ammonia occupies 22,400 cc. at S.T.P.).

(i) 0.01 N acid consumed by NH_3 gas

$$= (50.0 - 18.0) = 32.0 \text{ c.c.}$$

(ii) Wt of acid/litre = normality × eq wt

$$= 0.01 × 49 = 0.49 \text{ g}$$

(iii) 1000 c.c. acid solution contains 0.49 g acid

$$\therefore \quad 32.0 \text{ c.c.} \quad \cdots \quad \cdots \quad \cdots \frac{32}{1000} \times 0.49 = 0.01568 \text{ g acid}$$

(iv) $$2NH_3 + H_2SO_4 \longrightarrow (NH_4)_2SO_4$$
$$ 34 \text{ g} \quad\quad 98g$$

98 g of acid reacts with 34 g NH_3

$$\therefore \quad 0.01568 \text{ g} \quad \cdots \quad \cdots \quad \cdots \frac{0.01568}{98} \times 34$$

$$= 0.00544 \text{ g } NH_3$$

(v) Now, 17 g NH_3 occupies 22,400 c.c. at S.T.P.

$$\therefore \quad 0.00544 \text{ g} \quad \cdots \quad \cdots \frac{0.00544}{17} \times 22.400$$

$$= 7.2 \text{ c.c.}$$

The volume of NH_3 at S.T.P. in the given mixture is found to be 7.2 c.c.

Another example of titration method of gas analysis is provided by the determination of CO by using iodine pentoxide. On passing CO over I_2O_5 heated to 145°C, the following reaction takes place

$$I_2O_5 + 5CO \rightarrow I_2 + 5CO_2$$

The liberated iodine is passed through a standard $Na_2S_2O_3$ solution, and then the remaining thiosulphate is titrated with a standard solution of iodine. Knowing the amount of $Na_2S_2O_3$ consumed, the quantity of iodine produced in the above reaction can be found out and then the amount of CO can be calculated.

Example 20(iii)

A gas mixture containing N_2, O_2 and CO was passed over I_2O_5 at 145°C. The iodine vapour produced were passed through 30.0 c c. of 0.01N $Na_2S_2O_3$ solution. Later the residual $Na_2S_2O_3$ required 10.0 of 0.01N I_2 solution for complete reaction. Find out the volume of CO in the gas mixture. (Given that the molar volume of CO at S.T.P. is 22,400 c.c.).

(i) Volume of 0.01N $Na_2S_2O_3$ consumed

$$= (30.0 - 10.0) = 20.0 \text{ c c.}$$

(ii) $$2Na_2S_2O_3 \equiv I_2 \equiv 5CO$$

or, $$\frac{2}{5} Na_2S_2O_3 \equiv CO$$

or, $$\frac{2000}{5} \text{ c.c. N } Na_2S_2O_3 \equiv CO$$

or $$400 \text{ c.c. N } Na_2S_2O_3 \equiv 22,400 \text{ c.c. CO}$$

or $$400 \text{ c.c. } 0.01N \ Na_2S_2O_3 \equiv 224 \text{ c.c. CO}$$

or $$20 \text{ c.c. } 0.01 \ Na_2S_2O_3 \equiv 11.2 \text{ c.c. CO}$$

The given mixture contains 11.2 c.c. of CO at S.T.P.

The methods described in 20.1.A and 20.1.B are also known as *absorptiometric methods.*

20.1C PHYSICAL METHODS

In these methods are constitutent gases of a mixture are determined by measuring their physical properties such as thermal conductivity, refractive index, density, viscosity etc.

20.2 GAS-VOLUMETRIC OR GASOMETRIC METHODS

In a gas-volumetric or gasometric method, a liquid or a solid sample, to be analysed, is treated with an excess of such reagent which quantitatively liberates a gas. By measuring the volume of this gas, the quantity of the substance present in the given sample can be calculated. Gasometric methods are different from those of gas analysis as these are used for determining a liquid or a solid substance whereas in gas analysis we analyse a gaseous mixture However, since gasometric methods are also based on the measurement of volume of a gas, its technique and apparatus requirements are quite similar to those used in the methods of gas analysis. In this section we will briefly describe a few gasom etric methods.

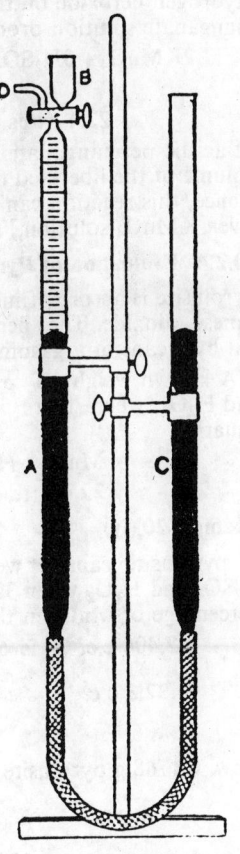

Fig. 20.3

20.2.1 Determination of Semicarbazide

A given sample solution of semicarbazide on treatment with lead peroxide produces nitrogen gas quantitavely i.e.. the volume of N_2 formed is proporponal to the amount of semicarbazide present in the sample solution. Hence by measuring the volume of the liberated N_2, the amount of semicarbazide can be found out bystoichiometric calculations. This method can be called azotometric method since it is based on the measurement of N_2 gas.

The measurement of the volume of nitrogen is done by means of Lunge nitrometer. This apparatus consists of a graduated tube A having a three-way tap at the upper end. The lower end of A is connected to another glasstube C (which is not graduated) by means of a long pressure rubber tubing This ungraduated tube C is called the levelling tube. Mercury is used as a confining liquid. The sample and reagentare mixed in a reaction bottle which is connected to Lunge gas volumeter through tube D (see Fig. 20.3).

20.2.2 Determination of Nitrates

When a nitrate (or a nitrite) is treated with an excess of con. H_2SO_4 and Hg, NO gas is librated in accordance with the equation

$$2HNO_3 + 3H_2SO_4 + 6Hg = 3Hg_2SO_4 + 4H_2O + 2NO$$

The liberated NO gas is measured by means of a Lunge volumeter. Now, according to above equation

$$2NO \equiv 2NO_3^-$$

or $$NO \equiv NO_3^- \qquad [\text{ionic wt} = 62]$$

∴ 22,400 c.c. NO gas $\equiv$ 62 g NO_3^- ion at S.T.P.

or 1 c.c. of NO $\equiv$ 0.002768 g of nitrate

20.2.3 Determination of Hydrogen Peroxide

Hydrogen peroxide on treatment with an excess of acidic potassium permanganate solution produces oxygen according to the equation

$$2KMnO_4 + 3H_2SO_4 + 5H_2O_2 = K_2SO_4 + 2MnSO_4 + 8H_2O + 5O_2$$
$$O_2 \equiv H_2O_2 \text{ (mol. wt} = 34)$$
$$22.4 \text{ litres of } O_2 \text{ gas} = 34 \text{ g } H_2O_2 \qquad \text{at S.T.P}$$

[If acidic permanganate sloution is treated with an *excess* of H_2O_2 then the volume of the liberated oxygen is proportional to the quantity of KMnO$_4$. Hence, this reaction can also be used for finding out the concentration of a given KMnO$_4$ solution,]

20.2.4 Evaluation of Pyrolusite

Pyrolusite is an ore of manganese, in which manganese is present as manganese dioxide. The percentage of manganese in pyrolusite can be found out by means of a gasometric method.

A known weight of pyrolusite sample is treated with an excess of H_2SO_4 and H_2O_2 when there is a quantitative liberation of O_2 as shown by the equation

$$MnO_2 + H_2SO_4 + H_2O_2 \longrightarrow MnSO_4 + 2H_2O + O_2$$
$$22.4 \text{ litre of } O_2 \equiv 86.94 \text{ g } MnO_2 \text{ at S.T.P.}$$

Example 20.(iv)

A pyrolusite sample weighing 0.1768 g was treated with an excess of H_2SO_4 and H_2O_2 when 32.3 c.c. of O_2 was liberated at N.T.P. Calculate the percentage of MnO_2 in the pyrolusite sample.

22,400 c.c. O_2 is obtained from 86.94 g MnO_2

∴ 32.3 c.c. ... ... $\dfrac{32.3}{22,400} \times 86.94$

$$= 0.1254 \text{ g Mn } O_2$$

Now, 0.1768 g pyrolusite sample contains 0.1253 g MnO_2

∴ 100 g ... ... $\dfrac{100}{0.1768} \times 0.1253$ g MnO_2

Thus the percentage of Mn O_2 in the pyrolysite sample will be 70.90.

20.2.5 Determination of Urea

When urea is treated with sodium hypobromite, nitrogen gas evolves.

$$CO(NH_2)_2 + 3NaOBr + 2NaOH = NaCO_3 + 3NaBr + 3H_2O + N_2$$

This reaction is incomplete and it has been empirically found that 1g of urea produces 357.0 c.c. N_2 gas. This relationship can be used for the gasometric determination of urea (see section 18.D.8).

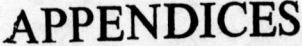

APPENDICES

Appendix—I. Table of Atomic Weights

Element	Symbol	Atomic No.	Atomic Weight
Actinium	Ac	89	[227]
Aluminium	Al	13	26·98
Americium	Am	95	[243]
Antimony	Sb	51	121·75
Argon	Ar	18	39·948
Arsenic	As	33	74·916
Astatine	At	85	[210]
Barium	Ba	56	137·34
Berkelium	Bk	97	[247]
Beryllium	Be	4	9·012
Bismuth	Bi	83	208.98
Boron	B	5	10.81
Bromine	Br	35	79.904
Cadmium	Cd	48	112·40
Calcium	Ca	20	40·08
Californium	Cf	98	[251]
Carbon	C	6	12·011
Cerium	Ce	58	140·12
Cesium	Cs	55	132·91
Chlorine	Cl	17	35·453
Chromium	Cr	24	52·0
Cobalt	Co	27	58·933
Copper	Cu	29	63·546
Curium	Cm	96	[247]
Dysprosium	Dy	66	162·50
Einsteinium	Es	99	[254]
Erbium	Er	68	167·26
Europium	Eu	63	152·0
Fermium	Fm	100	[257]
Fluorine	F	9	19·00
Francium	Fr	87	[223]
Gadolinium	Gd	64	157·25
Gallium	Ga	31	69·72
Germanium	Ge	32	72.60

Element	Symbol	Atomic No.	Atomic Weight
Gold	Au	79	197·0
Hafnium	Hf	72	178·50
Helium	He	2	4·003
Holmium	Ho	67	164·93
Hydrogen	H	1	1·008
Indium	In	49	114·82
Iodine	I	53	126·90
Iridium	Ir	77	192·22
Iron	Fe	26	55·85
Krypton	Kr	36	83·80
Lanthanum	La	57	138·91
Lawrencium	Lr	103	[260]
Lead	Pb	82	207·2
Lithium	Li	3	6·94
Lutetium	Lu	71	174·97
Magnesium	Mg	12	24·31
Manganese	Mn	25	54·94
Mendelevium	Md	101	[258]
Mercury	Hg	80	200·59
Molybdenum	Mo	42	95·94
Neodymium	Nd	60	144·24
Neon	Ne	10	20·18
Neptunium	Np	93	[237]
Nickel	Ni	28	58·70
Niobium	Nb	41	92·906
Nitrogen	N	7	14·007
Nobelium	No	102	[255]
Osmium	Os	76	190·2
Oxygen	O	8	16·0
Palladium	Pd	46	106·4
Phosphorus	P	15	30·974
Platinum	Pt	78	195·09
Plutonium	Pu	94	[244]

Element	Symbol	Atomic No.	Atomic Weight
Polonium	Po	84	[209]
Potassium	K	19	39·10
Praseodymium	Pr	59	140·908
Promethium	Pm	61	[145]
Protactinium	Pa	91	231·036
Radium	Ra	88	226·02
Radon	Rn	86	[222]
Rhenium	Re	75	186·21
Rhodium	Rh	45	102·91
Rubidium	Rb	37	85·47
Ruthenium	Ru	44	101·07
Samarium	Sm	62	150·4
Scandium	Sc	21	44·96
Selenium	Se	34	78·96
Silicon	Si	14	28·086
Silver	Ag	47	107·87
Sodium	Na	11	22·99
Strontium	Sr	38	87·62
Sulphur	S	16	32·06
Tantalum	Ta	73	180·95
Technetium	Tc	43	[97]
Tellurium	Te	52	127·60
Terbium	Tb	65	158·93
Thallium	Tl	81	204·37
Thorium	Th	90	232·04
Thulium	Tm	69	168·93
Tin	Sn	50	118·70
Titanium	Ti	22	47·90
Tungsten	W	74	183·85
Uranium	U	92	238·03
Vanadium	V	23	50·94
Xenon	Xe	54	131·30
Ytterbium	Yb	70	173·04
Yttrium	Y	39	88·91
Zinc	Zn	30	65·38
Zirconium	Zr	40	91·22

Note. Values in brackets refer to the isotope of longest known half-life for radioactive element.

Appendix II—Table of Formula Weights

AgBr	187·80
AgCNS	165·96
AgCl	143·34
Ag_2CrO_4	331·77
AgI	234·79
$AgNO_3$	169·89
Al_2O_3	101·96
$Al(OH)_3$	78·00
As_2O_3	197·82
As_2O_5	229·82
$BaCO_3$	197·37
$BaCl_2$	208·27
$BaCrO_4$	253·37
$Ba(OH)_2$	171·38
$BaSO_4$	233·43
Bi_2S_3	514·20
$CaCO_3$	100·09
CaC_2O_4	128·10
$Ca(OH)_2$	74·08
$CaSO_4$	136·15
$Ce(SO_4)_2$	332·26
$CuSO_4.5H_2O$	249·64
CuS	95·61
Fe_2O_3	159·70
$Fe(OH)_3$	106·87
$FeSO_4.7H_2O$	278·03
$FeSO_4.(NH_4)_2SO_4.6H_2O$	392·16
$Fe_2(SO_4)_3$	399·90
HBr	80·92
$H_2C_2O_4.2H_2O$ (oxalic)	126·07
$H.C_2H_3O_2$ (acetic)	60·05
$H.C_7H_5O_2$ (benzoic)	122·12

HCl	36·46
HClO$_4$	100·46
HNO$_3$	63·02
H.NH$_2$SO$_3$ (sulphamic)	97·10
H$_3$PO$_4$	98·00
H$_2$S	34·08
H$_2$SO$_3$	82·08
H$_2$SO$_4$	98·08
Hg(NO$_3$)$_2$	324·63
HgO	216·61
HgS	232·68
Hg$_2$Cl$_2$	472·13
KBr	119·02
KCl	74·55
KI	166·01
KIO$_3$	214·01
KBrO$_3$	167·02
KMnO$_4$	157·95
KOH	56·01
MgCO$_3$	84·32
MgNH$_4$PO$_4$	137·34
MgO	40·32
Mg$_2$P$_2$O$_7$	222·59
Na$_3$AsO$_3$	191·88
Na$_2$B$_4$O$_7$	201·28
NaBr	102·92
Na$_2$CO$_3$	106·0
Na$_2$C$_2$O$_4$	134·0
NaHCO$_3$	84.02
NaI	149·90
NaNO$_3$	85·00
NaOH	40·00
Na$_3$PO$_4$	163·95
Na$_2$SO$_3$	126·05
Na$_2$SO$_4$	142·05
NH$_3$	17·03
N$_2$H$_4$	32·05

$(NH_4)_2C_2O_4$	124·10
$PbCl_2$	278·13
$Pb(NO_3)_2$	331·23
$PbSO_4$	303·28
Sb_2S_3	339·72
SiO_2	60·09
$SnCl_2$	189·61
SnO_2	150·70
SO_2	64·07
SO_3	80·07
$SrCO_3$	147·64
SrC_2O_4	175·65
V_2O_5	181·90
$ZnBr_2$	225·21
ZnO	81·38
$Zn_2P_2O_7$	304·71
ZnS	97·45
$ZnBr_2$	225·21
$ZnSO_4$	161·45

Appendix III. Solubility Product Constant
(at room temperature)

Substance	Formula	Solubility Product
Aluminium hydroxide	$Al(OH)_3$	2×10^{-32}
Barium carbonate	$BaCO_3$	8.1×10^{-9}
Barium chromate	$BaCrO_4$	2.4×10^{-10}
Barium oxalate	BaC_2O_4	2.3×10^{-8}
Barium sulphate	$BaSO_4$	1.08×10^{-10}
Bismuth hydroxide	$BiO.OH$	4×10^{-10}
Bismuth sulphide	Bi_2S_3	1×10^{-97}
Cadmium hydroxide	$Cd(OH)_2$	5.9×10^{-15}
Cadmium oxalate	CdC_2O_4	1.5×10^{-8}
Cadmium sulphide	CdS	7.8×10^{-27}
Calcium carbonate	$CaCO_3$	8.7×10^{-9}
Calcium fluoride	CaF_2	4.0×10^{-11}
Calcium hydroxide	$Ca(OH)_2$	5.5×10^{-6}
Calcium oxalate	CaC_2O_4	2.6×10^{-9}
Calcium phosphate	$Ca_3(PO_4)_2$	2.0×10^{-29}
Calcium sulphate	$CaSO_4$	1.9×10^{-4}
Chromium (II) bydroxide	$Cr(OH)_2$	1.0×10^{-17}
Chromium (III) hydroxide	$Cr(OH)_3$	6×10^{-31}
Cobalt (II) hydroxide	$Co(OH)_2$	2×10^{-16}
Copper (I) iodide	CuI	5.1×10^{-12}
Copper (II) sulphide	CuS	9×10^{-36}
Copper (I) thiocyanate	$CuSCN$	4.8×10^{-15}
Iron (II) carbonate	$FeCO_3$	3.5×10^{-11}
Iron (II) hydroxide	$Fe(OH)_2$	8×10^{-16}
Iron (III) hydroxide	$Fe(OH)_3$	4×10^{-38}
Lead carbonate	$PbCO_3$	3.3×10^{-14}
Lead chloride	$PbCl_2$	1.6×10^{-5}
Lead chromate	$PbCrO_4$	1.8×10^{-14}
Lead iodide	PbI_2	7.1×10^{-9}
Lead oxalate	PbC_2O_4	4.8×10^{-10}
Lead sulphate	$PbSO_4$	1.6×10^{-8}
Lead sulphide	PbS	8×10^{-28}

Substance	Formula	Solubility Product
Magnesium ammonium phosphate	$MgNH_4PO_4$	2.5×10^{-13}
Magnesium carbonate	$MgCO_3$	1×10^{-5}
Magnesium fluoride	MgF_2	6.5×10^{-9}
Magnesium hydroxide	$Mg(OH)_2$	1.2×10^{-11}
Magnesium oxalate	MgC_2O_4	-1×10^{-8}
Manganese (II) hydroxide	$Mn(OH)_2$	1.9×10^{-13}
Mercury (I) chloride	Hg_2Cl_2	1.3×10^{-18}
Mercury (II) sulphide	HgS	4×10^{-53}
Mercury (I) thiocyanate	$Hg_2(SCN)_2$	3.0×10^{-20}
Nickel carbonate	$NiCO_3$	6.6×10^{-9}
Nickel hydroxide	$Ni(OH)_2$	6.5×10^{-18}
Nickel sulphide	NiS	3×10^{-19}
Silver bromide	$AgBr$	5.25×10^{-13}
Silver carbonate	Ag_2CO_3	8.1×10^{-12}
Silver chloride	$AgCl$	1.78×10^{-10}
Silver chromate	Ag_2CrO_4	2.45×10^{-12}
Silver cyanide	$AgCN$	5.0×10^{-12}
Silver iodide	AgI	8.31×10^{-17}
Silver oxalate	$Ag_2C_2O_4$	3.5×10^{-11}
Silver phosphate	Ag_3PO_4	1.3×10^{-20}
Silver sulphate	Ag_2SO_4	1.6×10^{-5}
Silver sulphide	Ag_2S	2×10^{-49}
Silver thiocyanate	$AgSCN$	1×10^{-12}
Strontium carbonate	$SrCO_3$	1.1×10^{-10}
Strontium chromate	$SrCrO_4$	3.6×10^{-5}
Strontium fluoride	SrF_2	2.8×10^{-9}
Strontium oxalate	SrC_2O_4	1.6×10^{-7}
Strontium sulphate	$SrSO_4$	3.8×10^{-7}
Tin (Ii) sulphide	SnS	1×10^{-25}
Zinc carbonate	$ZnCO_3$	1.4×10^{-11}
Zinc hydroxide	$Zn(OH)_2$	1.2×10^{-17}
Zinc oxalate	ZnC_2O_4	2.8×10^{-8}
Zinc phosphate	$Zn_3(PO_4)_2$	9.1×10^{-33}
Zinc sulphide	ZnS	1×10^{-21}

Appendix—IV Dissociation Constants for Acids and Bases
(at room temperature)

Acid/Base	Dissociation Equilibrium	Dissociation constant
Acetic	$CH_3COOH \rightleftharpoons CH_3COO^- + H^+$	$K = 1\cdot75 \times 10^{-5}$
Arsenic	$H_3AsO_4 \rightleftharpoons H_2AsO_4^- + H^+$	$K_1 = 6\cdot0 \times 10^{-3}$
	$H_2AsO_4^- \rightleftharpoons HAsO_4^{2-} + H^+$	$K_2 = 1\cdot0 \times 10^{-7}$
	$HAsO_4^{2-} \rightleftharpoons AsO_4^{3-} + H^+$	$K_3 = 3\cdot0 \times 10^{-12}$
Arsenious	$H_3AsO_3 \rightleftharpoons H_2AsO_3^- + H^+$	$K_1 = 6 \times 10^{-10}$
	$H_2AsO_3^- \rightleftharpoons HAsO_3^{2-} + H^+$	$K_2 = 3 \times 10^{-14}$
Benzoic	$C_7H_6O_2 \rightleftharpoons C_7H_5O_2^- + H^+$	$K = 6\cdot3 \times 10^{-5}$
Boric	$H_3BO_3 \rightleftharpoons H_2BO_3^- + H^+$	$K = 6\cdot4 \times 10^{-10}$
Bromoacetic	$Br. CH_2COOH \rightleftharpoons Br CH_2 COO^- + H^+$	$K = 1\cdot38 \times 10^{-3}$
Carbonic	$H_2CO_3 \rightleftharpoons HCO_3^- + H^+$	$K_1 = 4\cdot47 \times 10^{-7}$
	$HCO_3^- \rightleftharpoons CO_3^{2-} + H^+$	$K_2 = 4\cdot68 \times 10^{-11}$
Chloroacetic	$Cl CH_2 COOH \rightleftharpoons Cl CH_2 COO^- + H^+$	$K = 1\cdot54 \times 10^{-3}$
Ethylenediamine-tetraacetic (H_4Y)	$H_4Y \rightleftharpoons H_3Y^- + H^+$	$K_1 = 1\cdot00 \times 10^{-2}$
	$H_3Y^- \rightleftharpoons H_2Y^{2-} + H^+$	$K_2 = 2\cdot16 \times 10^{-3}$
	$H_2Y^{2-} \rightleftharpoons HY^{3-} + H^+$	$K_3 = 6\cdot92 \times 10^{-7}$
	$HY^{3-} \rightleftharpoons Y^{4-} + H^+$	$K_4 = 5\cdot50 \times 10^{-11}$
Formic	$HCOOH \rightleftharpoons HCOO^- + H^+$	$K = 1\cdot76 \times 10^{-4}$
Hydrogen sulphide	$H_2S \rightleftharpoons HS^- + H^+$	$K_1 = 9\cdot1 \times 10^{-8}$
	$HS^- \rightleftharpoons S^{2-} + H^+$	$K_2 = 1\cdot2 \times 10^{-15}$
Oxalic	$H_2C_2O_4 \rightleftharpoons HC_2O_4^- + H^+$	$K_1 = 6\cdot5 \times 10^{-2}$
	$HC_2O_4^- \rightleftharpoons C_2O_4^{2-} + H^+$	$K_2 = 6\cdot1 \times 10^{-5}$
Phenol	$C_6H_5OH \rightleftharpoons C_6H_5O^- + H^+$	$K = 1\cdot1 \times 10^{-10}$
Phosphoric	$H_3PO_4 \rightleftharpoons H_2PO_4^- + H^+$	$K_1 = 7\cdot5 \times 10^{-3}$
	$H_2PO_4^- \rightleftharpoons HPO_4^{2-} + H^+$	$K_2 = 6\cdot2 \times 10^{-8}$
	$HPO_4^{2-} \rightleftharpoons PO_4^{3-} + H^+$	$K_3 = 4\cdot8 \times 10^{-13}$
Succinic	$HOOC.CH_2.CH_2.COOH \rightleftharpoons HOOC.CH_2.CH_2.CH_2.COO^- + H^+$	$K_1 = 6\cdot2 \times 10^{-5}$
	$HOOC.CH_2.CH_2.COO^- \rightleftharpoons {}^-OOC.CH_2.CH_2.COO^- + H^+$	$K_2 = 2\cdot3 \times 10^{-6}$

Acid/Base	Dissociation Equilibrium	Dissociation constant
Sulphamic	$NH_2SO_3H \rightleftharpoons NH_2SO_3^- + H^+$	$K = 0.10$
Sulphuric	$H_2SO_4 \rightleftharpoons HSO_4^- + H^+$	$K_1 \gg 1$
	$HSO_4^- \rightleftharpoons SO_4^{2-} + H^+$	$K_2 = 1.2 \times 10^{-2}$
Sulphurous	$H_2SO_3 \rightleftharpoons HSO_3^- + H^+$	$K_1 = 1.7 \times 10^{-2}$
	$HSO_3^- \rightleftharpoons SO_3^{2-} + H^+$	$K_2 = 6.5 \times 10^{-8}$
Ammonia	$NH_3 + H_2O \rightleftharpoons NH_4^+ + OH^-$	$K = 1.80 \times 10^{-5}$
Aniline	$C_6H_5NH_2 + H_2O \rightleftharpoons C_6H_5NH_3^+ + OH^-$	$K = 4.0 \times 10^{-10}$
Ethylenedia-mine	$NH_2CH_2CH_2NH_2 + H_2O \rightleftharpoons NH_2 CH_2CH_2NH_3^+ + OH^-$	$K_1 = 8.5 \times 10^{-}$
	$NH_2CH_2CH_2NH_3^+ + H_2O \rightleftharpoons {}^+NH_3CH_2CH_2NH_3^+ + OH^-$	$K_2 = 7.1 \times 10^{-8}$
Hydrazine	$H_2NNH_2 + H_2O \rightleftharpoons H_2NNH_3^+ + OH^-$	$K = 1.3 \times 10^{-6}$
Hydroxylamine	$HONH_2 + H_2O \rightleftharpoons HONH_3^+ + OH^-$	$K = 9.1 \times 10^{-9}$
Methylamine	$CH_3NH_2 + H_2O \rightleftharpoons CH_3NH_3^+ + OH^-$	$K = 4.8 \times 10^{-4}$

Appendix—V Surface Tension of Some Common Liquids

Liquid	Surface Tension (Dynes cm^{-1} at 20C°)
Acetone	23.70
Benzene	28.85
Carbon tetrachloride	26.77
Chlorobenzene	33.20
Chloroform	27.10
Cyclohexane	25.30
Ethyl acetate	23.90
Ethyl alcohol	22.30
Ethyl ether	17.01
Glycol	47.70
n-Hexane	18.43
Methyl acetate	24.60
Methyl alcohol	22.61
Toluene	28.43
Water	72.75

Appendix—VI Viscosity Coefficients of Some Common Liquids

Liquid	Viscosity Coefficient (Centipoise at 20C°)
Carbon tetrachloride	0·969
Chloroform	0·580
Ethyl acetate	0·455
Ethyl alcohol	1·200
n-Heptane	0·409
n-Hexane	0·326
Methyl acetate	0·381
Methyl alcohol	0·597
Benzene	0·652
Toluene	0·590
Water	1·002

Appendix—VII Approximate Density of Some Common Substances

Substance	Density g/c.c.	Substance	Density g/c.c.
Air	0·0012	Lead	11·3
Alcohol	0·90	Mercury	13·6
Aluminium	2·7	Nickel	8·9
Brass	8·4	Platinum	21·4
Copper	8·9	Porcelain	2·4
Glass	2·6	Silver	10·5
Gold	19·3	Stainless steel	8·0
Iron	7·9	Water	1·0

Appendix VIII—Recording the Details of Weighing

Article weighed   ...   .   Crucible no. 1

Number of times weighing done   ...   4

Details of first weighing

Weights used :

20 g	—	—
10 g	1	10·0000
5 g	—	—
3 g	1	3·0000
2 g	—	—
1 g	—	—
500 mg	—	—
300 mg	1	0·3000
200 mg	—	—
100 mg	1	0·1000
50 mg	1	0·0500
30 mg	—	—
20 mg	—	—
10 mg	—	—
Rider position on the scale	5·3	0·0056

(1 small division =0·2 mg)

(Similarly record other

TOTAL   13·4556 g   weighings)

Appendix —IX Reporting Titrimetric Analysis

[Reagent used is a primary standard]

   (*i*) Weight of the reagent taken   ————

   (*ii*) Volume of the reagent solution ————

   (*iii*) Eq. wt. of the reagent   ————

   (*iv*) Normality of the reagent solution————-——

Titration of the sample solution with reagent solution

	I	II	III	IV
ml of sample solution	——	———	———	———
ml of reagent solution	——	———	———	———

X ml of sample solution$\equiv$Y ml of reagent solution

Normality of the sample solution   ————

[Reagent used is not a primary standard.]

Standardisation of reagent solution against a primary standard

   (*i*) Weight of the primary standard taken   ————

   (*ii*) Volume of the solution of primary standard ————

   (*iii*) Eq. wt. of the primary standard   ————

   (*iv*) Normality of the solution of primary standard————

Titration of reagent solution against primary standard solution

	I	II	III	IV
ml of reagent solution	——	———	———	——
ml of solution of primary standard	——	———	———	——

X_1 ml reagent solution$\equiv Y_1$ ml of solution of primary standard

Normality of reagent solution=————

Titration of sample solution with reagent solution

	I	II	III	IV
ml of sample solution	——	——	———	———
ml of reagent solution	——	——	———	———

X_2 ml sample solution$\equiv Y_2$ ml of reagent solution

Normality of sample solution————

Appendix—X;The use of Logarithms

Very large or very small numbers can be expressed conveniently in exponential form.

Example X (i).

3,560,000	may be written as $3·56 \times 10^6$
3,560	may be written as $3·56 \times 10^3$
0·356	may be written as $3·56 \times 10^{-1}$
0·0000356	may be written as $3·56 \times 10^{-5}$

The common logarithm (briefly called log) of a number is the power of 10 which will give that number.

Example X (ii)

$$\log \quad 10,000 = \log\ (10 \times 10 \times 10 \times 10) = \log 10^4 = 4$$

$$\log \quad 1,000 = \log (10 \times 10 \times 10) \quad = \log 10^3 = 3$$

$$\log \quad 100 = \log (10 \times 10) \quad = \log 10^2 = 2$$

$$\log \quad 10 = \log 10 \quad = \log 10^1 = 1$$

$$\log \quad 1 = \quad = \log 10^0 = 0$$

$$\log \quad 0·1 = \log \frac{1}{10} \quad = \log 10^{-1} = -1 \ (or\ \bar{1})$$

$$\log \quad 0·01 = \log\left(\frac{1}{10} \times \frac{1}{10} \right) \quad = \log 10^{-2} = -2$$

$$\log \quad 0·001 = \log\left(\frac{1}{10} \times \frac{1}{10} \times \frac{1}{10} \right) = \log 10^{-3} = -3$$

From the above example it is evident that log of any number from 1 to 10 will be between 0 and 1. Similarly, log value for a number from 10 to 100 will be between 1 and 2. The log value is not always in whole numbers. It usually comtains an integer called *characteristic* and a fraction called *mantissa*. The mantissa is obtained from a log table and the characteristic by noting the position of the decimal point.

Example X(iii)

Suppose we want to find out the log value for 35·68. In a four-figure log table, find out the horizontal line containing number 35. Note the number given under 6th column of the line, and add to it the number given in the 8th column in the proportional parts (maen difference).

The number under column 6, in the line containing 35 is 5514. The number under column 8 in the proportional parts is 10. Hence,. the mantissa will be 5514+10=5524. The decimal point in 35·68. is after two digits, hence the characteristic will be (2−1)=1. Thus. the log value of 35·68 will be 1·5524. Similarly, we can write :

$$\log 356\cdot 8 = 2\cdot 5524$$
$$\log 35\cdot 68 = 1\cdot 5524$$
$$\log 3\cdot 568 = 0\cdot 5524$$

$$\log 0\cdot 3568 = \bar{1}\cdot 5524$$

$$\log 0\cdot 03568 = \bar{2}\cdot 5524$$

If log value is given, we can find out the corresponding number. For example, we are given log value as $1\cdot 5524$ and we have to find out its corresponding number *i.e.*, antilog of $1\cdot 5524$. In the four-figure log table, in the horizontal line containing 35, the number under 6th column is 5514 and that under 7th column is 5527. Thus we know three digits of the number, *i.e.*, 356. In the same line, the 8th column under proportional parts shows 10 which on adding to 5514 gives 5524. So that we get the number 3568. Since in the log value $1\cdot 5524$, characteristic is 1, the decimal is placed after two digits, *i.e.*, antilog of $1\cdot 5524 = 35\cdot 68$.

MATHEMATICAL OPERATIONS WITH LOGARITHMS

(i) *Multiplication and Division*

The process of addition is much simpler than that of multiplication. If we make use of logrithmic values, the process of multiplication is reduced to that of addition. For example, we have to find out the value of the product 100×100. The actual multiplication is relatively difficult and time consuming. However, the result can be more quickly and conveniently obtained by expressing the numbers involved exponentially using the power of 10 *i.e.*, the log values as shown below.

$$100 \times 100 = 10^2 \times 10^2 = 10^{(2+2)} = 10^4 = 10,000.$$

The answer is 10,000. By writing 100 in the exponential form as 10^2, we are simply required to add the powers of 10 ($2+2=4$) to obtain the answer, which is much simpler to the actual multiplication of 100×100. In this example, the power of 10 is the log value, so that we can write :

$$\log 100 = \log 10^2 = 2\cdot 0000$$
$$\log 100 = \log 10^2 = 2\cdot 0000$$
$$\text{sum} = 4\cdot 0000$$

Antilog $(4\cdot 0000) = 10,000.$

Example X(*iv*)

$$43\cdot 26 \times 0\cdot 1016 \times 0\cdot 05301 = ?$$

$$\log 43\cdot26 = 1\cdot6361$$

$$\log 0\cdot1016 = \overline{1}\cdot0068$$

$$\log 0\cdot05301 = \overline{2}\cdot7244 \text{ or,}$$

$$\text{sum} = \overline{1}\cdot3673$$

Antilog $(\overline{1}\cdot3673) = 0\cdot2330$

[**Note.** Mantissa is always positive, characteristic can be positive or negative depending upon the position of the decimal.]

Example X(v)

$$\frac{0\cdot8436}{0\cdot2042} = ?$$

$$\log 0\cdot8436 = \overline{1}\cdot9261$$

$$\log 0\cdot2042 = \overline{1}\cdot3100$$

$$\text{difference} = 0\cdot6161$$

Antilog $(0\cdot6161) = 4\cdot131$

[Remember : $\log (a \times b) = \log a + \log b$

and $\qquad\qquad \log a/b = \log a - \log b$]

(ii) Powers and Roots

To raise a number to a given power, multiply the log of the number by the power expressed, then find the antilog. In general : $\log a^n = n \times \log a$.

Example X(vi)

$(32\cdot5)^3 = ?$

$\log 32\cdot5 = 1\cdot5119 : 3 \times 1\cdot5119 = 4\cdot5357$

Antilog $(4\cdot5357) = 3\cdot433 \times 10^4$.

To take roots, divide the log of the number by the root to be taken and then find the antilog. In general :

$$\log \sqrt[n]{a} = \frac{1}{n} \log a.$$

Example X(vii)

$$\sqrt[5]{924} = ?$$

$$\log 924 = 2\cdot9657 ; \quad \frac{2\cdot9657}{5} = 0\cdot5931$$

Antilog $(0\cdot5931) = 3\cdot918$

SUBJECT INDEX